Birkhäuser Advances in Infectious Diseases

BAID

Series Editors

Poxviruses

Edited by A. A. Mercer, A. Schmidt and O. Weber

Birkhäuser Verlag
Basel • Boston • Berlin

Editors

Andrew A. Mercer
Department of Microbiology
University of Otago
PO Box 56
700 Cumberland Street
Dunedin
New Zealand

Axel Schmidt
University Witten/Herdecke
Faculty of Medicine
Alfred-Herrhausen-Str. 50
58448 Witten
Germany

Olaf Weber
BAYER HEALTHCARE AG
Product-related Research
42096 Wuppertal
Germany

Library of Congress Control Number: 2006693300

Bibliographic information published by Die Deutsche Bibliothek
Die Deutsche Bibliothek lists this publication in the Deutsche Nationalbibliografie;
detailed bibliographic data is available in the internet at http://dnb.ddb.de

ISBN 3-7643-7556-6 Birkhäuser Verlag, Basel - Boston - Berlin

Part of Springer Science+Business Media
Printed on acid-free paper produced from chlorine-free pulp. TFC ∞
Cover illustration: see page 261. With the friendly permission of Robert Granados, Boyce Thompson Institute for Plant Research at Cornell University, Ithaca, NY
Printed in Germany
ISBN-10: 3-7643-7556-6
ISBN-13: 978-3-7643-7556-0
9 8 7 6 5 4 3 2 1

e-ISBN-10: 3-7643-7557-4
e-ISBN-13: 978-3-7643-7557-7
www. birkhauser.ch

Contents

List of contributors

Claudio L. Afonso, Southeast Poultry Research Laboratory, Agricultural Research Service, United States Department of Agriculture, Athens, GA 30605, USA

Andrea Ammon, European Centre for Disease Prevention and Control (ECDC), 17183 Stockholm, Sweden;
e-mail: Andrea.Ammon@ecdc.eu.int

Graciela Andrei, Rega Institute for Medical Research, K.U. Leuven, 3000 Leuven, Belgium

John W. Barrett, Robarts Research Institute and Department of Microbiology and Immunology, Schulich School of Medicine and Dentistry, The University of Western Ontario, 1400 Western Rd., London, ON N6G 2V4, Canada

Marie N. Becker, Department of Molecular Genetics and Microbiology, College of Medicine, P.O. Box 100266, University of Florida, Gainesville, FL 32610, USA

Clifford J. Bellone, Department of Molecular Microbiology and Immunology, Saint Louis University Health Sciences Center, St. Louis, MO 63104, USA; e-mail: bellonec@slu.edu

David Boyle, CSIRO Livestock Industries, Australian Animal Health Laboratory, 5 Portarlington Road, Geelong, Victoria 3220, Australia;
e-mail: david.boyle@csiro.au

Joachim Bugert, Department of Medical Microbiology, Cardiff University School of Medicine, Wales College of Medicine, Heath Park Cardiff CF14 4XN, UK; e-mail: bugertjj@cf.ac.uk

R. Mark Buller, Department of Molecular Microbiology and Immunology, Saint Louis University Health Sciences Center, St. Louis, MO 63104, USA

Inger K. Damon, Poxvirus Program, Division of Viral and Rickettsial Diseases, Centers for Disease Control and Prevention, MS G-18, Atlanta, GA 30333, USA; e-mail: iad7@cdc.gov

Erik De Clercq, Rega Institute for Medical Research, K.U. Leuven, 3000 Leuven, Belgium

Gustavo A. Delhon, Dept. of Pathobiology, College of Veterinary Medicine, University of Illinois, 2001 S. Lincoln Avenue, Urbana, IL 61802, USA; and Area of Virology, School of Veterinary Science, University of Buenos Aires, 1427 Buenos Aires, Argentina

Adama Diallo, Animal Production Unit, FAO/IAEA Agriculture and Biotechnology Laboratory, International Atomic Energy Agency, Wagrammerstrasse 5, P.O. Box 100, 1400 Vienna, Austria; e-mal: a.diallo@iaea.org

Sandra Essbauer, Bundeswehr Institute of Microbiology, Neuherbergstr. 11, 80937 München, Germany

Martin Exner, Institute of Hygiene and Public Health, Rheinische-Friedrich-Wilhelms-Universität Bonn, Sigmund-Freud-Str. 25, 53105 Bonn, Germany

Stephen Fleming, Department of Microbiology, University of Otago, PO Box 56, 700 Cumberland Street, Dunedin, New Zealand

Jürgen Gebel, Institute of Hygiene and Public Health, Rheinische-Friedrich-Wilhelms-Universität Bonn, Sigmund-Freud-Str. 25, 53105 Bonn, Germany; e-mail: Juergen.Gebel@ukb.uni-bonn.de

Lauren M. Handley, Department of Molecular Microbiology and Immunology, Saint Louis University Health Sciences Center, St. Louis, MO 63104, USA

Percy Knolle, Institute for Molecular Medicine and Experimental Immunology, Universitätsklinikum Bonn, Rheinische Friedrich-Wilhelms-Universität, Sigmund Freud Str. 25, 53105 Bonn, Germany

J. Paige Mackey, Department of Molecular Microbiology and Immunology, Saint Louis University Health Sciences Center, St. Louis, MO 63104, USA

Grant McFadden, Robarts Research Institute and Department of Microbiology and Immunology, Schulich School of Medicine and Dentistry, The University of Western Ontario, 1400 Western Rd., London, ON N6G 2V4, Canada; e-mail: mcfadden@robarts.ca.

Andrew A. Mercer, Department of Microbiology, University of Otago, PO Box 56, 700 Cumberland Street, Dunedin, New Zealand; e-mail: andy.mercer@stonebow.otago.ac.nz

Hermann Meyer, Bundeswehr Institute of Microbiology, Neuherbergstr. 11, 80937 München, Germany; e-mail: hermann1meyer@bundeswehr.org

Richard W. Moyer, Department of Molecular Genetics and Microbiology, College of Medicine, P.O. Box 100266, University of Florida, Gainesville, FL 32610, USA; e-mail: rmoyer@ufl.edu.

Steven H. Nazarian, Robarts Research Institute and Department of Microbiology and Immunology, Schulich School of Medicine and Dentistry, The University of Western Ontario, 1400 Western Rd., London, ON N6G 2V4, Canada

Martin Pfeffer, Bundeswehr Institute of Microbiology, Neuherbergstr. 11, 80937 München, Germany

Klaus Riedmann, Robert-Koch-Institut, Seestr. 10, 13353 Berlin, Germany

Daniel L. Rock, Department of Pathobiology, College of Veterinary Medicine, 2522 VMBSB, University of Illinois, 2001 S. Lincoln Avenue, Urbana, IL 61802, USA; e-mail: dlrock@uiuc.edu

Julia Sasse, Robert-Koch-Institut, Seestr. 10, 13353 Berlin, Germany

Axel Schmidt, Institute of Microbiology and Virology, University Witten/Herdecke, Stockumer Str. 10, 58448 Witten, Germany; e-mail: axel780961@aol.com

Barbara S. Schnierle, Paul-Ehrlich-Institut, Department of Virology, Paul-Ehrlich-Str. 51–59, 63225 Langen, Germany

Geoffrey L. Smith, Department of Virology, Faculty of Medicine, Imperial College London, St. Mary's Campus, Norfolk Place, London W2 1PG, UK; e-mail: glsmith@imperial.ac.uk

Robert Snoeck, Rega Institute for Medical Research, K.U. Leuven, 3000 Leuven, Belgium; e-mail: robert.snoeck@rega.kuleuven.ac.be

Yasemin Suezer, Paul-Ehrlich-Institut, Department of Virology, Paul-Ehrlich-Str. 51-59, 63225 Langen, Germany

Gerd Sutter, Paul-Ehrlich-Institut, Department of Virology, Paul-Ehrlich-Str. 51-59, 63225 Langen, Germany; e-mail: sutge@pei.de

Edan R. Tulman, Center of Excellence for Vaccine Research, University of Connecticut, Storrs, CT 06269, USA

Friedrich von Rheinbaben, Institute of Medical Microbiology and Virology, University Witten/Herdecke, Stockumer Str. 10, 58448 Witten, Germany; e-mail: axel780961@aol.com

Gerrit J. Viljoen, Animal Production and Health Section, FAO/IAEA Joint Division, International Atomic Energy Agency, Wagrammerstrasse 5, P.O. Box 100, 1400 Vienna, Austria; e-mail: gerrit.viljoen@iaea.org

Hans-Dieter Volk, Institute of Medical Immunology, Humboldt-Universität Berlin, Charité, Campus Mitte, 10098 Berlin, Germany

Olaf Weber, BAYER HEALTHCARE AG, Product-related Research, 42096 Wuppertal, Germany; e-mail: olaf.weber@bayerhealthcare.com

Preface

The study of poxviruses has a long and distinguished history that includes Jenner's founding work on smallpox vaccination. In the more than 200 years since that time we have seen the remarkable eradication of smallpox. It is difficult to overstate the significance of that achievement. It not only removed a disease that must rate as one of humankind's greatest scourges, but also demonstrated the effectiveness of the general principle of vaccination in our battles against disease.

This book begins with a review of smallpox and its causative agent, *Variola virus*. The vaccine used in the successful smallpox eradication campaign, vaccinia virus, is reviewed in the following chapter that describes its origin and its use as a vaccine, as well as the current understanding of the molecular biology and pathogenesis of this virus. *Vaccinia virus* is the most intensively studied poxvirus and the descriptions of the biology of this virus are relevant to all vertebrate poxviruses.

The eradication of smallpox has drawn attention to the potential threat posed by other orthopoxviruses that infect humans, particularly *Monkeypox virus*. A description of this virus is given in the third chapter. Jenner's original vaccine is believed to have been *Cowpox virus* and this virus is reviewed in the chapter by Essbauer and Meyer. Additional chapters are devoted to each of the recognized genera of the vertebrate poxviruses and a further chapter describes the subfamily of poxviruses infecting invertebrates. Together these provide a comprehensive review of the poxvirus family. Each of the chapters is written by specialists in the area and includes an emphasis on new and important developments.

The impact of poxviruses as pathogens is at least in part related to their expression of an impressive array of immunomodulators that block, subvert and redirect host responses to infection. This area is reviewed in the chapter by Nazarian and McFadden and a potential beneficial exploitation of such properties in immunotherapy is described by Weber and coauthors. Further discussion of the beneficial uses of poxviruses is presented in the following chapter, which reviews the use of recombinant poxviruses as delivery vehicles, and their potential to be used in the prevention and/or treatment of diverse infectious diseases and cancers.

The very real concern that smallpox might be used as a bioterrorism weapon has emphasized the need to review our knowledge of the correlates of immune protection, the features of established vaccines and the development of new generation vaccines with fewer adverse reactions. These topics are addressed in the chapter by Handley and coauthors. Similarly, the heightened awareness of the threat to human health posed by orthopoxviruses dictates that we consider options available for the diagnosis, therapy, handling and management of poxviral diseases. Each of these aspects is covered in the following four chapters, respectively.

The last chapter provides an opportunity to consider the impact of smallpox on a community and the historical developments of attempts to control this "the most terrible of all the ministers of death".

Dunedin, New Zealand, September 2006

Andrew Mercer
Axel Schmidt
Olaf Weber

Glossary

ADCC	antibody-dependent cell-mediated cytotoxicity
AFNOR	Association Francaise de Normalisation
AGID	agar immunodiffusion test
ALV	*Avian leukosis virus*
AMEV	*Amsacta moorei entomopoxvirus*
AP	alkaline phosphatase (stain)
APC	antigen-presenting cell
ATCC	American Type Culture Collection
ATI	acidophilic-type inclusion
BAC	bacterial artificial chromosome
BPSV	*Bovine papular stomatitis virus*
BTV	*Bluetongue virus*
CAM	chorioallantoic membrane(s)
CBP	chemokine binding protein
CCP	complement control protein
CDV	cidifovir
CEA	carcinoembryonic antigen
CEV	cell-associated enveloped virus
CF	complement fixation
CFA	complete Freund's adjuvant
ChPV	Chordopox virus
CL	Connaught Laboratories
cMGF	chicken myelomonocytic growth factor
CMI	cell-mediated immunity
CMV	cytomegalovirus
CNPV	*Canarypox virus*
CPE	cytopathic effect
CPXV	*Cowpox virus*
CRD	cysteine-rich domain
Crm	cytokine response modifier
CS	chondroitin sulphate
CTL	cytotoxic T lymphocyte
CV	Chordopox virus
DC	dendritic cell
DED	death effector domain
DIC	disseminated intravascular coagulation
DIVA	differentiation of infected from vaccinated animals

dUTP-UNG	deoxyuridine triphosphate/uracil-N-glycosylase
DVG	Deutsche Veterinärmedizinische Gesellschaft (German Society of Veterinary Medicine)
DVV	Deutsche Vereinigung zur Bekämpfung der Viruskrankheiten (German Society for the Control of Virus Diseases)
EBV	Epstein-Barr virus
ECTV	*Ectromelia virus*
EEA	early endosomal antigen
EEV	extracellular enveloped virus
EGF	epidermal growth factor
EGFR	epidermal growth factor receptor
EMCV	*Encephalomyocarditis virus*
EV	Entomopoxvirus
EV	extracellular virus
F	fusion
FADD	Fas-associated eath domain protein
FLICE	FADD-like IL-1β-converting enzyme
FWPV	*Fowlpox virus*
GAG	glycosaminoglycan
GIF	GM-CSF/IL-2 inhibitory factor
GM-CSF	granulocyte-macrophage colony-stimulating factor
GTPV	*Goatpox virus*
HA	haemagglutinin
HAART	highly active antiretroviral therapy
HAVE	*Heliothis armigera entomopoxvirus*
HBV	*Hepatitis B virus*
HCMV	human cytomegalovirus
HE	hematoxylin/eosin (staining)
HFV	*Hare fibroma virus*
HHV	human herpesvirus
HI	haemagglutination inhibiting/inhibition
HN	haemagglutinin-neuraminidase
HPAI	highly pathogenic avian influenza
hpi	hours post infection
HPV	*Human papillomavirus*
HS	heparin sulphate
HSV	herpes simplex virus
IATA	International Air Transport Association
IBDV	*Infectious bursal disease virus*
ICTV	International Committee on Taxonomy of Viruses
IFA	indirect immunofluorescene assay
ILC	IL-11 receptor α locus chemokine
IMP	inflammation modulatory protein
IMP	inosine 5'-monophosphate
IMV	intracellular mature virus

IRF	interferon regulatory factor
ISG	interferon-stimulated gene
ITR	inverted terminal repeat
IV	intracellular virus
JAK	Janus kinase
LPAI	low pathogenic avian influenza
LSDV	*Lumpy skin disease virus*
LT	lymphotoxin
LTR	long terminal repeat
MCV	*Molluscum contagiosum virus*
MDV	Marek's disease virus
MGF	myxoma growth factor
MMEV	*Melolontha melolontha entomopoxvirus*
MNF	myxoma nuclear factor
MOCV	*Molluscum contagiosum virus*
MPXV	*Monkeypox virus*
MSEV	*Melanoplus sanguinipes entomopoxvirus*
MV	*Myxoma virus*
MVA	modified vaccinia virus Ankara
MYXV	*Myxoma virus*
NDV	*Newcastle disease virus*
NK	natural killer (cell)
NP	nucleoprotein
NT	neutralization test
NYCBH	New York City Board of Health
OAS	2',5'-oligoadenylate synthetase
OB	occlusion body
OIE	Office International des Epizooties
OMP	orotidine 5'-monophosphate
OPV	orthopoxvirus
ORF	open reading frame
ORFV	*Orf virus*
OV	oncolytic virus
PBMC	peripheral blood mononuclear cells
PCPV	*Pseudocowpox virus*
PCR	polymerase chain reaction
PFU	plaque-forming unit
PGPV	*Pigeonpox virus*
PlGF	placental growth factor
POD	peroxidase (stain)
PPRV	*Peste des petits ruminants virus*
PPVO	Parapox ovis virus
PRNT	plaque reduction neutralization test
PrV	pseudorabies virus

PTP	permeability transition pore
PVNZ	*Parapoxvirus of red deer in New Zealand*
QAC	quaternary ammonium compounds
QUPV	*Quailpox virus*
r	recombinant
RAPD	random amplified polymorphic DNA analysis
REV	*Reticuloendotheliosis virus*
RFLP	restriction fragment length polymorphism
RKI	Robert Koch Institute
RVF	*Rabbit fibroma virus*
SAH	S-adenosylhomocysteine
SCR	short consensus repeat
SECRET	smallpox virus-encoded chemokine receptor
SFV	Shope fibroma virus
SGF	SFV growth factor
SLAM	signaling lymphocytic activation molecule
SPGF	smallpox growth factor
SPICE	smallpox inhibitor of complement enzymes (variola homolog of VCP)
SPPV	*Sheeppox virus*
SqFV	*Squirrel fibroma virus*
STAT	signal transducer and activator of transcription
SWPV	*Swinepox virus*
TAA	tumor-associated antigen
TANV	*Tanapox virus*
TCID	tissue culture infective dose
TGN	trans-Golgi network
TK	thymidine kinase
TKPV	*Turkeypox virus*
TNF	tumor necrosis factor
VACV	*Vaccinia virus*
VARV	*Variola virus*
VCP	vaccinia virus complement control protein
VEGF	vascular endothelial growth factor
VETF	VACV early transcription factor
VGF	vaccinia virus growth factor
VIG	vaccinia immune globulin
VITF	virus intermediate transcription factor
vMIP	viral macrophage-inflammatory protein
WPL	without protein load
WR	Western Reserve (vaccinia virus strain)
YLDV	*Yaba-like disease virus*
YMTV	*Yaba monkey tumor virus*

Taxonomic structure of the *Poxviridae* family

The type species of each genus is underlined.

Subfamily *Chordopoxvirinae*

Genus *Orthopoxvirus*

Camelpox virus (CMLV)
Cowpox virus (CPXV)
Ectromelia virus (Mousepox) (ECTV)
Monkeypox virus (MPXV)
Raccoonpox virus (RCNV)
Taterapox virus (GBLV)
<u>*Vaccinia virus* (VACV)</u>
Variola virus (VARV)
Volepox virus (VPXV)

Tentative species in the genus
Skunkpox virus
Uasin Gishu disease virus

Genus *Parapoxvirus*

Bovine papular stomatitis virus (BPSV)
<u>*Orf virus* (ORFV)</u>
Parapoxvirus of red deer in New Zealand (PVNZ)
Pseudocowpox virus (PCPV)

Tentative species in the genus
Auzduk disease virus (Camel contagious ecthyma virus)
Chamois contagious ecthyma virus
Sealpox virus

Genus *Avipoxvirus*

Canarypox virus (CNPV)
<u>*Fowlpox virus* (FWPV)</u>

Juncopox virus (JNPV)
Mynahpox virus (MYPV)
Pigeonpox virus (PGPV)
Psittacinepox virus (PSPV)
Quailpox virus (QUPV)
Sparrowpox virus (SRPV)
Starlingpox virus (SLPV)
Turkeypox virus (TKPV

Tentative species in the genus
Crowpox virus
Peacockpox virus
Penguinpox virus

Genus *Capripoxvirus*
Goatpox virus (GTPV)
Lumpy skin disease virus (LSDV)
Sheeppox virus (SPPV)

Genus *Leporipoxvirus*
Hare fibroma virus (FIBV)
Myxoma virus (MYXV)
Rabbit fibroma virus (SFV) (*Shope fibroma virus*)
Squirrel fibroma virus (SQFV)

Genus *Suipoxvirus*
Swinepox virus (SWPV)

Genus *Molluscipoxvirus*
Molluscum contagiosum virus (MOCV)

Tentative species in the genus
Unnamed viruses of horses, donkeys, chimpanzees

Genus *Yatapoxvirus*
Tanapox virus (TANV)
Yaba monkey tumor virus (YMTV)

Unassigned viruses in the subfamily
California harbor seal poxvirus
Cotia virus
Dolphin poxvirus
Embu virus
Grey kangaroo poxvirus
Marmoset poxvirus
Molluscum-like poxvirus
Mule deer poxvirus
Nile crocodile poxvirus
Quokka poxvirus
Red kangaroo poxvirus
Salanga poxvirus
Spectacled caiman poxvirus
Squirrel poxvirus
Yoka poxvirus

Subfamily *Entomopoxvirinae*

Genus *Alphaentomopoxvirus*
Anomala cuprea entomopoxvirus (ACEV)
Aphodius tasmaniae entomopoxvirus (ATEV)
Demodema boranensis entomopoxvirus (DBEV)
Dermolepida albohirtum entomopoxvirus (DAEV)
Figulus subleavis entomopoxvirus (FSEV)
Geotrupes sylvaticus entomopoxvirus (GSEV)
Melolontha melolontha entomopoxvirus (MMEV)

Genus *Betaentomopoxvirus* ("L" = lepidopteran, "O" = orthopteran)
Acrobasis zelleri entomopoxvirus "L" (AZEV)
Amsacta moorei entomopoxvirus "L" (AMEV)
Arphia conspersa entomopoxvirus "O" (ACOEV)
Choristoneura biennis entomopoxvirus "L" (CBEV)
Choristoneura conflicta entomopoxvirus "L" (CCEV)
Choristoneura diversuma entomopoxvirus "L" (CDEV)
Choristoneura fumiferana entomopoxvirus "L" (CFEV)
Chorizagrotis auxiliars entomopoxvirus "L" (CXEV)
Heliothis armigera entomopoxvirus "L" (HAEV)
Locusta migratoria entomopoxvirus "O" (LMEV)
Oedaleus senigalensis entomopoxvirus "O" (OSEV)
Operophtera brumata entomopoxvirus "L" (OBEV)
Schistocera gregaria entomopoxvirus "O" (SGEV)

Genus *Gammaentomopoxvirus*
Aedes aegypti entomopoxvirus (AAEV)
Camptochironomus tentans entomopoxvirus (CTEV)
Chironomus attenuatus entomopoxvirus (CAEV)
Chironomus luridus entomopoxvirus (CLEV)
Chironomus plumosus entomopoxvirus (CPEV)
Goeldichironomus holoprasimus entomopoxvirus (GHEV)

Unassigned viruses in the subfamily
Diachasmimorpha entomopoxvirus (DIEVV)
Melanoplus sanguinipes entomopoxvirus "O" (MSEV)

Poxviruses
ed. by Andrew A. Mercer, Axel Schmidt and Olaf Weber

Genus *Orthopoxvirus: Vaccinia virus*

Geoffrey L. Smith

Department of Virology, Faculty of Medicine, Imperial College London, St. Mary's Campus, Norfolk Place, London W2 1PG, UK

Abstract

Vaccinia virus (VACV) and *Cowpox virus* (CPXV) have played seminal roles in human medical and biological science. In 1796 Jenner used CPXV as the first human vaccine and, subsequently, widespread immunization with the related orthopoxvirus (OPV), VACV, led to the eradication of smallpox in 1980. VACV was the first animal virus to be purified and chemically analyzed. It was also the first virus to be genetically engineered and the recombinant viruses applied as a vaccine against other infectious diseases. Here the structure, genes and replication of VACV are reviewed and its phylogenetic relationship to other OPVs is described.

Introduction

Vaccinia virus (VACV) is a member of the *Orthopoxvirus* (OPV) genus of the *Poxviridae* and is the most intensively studied poxvirus. It is famous as the vaccine that was used to eradicate smallpox, a feat completed in 1977 that remains the greatest triumph for the World Health Organization (WHO) [1]. Yet despite VACV being the only vaccine to have eradicated a disease, its origin and natural history are unknown and VACV remains an enigma of virology [2].

Following the eradication of smallpox, VACV has continued to be studied intensively. This is due partly to its development as an expression vector [3, 4] and the potential to use recombinant VACVs as live vaccines against other infectious diseases [5, 6]. In addition, VACV represents a great model for studying transcription and DNA replication in a eukaryotic cell and how a virus interacts with the host cell and immune system. So, although it is now 28 years since the last case of smallpox, there are compelling reasons to continue to study this virus.

The origin of VACV

VACV is often confused with *Cowpox virus* (CPXV), but it is established that these are distinct virus species. The confusion arises from the fact that CPXV was the virus we believe Jenner used in 1796 when he introduced vaccination against smallpox with a virus taken (indirectly) from a cow [7]. However, Downie showed in 1939 that the smallpox vaccines in use in the 20th century were not CPXV but were a related virus that became known as VACV [8, 9]. So if Jenner had used CPXV in 1796, and this is uncertain because the original virus is not available for analysis, then VACV replaced CPXV as the smallpox vaccine sometime between that date and 1939. Anecdotal evidence suggests that this change occurred early during the 19th century [2]. Importantly, CPXV, VACV and *Variola virus* (VARV), the cause of smallpox, are all closely related immunologically, so that both VACV and CPXV are effective vaccines against smallpox [10].

The name given to VACV derives from the Latin word vacca for cow and would be appropriate for a virus from cows, but it is uncertain if VACV does originate from cows. Some argue it is more probable that VACV derives from horses [2]. If so, then logically its name should be equinia not vaccinia, and the terms that derive from vaccinia, such as vaccines, vaccination and vaccinated, should be replaced by equines, equination and equinated! But vaccinia, vaccines and vaccination are firmly established in our language and are unlikely to be dislodged.

Classification

VACV is a member of the OPV genus [10] that is one of eight *Chordopoxvirus* (ChPV) genera. Other OPVs include VARV, CPXV, *Monkeypox virus* (MPXV), *Ectromelia virus* (ECTV), *Camelpox virus* (CMLV), *Volepox virus*, *Raccoonpox virus*, *Uasin Gishu virus* and *Taterapox virus* (gerbilpox) (Tab. 1). All of these viruses are cross-reactive immunologically and cross-protective, so that prior infection by any member of the genus protects against subsequent infection by any other member of the genus. Genetic studies that analyzed the pattern of restriction enzyme cleavage sites in OPV genomes showed that the central part (~ 100 kb) of these genomes is highly conserved, whereas the terminal regions vary in both length and the pattern of restriction cleavage sites [11–13]. More recently, the sequencing of whole virus genomes (www.poxvirus.org) has confirmed this analysis and provided more accurate phylogenetic relationships (see below).

There are numerous VACV strains that differ in their biological properties and virulence in man or different animal models [1, 10, 14, 15] (Tab. 2). Of the 35 strains investigated by Wokatsch [15], seven were reported to derive from VARV: Dairen, Ikeda, Lister, LMC, Tashkent, Tian Tan (or Temple of Heaven) and Williamsport. The strains that were used most widely in the

Table 1. The orthopoxviruses

Species	Host range	Comments/origin
Vaccinia virus[a]	Broad	The smallpox vaccine, origin uncertain
Variola virus	Narrow (man only)	The cause of smallpox
Cowpox virus	Broad	Isolated from rodents in Europe and USSR
Camelpox virus	Narrow (camels only)	The cause of camelpox in Africa and Asia
Ectromelia virus	Narrow	The cause of mousepox. From Europe.
Monkeypox virus	Broad	Resident in rodents in West & Central Africa
Uasin Gishu virus	Medium	Isolated from horses in Kenya and Zambia
Taterapox virus	Narrow	Isolated from *Tatera kempi* (gerbil) in West Africa
Raccoonpox virus	Broad ?	From USA
Volepox virus	Broad ?	From USA

[a]Prototypic member of genus. Adapted from Fenner et al. [10]. Rabbitpox virus and buffalopox virus are considered to be strains of VACV.

smallpox eradication campaign were Lister, New York City Board of Health (NYCBH), EM-63 and Tian Tan [1]. These were selected because they had a better safety record than some other VACV strains such as Copenhagen, Tashkent and Bern that were more reactogenic in man [1, 16].

To make a bacteriologically sterile VACV preparation, Rivers in 1931 [17] passaged the NYCBH strain in cell culture and rabbit testes, and isolated attenuated derivatives CVI-78 and CVII. Later Kempe [18] used the CVI-78 strain for vaccination of children with eczema or with other contraindications of vaccination and observed milder reactions than with the traditional calf lymph vaccine. Towards the end of the smallpox eradication campaign additional attenuated VACV strains were produced, such as modified virus Ankara (MVA) in Germany [19] and LC16m8 (derived from strain Lister) in Japan [20]. More recently, other strains have been produced by genetic engineering. For instance, NYVAC was derived from strain Copenhagen by deletion of several nonessential genes [21], and a strain of VACV Lister was engineered that lacks an essential gene and is grown on a complementing cell line [22].

The most widely used laboratory VACV strains are Western Reserve (WR) and Copenhagen, and the latter was the first VACV strain to be sequenced [23]. VACV WR is not a licensed vaccine strain and was passaged through mouse brain [24]. It is virulent for mice and was described as neurovirulent, but, although virus does reach the brain after intranasal infection, its virulence correlates with virus replication in the lungs rather than brain [25].

Table 2. Some VACV strains[a]

Strain	Origin	Comments	Ref.
Ankara	Ankara, Turkey, 1954	Passed in equines and then in chorioallantoic membrane. Called chorioallantois vaccinia Ankara (CVA)	[26]
Aracatuba virus	Aracatuba, Brazil, 2003	Circulating in dairy herds and causing infection in man. Similar to Cantalago virus	[27]
BeAn 58058 virus (BAV)	Brazil, 2001	VACV strain isolated from wild animals. Less virulent than Lister	[28]
Bern	Swiss Serum and Vaccine Institute, Berne Switzerland, 1898	Used for vaccine production in Berne 1898–1962. Virulent strain, use in man discontinued	[29]
Buffalopox	Northern India, 1967	Circulating in buffalos in Northern India. Also found in Bangladesh, Pakistan, Egypt, Indonesia	[30, 31]
Connaught Laboratories (CL)	Connaught Laboratories, 1932	Probably derived from NYCBH strain. American Type Culture Collection (ATCC) VR 117	[14, 32]
Copenhagen	Copenhagen, Denmark	First VACV strain sequenced	[23]
CVI-78	Rockefeller Institute, New York, USA, 1931	Derived from NYCBH strain by passage in chick embryo fibroblasts and rabbit testes. Attenuated strain used to immunize eczematous children	[17, 18]
Dairen I	University of Tokyo, Japan, 1934	Isolated from patient in Tokyo with vesicular rash	[33, 34]
DI	National Institutes of Health, Tokyo, Japan, 1959	Derived form Dairen I strain by passage in chick embryos	[35, 36]
dVV-L	Baxter, BioScience / Vaccine Orth/ Donau, Austria, 2002	Derived from VACV Lister by deletion of the D4R gene encoding uracil DNA glycosidase. Replication defective virus grown on complementing cell line	[22, 37]
Ecuador	Institute of National Hygiene, Guayaquil, Ecuador, 1940	Derived from Massachusetts Department of Health, Boston, USA. Low virulence	[16, 38]
EM-63	Russia, 1963	Derived from strain Ecuador. Induced mild reactions in children. Used widely in smallpox eradication campaign	[39]
Gillard	Hall Institute, Melbourne, Australia, 1942	Derived from commercial vaccine taken by the US Army Medical Service to the Hall Institute, Melbourne, Australia in 1942. Passaged on chorioallantoic membrane	[14]
Hall Institute	Melbourne, Australia, 1934	Derivative of Pasteur Institute strain number 10 supplied to the Walter and Eliza Hall Institute	[14, 40]

Table 2. (continued)

Strain	Origin	Comments	Ref.
International Health Division (IHD)-J	New York City Department of Health, USA, 1954	Derived from the NYCBH strain. Passaged by intracerebral inoculation of mice and then passed once on CAM. ATCC VR 156	[24, 41]
International Health Division – White (IHD-W)	New York City Department of Health, USA, 1954	Derived from IHD strain, hemagglutinin negative	[42]
LC16m8	Japan, 1972	Attenuated strain derived from Lister. Used for smallpox vaccination in Japan since 1974	[20]
Lister	Lister Institute, Elsetree, London, UK, 1892	Isolated from Prussian soldier in Franco-Prussian war in 1870. Used in UK since 1892 at the Lister Institute. WHO approved International Smallpox Vaccine Reference strain. Used widely in smallpox eradication campaign	[43, 44]
Mill Hill	Established at Medical Research Council, Mill Hill, London, England	Supplied to Hall Institute Melbourne, Australia as preparation of elementary bodies from back of scarified rabbit	[14]
Modified virus Ankara (MVA)	Munich, Germany, 1971	Attenuated strain derived from Ankara strain by 572 passages in chick embryo fibroblasts	[19, 45, 46]
New York City Board of Health (NYCBH)	Taken from England to New York, USA, 1856	Loines brought strain from England in 1856. Developed at New York City Board of Health Laboratories. WHO approved vaccine strain. Used widely in smallpox eradication campaign	[17]
NYVAC	Albany, New York, 1992	Derived form Copenhagen by deletion or inactivation of 18 genes. Attenuated and host range restricted	[21]
Rabbitpox	Utrecht, Holland, 1941	Isolated from rabbits during outbreak of poxvirus infection in rabbit colony	[47]
SPAn232 virus (SPAnv)	South Eastern Brazil, 2002	Isolated from sentinel mice in the forest of Cotia, Sao Paulo, Brazil	[48]
Tashkent	Origin unknown	Virulent strain, use in man discontinued	[1, 49]
Tian Tan (Temple of Heaven)	China, 1926	Used as vaccine in China	[1]
Western Reserve	Western Reserve University, Cleveland Ohio, 1941	Derived from NYCBH USA by passage in mouse brain. Widely used laboratory strain. ATCC:VR-1354	[24]
Williamsport	Indiana University Medical Center, USA, 1951	Lethal for mice after intracerebral inoculation	[14, 50]

[a]Information taken from [1, 10, 14, 15] and other sources.

VACV strains MVA, LC16m8 and NYVAC are being studied intensively and developed as live vaccines against infectious disease and cancer. In addition, following the terrorist attacks in USA in 2001, there is a drive to produce additional safer smallpox vaccines, and MVA and LC16m8, in particular, are being investigated for this purpose.

Vaccination against smallpox with VACV

Although vaccination with VACV led to the eradication of smallpox, the vaccine had a poor safety record compared to other vaccines. In the USA in the late 1960s, vaccination with VACV strain NYCBH induced approximately one death per million vaccinees and there were other infrequent but serious complications [51]. The frequency of post-vaccination complications varied with the strain of VACV used [1] and, as noted above, the more reactogenic strains were replaced by those with a better safety profile. The frequency of all complications was greater during primary vaccination than revaccination [51]. The major types of complication noted were skin disorders, neurological conditions, systemic infection and progressive vaccinia.

Progressive vaccinia occurred in vaccinees with T cell immunological deficiency and had a grave prognosis. Virus would spread from the vaccination site in a slow progressive wave that was not controlled by the immune system and was usually fatal. Administration of vaccinia immune globulin (VIG) was recommended but not always effective.

Generalized vaccinia was caused by the systemic spread of the virus from the vaccination site with the appearance of skin lesions all over the body, which resembled an infection with VARV or MPXV. In most cases the virus was eventually cleared by the immune system and the patient recovered.

Vaccinia eczematum was a disease in those with skin disorders, such as eczema, and represented a serious infection that could be widely disseminated throughout the body. Eczema is considered a contraindication to smallpox vaccination and vaccinees should be especially careful to cover the vaccination site if household members have eczema.

In addition to these adverse reactions, there were rarer neurological complications of smallpox vaccination, such as encephalitis. These were not associated with any specific pre-disposing condition and the outcome was mixed. Some vaccinees recovered completely, some recovered with sequelae and some succumbed.

Lastly, vaccination also caused myocarditis in some vaccinees. This complication was largely overlooked during the vaccination program in the 1960s and 1970s, but was detected by more careful screening of vaccinees after the re-introduction of limited vaccination in USA in the 21st century, because of fear of bioterrorism with smallpox [52]. In most cases the patient recovered but there were very rare reports of heart failure following smallpox vaccination. In these rare cases it was difficult to ascertain

and mutagenesis of specific genes indicates that approximately half of the VACV genes are nonessential for virus replication in cell culture. However, these genes may affect the outcome of virus replication *in vivo*.

The VACV replication cycle

The replication cycle starts with the attachment of virions to a susceptible cell. Before going further, it is important to reiterate that there are two infectious forms of VACV, IMV and EEV, which are surrounded by different numbers of membranes and have different surface antigens (Fig. 1) [101]. Consequently, when considering virus entry it is essential to define which form of virus is being described.

The entry of both IMV and EEV has been reviewed recently [76]. For IMV, the entry process is topologically simple because it is surrounded by a single lipid envelope [77, 81] and so the virus core can gain entry into the cytosol after fusion of the virus membrane with the plasma membrane. Early electron micrographs provided evidence of fusion of the virus membrane with the plasma membrane and deposition of the virus antigens into the plasma membrane [102, 103]. Consistent with this, the entry of IMV was accompanied by transfer of lipid into the plasma membrane, indicating a fusion event [104]. However, subsequent reports claimed that the IMV was surrounded by at least two membranes [78, 79, 105] and these membranes were all shed outside the cell, followed by the core crossing the plasma membrane by an unexplained mechanism [106]. Claims of multiple IMV membranes that are shed outside the cell are inconsistent with the observations that (i) antibody specific to virus cores detected virus cores only inside the cell and not at the cell surface [107, 108], and (ii) there have been clear images of IMV entering the cell by fusion of a single membrane with the plasma membrane [102, 103, 109, 110].

There is also controversy over the receptors used for VACV binding to cells. An early claim that the epidermal growth factor receptor (EGFR) was used [111] was refuted [112]. Similarly, the claim that chemokine receptors were used by myxoma virus (MYXV) [113] was disproved [114]. Several proteins on the surface of IMV have been proposed as attachment proteins based on their ability to interact with cell surface glycosaminoglycans (GAGs). For instance, A27 binds cell surface heparan sulfate (HS) [115, 116], D8 binds chondroitin sulfate (CS) [117] and soluble H3 binds HS [118]. However, the significance of these findings is questionable because IMV with the *A27L* gene repressed [119] or deleted [120] remains infectious; similarly, an IMV double mutant lacking A27 and D8 is infectious [116]. Moreover, soluble CS did not inhibit IMV infectivity [115] and several other GAGs and polyanions had little effect on IMV infectivity on some cell types and none on others [109]. So the IMV receptor(s) remain unknown. However, it is established that the receptors used by IMV and EEV are different [121], and that a monoclonal antibody directed against a cell surface trypsin-sensitive antigen can block binding of the majority of IMV [122] but has no effect on EEV [121]. The antigen recognized by this antibody remains to be identified.

Enveloped viruses enter cells by fusion of the virus membrane with a cell membrane and this fusion is catalyzed by virus protein(s) in the virus membrane [123]. For many viruses this fusion machine is formed by a single virus glycoprotein that may be cleaved from a precursor into two subunits. In contrast, the fusion machine of VACV IMV is composed of a complex of eight separate proteins. These proteins, A28 [108], A21 [124], L5 [125], H2 [126], A16 [127], G3, G9 and A5 [128] are small, non-glycosylated proteins that are present in the IMV membrane. Proteins A21, A28, G3, H2 and L5 all have an N-terminal transmembrane domain and up to two disulfide bonds, whereas proteins J5, A16 and G9 all have a C-terminal transmembrane domain and four to ten predicted disulphide bonds [128]. Each of these proteins is conserved in all sequenced poxviruses, suggesting a common mechanism of entry. This fusion machine is essential for entry of both IMV and EEV, showing that both types of virus have a common fusion event during their entry (Fig. 3).

EEV is surrounded by two membranes and is therefore faced with a topological difficulty during entry into a cell. Fusion of the outer membrane with a cell membrane will only deliver an IMV particle into the cytosol. Unless the IMV membrane is also removed, replication cannot start. This difficulty has been resolved by the demonstration that the outer membrane of EEV is removed by a non-fusogenic mechanism that requires specific molecules on the surface of the cell and virus [110] (Fig. 3). Upon binding to a susceptible cell, the EEV outer membrane is disrupted at the point of contact enabling the IMV particle within to bind to the plasma membrane. It can then fuse and enter the cell like a free IMV particle. After its disruption, the EEV membrane remains over the IMV particle as a shroud and continues to protect the IMV particle from antibody. The EEV membrane, and the antigens it contains, remain outside the cell.

The cell surface molecules required for disruption of the EEV membrane are GAGs and the greater the negative charge and larger the molecule, the more effectively the EEV membrane is disrupted. Interestingly, cells lacking cell surface HS and CS are still able to bind EEV particles, but membrane disruption does not take place under the conditions measured. Genetic studies showed that EEV surface proteins A34 and B5, which form a complex [129], are required for membrane rupture [110]. The mechanism by which the EEV outer membrane is shed seems unique in virology, for hitherto, all known enveloped viruses were thought to shed their membranes by fusion [130].

After a virus core has entered the cytoplasm, it is transported on microtubules deeper into the cell to sites near the nucleus [131]. The proteins on the core surface needed for this transportation have not been identified.

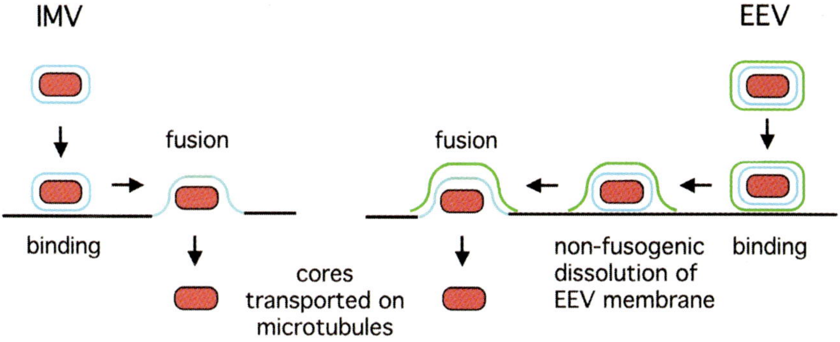

Figure 3. The entry of VACV IMV and EEV. IMV binds to an unidentified cell surface receptor and fuses with the plasma membrane enabling release of the core into the cytoplasm. EEV binds to the cell surface and glycosaminoglycans mediate non-fusogenic disruption of the EEV outer membrane. The internal IMV particle then binds to the cell surface and enters as for IMV.

Virus transcription

VACV genes are transcribed by the virus-encoded, multi-subunit, DNA-dependent RNA polymerase that is packaged in the virus core [83, 132]. mRNAs are polyadenylated [133] and have a 5' methylated cap [134, 135]. Transcription is divided into three classes: early, intermediate and late, with expression of each gene class dependent upon prior expression of proteins of the preceding class (for review see [136]). The presence of a complete transcriptional system within the VACV core, including a capping enzyme [134], polyA polymerase [133], early transcription initiation factor [137, 138] and early transcription termination factor [139], enables early mRNAs to be synthesized immediately after infection without host protein synthesis. Early mRNAs are complementary to approximately one half of the VACV genome [140, 141].

Early VACV promoters are quite short (~30 bp) and rich in A^{+}T [142]. These promoters are not recognized by the RNA polymerase II of host cells, and the VACV RNA polymerase also does not recognize promoters from cells that are transcribed by host DNA-dependent RNA polymerase II. Transcription of early VACV genes is terminated approximately 30 nucleotides downstream of a sequence TTTTTNT (where N represents any nucleotide) [143], although this signal is recognized in RNA as UUUUUNU [144]. The termination of transcription at this sequence is not 100% efficient so that some transcripts are longer than a single ORF.

Early virus transcripts are extruded from the partially uncoated cores, possibly *via* the pores in the core surface identified by cryo-electron tomog-

Table 3. Vaccinia virus enzymes for DNA precursor synthesis

Enzyme	Gene	Comment	References
Ribonucleotide reductase	*F4L, I4L*	Heterodimer, nonessential, contributes to virulence	[174–178]
Thymidine kinase	*J2R*	Expressed early, homotetramer, non-essential, contributes to virulence	[179–183]
Thymidylate kinase	*A48R*	Expressed early, nonessential	[184, 185]
dUTPase	*F2L*	Originally called pseudo-protease, expressed early, nonessential	[186–189]
Guanylate kinase	*A57R*	Incomplete gene in VACV and VARV	[190, 191]

raphy [82], and were reported to co-localize with microtubules [145]. Early genes encode proteins that aid evasion of the host response to infection (considered in the accompanying chapter by Grant McFadden), enzymes to increase the size of the nucleoside pools (see Tab. 3) and enzymes for virus nucleic acid synthesis, such as DNA polymerase (see below).

After early proteins have been expressed, the virus core is uncoated further and the DNA genome is released for replication. Once DNA replication starts, the pattern of transcription changes and intermediate genes are transcribed [146]. Intermediate genes encoded on plasmids can be transcribed in the absence of virus DNA replication [146], suggesting DNA replication may dilute out an inhibitory factor on virus genomes. The intermediate promoters are functionally distinct [147] and their recognition by the VACV RNA polymerase requires virus intermediate transcription factors (VITFs). These include the capping enzyme [148], VITF-1, VITF-2, and VITF-3. VITF-1 is a 30-kDa protein that is also a component of the RNA polymerase (gene *E4L*) [149], VITF-3 is a heterodimer composed of the A8 and A23 proteins [150] and VITF-2 is a host factor [151]. Intermediate genes are less numerous than early (or late) genes and some encode late transcription factors [152].

Late transcription requires prior expression of both early and intermediate proteins and the replication of virus DNA. Late promoters contain the sequence TAAAT(G) or TAAAAT(G) at the site of transcriptional initiation [153] and have been defined by mutagenesis [154]. Late transcription factors are encoded by the *A1L*, *A2L*, and *G8R* intermediate genes, an early gene [155, 156] and a host factor [157, 158]. In general, late genes encode structural proteins that form new virions, additional virulence factors that aid virus escape from the immune system, or enzymes that are packaged into new virions to initiate transcription in the next infected cell. Late mRNAs have two unusual features: first, there is a polyA sequence of unknown function at the 5' end of the mRNA immediately downstream of the cap structure and upstream of the AUG codon [159, 160]; second, the mRNAs are long and heterogeneous in length [161] due to a failure to terminate at specific sites (the early termination sequence is no longer recognized by the virus RNA polymerase).

DNA replication

DNA replication begins after the expression of early proteins and may be evident within 2 h after infection at high multiplicity [162]. The VACV proteins needed for DNA replication include DNA polymerase [163] (gene *E9L*), DNA processivity factor (gene *A20R*) [164], a serine-threonine protein kinase (gene *B1R*) [165, 166], nucleic acid-independent nucleoside triphosphatase (gene *D5R*) [167] and uracil DNA glycosylase (gene *D4R*) [168] (for review see Moss 2001 [169]). VACV also encodes a DNA ligase (gene *A50R*) [170, 171]. Surprisingly, this enzyme is not essential for virus replication [91, 172]. However, a DNA ligase negative mutant was attenuated *in vivo* and showed enhanced sensitivity to DNA damaging agents [173].

In addition to these enzymes involved in DNA replication, VACV encodes several enzymes involved in the synthesis of DNA precursors (Tab. 3). These are all nonessential for virus replication and, where tested, have been shown to promote virulence. The ribonucleotide reductase and thymidine kinase enzymes are closely related to their mammalian orthologues and show 70–80% amino acid identity.

DNA replication starts with the introduction of a nick into one of the DNA strands near the terminal hairpin (Fig. 4). Unfolding of the hairpin allows DNA polymerase to copy the hairpin and elongate to the end of the template. Then the two strands separate and the nascent DNA refolds into a hairpin enabling the DNA polymerase to continue to elongate down the length of the genome. Eventually concatemeric molecules are produced. These are resolved by nicking with specific nucleases into unit length monomers that are packaged into new virions. Resolution of the concatemers requires late gene expression [192] and at least three virus proteins: DNA topoisomerase I (gene *H7R*) [193, 194] that can resolve Holliday junctions; a DNase with nicking joining activity (gene *K4L*) that can cleave concatemeric junction fragments [195]; and a Holliday junction resolvase encoded by gene *A22R* [196, 197]. During virus morphogenesis the DNA genome is packaged into virions by the A32 protein [198]. It has been estimated that approximately 10 000 copies of the virus genome are produced per cell and approximately half of these are packaged [162, 199].

Morphogenesis

For an overview of virus morphogenesis, see [101] (Fig. 5). Virus replication occurs in cytoplasmic factories in which the first structures visible by elec-

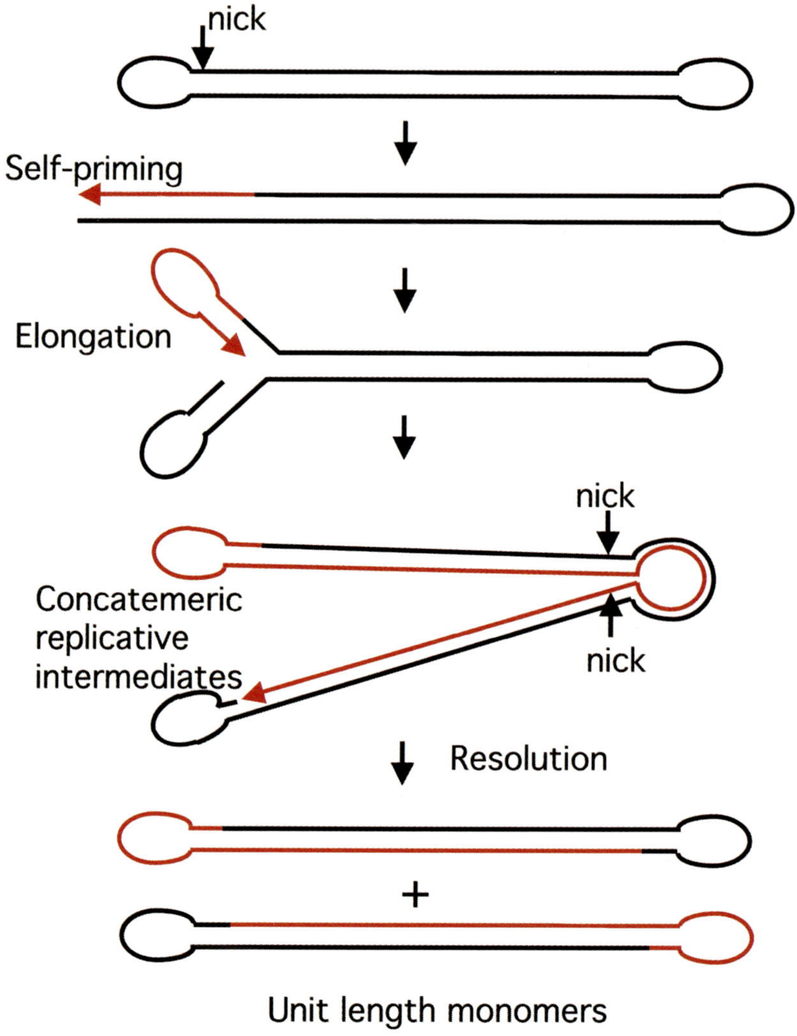

Figure 4. Schematic depiction of VACV DNA replication. The linear dsDNA molecule with terminal hairpins is nicked near one hairpin enabling extension to the end of the template. After refolding of the terminal hairpin, elongation continues to produce concatemeric DNA intermediates that are resolved into unit length monomers. Newly synthesized DNA is shown in red, and parental DNA in black.

tron microscopy are crescent shaped and are composed of virus protein and host-derived lipid. Crescents associate with the virus DNA/protein complex and become a sealed oval or spherical particle called immature virus (IV). IV matures into an electron-dense IMV by proteolytic cleavage of some capsid proteins and condensation. Subsequently, IMV particles are trans-

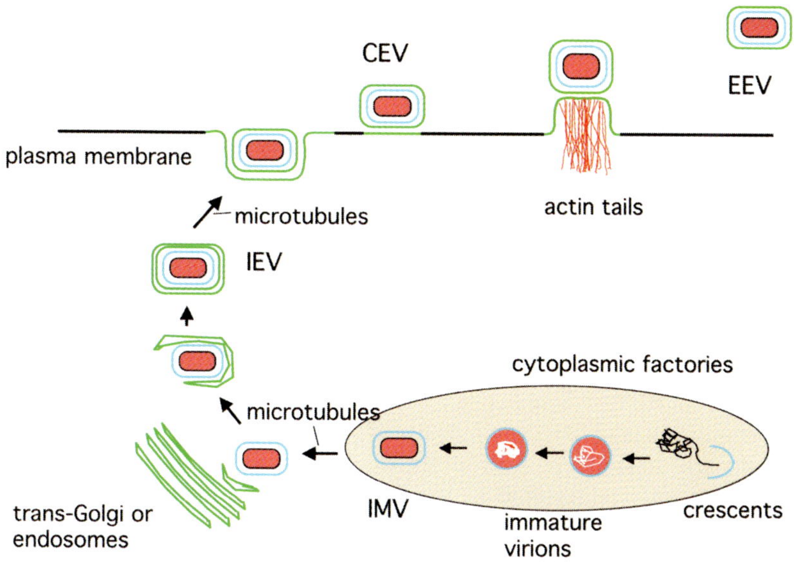

Figure 5. The pathway of VACV morphogenesis. A virus crescent forms in cytoplasmic factories and grows to form immature virus (IV). IV condenses and matures into IMV that is transported on microtubules from the virus factory to sites where it is wrapped by additional intracellular membranes to form intracellular enveloped virus (IEV). IEV is transported to the cell periphery on microtubules and is exposed on the cell surface by exocytosis as cell-associated enveloped virus (CEV). CEV may induce formation of an actin tail or be released as EEV. Adapted and reproduced from Smith et al. [101] with permission from the Society for General Microbiology.

ported from the virus factory on microtubules, wrapped by intracellular membranes to form intracellular enveloped virions (IEVs) and transported to the cell surface on microtubules. Here, the IEV outer membrane fuses with the plasma membrane to expose a virion on the cell surface by exocytosis. This virion is called cell-associated enveloped virus (CEV) and, if it is released from the cell, it is termed EEV.

The number and origin of lipid membranes in the virus crescent has been disputed. Early reports claimed that these were a single lipid bilayer that was synthesized *de novo* in the cytoplasm [77, 200, 201]. Later, this view was challenged and it was reported that these structures represented a double lipid bilayer that was derived from and continuous with the intermediate compartment within the endoplasmic reticulum and Golgi stack [78]. Other studies supported this hypothesis [79, 105, 202]. However, these reports lacked unequivocal images showing two lipid membranes in the nascent crescent membrane or the IMV particle and freeze fracture studies also failed to show evidence of two membranes [79, 203]. On the other hand, the thickness of the crescent membrane and the IMV membrane were each 5 nm, the same as cellular membranes measured by the same technique in the same cell [81]. Moreover, tilt series analysis and serial sectioning of samples showed no continuity with cellular membranes [81]. Lastly, unequivocal evidence for a single membrane was provided by electron micrographs that showed fusion of the virus membrane with the plasma membrane and the absence of any other virus membrane [109, 110]. The challenge now is to understand how a single membrane can be produced in the cytoplasm.

Studies of morphogenesis have utilized drugs, conditional lethal mutants and electron microscopy, and have defined several stages in virion development. The earliest stage of crescent membrane formation requires the F10 protein kinase [204, 205] and the H5 protein [206]. Two other proteins needed early in crescent formation are A14 and A17. These form a complex and are phosphorylated by the F10 kinase. Interestingly, without these proteins tubular vesicles accumulate near the factories [207–210]. The G5 protein is also needed for membrane formation and for A17 phosphorylation and cleavage [211]. Membrane formation is inhibited reversibly by the drug rifampicin [201, 212] and genetic studies, using viruses resistant to this drug, showed that the D13 protein was the drug target [213, 214]. Repression of the *D13L* gene inhibited virus morphogenesis at the same stage as rifampicin [215]. Recently, the D13 65-kDa protein was shown to form trimers that assemble into a lattice on the external side of the crescent membrane and may provide a scaffold for membrane assembly [216]. A mutation in the D13 protein enabled lattice formation but the crescent did not form. Instead, the D13 lattice formed back-to-back protein layers [216]. The A11 protein is also needed for the formation of crescents, but is not part of the mature virion [217]. A11 binds the DNA packaging protein A32, is phosphorylated and is needed for the proteolytic cleavage of several capsid proteins [217].

The next stage of morphogenesis requires interaction of the virus membrane with the viroplasm containing the DNA genome. This process requires the A30 [218] and G7 proteins [219], which interact. The packaging of DNA into virions requires the A32 protein, without which sealed IVs can form. These can complete the morphogenic pathway but they lack the DNA genome [198].

Proteins A9 [220], L1 [221, 222] and H3 [223, 224] each form part of the IMV surface and are required for the conversion of IV to IMV. Similarly, core proteins F17 [225] and I1 [226] are needed for maturation of IV to IMV. Maturation is associated with cleavage of several capsid proteins [227] at an AGA/S motif [228] and if this cleavage is inhibited, maturation is arrested [229].

The IMV membrane contains many proteins. As mentioned above, eight of these form a complex and are conserved in all poxviruses sequenced

[128]. These proteins are grouped into two classes. Proteins A16, G9 and J5 all contain a C-terminal, membrane-spanning, hydrophobic domain and a Cys-rich domain on the virion surface with intramolecular disulfide bonds. The latter domain shares sequence similarity between these proteins suggesting they were produced by gene duplication events. The second group of proteins A21, A28, H2, L5, and G3 all have a hydrophobic domain at or near the N terminus and are unrelated in sequence. These also contain Cys residues, although these are fewer than those in the other group. Genetic studies have shown that in the absence of any one of these proteins, the protein complex is either present in lower amounts or is less stable. In the absence of proteins A21 [124], A28 [108], H2 [126], L5 [125] and A16 [127], virus morphogenesis is normal but virions lack infectivity, due to a defect in entry (see above).

Other proteins on the IMV surface include D8 [230], L1 [221, 222], H3 [118, 224], A27 [231], A14 [209], A14.5 [232] and A17 [207, 233–235]. It is notable that all these proteins are not glycosylated. A27 is associated with the IMV surface *via* interactions with other IMV membrane proteins, whereas most other IMV surface proteins are integral membrane proteins. The A27 [236], H3 [237] and L1 [238] are targets for antibodies that neutralize IMV infectivity.

The presence of so many disulfide bonds on the surface of IMV particles posed the question, "How can such bonds be established in the cytoplasm?", a reducing environment. This problem was solved by the discovery that VACV encodes its own thiol oxidoreductase system [239] that is composed of proteins E10 [240, 241], G4 [242] and A2.5 [243]. These proteins are essential for virus morphogenesis and establish disulfide bonds in several IMV membrane proteins.

Transport and wrapping of IMV particles

After the formation of IMV, virions are transported away from virus factories on microtubules [120, 244] to sites within the cytoplasm where they are wrapped by membrane cisternae derived from either the *trans*-Golgi network [86, 245] or endosomes [87]. Three VACV proteins have been identified that are needed for this wrapping. One of these, A27, is present as a trimer on the IMV surface [231] and when it is repressed [119] or deleted [120] wrapping is inhibited. The other two proteins, F13 [246] and B5 [68, 69], are incorporated into the wrapping membranes.

In the absence of F13, wrapping is inhibited, virus dissemination to the cell periphery is reduced and the yield of EEV is reduced approximately 100-fold [247]. The phenotype of virus lacking F13 is similar to that of infected cells treated with drugs IMCBH [248] or ST-246 [249], and IMCBH-resistant VACV strains contain a mutation in the F13 protein [250]. The F13 protein shows amino acid similarity to phospholipases [251], and has phospholipase activity [252, 253]. It is located on the cytosolic face of the wrapping membranes [254] and is acylated [245, 255], a modification needed for correct targeting to the wrapping membranes [256]. The phospholipase activity of F13 is required for wrapping of IMV by post-Golgi vesicles [257], for targeting of B5 to these vesicles [258] and for enveloped virus formation [259].

Gene *B5R* encodes a 42-kDa type I transmembrane protein that is related to complement control proteins and is expressed on the surface of EEV [66, 68, 69]. A 35-kDa proteolytic fragment is also secreted from infected cells [260]. Deletion of the B5R gene caused a failure to wrap IMV to IEV, lack of dissemination of virus to the cell surface and a small plaque phenotype [261–263]. The B5 deletion mutant is also highly attenuated [261]. B5 also interacts with another EEV protein A34 [129].

Transport of IEV to the cell surface

After IEVs are formed they are transported to the cell surface. Originally this process was reported to be due to the polymerization of actin on IEVs [264], but in fact, IEVs are transported on microtubules [265–268]. Microtubule-based transport of IEVs was reported to require proteins A36 [267, 269] and F12 [270]. However, although A36 binds the microtubule-motor protein kinesin [271], virions are still transported to the cell surface without A36 [272–275]. In contrast, in the absence of F12, they are not [275, 276]. Kinetic measurements indicated that without A36 the transport of IEV was delayed and the length of movement of individual IEV particles on microtubules was reduced [275]. Nonetheless, without A36, IEV still move on microtubules and, therefore, at least one other protein must mediate interaction of IEV with microtubule motors. A good candidate is the F12 protein because in its absence IEV are not transported to the cell periphery [275, 276].

Actin tail formation from the cell surface

Once an IEV reaches the cell periphery, the outer membrane fuses with the plasma membrane to expose a virion on the surface by endocytosis. The cell surface CEV particle can then induce actin tail formation from the cytosolic face of the plasma membrane beneath the CEV particle. The presence of virus-induced cell surface projections had been noted in early studies [277, 278]. Virus proteins required for actin tail polymerization include B5, F13, F12, A36, A34 and A33. In the absence of B5, F13 and F12, the defect can be attributed to morphogenesis being arrested prior to formation of CEV. The presence of the A36 protein, however, is essential for actin polymerization at the cell surface [272, 273, 279]. A36 accumulates on the cytosolic face of the plasma membrane beneath CEV particles [274] where specific tyrosine phosphorylation of this protein initiates a chain of reactions leading to polymerization of actin [279, 280]. It was proposed that B5-induced signaling from the outside of the cell via src tyrosine kinase [281] was needed to initiate this cascade of events. Drugs that block this pathway are effective at combating infections caused by OPVs [282]. The requirement for protein A33 may reflect its role as a chaperone for correct A36 transport [283]. Similarly, A34 may be required indirectly, through its interaction with B5 [129].

The importance of actin tails for cell-to-cell spread of virus is illustrated by the fact that all mutants unable to make actin tails form a small plaque and, where tested, have been shown to be attenuated *in vivo* (for reviews see [101, 284, 285]).

VACV may spread from cell to cell in several ways in tissue culture [101]. First, released EEV may bind to either adjacent or distal cells. Convection-mediated spread of EEV in a unidirectional manner to distal cells [286] gives rise to the characteristic comet-shaped plaques [287]. Comets are more pronounced with strains of virus that release greater amounts of EEV [288]. The formation of comet tails (formed by secondary plaques) is inhibited by antibody directed to EEV [287], but the size of the primary plaque is reduced only slightly [286]. This indicates that virus can spread from cell to cell in an antibody-resistant manner. This spread may or may not utilize actin tails, as illustrated by a mutant lacking the A56 protein, which does make actin tails, and a mutant lacking the A36 protein, which does not [286]. VACV may also spread from cell to cell by an antibody-sensitive pathway. This was illustrated by a mutant lacking the A33 protein, which formed plaques that are inhibited by EEV antibody [286]. Therefore, the A33 protein contributes to the spread of EEV from cell to cell in an antibody-resistant manner. Another mechanism of spread involves VACV-induced motility of infected cells [289] that requires the F11 protein [290].

Release of EEV

EEV is released from infected cells before cell lysis, whereas IMV is released only after cell lysis. The amount of EEV released varies with the VACV strain [288] and the cell type [291]. The EEV envelope contains several proteins that are absent from IMV [292] and these were mapped to the *B5R* [68, 69], *A33R* [293], *A34R* [294], *A56R* [295], *F13L* [246] and *K2R* [296] genes, although the last study was done with CPXV, not VACV. Deletion or mutation of several of these proteins influences the production or release of EEV (Tab. 4). Without B5 or F13, the yield of EEV drops 5–10- or 100-fold, respectively, due to inhibition of IEV formation. Similarly, without F12 there is a 7–10-fold reduction in CEV due to the failure of IEV

Table 4. Properties of virus mutants lacking genes encoding IEV- and EEV-specific proteins

Virus mutant lacking	Plaque size	Actin tails	IEV	EEV	References
A33	Small	No	Yes	↑ × 3	[297]
A34	Small	No	Few	↑ × 25[a]	[298]
A56	Fusogenic	Yes	Yes	Normal	[101]
B5	Small	Very few	Very few	↓ × 5–10	[261, 262]
F13	Tiny	No	No	↓ × 100	[278]
A36	Tiny	No	Yes	↓ 5	[272, 273, 302]
F12	Tiny	Very few	Yes	No	[270, 276]

[a] Specific infectivity reduced fivefold.

to be transported to the cell surface [276]. Loss of the A56 protein (hemagglutinin) does not affect EEV formation. In contrast, loss of A33 [297] or A34 [298] caused an increase in EEV release, although in the latter case there was a 5-fold reduction in specific infectivity [298]. The role of the A34 protein in release of EEV was demonstrated earlier in a report showing that a K151D mutation in the C-type lectin-like domain caused enhanced EEV release [299]. Other mutations that affect EEV release include truncations of the A33 protein and a P185S mutation in B5 [300, 301].

Phylogenetic comparisons of OPV genes

The availability of sequence data from many poxviruses, see www.poxvirus.org, has enabled bioinformatic analysis of genes that are conserved between different viruses and the establishment of phylogenetic trees. A phylogenetic tree of the ChPVs, other than parapoxviruses, [100] (Fig. 6a) showed that the *Avipoxvirus* genus, exemplified by fowlpox virus (FWPV), was the most divergent genus with the largest genome and the greatest number of genes unique to a specific genus. The *Molluscipoxvirus* genus (containing a single member, molluscum contagiosum virus, MOCV) was the next most divergent group with many unique genes and a collection of immunodulatory proteins quite distinct from other ChPVs. Subsequent analysis of proteins of the *Parapoxvirus* genus showed that this genus forms a divergent group of viruses in a manner similar to, but distinct from, MOCV [303, 304]. The *Suipoxvirus*, *Leporipoxvirus*, *Yatapoxvirus* and *Capripoxvirus* genera formed a subgroup with slightly smaller genomes and some other features, such as the presence of a gene related to VACV *C7L* within the central region of the genome, that distinguish these viruses from the OPV genus. Lastly, the OPV genus is a group of closely related viruses that have genomes of approximately 200 kb and are now considered in more detail.

Overall, the degree of relatedness of the OPVs is higher than within other genera. For instance, the leporipoxviruses, *Shope fibroma virus* (SFV) and MYXV are more divergent (Fig. 6a). The close relatedness of OPVs is also illustrated by analysis of the central 100 kb of their genome where the gene content, order and sequence are highly conserved. For instance, CMPL strain CMS and VARV Bangladesh 1975 differ in length by only 82 nucleotides over this 100 kb region [92]. Within the OPVs, the greatest difference in length in this region is between MPXV Zaire (shortest) and CPXV Brighton Red (longest) and is only 382 nucleotides [100]. Figure 6b shows a phylogenetic tree of selected viruses from the OPV genus [100]. This tree shows, firstly, that VARV and CMLV are closely related species and represent one branch of the unrooted tree. Secondly, MPXV is quite distinct from VARV genetically, despite causing a similar disease in man. Recently, comparison of the sequence of the MPXV strain that caused an epidemic in USA in 2003 (that originated from West Africa) with the strain from Zaire in Central Africa showed that there are two distinct MPXV clades [305]. The former had lower virulence in man and there were no fatalities reported from the outbreak in USA [306]. The phylogenetic tree also showed that, whereas all other strains of a particular virus species cluster together, strains of CPXV were divergent, suggesting that these viruses should be re-classified as separate species [100].

There are 89 genes that are conserved in all sequenced ChPVs. Originally, 90 genes were identified [99, 100], but the sequences of the parapoxviruses *Orf virus* and *Bovine papular stomatitis virus* [303] showed that genes equivalent to VACV Copenhagen *F15L* and *D9R* are absent from these viruses. The recognition of one extra gene, *A2.5L* [243], which was not classified originally because of its small size, made the current number of conserved genes 89. These are all located in the central region of the genome (Fig. 2), and encode proteins that have essential functions in virus replication, such as entry, transcription, or assembly. These 89 genes have a conserved arrangement and orientation, except in avipoxviruses where blocks of genes are inverted compared to other ChPVs [100]. At least one function has now been established for 78 out of these 89 genes. These genes presumably represent the core genome of an ancestral poxvirus from which the poxviruses known today have evolved. During evolution of these viruses with their hosts, additional genes were acquired that give the individual viruses their specific host range, virulence and tropism. These genes are located near the genome termini and are variable in number, type and sequence. An interesting feature of these genes is that with very few exceptions they are transcribed outwards towards the genome termini. It has been suggested that such arrangement might reduce dsRNA formation and so minimize induction of IFN [307].

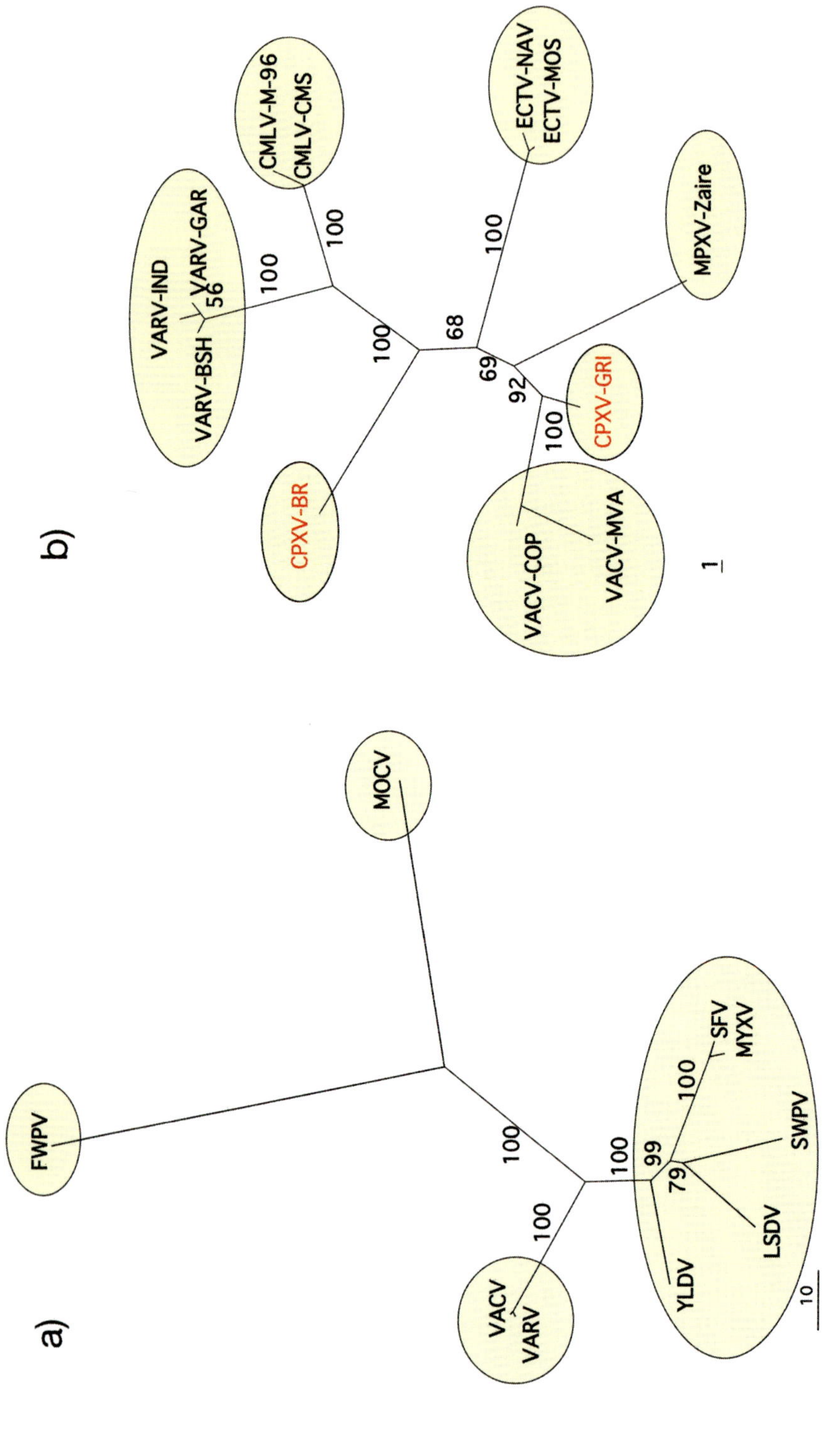
a)
FWPV
MOCV
VACV
VARV
100
100
100
99
79
SFV
MYXV
SWPV
LSDV
YLDV
10
b)
VARV-IND
VARV-GAR
VARV-BSH
56
100
CMLV-M-96
CMLV-CMS
100
100
68
ECTV-NAV
ECTV-MOS
100
MPXV-Zaire
69
92
CPXV-GRI
100
CPXV-BR
VACV-COP
VACV-MVA
1

Vaccinia virus pathogenesis

The need to create more attenuated VACV strains has prompted several groups to investigate VACV genes contributing to virus virulence. These are numerous and are located throughout the genome, although concentrated in the terminal regions [75]. The proteins encoded by these genes can be classified into groups according to function. The first group include genes encoding enzymes that enhance virus replication by increasing the size of nucleoside triphosphate precursors for nucleic acid synthesis. Several such enzymes are listed in Table 3. The second group includes proteins that aid virus spread from cell to cell, but which are not required for production of IMV. These proteins include those of the IEV and EEV envelope B5, F12, F13, A33, A34 and A36 (see Tab. 4). Without these proteins, normal amounts of IMV can be made but the virus is highly attenuated due to a failure to spread efficiently from the infected cell. The third group includes proteins that counteract the host response to infection and have been termed immunomodulators. These may either function inside the cell to inhibit apoptosis or signaling cascades leading to induction of pro-inflammatory host proteins, or they may be secreted from the cell and function by binding to and neutralizing host complement factors, cytokines, chemokines or IFNs. The immunomodulators are reviewed in another chapter of this book by Nazarian and McFadden.

Several models have been developed for studying VACV pathogenesis in mice. The most widely used model is an intranasal infection of BALB/c mice that gives a systemic infection [49, 308]. The outcome of infection by this route depends on the virus dose administered as well as the age of animals infected. The severity of the infection is monitored by weight loss, signs

Figure 6. Phylogenetic relationships of poxviruses. (a) Unrooted phylogenetic tree showing the relationships of ChPVs. The amino acid sequences of 17 poxvirus proteins (VACV-COP E9, I7, I8, G9, J3, J6, H2, H4, H6, D1, D5, D6, D11, D13, A7, A16 and A24) were aligned and a maximum-likelihood tree was obtained as described previously [100]. The bootstrap values from 1000 replica samplings and the divergence scale (substitutions/site) are indicated. (b) Unrooted phylogenetic tree of 12 OPVs obtained by a maximum likelihood method using protein sequences. The amino acid sequences of 12 proteins (VACV-COP C6, C7, N1, K2, F2, F4, F6, F8, A56, B1, B5 and B15) encoded in the terminal regions of the genomes were aligned and the maximum-likelihood tree was obtained as described previously [100]. The bootstrap values from 1000 replica samplings and the divergence scale (substitutions/site) are indicated. The two CPXV strains do not cluster together and are shown in red. VACV, vaccinia virus; VARV, variola virus; MOCV, molluscum contagiosum virus; FWPV, fowlpox virus; SFV, Shope fibroma virus; MYXV, myxoma virus; YLDV, Yaba-like disease virus; LSDV, lumpy skin disease virus; SWPX, swinepox virus; VACV-COP, vaccinia virus strain Copenhagen; VACV-MVA, vaccinia virus strain modified virus Ankara; MPXV-Zaire, monkeypox virus strain Zaire; ECTV-NAV, ectromelia virus strain Naval; ECTV-MOS, ectromelia virus strain Moscow; CMLV-CMS, camelpox virus strain CMS; CMLV-M-96, camelpox virus strain M-96; VARV-India, variola major virus strain India; VARV-BSH, variola major virus strain Bangladesh 1975; VARV-GAR; variola minor virus strain Garcia. Adapted and reproduced from Gubser et al. [100] with permission from the Society for General Microbiology.

of illness, such as arched back, ruffled fur, mobility and piloerection [309] and by virus titers in different organs [310, 311]. The disease is attributable to pneumonia, rather than to virus spread to and replication in other organs such as the brain [25].

A second mouse model utilizes infection by the intradermal route into the ear pinnae [312, 313]. This results in a localized, mild infection in which the animals show no systemic signs of illness and in which virus does not spread from the inoculation site. The severity of infection is measured by the size of the infected lesion and the virus titer within it. An attractive feature of this model, in addition to the mild nature of the infection, is the ability to quantify and analyze the cell populations that have migrated into the infected ear by fluorescence activated cell sorting [314, 315]. This model was used to measure the virulence of several smallpox vaccine strains, and showed that the virulence observed [313] was consistent with the virulence of the viruses in man during smallpox vaccination [1].

Both the intradermal and intranasal models of infection have useful features, and the consequence of knocking out a specific gene may vary in the different models. Other models such as intracranial and intraperitoneal injection have been used by some investigators but are more severe and do not represent natural routes of infection.

Acknowledgements

I thank Kim L. Roberts, Claire M. Midgley and Aodhnait Fahy for critical reading of the manuscript. Work in the author's laboratory has been supported by the UK Medical Research Council, the Wellcome Trust, Biotechnology and Biological Sciences Research Council and the European Community. The author is a Wellcome Trust Principal Research Fellow.

References

1 Fenner F, Anderson DA, Arita I, Jezek Z, Ladnyi ID (1988) *Smallpox and Its Eradication*. World Health Organisation, Geneva

2 Baxby D (1981) *Jenner's Smallpox Vaccine. The Riddle of the Origin of Vaccinia Virus*. Heinemann, London

3 Mackett M, Smith GL, Moss B (1982) Vaccinia virus: a selectable eukaryotic cloning and expression vector. *Proc Natl Acad Sci USA* 79: 7415–7419

4 Panicali D, Paoletti E (1982) Construction of poxviruses as cloning vectors: insertion of the thymidine kinase gene from herpes simplex virus into the DNA of infectious vaccinia virus. *Proc Natl Acad Sci USA* 79: 4927–4931

5 Smith GL, Mackett M, Moss B (1983) Infectious vaccinia virus recombinants that express hepatitis B virus surface antigen. *Nature* 302: 490–495

6 Panicali D, Davis SW, Weinberg RL, Paoletti E (1983) Construction of live vaccines by using genetically engineered poxviruses: Biological activity of recom-

binant vaccinia virus expressing influenza virus hemagglutinin. *Proc Natl Acad Sci USA* 80: 5364–5368
7 Jenner E (1798) *An Enquiry into the Causes and Effects of Variolae Vaccinae, a Disease Discovered in some Western Countries of England, particularly Gloucestershire, and known by the Name of Cow Pox*. Reprinted by Cassell, 1896, London
8 Downie AW (1939) Immunological relationship of the virus of spontaneous cowpox to vaccinia virus. *Br J Exp Pathol* 20: 158–176
9 Downie AW (1939) A study of the lesions produced experimentally by cowpox virus. *J Pathol Bacteriol* 48: 361–379
10 Fenner F, Wittek R, Dumbell KR (1989) *The Orthopoxviruses*. Academic Press, London
11 Wittek R, Menna A, Schumperli D, Stoffel S, Muller HK, Wyler R (1977) HindIII and SstI restriction sites mapped on rabbit poxvirus and vaccinia virus DNA. *J Virol* 23: 669–678
12 Mackett M, Archard LC (1979) Conservation and variation in Orthopoxvirus genome structure. *J Gen Virol* 45: 683–701
13 Esposito JJ, Knight JC (1985) Orthopoxvirus DNA: a comparison of restriction profiles and maps. *Virology* 143: 230–251
14 Fenner F (1958) The biological characters of several strains of vaccinia, cowpox and rabbitpox viruses. *Virology* 5: 502–529
15 Wokatsch R (1972) Vaccinia virus. In: M Majer, SA Plotkin (eds): *Strains of human viruses*. Karger, Basel, 241–257
16 Polak MF, Beunders BJW, Werff AR, Van der Sanders EW, Klaveren JN, Van Brans LM (1963) A comparative study of clinical reactions observed after application of several smallpox vaccines in primary vaccination of young adults. *Bull World Health Organ* 29: 311–322
17 Rivers TM (1931) Cultivation of vaccine virus for Jennerian prophylaxis in man. *J Exp Med* 54: 453–461
18 Kempe CH (1968) Smallpox vaccination of eczema patients with attenuated live vaccinia virus. *Yale J Biol Med* 41: 1–12
19 Stickl H, Hochstein-Mintzel V (1971) [Intracutaneous smallpox vaccination with a weak pathogenic vaccinia virus ("MVA virus")]. *Muench Med Wochenschr* 113: 1149–1153
20 Hashizume S, Yoshizawa H, Morita M, Suzuki K (1985) Properties of attenuated mutant of vaccinia virus, LC16m8, derived from Lister strain. In: GV Quinnan (eds): *Vaccinia Viruses as Vectors for Vaccine Antigens*. Elsevier Science, New York, 87–99
21 Tartaglia J, Perkus ME, Taylor J, Norton EK, Audonnet JC, Cox WI, Davis SW, van der Hoeven J, Meignier B, Riviere M et al (1992) NYVAC: a highly attenuated strain of vaccinia virus. *Virology* 188: 217–232
22 Ober BT, Bruhl P, Schmidt M, Wieser V, Gritschenberger W, Coulibaly S, Savidis-Dacho H, Gerencer M, Falkner FG (2002) Immunogenicity and safety of defective vaccinia virus Lister: comparison with modified vaccinia virus Ankara. *J Virol* 76: 7713–7723
23 Goebel SJ, Johnson GP, Perkus ME, Davis SW, Winslow JP, Paoletti E (1990)

The complete DNA sequence of vaccinia virus. *Virology* 179: 247–266, 517–263
24 Parker RF, Bronson LH, Green RH (1941) Further studies on the infectious unit of vaccinia. *J Exp Med* 74: 268–281
25 Law M, Putz MM, Smith GL (2005) An investigation of the therapeutic value of vaccinia-immune IgG in a mouse pneumonia model. *J Gen Virol* 86: 991–1000
26 Herrlich A, Mayr A (1954) [Comparative experimental works on cowpox virus vaccines.] [Translated from German]. *Arch Hyg Bakteriol* 138: 479–504
27 de Souza Trindade G, da Fonseca FG, Marques JT, Nogueira ML, Mendes LC, Borges AS, Peiro JR, Pituco EM, Bonjardim CA, Ferreira PC et al (2003) Aracatuba virus: a vaccinia-like virus associated with infection in humans and cattle. *Emerg Infect Dis* 9: 155–160
28 Marques JT, Trindade GD, Da Fonseca FG, Dos Santos JR, Bonjardim CA, Ferreira PC, Kroon EG (2001) Characterization of ATI, TK and IFN-alpha/betaR genes in the genome of the BeAn 58058 virus, a naturally attenuated wild Orthopoxvirus. *Virus Genes* 23: 291–301
29 Kunert H, Wolff I (1960) Comparative studies on the virulence of the vaccine virus strains Berlin and Bern. *Arch Hyg Bakteriol* 144: 37–47
30 Lal SM, Singh IP (1973) Buffalopox – a review. *Trop Anim Health Prod* 9: 107–112
31 Dumbell K, Richardson M (1993) Virological investigations of specimens from buffaloes affected by buffalopox in Maharashtra State, India between 1985 and 1987. *Arch Virol* 128: 257–267
32 Cragie J (1932) The nature of the vaccinia virus flocculation reaction and observation of the elementary bodies of vaccinia. *Br J Exp Pathol* 13: 259–268
33 Harada K, Matumoto M (1962) Antigenic relationship between mammalian and avian pox viruses as revealed by complement fixation reaction. Jpn *J Exp Med* 32: 369–385
34 Oda M (1965) Rescue of dermovaccinia abortive infection by neurovaccinia virus in L cells. *Virology* 25: 664–666
35 Tagaya I, Kitamura T, Sano Y (1961) A new mutant of dermovaccinia virus. *Nature* 192: 381–382
36 Kitamura T (1963) Reactivation of protease-inactivated vaccinia virus. *Virology* 21: 286–289
37 Coulibaly S, Bruhl P, Mayrhofer J, Schmid K, Gerencer M, Falkner FG (2005) The nonreplicating smallpox candidate vaccines defective vaccinia Lister (dVV-L) and modified vaccinia Ankara (MVA) elicit robust long-term protection. *Virology* 341: 91–101
38 Polak MF, Swart-Vanderhoeven JT, Smeenk C, Pel JZ, Van S, Pasdeloup F (1964) [Comparison of 2 vaccinia strains in vaccination of infants]. *Ned Tijdschr Geneeskd* 108: 459–464
39 Marennikova SS, Chimishkyan KL, Maltseva NN, Shelukhina EMF, Fedorov VV (1969) Characteristics of virus strains for production of smallpox vaccines. In: B Gusic (ed): *Proceedings of the Symposium on Smallpox*. Yugoslav Academy of Sciences and Arts, Zagreb, 65–69
40 Koegh EV (1936) Titration of vaccinia virus on the chorioallantoic membrane

of the chick embryo and its application to immunological studies of neuro-vaccinia. *J Pathol Bacteriol* 43: 441–454
41 Thompson RA, Minton SA Jr, Officer LE, Hutchings GH (1953) Effect of heterocyclic and other thiocarbazones on vaccinia infection in the mouse. *J Immunol* 70: 229–234
42 Ichihashi Y, Dales S (1971) Biogenesis of poxviruses: interrelationship between hemagglutinin production and polykaryocytosis. *Virology* 46: 533–543
43 Horgan ES, Haseeb MA (1939) Cross immunity experiments in monkeys between variola, alstrim and vaccinia. *J Hyg* 39: 615–637
44 Morikawa S, Sakiyama T, Hasegawa H, Saijo M, Maeda A, Kurane I, Maeno G, Kimura J, Hirama C, Yoshida T et al (2005) An attenuated LC16m8 smallpox vaccine: analysis of full-genome sequence and induction of immune protection. *J Virol* 79: 11873–11891
45 Mayr A (1976) [TC marker of the attenuated vaccinia vaccide strain "MVA" in human cell cultures and protective immunization against orthopox diseases in animals]. *Zentralbl Veterinarmed* B 23: 417–430
46 Antoine G, Scheiflinger F, Dorner F, Falkner FG (1998) The complete genomic sequence of the modified vaccinia Ankara strain: comparison with other orthopoxviruses. *Virology* 244: 365–396
47 Jansen J (1946) Immunity in rabbit plague-immunological relationship with cowpox. *Antonie van Leeuwenhowek J Microbiol Serol* 11: 139–167
48 da Fonseca FG, Trindade GS, Silva RL, Bonjardim CA, Ferreira PC, Kroon EG (2002) Characterization of a vaccinia-like virus isolated in a Brazilian forest. *J Gen Virol* 83: 223–228
49 Turner GS (1967) Respiratory infection of mice with vaccinia virus. *J Gen Virol* 1: 399–402
50 Minton SA Jr, Officer JE, Thompson RL (1953) Effect of thiosemicarbazones and dichlorophenoxy thiouracil on multiplication of a recently isolated strain of variola-vaccinia virus in the brain of the mouse. *J Immunol* 70: 222–228
51 Lane JM, Ruben FL, Neff JM, Millar JD (1969) Complications of smallpox vaccination, 1968. National surveillance in the United States. *N Engl J Med* 281: 1201–1208
52 Chen RT, Lane JM (2003) Myocarditis: the unexpected return of smallpox vaccine adverse events. *Lancet* 362: 1345–1346
53 Meyer H, Sutter G, Mayr A (1991) Mapping of deletions in the genome of the highly attenuated vaccinia virus MVA and their influence on virulence. *J Gen Virol* 72: 1031–1038
54 Sutter G, Moss B (1992) Nonreplicating vaccinia vector efficiently expresses recombinant genes. *Proc Natl Acad Sci USA* 89: 10847–10851
55 Carroll MW, Moss B (1997) Host range and cytopathogenicity of the highly attenuated MVA strain of vaccinia virus: propagation and generation of recombinant viruses in a nonhuman mammalian cell line. *Virology* 238: 198–211
56 Okeke MI, Nilssen O, Traavik T (2006) Modified vaccinia virus Ankara multiplies in rat IEC-6 cells and limited production of mature virions occurs in other mammalian cell lines. *J Gen Virol* 87: 21–27
57 Mayr A, Stickl H, Muller HK, Danner K, Singer H (1978) [The smallpox vaccination strain MVA: marker, genetic structure, experience gained with the

parenteral vaccination and behavior in organisms with a debilitated defence mechanism (author's transl)]. *Zentralbl Bakteriol B* 167: 375–390
58 Cebere I, Dorrell L, McShane H, Simmons A, McCormack S, Schmidt C, Smith C, Brooks M, Roberts JE, Darwin SC et al (2006) Phase I clinical trial safety of DNA- and modified virus Ankara-vectored human immunodeficiency virus type 1 (HIV-1) vaccines administered alone and in a prime-boost regime to healthy HIV-1-uninfected volunteers. *Vaccine* 24: 417–425
59 Stickl H, Hochstein-Mintzel V, Mayr A, Huber HC, Schafer H, Holzner A (1974) [MVA vaccination against smallpox: clinical tests with an attenuated live vaccinia virus strain (MVA) (author's transl)]. *Dtsch Med Wochenschr* 99: 2386–2392
60 Drexler I, Staib C, Kastenmuller W, Stevanovic S, Schmidt B, Lemonnier FA, Rammensee HG, Busch DH, Bernhard H, Erfle V et al (2003) Identification of vaccinia virus epitope-specific HLA-A*0201-restricted T cells and comparative analysis of smallpox vaccines. *Proc Natl Acad Sci USA* 100: 217–222
61 Earl PL, Americo JL, Wyatt LS, Eller LA, Whitbeck JC, Cohen GH, Eisenberg RJ, Hartmann CJ, Jackson DL, Kulesh DA et al (2004) Immunogenicity of a highly attenuated MVA smallpox vaccine and protection against monkeypox. *Nature* 428: 182–185
62 Staib C, Drexler I, Sutter G (2004) Construction and isolation of recombinant MVA. *Methods Mol Biol* 269: 77–100
63 Blanchard TJ, Alcami A, Andrea P, Smith GL (1998) Modified vaccinia virus Ankara undergoes limited replication in human cells and lacks several immunomodulatory proteins: implications for use as a human vaccine. *J Gen Virol* 79: 1159–1167
64 Staib C, Kisling S, Erfle V, Sutter G (2005) Inactivation of the viral interleukin 1{beta} receptor improves CD8+ T-cell memory responses elicited upon immunization with modified vaccinia virus Ankara. *J Gen Virol* 86: 1997–2006
65 Clark RH, Kenyon JC, Bartlett NW, Tscharke DC, Smith GL (2006) Deletion of gene A41L enhances vaccinia virus immunogenicity and vaccine efficacy. *J Gen Virol* 87: 29–38
66 Takahashi-Nishimaki F, Funahashi S, Miki K, Hashizume S, Sugimoto M (1991) Regulation of plaque size and host range by a vaccinia virus gene related to complement system proteins. *Virology* 181: 158–164
67 Takahashi-Nishimaki F, Suzuki K, Morita M, Maruyama T, Miki K, Hashizume S, Sugimoto M (1987) Genetic analysis of vaccinia virus Lister strain and its attenuated mutant LC16m8: production of intermediate variants by homologous recombination. *J Gen Virol* 68: 2705–2710
68 Engelstad M, Howard ST, Smith GL (1992) A constitutively expressed vaccinia gene encodes a 42-kDa glycoprotein related to complement control factors that forms part of the extracellular virus envelope. *Virology* 188: 801–810
69 Isaacs SN, Wolffe EJ, Payne LG, Moss B (1992) Characterization of a vaccinia virus-encoded 42-kilodalton class I membrane glycoprotein component of the extracellular virus envelope. *J Virol* 66: 7217–7224
70 Galmiche MC, Goenaga J, Wittek R, Rindisbacher L (1999) Neutralizing and protective antibodies directed against vaccinia virus envelope antigens. *Virology* 254: 71–80

71 Law M, Smith GL (2001) Antibody neutralization of the extracellular enveloped form of vaccinia virus. *Virology* 280: 132–142
72 Bell E, Shamim M, Whitbeck JC, Sfyroera G, Lambris JD, Isaacs SN (2004) Antibodies against the extracellular enveloped virus B5R protein are mainly responsible for the EEV neutralizing capacity of vaccinia immune globulin. *Virology* 325: 425–431
73 Putz MM, Midgley CM, Law M, Smith GL (2006) Quantification of antibody responses against multiple antigens of the two infectious forms of *Vaccinia virus* provides a benchmark for smallpox vaccination. *Nat Med; in press*
74 Kidokoro M, Tashiro M, Shida H (2005) Genetically stable and fully effective smallpox vaccine strain constructed from highly attenuated vaccinia LC16m8. *Proc Natl Acad Sci USA* 102: 4152–4157
75 Seet BT, Johnston JB, Brunetti CR, Barrett JW, Everett H, Cameron C, Sypula J, Nazarian SH, Lucas A, McFadden G (2003) Poxviruses and immune evasion. *Annu Rev Immunol* 21: 377–423
76 Moss B (2006) Poxvirus entry and membrane fusion. *Virology* 344: 48–54
77 Dales S, Siminovitch L (1961) The development of vaccinia virus in Earle's L strain cells as examined by electron microscopy. *J Biophys Biochem Cytol* 10: 475–503
78 Sodeik B, Doms RW, Ericsson M, Hiller G, Machamer CE, van ,t Hof W, van Meer G, Moss B, Griffiths G (1993) Assembly of vaccinia virus: role of the intermediate compartment between the endoplasmic reticulum and the Golgi stacks. *J Cell Biol* 121: 521–541
79 Risco C, Rodriguez JR, Lopez-Iglesias C, Carrascosa JL, Esteban M, Rodriguez D (2002) Endoplasmic reticulum-Golgi intermediate compartment membranes and vimentin filaments participate in vaccinia virus assembly. *J Virol* 76: 1839–1855
80 Roos N, Cyrklaff M, Cudmore S, Blasco R, Krijnse-Locker J, Griffiths G (1996) A novel immunogold cryoelectron microscopic approach to investigate the structure of the intracellular and extracellular forms of vaccinia virus. *EMBO J* 15: 2343–2355
81 Hollinshead M, Vanderplasschen A, Smith GL, Vaux DJ (1999) Vaccinia virus intracellular mature virions contain only one lipid membrane. *J Virol* 73: 1503–1517
82 Cyrklaff M, Risco C, Fernandez JJ, Jimenez MV, Esteban M, Baumeister W, Carrascosa JL (2005) Cryo-electron tomography of vaccinia virus. *Proc Natl Acad Sci USA* 102: 2772–2777
83 Munyon W, Paoletti E, Grace JT Jr (1967) RNA polymerase activity in purified infectious vaccinia virus. *Proc Natl Acad Sci USA* 58: 2280–2287
84 Morgan C (1976) Vaccinia virus reexamined: development and release. *Virology* 73: 43–58
85 Dubochet J, Adrian M, Richter K, Garces J, Wittek R (1994) Structure of intracellular mature vaccinia virus observed by cryoelectron microscopy. *J Virol* 68: 1935–1941
86 Schmelz M, Sodeik B, Ericsson M, Wolffe EJ, Shida H, Hiller G, Griffiths G (1994) Assembly of vaccinia virus: the second wrapping cisterna is derived from the trans Golgi network. *J Virol* 68: 130–147

87 Tooze J, Hollinshead M, Reis B, Radsak K, Kern H (1993) Progeny vaccinia and human cytomegalovirus particles utilize early endosomal cisternae for their envelopes. *Eur J Cell Biol* 60: 163–178
88 Berns KI, Silverman C (1970) Natural occurrence of cross-linked vaccinia virus deoxyribonucleic acid. *J Virol* 5: 299–304
89 Baroudy BM, Venkatesan S, Moss B (1982) Incompletely base-paired flip-flop terminal loops link the two DNA strands of the vaccinia virus genome into one uninterrupted polynucleotide chain. *Cell* 28: 315–324
90 Garon CF, Barbosa E, Moss B (1978) Visualization of an inverted terminal repetition in vaccinia virus DNA. *Proc Natl Acad Sci USA* 75: 4863–4867
91 Colinas RJ, Goebel SJ, Davis SW, Johnson GP, Norton EK, Paoletti E (1990) A DNA ligase gene in the Copenhagen strain of vaccinia virus is nonessential for viral replication and recombination. *Virology* 179: 267–275
92 Gubser C, Smith GL (2002) The sequence of camelpox virus shows it is most closely related to variola virus, the cause of smallpox. *J Gen Virol* 83: 855–872
93 Massung RF, Liu LI, Qi J, Knight JC, Yuran TE, Kerlavage AR, Parsons JM, Venter JC, Esposito JJ (1994) Analysis of the complete genome of smallpox variola major virus strain Bangladesh-1975. *Virology* 201: 215–240
94 Pickup DJ, Ink BS, Parsons BL, Hu W, Joklik WK (1984) Spontaneous deletions and duplications of sequences in the genome of cowpox virus. *Proc Natl Acad Sci USA* 81: 6817–6821
95 Wittek R, Moss B (1980) Tandem repeats within the inverted terminal repetition of vaccinia virus DNA. *Cell* 21: 277–284
96 Baroudy BM, Moss B (1982) Sequence homologies of diverse length tandem repetitions near ends of vaccinia virus genome suggest unequal crossing over. *Nucleic Acids Res* 10: 5673–5679
97 Merchlinsky M, Moss B (1989) Nucleotide sequence required for resolution of the concatemer junction of vaccinia virus DNA. *J Virol* 63: 4354–4361
98 Merchlinsky M (1990) Mutational analysis of the resolution sequence of vaccinia virus DNA: essential sequence consists of two separate AT-rich regions highly conserved among poxviruses. *J Virol* 64: 5029–5035
99 Upton C, Slack S, Hunter AL, Ehlers A, Roper RL (2003) Poxvirus orthologous clusters: toward defining the minimum essential poxvirus genome. *J Virol* 77: 7590–7600
100 Gubser C, Hué S, Kellam P, Smith GL (2004) Poxvirus genomes: a phylogenetic analysis. *J Gen Virol* 85: 105–117
101 Smith GL, Vanderplasschen A, Law M (2002) The formation and function of extracellular enveloped vaccinia virus. *J Gen Virol* 83: 2915–2931
102 Armstrong JA, Metz DH, Young MR (1973) The mode of entry of vaccinia virus into L cells. *J Gen Virol* 21: 533–537
103 Chang A, Metz DH (1976) Further investigations on the mode of entry of vaccinia virus into cells. *J Gen Virol* 32: 275–282
104 Doms RW, Blumenthal R, Moss B (1990) Fusion of intra- and extracellular forms of vaccinia virus with the cell membrane. *J Virol* 64: 4884–4892
105 Griffiths G, Wepf R, Wendt T, Locker JK, Cyrklaff M, Roos N (2001) Structure and assembly of intracellular mature vaccinia virus: isolated-particle analysis. *J Virol* 75: 11034–11055

106 Locker JK, Kuehn A, Schleich S, Rutter G, Hohenberg H, Wepf R, Griffiths G (2000) Entry of the two infectious forms of vaccinia virus at the plasma membane is signaling-dependent for the IMV but not the EEV. *Mol Biol Cell* 11: 2497–2511
107 Vanderplasschen A, Hollinshead M, Smith GL (1998) Intracellular and extracellular vaccinia virions enter cells by different mechanisms. *J Gen Virol* 79: 877–887
108 Senkevich TG, Ward BM, Moss B (2004) Vaccinia virus entry into cells is dependent on a virion surface protein encoded by the A28L gene. *J Virol* 78: 2357–2366
109 Carter GC, Law M, Hollinshead M, Smith GL (2005) The entry of the vaccinia virus intracellular mature virion and its interactions with glycosaminoglycans. *J Gen Virol* 86: 1279–1290
110 Law M, Carter GC, Roberts KL, Hollinshead M, Smith GL (2006) Ligand-induced and non-fusogenic dissolution of a virus membrane. *Proc Natl Acad Sci USA* 103: 5989–5994
111 Eppstein DA, Marsh YV, Schreiber AB, Newman SR, Todaro GJ, Nestor JJ Jr (1985) Epidermal growth factor receptor occupancy inhibits vaccinia virus infection. *Nature* 318: 663–665
112 Hugin AW, Hauser C (1994) The epidermal growth factor receptor is not a receptor for vaccinia virus. *J Virol* 68: 8409–8412
113 Lalani AS, Masters J, Zeng W, Barrett J, Pannu R, Everett H, Arendt CW, McFadden G (1999) Use of chemokine receptors by poxviruses. *Science* 286: 1968–1971
114 Masters J, Hinek AA, Uddin S, Platanias LC, Zeng W, McFadden G, Fish EN (2001) Poxvirus infection rapidly activates tyrosine kinase signal transduction. *J Biol Chem* 276: 48371–48375
115 Chung CS, Hsiao JC, Chang YS, Chang W (1998) A27L protein mediates vaccinia virus interaction with cell surface heparan sulfate. *J Virol* 72: 1577–1585
116 Hsiao JC, Chung CS, Chang W (1998) Cell surface proteoglycans are necessary for A27L protein-mediated cell fusion: identification of the N-terminal region of A27L protein as the glycosaminoglycan-binding domain. *J Virol* 72: 8374–8379
117 Hsiao JC, Chung CS, Chang W (1999) Vaccinia virus envelope D8L protein binds to cell surface chondroitin sulfate and mediates the adsorption of intracellular mature virions to cells. *J Virol* 73: 8750–8761
118 Lin CL, Chung CS, Heine HG, Chang W (2000) Vaccinia virus envelope H3L protein binds to cell surface heparan sulfate and is important for intracellular mature virion morphogenesis and virus infection *in vitro* and *in vivo*. *J Virol* 74: 3353–3365
119 Rodriguez JF, Smith GL (1990) IPTG-dependent vaccinia virus: identification of a virus protein enabling virion envelopment by Golgi membrane and egress. *Nucleic Acids Res* 18: 5347–5351
120 Ward BM (2005) Visualization and characterization of the intracellular movement of vaccinia virus intracellular mature virions. *J Virol* 79: 4755–4763
121 Vanderplasschen A, Smith GL (1997) A novel virus binding assay using confo-

cal microscopy: demonstration that the intracellular and extracellular vaccinia virions bind to different cellular receptors. *J Virol* 71: 4032–4041
122 Chang W, Hsiao JC, Chung CS, Bair CH (1995) Isolation of a monoclonal antibody which blocks vaccinia virus infection. *J Virol* 69: 517–522
123 Young JAT (2001) Virus entry and uncoating. In: DM Knipe, PM Howley (eds): *Fields Virology*. Lippincott-Raven Publishers, Philadephia, 87–103
124 Townsley AC, Senkevich TG, Moss B (2005) Vaccinia virus A21 virion membrane protein is required for cell entry and fusion. *J Virol* 79: 9458–9469
125 Townsley AC, Senkevich TG, Moss B (2005) The product of the vaccinia virus L5R gene is a fourth membrane protein encoded by all poxviruses that is required for cell entry and cell-cell fusion. *J Virol* 79: 10988–10998
126 Senkevich TG, Moss B (2005) Vaccinia virus H2 protein is an essential component of a complex involved in virus entry and cell-cell fusion. *J Virol* 79: 4744–4754
127 Ojeda S, Senkevich TG, Moss B (2006) Entry of vaccinia virus and cell-cell fusion require a highly conserved cysteine-rich membrane protein encoded by the A16L gene. *J Virol* 80: 51–61
128 Senkevich TG, Ojeda S, Townsley A, Nelson GE, Moss B (2005) Poxvirus multiprotein entry-fusion complex. *Proc Natl Acad Sci USA* 102: 18572–18577
129 Röttger S, Frischknecht F, Reckmann I, Smith GL, Way M (1999) Interactions between vaccinia virus IEV membrane proteins and their roles in IEV assembly and actin tail formation. *J Virol* 73: 2863–2875
130 Earp LJ, Delos SE, Park HE, White JM (2005) The many mechanisms of viral membrane fusion proteins. *Curr Top Microbiol Immunol* 285: 25–66
131 Carter GC, Rodger G, Murphy BJ, Law M, Krauss O, Hollinshead M, Smith GL (2003) Vaccinia virus cores are transported on microtubules. *J Gen Virol* 84: 2443–2458
132 Kates JR, McAuslan BR (1967) Poxvirus DNA-dependent RNA polymerase. *Proc Natl Acad Sci USA* 58: 134–141
133 Kates J, Beeson J (1970) Ribonucleic acid synthesis in vaccinia virus. II. Synthesis of polyriboadenylic acid. *J Mol Biol* 50: 19–33
134 Wei CM, Moss B (1974) Methylation of newly synthesized viral messenger RNA by an enzyme in vaccinia virus. *Proc Natl Acad Sci USA* 71: 3014–3018
135 Wei CM, Moss B (1975) Methylated nucleotides block 5'-terminus of vaccinia virus messenger RNA. *Proc Natl Acad Sci USA* 72: 318–322
136 Broyles SS (2003) Vaccinia virus transcription. *J Gen Virol* 84: 2293–2303
137 Yuen L, Davison AJ, Moss B (1987) Early promoter-binding factor from vaccinia virions. *Proc Natl Acad Sci USA* 84: 6069–6073
138 Broyles SS, Moss B (1988) DNA-dependent ATPase activity associated with vaccinia virus early transcription factor. *J Biol Chem* 263: 10761–10765
139 Shuman S, Broyles SS, Moss B (1987) Purification and characterization of a transcription termination factor from vaccinia virions. *J Biol Chem* 262: 12372–12380
140 Paoletti E, Grady LJ (1977) Transcriptional complexity of vaccinia virus *in vivo* and *in vitro*. *J Virol* 23: 608–615
141 Boone RF, Moss B (1978) Sequence complexity and relative abundance of vaccinia virus mRNA's synthesized *in vivo* and *in vitro*. *J Virol* 26: 554–569

142 Davison AJ, Moss B (1989) Structure of vaccinia virus early promoters. *J Mol Biol* 210: 749–769
143 Yuen L, Moss B (1987) Oligonucleotide sequence signaling transcriptional termination of vaccinia virus early genes. *Proc Natl Acad Sci USA* 84: 6417–6421
144 Shuman S, Moss B (1988) Factor-dependent transcription termination by vaccinia virus RNA polymerase. Evidence that the cis-acting termination signal is in nascent RNA. *J Biol Chem* 263: 6220–6225
145 Mallardo M, Schleich S, Krijnse Locker J (2001) Microtubule-dependent organization of vaccinia virus core-derived early mRNAs into distinct cytoplasmic structures. *Mol Biol Cell* 12: 3875–3891
146 Vos JC, Stunnenberg HG (1988) Derepression of a novel class of vaccinia virus genes upon DNA replication. *EMBO J* 7: 3487–3492
147 Baldick CJ Jr, Keck JG, Moss B (1992) Mutational analysis of the core, spacer, and initiator regions of vaccinia virus intermediate-class promoters. *J Virol* 66: 4710–4719
148 Harris N, Rosales R, Moss B (1993) Transcription initiation factor activity of vaccinia virus capping enzyme is independent of mRNA guanylylation. *Proc Natl Acad Sci USA* 90: 2860–2864
149 Rosales R, Harris N, Ahn BY, Moss B (1994) Purification and identification of a vaccinia virus-encoded intermediate stage promoter-specific transcription factor that has homology to eukaryotic transcription factor SII (TFIIS) and an additional role as a viral RNA polymerase subunit. *J Biol Chem* 269: 14260–14267
150 Sanz P, Moss B (1999) Identification of a transcription factor, encoded by two vaccinia virus early genes, that regulates the intermediate stage of viral gene expression. *Proc Natl Acad Sci USA* 96: 2692–2697
151 Rosales R, Sutter G, Moss B (1994) A cellular factor is required for transcription of vaccinia viral intermediate-stage genes. *Proc Natl Acad Sci USA* 91: 3794–3798
152 Keck JG, Baldick CJ Jr, Moss B (1990) Role of DNA replication in vaccinia virus gene expression: a naked template is required for transcription of three late trans-activator genes. *Cell* 61: 801–809
153 Rosel JL, Earl PL, Weir JP, Moss B (1986) Conserved TAAATG sequence at the transcriptional and translational initiation sites of vaccinia virus late genes deduced by structural and functional analysis of the HindIII H genome fragment. *J Virol* 60: 436–449
154 Davison AJ, Moss B (1989) Structure of vaccinia virus late promoters. *J Mol Biol* 210: 771–784
155 Wright CF, Coroneos AM (1993) Purification of the late transcription system of vaccinia virus: identification of a novel transcription factor. *J Virol* 67: 7264–7270
156 Kovacs GR, Rosales R, Keck JG, Moss B (1994) Modification of the cascade model for regulation of vaccinia virus gene expression: purification of a prereplicative, late-stage-specific transcription factor. *J Virol* 68: 3443–3447
157 Wright CF, Hubbs AE, Gunasinghe SK, Oswald BW (1998) A vaccinia virus late transcription factor copurifies with a factor that binds to a viral late pro-

moter and is complemented by extracts from uninfected HeLa cells. *J Virol* 72: 1446–1451
158 Gunasinghe SK, Hubbs AE, Wright CF (1998) A vaccinia virus late transcription factor with biochemical and molecular identity to a human cellular protein. *J Biol Chem* 273: 27524–27530
159 Bertholet C, Van Meir E, ten Heggeler-Bordier B, Wittek R (1987) Vaccinia virus produces late mRNAs by discontinous synthesis. *Cell* 50: 153–162
160 Schwer B, Visca P, Vos JC, Stunnenberg HG (1987) Discontinuous transcription or RNA processing of vaccinia virus late messengers results in a 5' poly(A) leader. *Cell* 50: 163–169
161 Cooper JA, Wittek R, Moss B (1981) Extension of the transcriptional and translational map of the left end of the vaccinia virus genome to 21 kilobase pairs. *J Virol* 39: 733–745
162 Salzman NP (1960) The rate of formation of vaccinia deoxyribonucleic acid and vaccinia virus. *Virology* 10: 150–152
163 Challberg MD, Englund PT (1979) Purification and properties of the deoxyribonucleic acid polymerase induced by vaccinia virus. *J Biol Chem* 254: 7812–7819
164 Klemperer N, McDonald W, Boyle K, Unger B, Traktman P (2001) The A20R protein is a stoichiometric component of the processive form of vaccinia virus DNA polymerase. *J Virol* 75: 12298–12307
165 Lin S, Chen W, Broyles SS (1992) The vaccinia virus B1R gene product is a serine/threonine protein kinase. *J Virol* 66: 2717–2723
166 Banham AH, Smith GL (1992) Vaccinia virus gene B1R encodes a 34-kDa serine/threonine protein kinase that localizes in cytoplasmic factories and is packaged into virions. *Virology* 191: 803–812
167 Evans E, Klemperer N, Ghosh R, Traktman P (1995) The vaccinia virus D5 protein, which is required for DNA replication, is a nucleic acid-independent nucleoside triphosphatase. *J Virol* 69: 5353–5361
168 Millns AK, Carpenter MS, DeLange AM (1994) The vaccinia virus-encoded uracil DNA glycosylase has an essential role in viral DNA replication. *Virology* 198: 504–513
169 Moss B (2001) Poxviridae: the viruses and their replication. In: BN Fields, DM Knipe, PM Howley, RM Chanock, J Melnick, TP Monath, B Roizman, SE Straus (eds): *Virology*. Lippincott-Raven Publishers, Philadelphia, 2849–2883
170 Kerr SM, Smith GL (1989) Vaccinia virus encodes a polypeptide with DNA ligase activity. *Nucleic Acids Res* 17: 9039–9050
171 Smith GL, Chan YS, Kerr SM (1989) Transcriptional mapping and nucleotide sequence of a vaccinia virus gene encoding a polypeptide with extensive homology to DNA ligases. *Nucleic Acids Res* 17: 9051–9062
172 Kerr SM, Smith GL (1991) Vaccinia virus DNA ligase is nonessential for virus replication: recovery of plasmids from virus-infected cells. *Virology* 180: 625–632
173 Kerr SM, Johnston LH, Odell M, Duncan SA, Law KM, Smith GL (1991) Vaccinia DNA ligase complements *Saccharomyces cerevisiae* cdc9, localizes in cytoplasmic factories and affects virulence and virus sensitivity to DNA damaging agents. *EMBO J* 10: 4343–4350

174 Slabaugh MB, Mathews CK (1984) Vaccinia virus-induced ribonucleotide reductase can be distinguished from host cell activity. *J Virol* 52: 501–506
175 Slabaugh M, Roseman N, Davis R, Mathews C (1988) Vaccinia virus-encoded ribonucleotide reductase: sequence conservation of the gene for the small subunit and its amplification in hydroxyurea-resistant mutants. *J Virol* 62: 519–527
176 Tengelsen LA, Slabaugh MB, Bibler JK, Hruby DE (1988) Nucleotide sequence and molecular genetic analysis of the large subunit of ribonucleotide reductase encoded by vaccinia virus. *Virology* 164: 121–131
177 Child SJ, Palumbo GJ, Buller RM, Hruby DE (1990) Insertional inactivation of the large subunit of ribonucleotide reductase encoded by vaccinia virus is associated with reduced virulence *in vivo*. *Virology* 174: 625–629
178 Howell ML, Sanders-Loehr J, Loehr TM, Roseman NA, Mathews CK, Slabaugh MB (1992) Cloning of the vaccinia virus ribonucleotide reductase small subunit gene. Characterization of the gene product expressed in *Escherichia coli*. *J Biol Chem* 267: 1705–1711
179 Bajszar G, Wittek R, Weir JP, Moss B (1983) Vaccinia virus thymidine kinase and neighboring genes: mRNAs and polypeptides of wild-type virus and putative nonsense mutants. *J Virol* 45: 62–72
180 Hruby DE, Maki RA, Miller DB, Ball LA (1983) Fine structure analysis and nucleotide sequence of the vaccinia virus thymidine kinase gene. *Proc Natl Acad Sci USA* 80: 3411–3415
181 Black ME, Hruby DE (1992) Site-directed mutagenesis of a conserved domain in vaccinia virus thymidine kinase. Evidence for a potential role in magnesium binding. *J Biol Chem* 267: 6801–6806
182 Black ME, Hruby DE (1992) A single amino acid substitution abolishes feedback inhibition of vaccinia virus thymidine kinase. *J Biol Chem* 267: 9743–9748
183 Buller RM, Smith GL, Cremer K, Notkins AL, Moss B (1985) Decreased virulence of recombinant vaccinia virus expression vectors is associated with a thymidine kinase-negative phenotype. *Nature* 317: 813–815
184 Smith GL, de Carlos A, Chan YS (1989) Vaccinia virus encodes a thymidylate kinase gene: sequence and transcriptional mapping. *Nucleic Acids Res* 17: 7581–7590
185 Hughes SJ, Johnston LH, de Carlos A, Smith GL (1991) Vaccinia virus encodes an active thymidylate kinase that complements a cdc8 mutant of *Saccharomyces cerevisiae*. *J Biol Chem* 266: 20103–20109
186 Slabaugh MB, Roseman NA (1989) Retroviral protease-like gene in the vaccinia virus genome. *Proc Natl Acad Sci USA* 86: 4152–4155
187 McGeoch DJ (1990) Protein sequence comparisons show that the ‚pseudoproteases' encoded by poxviruses and certain retroviruses belong to the deoxyuridine triphosphatase family. *Nucleic Acids Res* 18: 4105–4110
188 Broyles SS (1993) Vaccinia virus encodes a functional dUTPase. *Virology* 195: 863–865
189 Perkus ME, Goebel SJ, Davis SW, Johnson GP, Norton EK, Paoletti E (1991) Deletion of 55 open reading frames from the termini of vaccinia virus. *Virology* 180: 406–410
190 Smith GL, Chan YS, Howard ST (1991) Nucleotide sequence of 42 kbp of vac-

cinia virus strain WR from near the right inverted terminal repeat. *J Gen Virol* 72: 1349–1376
191 Aguado B, Selmes IP, Smith GL (1992) Nucleotide sequence of 21.8 kbp of variola major virus strain Harvey and comparison with vaccinia virus. *J Gen Virol* 73: 2887–2902
192 DeLange AM (1989) Identification of temperature-sensitive mutants of vaccinia virus that are defective in conversion of concatemeric replicative intermediates to the mature linear DNA genome. *J Virol* 63: 2437–2444
193 Shuman S, Moss B (1987) Identification of a vaccinia virus gene encoding a type I DNA topoisomerase. *Proc Natl Acad Sci USA* 84: 7478–7482
194 Klemperer N, Traktman P (1993) Biochemical analysis of mutant alleles of the vaccinia virus topoisomerase I carrying targeted substitutions in a highly conserved domain. *J Biol Chem* 268: 15887–15899
195 Eckert D, Williams O, Meseda CA, Merchlinsky M (2005) Vaccinia virus nicking-joining enzyme is encoded by K4L (VACWR035). *J Virol* 79: 15084–15090
196 Garcia AD, Aravind L, Koonin EV, Moss B (2000) Bacterial-type DNA holliday junction resolvases in eukaryotic viruses. *Proc Natl Acad Sci USA* 97: 8926–8931
197 Garcia AD, Moss B (2001) Repression of vaccinia virus Holliday junction resolvase inhibits processing of viral DNA into unit-length genomes. *J Virol* 75: 6460–6471
198 Cassetti MC, Merchlinsky M, Wolffe EJ, Weisberg AS, Moss B (1998) DNA packaging mutant: repression of the vaccinia virus A32 gene results in noninfectious, DNA-deficient, spherical, enveloped particles. *J Virol* 72: 5769–5780
199 Joklik WK, Becker Y (1964) The replication and coating of vaccinia DNA. *J Mol Biol* 10: 452–474
200 Dales S, Mosbach EH (1968) Vaccinia as a model for membrane biogenesis. *Virology* 35: 564–583
201 Grimley PM, Rosenblum EN, Mims SJ, Moss B (1970) Interruption by Rifampin of an early stage in vaccinia virus morphogenesis: accumulation of membranes which are precursors of virus envelopes. *J Virol* 6: 519–533
202 Griffiths G, Roos N, Schleich S, Locker JK (2001) Structure and assembly of intracellular mature vaccinia virus: thin-section analyses. *J Virol* 75: 11056–11070
203 Heuser J (2005) Deep-etch EM reveals that the early poxvirus envelope is a single membrane bilayer stabilized by a geodetic "honeycomb" surface coat. *J Cell Biol* 169: 269–283
204 Traktman P, Caligiuri A, Jesty SA, Liu K, Sankar U (1995) Temperature-sensitive mutants with lesions in the vaccinia virus F10 kinase undergo arrest at the earliest stage of virion morphogenesis. *J Virol* 69: 6581–6587
205 Wang S, Shuman S (1995) Vaccinia virus morphogenesis is blocked by temperature-sensitive mutations in the F10 gene, which encodes protein kinase 2. *J Virol* 69: 6376–6388
206 DeMasi J, Traktman P (2000) Clustered charge-to-alanine mutagenesis of the vaccinia virus H5 gene: isolation of a dominant, temperature-sensitive mutant with a profound defect in morphogenesis. *J Virol* 74: 2393–2405
207 Wolffe EJ, Moore DM, Peters PJ, Moss B (1996) Vaccinia virus A17L open

reading frame encodes an essential component of nascent viral membranes that is required to initiate morphogenesis. *J Virol* 70: 2797–2808
208 Rodriguez JR, Risco C, Carrascosa JL, Esteban M, Rodriguez D (1997) Characterization of early stages in vaccinia virus membrane biogenesis: implications of the 21-kilodalton protein and a newly identified 15-kilodalton envelope protein. *J Virol* 71: 1821–1833
209 Rodriguez JR, Risco C, Carrascosa JL, Esteban M, Rodriguez D (1998) Vaccinia virus 15-kilodalton (A14L) protein is essential for assembly and attachment of viral crescents to virosomes. *J Virol* 72: 1287–1296
210 Traktman P, Liu K, DeMasi J, Rollins R, Jesty S, Unger B (2000) Elucidating the essential role of the A14 phosphoprotein in vaccinia virus morphogenesis: construction and characterization of a tetracycline-inducible recombinant. *J Virol* 74: 3682–3695
211 da Fonseca FG, Weisberg AS, Caeiro MF, Moss B (2004) Vaccinia virus mutants with alanine substitutions in the conserved G5R gene fail to initiate morphogenesis at the nonpermissive temperature. *J Virol* 78: 10238–10248
212 Moss B, Rosenblum EN, Katz E, Grimley PM (1969) Rifampicin: a specific inhibitor of vaccinia virus assembly. *Nature* 224: 1280–1284
213 Tartaglia J, Piccini A, Paoletti E (1986) Vaccinia virus rifampicin-resistance locus specifies a late 63,000 Da gene product. *Virology* 150: 45–54
214 Baldick CJ Jr, Moss B (1987) Resistance of vaccinia virus to rifampicin conferred by a single nucleotide substitution near the predicted NH2 terminus of a gene encoding an Mr 62,000 polypeptide. *Virology* 156: 138–145
215 Zhang Y, Moss B (1992) Immature viral envelope formation is interrupted at the same stage by lac operator-mediated repression of the vaccinia virus D13L gene and by the drug rifampicin. *Virology* 187: 643–653
216 Szajner P, Weisberg AS, Lebowitz J, Heuser J, Moss B (2005) External scaffold of spherical immature poxvirus particles is made of protein trimers, forming a honeycomb lattice. *J Cell Biol* 170: 971–981
217 Resch W, Weisberg AS, Moss B (2005) Vaccinia virus nonstructural protein encoded by the A11R gene is required for formation of the virion membrane. *J Virol* 79: 6598–6609
218 Szajner P, Weisberg AS, Wolffe EJ, Moss B (2001) Vaccinia virus A30L protein is required for association of viral membranes with dense viroplasm to form immature virions. *J Virol* 75: 5752–5761
219 Szajner P, Jaffe H, Weisberg AS, Moss B (2003) Vaccinia virus G7L protein interacts with the A30L protein and is required for association of viral membranes with dense viroplasm to form immature virions. *J Virol* 77: 3418–3429
220 Yeh WW, Moss B, Wolffe EJ (2000) The vaccinia virus A9L gene encodes a membrane protein required for an early step in virion morphogenesis. *J Virol* 74: 9701–9711
221 Ravanello MP, Hruby DE (1994) Characterization of the vaccinia virus L1R myristylprotein as a component of the intracellular virion envelope. *J Gen Virol* 75: 1479–1483
222 Ravanello MP, Hruby DE (1994) Conditional lethal expression of the vaccinia virus L1R myristylated protein reveals a role in virion assembly. *J Virol* 68: 6401–6410

223 da Fonseca FG, Wolffe EJ, Weisberg A, Moss B (2000) Effects of deletion or stringent repression of the H3L envelope gene on vaccinia virus replication. *J Virol* 74: 7518–7528
224 da Fonseca FG, Wolffe EJ, Weisberg A, Moss B (2000) Characterization of the vaccinia virus H3L envelope protein: topology and posttranslational membrane insertion via the C-terminal hydrophobic tail. *J Virol* 74: 7508–7517
225 Zhang YF, Moss B (1991) Vaccinia virus morphogenesis is interrupted when expression of the gene encoding an 11-kilodalton phosphorylated protein is prevented by the *Escherichia coli* lac repressor. *J Virol* 65: 6101–6110
226 Klemperer N, Ward J, Evans E, Traktman P (1997) The vaccinia virus I1 protein is essential for the assembly of mature virions. *J Virol* 71: 9285–9294
227 Moss B, Rosenblum EN (1973) Protein cleavage and poxvirus morphogenesis: tryptic peptide analysis of core precursors accumulated by blocking assembly with rifampicin. *J Mol Biol* 81: 267–269
228 Lee P, Hruby DE (1994) Proteolytic cleavage of vaccinia virus virion proteins. Mutational analysis of the specificity determinants. *J Biol Chem* 269: 8616–8622
229 Katz E, Moss B (1970) Formation of a vaccinia virus structural polypeptide from a higher molecular weight precursor: inhibition by rifampicin. *Proc Natl Acad Sci USA* 66: 677–684
230 Niles EG, Seto J (1988) Vaccinia virus gene D8 encodes a virion transmembrane protein. *J Virol* 62: 3772–3778
231 Rodriguez JF, Esteban M (1987) Mapping and nucleotide sequence of the vaccinia virus gene that encodes a 14-kilodalton fusion protein. *J Virol* 61: 3550–3554
232 Betakova T, Wolffe EJ, Moss B (2000) The vaccinia virus A14.5L gene encodes a hydrophobic 53-amino-acid virion membrane protein that enhances virulence in mice and is conserved among vertebrate poxviruses. *J Virol* 74: 4085–4092
233 Rodriguez D, Rodriguez JR, Esteban M (1993) The vaccinia virus 14-kilodalton fusion protein forms a stable complex with the processed protein encoded by the vaccinia virus A17L gene. *J Virol* 67: 3435–3440
234 Rodriguez D, Esteban M, Rodriguez JR (1995) Vaccinia virus A17L gene product is essential for an early step in virion morphogenesis. *J Virol* 69: 4640–4648
235 Wallengren K, Risco C, Krijnse-Locker J, Esteban M, Rodriguez D (2001) The A17L gene product of vaccinia virus is exposed on the surface of IMV. *Virology* 290: 143–152
236 Rodriguez JF, Janeczko R, Esteban M (1985) Isolation and characterization of neutralizing monoclonal antibodies to vaccinia virus. *J Virol* 56: 482–488
237 Davies DH, McCausland MM, Valdez C, Huynh D, Hernandez JE, Mu Y, Hirst S, Villarreal L, Felgner PL, Crotty S (2005) Vaccinia virus H3L envelope protein is a major target of neutralizing antibodies in humans and elicits protection against lethal challenge in mice. *J Virol* 79: 11724–11733
238 Ichihashi Y, Oie M (1996) Neutralizing epitope on penetration protein of vaccinia virus. *Virology* 220: 491–494
239 Senkevich TG, White CL, Koonin EV, Moss B (2002) Complete pathway for protein disulfide bond formation encoded by poxviruses. *Proc Natl Acad Sci USA* 99: 6667–6672

240 Senkevich TG, Weisberg AS, Moss B (2000) Vaccinia virus E10R protein is associated with the membranes of intracellular mature virions and has a role in morphogenesis. *Virology* 278: 244–252
241 Senkevich TG, White CL, Koonin EV, Moss B (2000) A viral member of the ERV1/ALR protein family participates in a cytoplasmic pathway of disulfide bond formation. *Proc Natl Acad Sci USA* 97: 12068–12073
242 White CL, Senkevich TG, Moss B (2002) Vaccinia virus G4L glutaredoxin is an essential intermediate of a cytoplasmic disulfide bond pathway required for virion assembly. *J Virol* 76: 467–472
243 Senkevich TG, White CL, Weisberg A, Granek JA, Wolffe EJ, Koonin EV, Moss B (2002) Expression of the vaccinia virus A2.5L redox protein is required for virion morphogenesis. *Virology* 300: 296–303
244 Sanderson CM, Hollinshead M, Smith GL (2000) The vaccinia virus A27L protein is needed for the microtubule-dependent transport of intracellular mature virus particles. *J Gen Virol* 81: 47–58
245 Hiller G, Weber K (1985) Golgi-derived membranes that contain an acylated viral polypeptide are used for vaccinia virus envelopment. *J Virol* 55: 651–659
246 Hirt P, Hiller G, Wittek R (1986) Localization and fine structure of a vaccinia virus gene encoding an envelope antigen. *J Virol* 58: 757–764
247 Blasco R, Moss B (1991) Extracellular vaccinia virus formation and cell-to-cell virus transmission are prevented by deletion of the gene encoding the 37,000-Dalton outer envelope protein. *J Virol* 65: 5910–5920
248 Hiller G, Eibl H, Weber K (1981) Characterization of intracellular and extracellular vaccinia virus variants: N1-isonicotinoyl-N2-3-methyl-4-chlorobenzoylhydrazine interferes with cytoplasmic virus dissemination and release. *J Virol* 39: 903–913
249 Yang G, Pevear DC, Davies MH, Collett MS, Bailey T, Rippen S, Barone L, Burns C, Rhodes G, Tohan S et al (2005) An orally bioavailable antipoxvirus compound (ST-246) inhibits extracellular virus formation and protects mice from lethal orthopoxvirus challenge. *J Virol* 79: 13139–13149
250 Schmutz C, Payne LG, Gubser J, Wittek R (1991) A mutation in the gene encoding the vaccinia virus 37,000-M(r) protein confers resistance to an inhibitor of virus envelopment and release. *J Virol* 65: 3435–3442
251 Ponting CP, Kerr ID (1996) A novel family of phospholipase D homologues that includes phospholipid synthases and putative endonucleases: identification of duplicated repeats and potential active site residues. *Protein Sci* 5: 914–922
252 Baek SH, Kwak JY, Lee SH, Lee T, Ryu SH, Uhlinger DJ, Lambeth JD (1997) Lipase activities of p37, the major envelope protein of vaccinia virus. *J Biol Chem* 272: 32042–32049
253 Sung TC, Roper RL, Zhang Y, Rudge SA, Temel R, Hammond SM, Morris AJ, Moss B, Engebrecht J, Frohman MA (1997) Mutagenesis of phospholipase D defines a superfamily including a trans-Golgi viral protein required for poxvirus pathogenicity. *EMBO J* 16: 4519–4530
254 Schmutz C, Rindisbacher L, Galmiche MC, Wittek R (1995) Biochemical analysis of the major vaccinia virus envelope antigen. *Virology* 213: 19–27
255 Grosenbach DW, Hansen SG, Hruby DE (2000) Identification and analysis of vaccinia virus palmitylproteins. *Virology* 275: 193–206

256 Grosenbach DW, Hruby DE (1998) Analysis of a vaccinia virus mutant expressing a nonpalmitylated form of p37, a mediator of virion envelopment. *J Virol* 72: 5108–5120
257 Husain M, Moss B (2002) Similarities in the induction of post-Golgi vesicles by the vaccinia virus F13L protein and phospholipase D. *J Virol* 76: 7777–7789
258 Husain M, Moss B (2001) Vaccinia virus F13L protein with a conserved phospholipase catalytic motif induces colocalization of the B5R envelope glycoprotein in post-Golgi vesicles. *J Virol* 75: 7528–7542
259 Roper RL, Moss B (1999) Envelope formation is blocked by mutation of a sequence related to the HKD phospholipid metabolism motif in the vaccinia virus F13L protein. *J Virol* 73: 1108–1117
260 Martinez-Pomares L, Stern RJ, Moyer RW (1993) The ps/hr gene (B5R open reading frame homolog) of rabbitpox virus controls pock color, is a component of extracellular enveloped virus, and is secreted into the medium. *J Virol* 67: 5450–5462
261 Engelstad M, Smith GL (1993) The vaccinia virus 42-kDa envelope protein is required for the envelopment and egress of extracellular virus and for virus virulence. *Virology* 194: 627–637
262 Wolffe EJ, Isaacs SN, Moss B (1993) Deletion of the vaccinia virus B5R gene encoding a 42-kilodalton membrane glycoprotein inhibits extracellular virus envelope formation and dissemination. *J Virol* 67: 4732–4741
263 Herrera E, Lorenzo MM, Blasco R, Isaacs SN (1998) Functional analysis of vaccinia virus B5R protein: essential role in virus envelopment is independent of a large portion of the extracellular domain. *J Virol* 72: 294–302
264 Cudmore S, Cossart P, Griffiths G, Way M (1995) Actin-based motility of vaccinia virus. *Nature* 378: 636–638
265 Hollinshead M, Rodger G, Van Eijl H, Law M, Hollinshead R, Vaux DJ, Smith GL (2001) Vaccinia virus utilizes microtubules for movement to the cell surface. *J Cell Biol* 154: 389–402
266 Ward BM, Moss B (2001) Vaccinia virus intracellular movement is associated with microtubules and independent of actin tails. *J Virol* 75: 11651–11663
267 Rietdorf J, Ploubidou A, Reckmann I, Holmstrom A, Frischknecht F, Zettl M, Zimmermann T, Way M (2001) Kinesin-dependent movement on microtubules precedes actin-based motility of vaccinia virus. *Nat Cell Biol* 3: 992–1000
268 Geada MM, Galindo I, Lorenzo MM, Perdiguero B, Blasco R (2001) Movements of vaccinia virus intracellular enveloped virions with GFP tagged to the F13L envelope protein. *J Gen Virol* 82: 2747–2760
269 Ward BM, Moss B (2001) Visualization of intracellular movement of vaccinia virus virions containing a green fluorescent protein-B5R membrane protein chimera. *J Virol* 75: 4802–4813
270 Zhang WH, Wilcock D, Smith GL (2000) Vaccinia virus F12L protein is required for actin tail formation, normal plaque size, and virulence. *J Virol* 74: 11654–11662
271 Ward BM, Moss B (2004) Vaccinia virus A36R membrane protein provides a direct link between intracellular enveloped virions and the microtubule motor kinesin. *J Virol* 78: 2486–2493
272 Sanderson CM, Frischknecht F, Way M, Hollinshead M, Smith GL (1998) Roles

of vaccinia virus EEV-specific proteins in intracellular actin tail formation and low pH-induced cell-cell fusion. *J Gen Virol* 79: 1415–1425
273 Wolffe EJ, Weisberg AS, Moss B (1998) Role for the vaccinia virus A36R outer envelope protein in the formation of virus-tipped actin-containing microvilli and cell-to-cell virus spread. *Virology* 244: 20–26
274 van Eijl H, Hollinshead M, Smith GL (2000) The vaccinia virus A36R protein is a type Ib membrane protein present on intracellular but not extracellular enveloped virus particles. *Virology* 271: 26–36
275 Herrero-Martinez E, Roberts KL, Hollinshead M, Smith GL (2005) Vaccinia virus intracellular enveloped virions move to the cell periphery on microtubules in the absence of the A36R protein. *J Gen Virol* 86: 2961–2968
276 van Eijl H, Hollinshead M, Rodger G, Zhang WH, Smith GL (2002) The vaccinia virus F12L protein is associated with intracellular enveloped virus particles and is required for their egress to the cell surface. *J Gen Virol* 83: 195–207
277 Hiller G, Weber K, Schneider L, Parajsz C, Jungwirth C (1979) Interaction of assembled progeny pox viruses with the cellular cytoskeleton. *Virology* 98: 142–153
278 Blasco R, Cole NB, Moss B (1991) Sequence analysis, expression, and deletion of a vaccinia virus gene encoding a homolog of profilin, a eukaryotic actin-binding protein. *J Virol* 65: 4598–4608
279 Frischknecht F, Moreau V, Rottger S, Gonfloni S, Reckmann I, Superti-Furga G, Way M (1999) Actin-based motility of vaccinia virus mimics receptor tyrosine kinase signalling. *Nature* 401: 926–929
280 Scaplehorn N, Holmstrom A, Moreau V, Frischknecht F, Reckmann I, Way M (2002) Grb2 and Nck act cooperatively to promote actin-based motility of vaccinia virus. *Curr Biol* 12: 740–745
281 Newsome TP, Scaplehorn N, Way M (2004) Src mediates a switch from microtubule- to actin-based motility of vaccinia virus. *Science* 306: 124–129
282 Reeves PM, Bommarius B, Lebeis S, McNulty S, Christensen J, Swimm A, Chahroudi A, Chavan R, Feinberg MB, Veach D et al (2005) Disabling poxvirus pathogenesis by inhibition of Abl-family tyrosine kinases. *Nat Med* 11: 731–739
283 Ward BM, Weisberg AS, Moss B (2003) Mapping and functional analysis of interaction sites within the cytoplasmic domains of the vaccinia virus A33R and A36R envelope proteins. *J Virol* 77: 4113–4126
284 Smith GL, Murphy BJ, Law M (2003) Vaccinia virus motility. *Annu Rev* Microbiol 57: 323–342
285 Smith GL, Law M (2004) The exit of Vaccinia virus from infected cells. *Virus Res* 106: 189–197
286 Law M, Hollinshead R, Smith GL (2002) Antibody-sensitive and antibody-resistant cell-to-cell spread by vaccinia virus: role of the A33R protein in antibody-resistant spread. *J Gen Virol* 83: 209–222
287 Boulter EA, Appleyard G (1973) Differences between extracellular and intracellular forms of poxvirus and their implications. *Prog Med Virol* 16: 86–108
288 Payne LG (1980) Significance of extracellular enveloped virus in the *in vitro* and *in vivo* dissemination of vaccinia. *J Gen Virol* 50: 89–100

289 Sanderson CM, Way M, Smith GL (1998) Virus-induced cell motility. *J Virol* 72: 1235–1243
290 Valderrama F, Cordeiro JV, Schleich S, Frischknecht F, Way M (2006) Vaccinia virus-induced cell motility requires F11L-mediated inhibition of RhoA signaling. *Science* 311: 377–381
291 Payne LG (1979) Identification of the vaccinia hemagglutinin polypeptide from a cell system yielding large amounts of extracellular enveloped virus. *J Virol* 31: 147–155
292 Payne L (1978) Polypeptide composition of extracellular enveloped vaccinia virus. *J Virol* 27: 28–37
293 Roper RL, Payne LG, Moss B (1996) Extracellular vaccinia virus envelope glycoprotein encoded by the A33R gene. *J Virol* 70: 3753–3762
294 Duncan SA, Smith GL (1992) Identification and characterization of an extracellular envelope glycoprotein affecting vaccinia virus egress. *J Virol* 66: 1610–1621
295 Shida H (1986) Nucleotide sequence of the vaccinia virus hemagglutinin gene. *Virology* 150: 451–462
296 Brum LM, Turner PC, Devick H, Baquero MT, Moyer RW (2003) Plasma membrane localization and fusion inhibitory activity of the cowpox virus serpin SPI-3 require a functional signal sequence and the virus encoded hemagglutinin. *Virology* 306: 289–302
297 Roper RL, Wolffe EJ, Weisberg A, Moss B (1998) The envelope protein encoded by the A33R gene is required for formation of actin-containing microvilli and efficient cell-to-cell spread of vaccinia virus. *J Virol* 72: 4192–4204
298 McIntosh AA, Smith GL (1996) Vaccinia virus glycoprotein A34R is required for infectivity of extracellular enveloped virus. *J Virol* 70: 272–281
299 Blasco R, Sisler JR, Moss B (1993) Dissociation of progeny vaccinia virus from the cell membrane is regulated by a viral envelope glycoprotein: effect of a point mutation in the lectin homology domain of the A34R gene. *J Virol* 67: 3319–3325
300 Katz E, Wolffe E, Moss B (2002) Identification of second-site mutations that enhance release and spread of vaccinia virus. *J Virol* 76: 11637–11644
301 Katz E, Ward BM, Weisberg AS, Moss B (2003) Mutations in the vaccinia virus A33R and B5R envelope proteins that enhance release of extracellular virions and eliminate formation of actin-containing microvilli without preventing tyrosine phosphorylation of the A36R protein. *J Virol* 77: 12266–12275
302 Parkinson JE, Smith GL (1994) Vaccinia virus gene A36R encodes a M(r) 43-50 K protein on the surface of extracellular enveloped virus. *Virology* 204: 376–390
303 Delhon G, Tulman ER, Afonso CL, Lu Z, de la Concha-Bermejillo A, Lehmkuhl HD, Piccone ME, Kutish GF, Rock DL (2004) Genomes of the parapoxviruses ORF virus and bovine papular stomatitis virus. *J Virol* 78: 168–177
304 Tikkanen MK, McInnes CJ, Mercer AA, Buttner M, Tuimala J, Hirvela-Koski V, Neuvonen E, Huovilainen A (2004) Recent isolates of parapoxvirus of Finnish reindeer (*Rangifer tarandus tarandus*) are closely related to bovine pseudocowpox virus. *J Gen Virol* 85: 1413–1418
305 Likos AM, Sammons SA, Olson VA, Frace AM, Li Y, Olsen-Rasmussen M,

Davidson W, Galloway R, Khristova ML, Reynolds MG et al (2005) A tale of two clades: monkeypox viruses. *J Gen Virol* 86: 2661–2672
306 Chen N, Li G, Liszewski MK, Atkinson JP, Jahrling PB, Feng Z, Schriewer J, Buck C, Wang C, Lefkowitz EJ et al (2005) Virulence differences between monkeypox virus isolates from West Africa and the Congo basin. *Virology* 340: 46–63
307 Smith GL, Symons JA, Alcamí A (1998) Poxviruses: interfering with interferon. Semin Virol 8: 409–418
308 Williamson JD, Reith RW, Jeffrey LJ, Arrand JR, Mackett M (1990) Biological characterization of recombinant vaccinia viruses in mice infected by the respiratory route. *J Gen Virol* 71: 2761–2767
309 Alcami A, Smith GL (1992) A soluble receptor for interleukin-1 beta encoded by vaccinia virus: a novel mechanism of virus modulation of the host response to infection. *Cell* 71: 153–167
310 Lee MS, Roos JM, McGuigan LC, Smith KA, Cormier N, Cohen LK, Roberts BE, Payne LG (1992) Molecular attenuation of vaccinia virus: mutant generation and animal characterization. *J Virol* 66: 2617–2630
311 Symons JA, Alcami A, Smith GL (1995) Vaccinia virus encodes a soluble type I interferon receptor of novel structure and broad species specificity. *Cell* 81: 551–560
312 Tscharke DC, Smith GL (1999) A model for vaccinia virus pathogenesis and immunity based on intradermal injection of mouse ear pinnae. *J Gen Virol* 80: 2751–2755
313 Tscharke DC, Reading PC, Smith GL (2002) Dermal infection with vaccinia virus reveals roles for virus proteins not seen using other inoculation routes. *J Gen Virol* 83: 1977–1986
314 Reading PC, Smith GL (2003) A kinetic analysis of immune mediators in the lungs of mice infected with vaccinia virus and comparison with intradermal infection. *J Gen Virol* 84: 1973–1983
315 Jacobs N, Chen RA-J, Gubser C, Najarro P, Smith GL (2006) Intradermal immune response after infection with Vaccinia virus. *J Gen Virol* 87: 1157–1161
316 Lee H-J, Essani K, Smith GL (2001) The genome sequence of Yaba-like disease virus, a yatapoxvirus. *Virology* 281: 170–192

Poxviruses
ed. by Andrew A. Mercer, Axel Schmidt and Olaf Weber

Genus *Orthopoxvirus: Variola virus*

Inger K. Damon

Poxvirus Program, Division of Viral and Rickettsial Diseases, Centers for Disease Control and Prevention, Atlanta, GA 30333, USA

The findings and conclusions in this report are those of the author and do not necessarily represent the views of the Centers for Disease Control and Prevention.

Abstract

Variola major virus caused the human disease smallpox; interpretations of the historic record indicate that the initial introduction of disease in a naïve population had profound effects on its demographics. Smallpox was declared eradicated by the World Health Organization (WHO) in 1980. This chapter reviews epidemiological, clinical and pathophysiological observations of disease, and review some of the more recent observations on the microbiology of *Variola virus*.

Taxonomy and history

The orthopoxvirus *Variola virus* is the only member species of the *Orthopoxvirus* genus which, as we understand the virus, is a solely human pathogen. Using genomic comparison, *Variola virus* has been shown to be most closely related to *Taterapox virus*, an orthopoxvirus found in one gerbil species in West Africa (of which there is one known isolate), and *Camelpox virus* [1, 2]. *Camelpox virus* is similarly unique amongst orthopoxviruses in that it is believed to be solely a pathogen of dromedary camels. The majority of other orthopoxviruses have broad host ranges, and many are believed to, or known to, have rodent reservoir hosts. At least two types of *Variola virus* have been clearly described that have distinct biological and genetic properties and different human clinical and epidemiological manifestations. These have been described as variola major and variola alastrim minor. Another variant of virus has been suggested, "intermedius", from examination of biological properties of ceiling temperatures of growth on chorioallantoic membranes (CAM) of embryonated eggs and correlation with age-adjusted case fatality rates; some investigators felt there was an intermediate biological phenotype and case fatality rate associated with these viruses. Other forms of disease with low case fatality rates had also been described in Africa, and termed "African minor"; in general, viruses obtained from cases associated with these outbreaks did not show biological properties distinguishing them from variola major.

Comprehensive, scholarly reviews of the history of smallpox and history of efforts to control the disease are available [3, 4], and will not be repeated here. The origin of smallpox is unknown, but it is likely an ancient disease. Based on visual inspection of the mummified head of Ramses V, from 1160 B.C. it appeared that he died from smallpox. Notably, there is no record of smallpox in the Bible, and no description of smallpox in the early Greek and Roman literature [3]. Dixon cites historic work that describes smallpox in China in 1122 B.C., and the introduction of the practice of inoculation in 590 B.C. using intranasal exposure to virus [3]. Henderson cites literature that identifies the practice of inoculation being used in India, before 1000 A.D., then spreading to China, Africa, western Asia and later Europe and North America in the 18th century [5]. Inoculation, using scabs from recovered patients, introduced variola virus either *via* the skin or nasal passages. Infection acquired *via* these routes, utilizing a skilled administrator, was less severe than that acquired *via* natural infection; although the individual could still transmit disease, the chance of death was about one-tenth that predicted if infection had been *via* natural exposure [5]. The name variola was first used by the Bishop Marius of Avenches, in Switzerland, in the 6th century and was derived from the Latin *varius* (spotted) or *varus* (pimple). In the 10th century, the Anglo-Saxon word poc or pocca (bag or pouch) and later pockes was used to describe a rash illness; by the 15th century, smallpox was used to differentiate the illness from syphilis, or the great pox [6].

The written description of vaccination, using pustular material from a human cowpox virus lesion, and its subsequent protection against variola virus challenge was described by Edward Jenner [7, 8] at the end of the 18th century. Vaccination gradually replaced the practice of inoculation or variolation, and was introduced by the Spanish in the New world [9], although variolation was used by certain populations even in the 20th century [4]. The exact origin of *Vaccinia virus*, which replaced the use of *Cowpox virus* as vaccine, is uncertain [10, 11].

The generation and use of more stable preparations of vaccinia virus, through freeze-drying [12], permitted use of the vaccine outside the cold-chain. Worldwide efforts, under the auspices of the WHO, led to the declaration of the eradication of human smallpox in 1980. The last naturally occurring cases were in 1977; two cases related to a laboratory were reported in 1978 [4]. Routine vaccination largely ceased in 1980, and the stocks of variola virus were voluntarily consolidated in two WHO Collaborating Center repositories. With current concerns that possible undeclared stocks of *Variola virus* exist, and the potential for their malevolent use, research into smallpox diagnostics, therapeutics and vaccines has been revitalized [13–15].

Epidemiology, disease, pathology

Unlike the majority of orthopoxviruses, the smallpox-causing *Variola virus* is a solely human disease pathogen. Nonhuman primates can be infected, and have transmitted disease, via respiratory and transcutaneous routes, to other member species within laboratory settings [16–18]. However, natural infection of animals other than humans was not recorded. Quantitative epidemiological studies were largely conducted during the last 50 years of naturally occurring smallpox. Virus was transmitted person to person; large respiratory droplets are believed to be the common source of infectious exposure [19–21]. Amongst contacts of cases the duration, frequency, and proximity of contact were all factors associated with disease acquisition. Household contacts were at greater risk than casual contacts. The extent of contact within a household also correlated with the likelihood of disease acquisition [22, 23]; in one study those with constant contact were more likely to acquire disease (26.8%) than those who left the home during the day (6.3%) [22]. Health care workers were also at risk for disease acquisition [24]. In a few notable outbreaks, airborne transmission of smaller aerosol droplets is believed to have resulted in infection [25]. These studies also suggested that the infectious dose was low. Transmission via fomites or contact with the infectious material from the rash also occurred [19, 26]. In household settings, secondary attack rates in unvaccinated contacts ranged from 37% to 88% [4, 20]. The density of populations also was important in determining the extent of individual outbreaks [27, 28], and the periodicity of outbreaks [29].

Vaccination with *Vaccinia virus* was demonstrated to be effective at prevention of disease acquisition. Within settings known to be associated with high-risk exposures, such as the household, the secondary attack rates in vaccinated contacts was appreciably lower than that seen in unvaccinated contacts. Aggregate data, collected during the smallpox eradication campaign, suggest a secondary attack rate of 58.4% in unvaccinated close or household contacts, and a secondary attack rate of 3.8% in previously vaccinated close or household contacts [4]. Case fatality rates for variola major varied with the type of disease manifest, but aggregate rates of 10–30% in various outbreaks have been recorded. If disease was acquired, severity was ameliorated if a previous vaccination scar was present; this was considered to be evidence of a "take", although in some cases the scar may have represented a bacterial superinfection. A study of hospitalized patients demonstrated that overall, the case fatality rate was 35.5% for unvaccinated case patients, and only 6.3% for vaccinated case patients [30]. Morbidity and mortality generally correlated with rash burden, and was also more severe in children and pregnant women [23, 31]. With the exception of the pregnant host, or the host who acquired the flat or hemorrhagic form of smallpox (see below), previous vaccination appeared to modify the disease course; 83.7% of previously vaccinated hospitalized patients presented with modified or discrete forms of smallpox (described below). In contrast, only 44.2% of unvaccinated hospitalized patients presented with these forms of disease. Variola alastrim minor, a variant of variola virus with a case fatality rate of < 1%, manifests with apparently similar epidemiological rates and characteristics of human to human transmission, but far less morbidity and mortality.

Environmental factors also likely contributed to the observed seasonality; the incidence of disease was highest in winter and early spring. The stability of the virus is enhanced at lower temperature and humidity [32], conditions present in these seasons. Case patients are most infectious from the time of rash onset through the first week of rash; this correlates with the magnitude of infectious viral particles that can be found in oropharyngeal secretions [33–35] during illness.

Disease

Naturally acquired variola virus infection caused a systemic illness characterized by fever and a distinctive rash. The WHO categorized eight types of smallpox; their classification was largely based on the clinical categorization of disease seen in India [30] (Tab. 1). The classic description of smallpox describes the ordinary forms of illness that were the most common clinical presentations. After an asymptomatic incubation period of 10–14 days (range, 7–17), fever quickly rose to about 103°F (38°–40°C) and sometimes dermal petechiae were manifest. Associated constitutional symptoms included backache, headache, vomiting, and prostration. Within 1 or 2 days after incubation, a systemic rash appeared that was characteristically centrifugally distributed (i.e., lesions were present in greater numbers on the oral mucosa, face, and extremities than on the trunk). The fever typically abated as the rash presented. Lesions commonly manifested on the palms and soles. The rash lesions were initially macular and then advanced to the papular stage, enlarging and progressing to a vesicle by days 4 to 5 and a pustule by day 7. When lesions became pustular, the fever typically returned. Lesions became encrusted and scabby by day 14 and then sloughed off. Skin lesions, at the vesicular and pustular stages, were deep seated and lesions were in the same stage of development in any one area of the body. Images of the classic presentation of ordinary smallpox are depicted in Figure 1. The ordinary type was subgrouped into three categories, which were based on the extent of rash on the face and the body: confluent, semi-confluent, and discrete. In ordinary confluent disease, no area of skin was visible

Table 1

WHO smallpox type	Clinical definition
Variola sine eruptione	Fever, no rash
Modified	Like ordinary, accelerated course
Ordinary discrete	Fever, rash, areas normal skin between pustules even on face
Ordinary semiconfluent	Fever, rash, pustules confluent on face, discrete elsewhere
Ordinary confluent	Fever, rash, pustules confluent on face and forearms
Flat	Fever, erythema and edema of skin, vesicles soft, flat and bullous
Hemorrhagic, early	Fever (persistent), hemorrhages and petechiae, purpuric rash at illness onset
Hemorrhagic, late	Fever (persistent), rash, hemorrhage into the base of vesicles late in illness

between vesiculopustular rash lesions on the trunk or the face. In ordinary semi-confluent and discrete disease, patches of normal skin were visible between rash lesions on the trunk and face, respectively, the remaineder experienced the more severe forms described below. Less severe manifestations (modified smallpox or variola sine eruptione) occurred in some unvaccinated, and more commonly in vaccinated, individuals. In a study of 3544 unvaccinated hospitalized smallpox cases, modified, discrete, semi-confluent or confluent ordinary disease was observed in 1.7%, 42.1%, 23.9% and 22.8% of patients, respectively, the remainder experiences the more severe forms described below. In the same study, the mortality rate correlated with rash burden; case fatality rates were 0%, 9.3%, 37.0% and 62.0%, respectively [30].

Variola major smallpox was differentiated into four main clinical types: (i) ordinary smallpox (~90% of cases) produced viremia, fever, prostration, and rash; mortality rates were generally proportional to the extent of rash and ranged, using the WHO classification, from less than 10% for ordinary discrete to 50–75% for the rarer ordinary confluent presentation; (ii) (vaccine) modified smallpox (5% of cases) produced a mild prodrome with few skin lesions in previously vaccinated people and had a mortality rate well under 10%; (iii) flat smallpox (~5% of hospitalized cases) produced slowly developing lesions that were difficult to ascertain because, at the vesicular stage, they appeared flush with the (edematous) skin, and was almost always fatal; and (iv) hemorrhagic smallpox (< 1% of cases) induced bleeding into the skin and the mucous membranes, and was invariably fatal. A discrete type of the ordinary form, with typical febrile prodrome and rash, resulted from alastrim variola minor infection [4]. Individuals with this form of disease were not nearly as moribund or "toxemic" as were individuals with variola major infection.

The most severe forms of smallpox, the flat and hemorrhagic presentations, did not appear to be dependent on the strain of variola virus circulat-

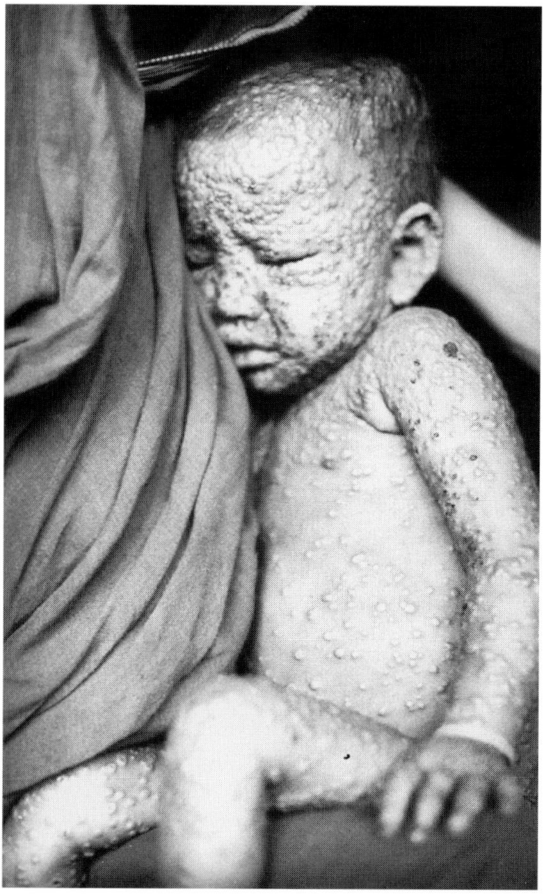

Figure 1. Young Bangladesh child, photographed in 1975, with ordinary confluent disease. From Public Health Information Library, image number 7735. http://phil.cdc.gov/phil/home.asp. Donated by CDL/WHO/Stanley Foster MD, MPH.

ing in an outbreak; contacts of hemorrhagic disease cases did not necessarily develop hemorrhagic disease. Defects in the host immune response are believed responsible for these forms of disease. Prior vaccination was not necessarily protective against the hemorrhagic forms of disease, but was suggested to be protective against flat forms of disease [30, 36–38]. Pregnant women were also prone to develop hemorrhagic forms of disease; an increase in cortisone levels present during pregnancy was suggested to be one of the host factors responsible [31, 38]. Administration of cortisone to nonhuman primates challenged with variola virus led to severe disease presentations with hemorrhagic features and worse outcomes [39]. In studies of viremia during illness, as detected by growth of virus on CAM, viremia was only routinely seen during illness in hemorrhagic forms of disease [40–42]; evaluation of the host's sera demonstrated minimal antibody response to virus.

In flat smallpox, illness was heralded by the abrupt onset of fever to 38.3–38.9°C, and the appearance of a rash after 3–4 days. The oral enanthema was often confluent, and sloughing of rectal mucosal membranes was also reported. At the papulovesicular stage of disease, lesions appeared as small indentations (day 6) with hemorrhages in the bases, and were surrounded by an erythematous ring. By days 7 or 8, the lesions appeared flat. Bullous lesions, which would slough, were reported. Fever persisted throughout the disease course, and respiratory complications were often observed by days 7 or 8 of illness. Thrombocytopenia, neutropenia and lymphocytosis were reported [3].

In hemorrhagic forms of smallpox, the timing of appearance of hemorrhagic manifestations led to the nomenclature of early and late forms. In addition, pathology studies support different pathogenic manifestations. These manifestations of smallpox were more prevalent in adults than in children. In early hemorrhagic disease, illness began with fever and typical prodromal symptoms; the fever never abated. Early after fever onset, petechiae and purpuric rashes became apparent; subconjunctival hemorrhages, hematuria, and vaginal bleeding were also seen. Patients usually died by day 6 of illness, well before any classic vesiculopustular rash was evident. In late hemorrhagic disease, after fever onset, typical maculopapular lesions developed, but the fever did not abate. The lesion evolved slowly, and areas of hemorrhage were evident at the base of the lesions. In some cases the lesions remained flat, in others the lesions vesiculated. Bleeding occurred in the mucous membranes, thrombocytopenia was profound, and death occurred between days 8 and 10 of illness.

Pathogenesis and pathology

Much of what is described about the pathogenesis of smallpox comes from experimental studies of variola virus infection of nonhuman primates, or the closely related orthopoxviruses *Monkeypox virus*, *Ectromelia virus* and *Rabbitpox virus* systemic infections of susceptible hosts. These studies, in addition to clinical diagnostic studies of human smallpox patients, or autopsy data from deceased smallpox patients, comprise our understanding of the pathogenesis of human smallpox.

The majority of infections were initiated by inhalation of respiratory droplets and implantation of virus on the oropharyngeal and respiratory mucosa. No primary localized site of infection was evident if the route of exposure was *via* inhalation. Disease could also be introduced through suspensions of virus obtained from scabs of patients which were introduced percutaneously and constituted the practice of variolation. In these cases (when skillfully administered), illness was usually less virulent, a localized primary infectious lesion was present, and the asymtomatic incubation period shorter.

After entry, in the model of pathogenesis that has been developed, virus moves to local lymph nodes, and then disseminates to the reticuloendothelial system to further replicate. At this time, the individual is asymptomatic. After 10–14 days, the secondary viremia occurs, which heralds the prodrome of symptomatic illness. During this time virus seeds the oropharynx and epidermis; the absence of a keratinized structure in the mucosa of the oropharynx leads to ulceration and release of virus in the saliva; virus replicates in the epidermis to cause the characteristic macular, papular, and vesicular eruptions of smallpox.

Recent studies of intravenous (i.v.) variola virus infection of cynomolgus monkeys provides a model of illness that resembles some aspects of types of clinical smallpox that had higher case fatality rates, and thus may provide additional information about the pathophysiological processes leading to fatal outcomes [43]. In this model, high doses of variola virus were administered (10^9 infectious particles) and a few days after infection, virus was recoverable in the oropharynx, centrifugally distributed vesicular lesions were evident, and death ensued 3–10 days postinfection. High levels of type I IFNs, IL-6, and IFN-γ, as well as D-dimers and thrombocytopenia suggestive of disseminated intravascular coagulation (DIC), and nitric oxide, were measurable in the plasma. Apoptosis with loss of T cells in lymphoid organs was also observed [43]. These findings are consistent with those seen in sepsis syndrome. Of note, TNF-α levels were minimal in the infected animals. Evaluation of host transcriptional responses in this variola virus infection model, using RNA extracted from peripheral blood mononuclear cells (PBMCs) isolated during infection, indicated a notable decrease in the expression of genes regulated by NF-κB and TNF-α. This is in contrast to what had been seen in bacterial infection of human PBMCs [44]; the function of the TNF receptor homologue of variola virus (see below) may be in part responsible for these findings.

In humans, it is the rash that has been extensively studied during smallpox disease pathogenesis. The viral lesion primarily develops in the epidermis, although early changes of capillary dilation, endothelial cell swelling and perivascular cuffing with lymphocytes, macrophages, plasma cells and eosinophils are seen in the papillary layer of the dermis prior to development of the rash lesion. Subsequently, within the epidermis, the cells of the Malpighian layer swell and vacuolate to undergo ballooning degeneration. B-type inclusions can be seen in the cytoplasm. The cytoplasm continues to enlarge, loss of nuclear material is noted and coalescence of vacuoles *via* cell rupture creates reticulating degeneration of the middle and upper layers of the stratum spinosum. In the next stages, the vesicle is formed. Cells of the lower stratum spinosum and basal layer exhibit nuclear condensation, and nuclei fragmentation. The cavity of the vesicle (later the pustule) thus develops adjacent to the dermis, permitting the "deep-seated" feel of the smallpox pustular lesions. The cavity retains some cellular remnants, which create a multi-loculated appearance, also adding to the firmness of the lesion. When polymorphonuclear cells move into the cavity, pustulation occurs. High titers of virus are found within the lesions [45]. In mucosal surfaces, the absence of a horny layer allows the necrosis caused by proliferation of virus within the epithelium, creating ulcers and leading to liberation of large quantities of virus into the oropharynx [34].

Evaluation of other organs in human smallpox has been done in select autopsy cases. Some observations indicate that liver and spleen do not show evidence of extensive viral replication and necrosis, in contrast to that seen in ectromelia virus infection of susceptible mice. Mild pathological changes are seen in the lungs, although cowpox infection of felines appears to cause severe bronchopneumonia [46], and focal areas of consolidation were noted in rabbitpox virus infection of rabbits, in addition to subpleural nodules [47].

Genome

A number of variola virus genomes have now been sequenced (Tab. 2) [1]. The genome size is ~185 000–186 000 base pairs, with 33.7% G + C, and 197–207 open reading frames (ORFs) of > 50 amino acids in the putative protein. These ORF predictions are inclusive of homologues which may be fragmented with respect to another orthopoxvirus counterparts. The general structure of the genome is analogous to that of other orthopoxviruses; the central region includes genes that encode proteins involved in the viral life cycle and virion morphogenesis; regions of nucleic acid on the left and right ends of the genome encode proteins believed, or predicted, to be involved in evasion of the host immune response or in viral host range. These regions are more variable across orthopoxvirus genomes.

The current availability of sequence information suggests that there are three distinctive groupings of *Variola virus*. One grouping comprises the strains identified as variola major by outbreak case fatality rates and biological properties. This group also includes those strains associated with very low case fatality rates in Africa (also known as African minor). Another group includes those strains identified by <1% outbreak-related case fatality rates and biological properties classified as variola alastrim minor. The last group contains isolates from West Africa, which had been included in later descriptions of *Variola virus* with age-adjusted intermediate case fatality rates and intermediate biological properties.

Many different analyses have been performed in an attempt to predict genes that may be important in defining the particular host range of *Variola virus*, and varying pathogenicity of the virus for the human host [48–59]. These studies have, in general, focused on genes predicted to be involved in evasion of the host immune response, which are present in orthopoxviruses

Table 2. Variola isolates sequenced as of 2006 (adapted from [1])

Acronym identifier Variola virus	Repository record Variola virus	Year isolated	Sample origin	Putative ORFs	accession number
BEN68_59	V68-59, Dahomey	1968	Benin	205	DQ441416
BOT72_143	V72-143	1972	Botswana	203	DQ441417
BOT73_225	V73-225	1973	Botswana	201	DQ441418
CNG70_46	V70-46 Kinshasa	1970	Congo region	203	DQ437583
CNG70_227	V74-227 Gispen Congo 9	1970	Congo region	200	DQ441423
ETH72_16	Eth16 R14-1X-72 Addis	1972	Ethiopia	202	DQ441424
ETH72_17	Eth17 R14-1X-72 Addis	1972	Ethiopia	201	DQ441425
GUI69_005	V69-005 Guinea	1969	Guinea	204	DQ441426
NIG69_001	import from Nigeria	1969	Niger	205	DQ441434
SAF65_102	102 Natal, Ingwavuma	1965	South Africa	200	DQ441435
SAF65_103	103 T'vaal, Nelspruit	1965	South Africa	202	DQ441436
SLN68_258	V68-258	1969	Sierra Leone	204	DQ441437
SOM77_ali	V77-2479 last case	1977	Somalia	202	DQ437590
SUD47_jub	Juba	1947	Sudan	201	DQ441440
TAN65_kem	Kembula	1965	Tanzania	198	DQ441443
AFG70_vlt4	Variolator 4	1970	Afghanistan	203	DQ437580
BSH74_nur	Nur Islam	1974	Bangladesh	196	DQ441420
BSH74_shz	Shahzaman	1974	Bangladesh	197	DQ441421
BSH74_sol	Solaiman	1974	Bangladesh	197	DQ441422
BSH75_banu	V75-550 resequence	1975	Bangladesh	201	DQ437581
CHN48_horn	China Horn Sabin lab	1948	China	204	DQ437582
IND53_mad	Kali-Muthu-Madras	1953	India	201	DQ441427
IND53_ndel	New Delhi	1953	India	201	DQ441428
IND64_vel4	7124 Vellore	1964	India	205	DQ437585
IND64_vel5	7125 Vellore	1964	India	202	DQ437586
IND67_mah	Vector Maharastra E6	1967	India	198	X69198
IRN72_tbrz	Iran 2602 Tabriz	1972	Iran	203	DQ437587
JAP46_yam	Yamada MS-2A Tokyo	1946	Japan	203	DQ441429

Table 2 (continued)

Acronym identifier Variola virus	Repository record Variola virus	Year isolated	Sample origin	Putative ORFs	accession number
JAP51_hrpr	Harper Masterseed	1951	Japan	202	DQ441430
JAP51_stwl	Stillwell Masterseed	1951	Japan	201	DQ441431
KOR47_lee	Lee Masterseed	1947	Korea	203	DQ441432
KUW67_1629	K1629	1967	Kuwait	199	DQ441433
NEP73_175	V73-175	1973	Nepal	202	DQ437588
PAK69_lah	Rafiq Lahore	1969	Pakistan	203	DQ437589
SUM70_222	V70-222	1970	Sumatra	202	DQ437591
SUM70_228	V70-228	1970	Sumatra	199	DQ441442
SYR72_119	V72-119	1972	Syria	203	DQ437592
GER58_hdlg	Heidelberg from India	1958	Germany	201	DQ437584
UNK44_harv	Harvey Middlesex	1944	UK	203	DQ441444
UNK46_hind	Hinden	1946	UK	198	DQ441445
UNK47_hig	Higgins Staffordshire	1947	UK	200	DQ441446
UNK52_but	Butler alastrim	1952	UK	207	DQ441447
YUG72_164	Yugoslavia from Iraq	1972	Yugoslavia	201	DQ441448
BRZ66_39	V66-39 alastrim	1966	Brazil	207	DQ441419
BRZ66_gar	Garcia alastrim	1966	Brazil	207	Y16780

that cause systemic disease (*Variola virus* and *Monkeypox virus*) or absent in those causing localized disease (*Vaccinia virus* and *Cowpox virus*) in the human host. The orthopoxviruses have developed a number of strategies to evade the host immune system, and these have been periodically reviewed [60–66] (see also chapter by Nazarian/McFadden). These include mechanisms to interfere with antiviral effects of IFN, minimize the inflammatory response, inhibit apoptosis and diminish innate complement-mediated immunity. Specific viral proteins are predicted to modulate a number of host proteins including complement cascade proteins, chemokines, NF-κB, IL-1β, IFN-α, IFN-β, IFN-γ, and TNF. The potential significance of differences between variola virus proteins and orthopoxviral counterparts predicted to be involved in interaction with these host proteins has been extensively reviewed. The general consensus is that it is difficult to be certain about the relative importance of the various observations of differences that have been made, and about which variola viral proteins and host responses may, together, interact to create the manifestations of human smallpox. Genome-based predictions of ORFs potentially affecting the characteristic pathogenesis of smallpox primarily exist in the left and right ends of the genome.

Notably, the variola viral homologue of the IL-1β receptor is predicted to be fragmented, and therefore not expressed by variola virus. Deletion of the IL-1β receptor gene in vaccinia virus has been shown to potentiate the febrile response, and weight loss in a murine model of intranasal infection.

To date only a handful of variola virus proteins have been studied directly. These have been expressed in non-orthopoxvirus systems, and then used in *in vitro* systems to compare their properties with those of a counterpart orthopoxvirus protein. The variola virus chemokine binding protein binds β-chemokines, but not α-chemokines, similar to other orthopoxviral homologues [67].

The variola virus homologue, smallpox inhibitor of complement enzyme (SPICE) of the vaccinia virus complement control protein (VCP) has been well studied *in vitro*. The homologues differ by 11 amino acids. The vaccinia virus protein has been demonstrated to interfere with the classical and alternate complement activation pathways, as has the variola virus protein [68–71], and is considered a virulence factor [70]. The variola virus homologue is more potent than the VCP at inactivation of human C3b and C4b, and is more human complement specific than VCP. SPICE inhibited human and baboon complement better than dog or guinea pig complement; the opposite was true for VCP [68]. This finding has been suggested to be one aspect of the human host tropism of *Variola virus* [59]. Additional detailed studies have looked at functional models of protein interaction with complement [72].

Vaccinia growth factor (VGF) has been demonstrated to be a virulence factor [73, 74]. The EGF domain of the variola virus homologue of VGF, expressed from the variola virus D4R ORF and named "smallpox growth factor" (SPGF), was evaluated for its biochemical properties. This 50-amino acid peptide, which has three amino acid differences with respect to its vaccinia virus counterpart, demonstrated subnanomolar specific binding to erbB1, and induced proliferation of human keratinocytes. Two monoclonal antibodies generated against the variola virus protein EGF domain efficiently blocked binding of SPGF to erbB1, but demonstrated diminished or absent ability to bind VGF. The former monoclonal antibody, when co-administered with a monoclonal anti-L1R (that neutralizes intracellular mature virions) in an intranasal vaccinia virus challenge of mice, enhanced clearance of vaccinia virus from mouse lung after day 6 of infection, apparently through augmentation of T cell responses, and potentially diminish the cytokine dysregulation induced by erbB1 stimulation [75].

Some poxviruses express a protein (IL-18BP) with the functional capability to bind to and to inhibit IL-18. Animal models using ectromelia or vaccinia viruses in which the IL-18BP is knocked out demonstrate attenuated virulence, and host responses including enhanced levels of IFN-γ, and enhanced NK cell and T cell activity [76–78]. The variola virus IL-18BP protein has been expressed, and is able to inhibit IL-18 activity; the affinity of the protein is higher for murine IL-18 than that for human IL-18. Of uncertain importance is the recognition that the variola virus protein, but not the ectromelia virus protein, has the ability to bind to glycosaminoglycans [76, 79].

Recent studies of the variola virus-expressed TNF binding protein (crmB, a product of the G2R ORF) demonstrated that the variola virus-expressed protein binds to and inhibits human TNF and human lymphotoxin-α, although less efficiently for the latter. In these studies, as with that seen with IL-18BP, the affinity of the variola virus protein was higher for, and demonstrated better inhibition of, the mouse or rat species host protein (in this case TNF). Additionally, the C-terminal domain of the crmB gene is able to bind and to inhibit the action of select chemokines predicted to potentially be involved in recruitment of an inflammatory response at critical steps in the predicted pathogenesis of viral dissemination. This domain, termed smallpox virus-encoded chemokine receptor (SECRET), is also found in the orthopoxvirus gene crmD (not present in the variola genome), and in three other secreted ectromelia virus or cowpox virus proteins [80].

The variola virus homologue of the ectromelia virus p28 protein has been synthesized and demonstrated to also have E3 ubiquitin ligase activity [81]. Although the predicted protein has ~95% amino acid identity across orthopoxviruses, the gene is truncated in vaccinia virus strains. The potential effects on virulence and apoptosis inhibition, demonstrated for the ectromelia virus protein [51, 82, 83], have not been evaluated for the variola virus protein.

References

1 Esposito JJ, Sammons SA, Frace AM, Osborne JD, Olsen-Rasmussen M, Zhang M, Govil D, Damon IK, Kline R, Laker M et al (2006) Genome sequence diversity and clues to the evolution of *Variola virus. Science* 313: 807–812

2 Gubser C, SmithGL (2002) The sequence of camelpox virus shows it is most closely related to variola virus, the cause of smallpox. *J Gen Virol* 83: 855–872

3 Dixon CW (1962) *Smallpox*. J. & A. Churchill, London

4 Fenner F, Henderson DA, Arita I, Jezek Z, Ladnyi ID (1988) *Smallpox and its Eradication*. World Health Organization, Geneva

5 Henderson DA, Moss B (1999) Smallpox and Vaccinia. In: S Plotkin, W Orenstein (eds): *Vaccines*. Saunders, New York, 74–97

6 Creighton C (1894) *History of Epidemics in Britain*. Cambridge University Press, London

7 Jenner E (1798) *An enquiry into the causes and effects of variolae vaccinae,*

a disease discovered in some of the western couties of England, particularly Gloucerstershire, and known by the name of cowpox. Samson Low, London
8 Jenner E (1799) *Further observations on the variolae vaccinae*. Samson Low, London
9 Franco-Paredes C, Lammoglia L, Santos-Preciado JI (2005) The Spanish royal philanthropic expedition to bring smallpox vaccination to the New World and Asia in the 19th century. *Clin Infect Dis* 41: 1285–1289
10 Baxby D (1999) The orgins of vaccinia virus – an even shorter rejoinder. *Soc Hist Med* 12: 139
11 Baxby D (1999) Edward Jenner's Inquiry; a bicentenary analysis. *Vaccine* 17: 301–307
12 Collier LH (1954) The preservation of vaccinia virus. *Bacteriol Rev* 18: 74–86
13 National Research Council (1999) *Assessment of Future Needs for Live Variola Virus*. NAS Press, Washington, D.C.
14 Leduc JW, Damon I, Relman DA, Huggins J, Jahrling PB (2002) Smallpox research activities: U.S. interagency collaboration, 2001. *Emerg Infect Dis* 8: 743–745
15 Leduc JW, Jahrling PB (2001) Strengthening national preparedness for smallpox: an update. *Emerg Infect Dis* 7: 155–157
16 Noble J Jr, Rich JA (1969) Transmission of smallpox by contact and by aerosol routes in *Macaca irus*. *Bull World Health Organ* 40: 279–286
17 Kalter SS, Rodriguez AR, Cummins LB, Heberling RL, Foster SO (1979) Experimental smallpox in chimpanzees. *Bull World Health Organ* 57: 637–641
18 Heberling RL, Kalter SS, Rodriguez AR (1976) Poxvirus infection of the baboon (*Papio cynocephalus*). *Bull World Health Organ* 54: 285–294
19 Downie AW, Meiklejohn M, St Vincent L, Rao AR, Sundara Babu BV, Kempe CH (1965) The recovery of smallpox virus from patients and their environment in a smallpox hospital. *Bull World Health Organ* 33: 615–622
20 Mack TM, Thomas DB, Muzaffar KM (1972) Epidemiology of smallpox in West Pakistan. II. Determinants of intravillage spread other than acquired immunity. *Am J Epidemiol* 95: 169–177
21 Mack TM, Thomas DB, Ali A, Muzaffar KM (1972) Epidemiology of smallpox in West Pakistan. I. Acquired immunity and the distribution of disease. *Am J Epidemiol* 95: 157–168
22 Heiner GG, Fatima N, McCrumb FR Jr (1971) A study of intrafamilial transmission of smallpox. *Am J Epidemiol* 94: 316–326
23 Rao AR, Jacob ES, Kamalakshi S, Appaswamy S, Bradbury (1968) Epidemiological studies in smallpox. A study of intrafamilial transmission in a series of 254 infected families. *Indian J Med Res* 56: 1826–1854
24 Mack TM (1972) Smallpox in Europe, 1950–1971. *J Infect Dis* 125: 161–169
25 Wehrle PF, Posch J, Richter KH, Henderson DA (1970) An airborne outbreak of smallpox in a German hospital and its significance with respect to other recent outbreaks in Europe. *Bull World Health Organ* 43: 669–679
26 Stallybrass CO (1931) *The principles of epidemiology and the process of infection*. Routledge, London, 329
27 Thomas DB, McCormack WM, Arita I, Khan MM, Islam S, MackTM (1971) Endemic smallpox in rural East Pakistan. I. Methodology, clinical and epide-

miologic characteristics of cases, and intervillage transmission. *Am J Epidemiol* 93: 361–372
28 Arita I, Wickett JF, Fenner F (1986) Impact of population density on immunization programs. *J Hyg Camb* 96: 459–466
29 Duncan SR, Scott S, Duncan CJ (1993) An hypothesis for the periodicity of smallpox epidemics as revealed by time series analysis. *J Theor Biol* 160: 231–248
30 Rao AR (1972) *Smallpox*. The Kothari Book Depot, Bombay
31 Rao AR, Prahlad I, Swaminathan M, Lakshmi A (1963) Pregnancy and smallpox. *J Indian Med Assoc* 40: 353–363
32 Harper GJ (1961) Airborne micro-organisms: survival tests with four viruses. *J Hyg (Lond)* 59: 479–486
33 Kitamura T, Aoyama Y, Kurata T, Arita M, Imagawa Y (1977) Virological studies of smallpox in an endemic area. II. Virus content of clinical specimens and typing of virus isolates. *Jpn J Med Sci Biol* 30: 229–239
34 Sarkar JK, Mitra AC, Mukherjee MK, De SK, Mazumdar DG (1973) Virus excretion in smallpox. 1. Excretion in the throat, urine, and conjunctiva of patients. *Bull World Health Organ* 48: 517–522
35 Downie AW, St Vincent L, Meiklejohn G, Ratnakannan NR, RaoAR, Krishnan GN, Kempe CH (1961) Studies on the virus content of mouth washings in the acute phase of smallpox. *Bull World Health Organ* 25: 49–53
36 Downie AW, Fedson DS, Saint VL, Rao AR, Kempe CH (1969) Haemorrhagic smallpox. *J Hyg (Lond)* 67: 619–629
37 Sarkar JK, Mitra AC, Chakravarty MS (1972) Relationship of clinical severity, antibody level, and previous vaccination state in smallpox. *Trans R Soc Trop Med Hyg* 66: 789–792
38 Rao AR (1964) Haemorrhagic smallpox: a study of 240 cases. *J Indian Med Assoc* 43: 224–229
39 Rao AR, Sukumar MS, Kamalakshi S, Paramasivam TV, Parasuraman TA, Shantha M (1968) Experimental variola in monkeys. I. Studies on disease enhancing property of cortisone in smallpox. A preliminary report. *Indian J Med Res* 56: 1855–1865
40 Downie AW, McCarthy K, Macdonald A, Maccallum FO, Macrae AE (1953) Virus and virus antigen in the blood of smallpox patients; their significance in early diagnosis and prognosis. *Lancet* 265: 164–166
41 Downie AW, McCarthy K, Macdonald A (1950) Viraemia in smallpox. *Lancet* 2: 513–514
42 Downie AW, Fedson DS, Saint VL, Rao AR, Kempe CH (1969) Haemorrhagic smallpox. *J Hyg (Lond)* 67: 619–629
43 Jahrling PB, Hensley LE, Martinez MJ, Leduc JW, Rubins KH, Relman DA, Huggins JW (2004) Exploring the potential of variola virus infection of cynomolgus macaques as a model for human smallpox. *Proc Natl Acad Sci USA* 101: 15196–15200
44 Rubins KH, Hensley LE, Jahrling PB, Whitney AR, Geisbert TW, Huggins JW, Owen A, Leduc JW, Brown PO, Relman DA (2004) The host response to smallpox: analysis of the gene expression program in peripheral blood cells in a nonhuman primate model. *Proc Natl Acad Sci USA* 101: 15190–15195

45 Bras G (1952) The morbid anatomy of smallpox. *Doc Med Geogr Trop* 4: 303

46 Marennikova S, Maltseva MN, Korneeva VI, Garanina NM (1977) Pox outbreak among carnivora (Felidae) and Endentata. *J Infect Dis* 135: 358

47 Greene HSN (1934) Rabbitpox. II. Pathology of the epidemic disease. *J Exp Med* 60: 427

48 Smith GL (1993) Vaccinia virus glycoproteins and immune evasion. The sixteenth Fleming Lecture. *J Gen Virol* 74: 1725–1740

49 Shchelkunov SN (1995) Functional organization of variola major and vaccinia virus genomes. *Virus Genes* 10: 53–71

50 Massung RF, Esposito JJ, Liu LI, Qi J, Utterback TR, Knight JC, Aubin L, Yuran TE, Parsons JM, Loparev VN et al (1993) Potential virulence determinants in terminal regions of variola smallpox virus genome. *Nature* 366: 748–751

51 Senkevich TG, Koonin EV, Buller RM (1994) A poxvirus protein with a RING zinc finger motif is of crucial importance for virulence. *Virology* 198: 118–128

52 Shchelkunov SN, Resenchuk SM, Totmenin AV, Blinov VM, Marennikova SS, Sandakhchiev LS (1993) Comparison of the genetic maps of variola and vaccinia viruses. *FEBS Lett* 327: 321–324

53 Alcami A, Smith GL (1993) Comment on the paper by Shchelkunov et al (1993) *FEBS Lett*ers 319, 80–83. Two genes encoding poxvirus cytokine receptors are disrupted or deleted in variola virus. *FEBS Lett* 335: 136–137

54 Buller RM, Palumbo GJ (1991) Poxvirus pathogenesis. *Microbiol Rev* 55: 80–122

55 Chen N, Li G, Liszewski MK, Atkinson JP, Jahrling PB, Feng Z, Schriewer J, Buck C, Wang C, Lefkowitz EJ et al (2005) Virulence differences between monkeypox virus isolates from West Africa and the Congo basin. *Virology* 340: 46–63

56 McFadden G (2005) Poxvirus tropism. *Nat Rev Microbiol* 3: 201–213

57 Jahrling PB, Fritz EA, Hensley LE (2005) Countermeasures to the bioterrorist threat of smallpox. *Curr Mol Med* 5: 817–826

58 Massung RF, Loparev VN, Knight JC, Totmenin AV, Chizhikov VE, Parsons JM, Safronov PF, Gutorov VV, Shchelkunov SN, Esposito JJ (1996) Terminal region sequence variations in variola virus DNA. *Virology* 221: 291–300

59 Dunlop LR, Oehlberg KA, Reid JJ, Avci D, Rosengard AM (2003) *Variola virus* immune evasion proteins. *Microbes Infect* 5: 1049–1056

60 Esteban DJ, Buller RM (2005) Ectromelia virus: the causative agent of mousepox. *J Gen Virol* 86: 2645–2659

61 Barry M, McFadden G (1997) Virus encoded cytokines and cytokine receptors. Parasitology 115 Suppl: S89–100

62 Cao JX, McFadden G (2001) Characterization of the myxoma virus M118L protein: a novel essential poxvirus IMV-associated protein. *Virus Genes* 23: 303–313

63 Everett H, McFadden G (2002) Poxviruses and apoptosis: a time to die. *Curr Opin Microbiol* 5: 395–402

64 Johnston JB, McFadden G (2004) Technical knockout: understanding poxvirus pathogenesis by selectively deleting viral immunomodulatory genes. *Cell Microbiol* 6: 695–705

65 Johnston JB, McFadden G (2003) Poxvirus immunomodulatory strategies: current perspectives. *J Virol* 77: 6093–6100

66 Lalani AS, Masters J, Zeng W, Barrett J, Pannu R, Everett H, Arendt CW, McFadden G (1999) Use of chemokine receptors by poxviruses. *Science* 286: 1968–1971

67 Smith CA, Smith TD, Smolak PJ, Friend D, Hagen H, Gerhart M, Park L, Pickup DJ, Torrance D, Mohler K et al (1997) Poxvirus genomes encode a secreted, soluble protein that preferentially inhibits beta chemokine activity yet lacks sequence homology to known chemokine receptors. *Virology* 236: 316–327

68 Rosengard AM, Liu Y, Nie Z, Jimenez R (2002) *Variola virus* immune evasion design: expression of a highly efficient inhibitor of human complement. *Proc Natl Acad Sci USA* 99: 8808–8813

69 Rosengard AM, Alonso LC, Korb LC, Baldwin WM III, Sanfilippo F, Turka LA, Ahearn JM (1999) Functional characterization of soluble and membrane-bound forms of vaccinia virus complement control protein (VCP). *Mol Immunol* 36: 685–697

70 Isaacs SN, Kotwal GJ, Moss B (1992) Vaccinia virus complement-control protein prevents antibody-dependent complement-enhanced neutralization of infectivity and contributes to virulence. *Proc Natl Acad Sci USA* 89: 628–632

71 Kotwal GJ, Isaacs SN, McKenzie R, Frank MM, Moss B (1990) Inhibition of the complement cascade by the major secretory protein of vaccinia virus. *Science* 250: 827–830

72 Sfyroera G, Katragadda M, Morikis D, Isaacs SN, Lambris JD (2005) Electrostatic modeling predicts the activities of orthopoxvirus complement control proteins. *J Immunol* 174: 2143–2151

73 Buller RM, Chakrabarti S, Moss B, Fredrickson T (1988) Cell proliferative response to vaccinia virus is mediated by VGF. *Virology* 164: 182–192

74 Buller RM, Chakrabarti S, Cooper JA, Twardzik DR, Moss B (1988) Deletion of the vaccinia virus growth factor gene reduces virus virulence. *J Virol* 62: 866–874

75 Kim M, Yang H, Kim SK, Reche PA, Tirabassi RS, Hussey RE, Chishti Y, Rheinwald JG, Morehead TJ, Zech T et al (2004) Biochemical and functional analysis of smallpox growth factor (SPGF) and anti-SPGF monoclonal antibodies. *J Biol Chem* 279: 25838–25848

76 Born TL, Morrison LA, Esteban DJ, VandenBos T, Thebeau LG, Chen N, Spriggs MK, Sims JE, Buller RM (2000) A poxvirus protein that binds to and inactivates IL-18, and inhibits NK cell response. *J Immunol* 164: 3246–3254

77 Symons JA, Adams E, Tscharke DC, Reading PC, Waldmann H, Smith GL (2002) The vaccinia virus C12L protein inhibits mouse IL-18 and promotes virus virulence in the murine intranasal model. *J Gen Virol* 83: 2833–2844

78 Reading PC, Smith GL (2003) Vaccinia virus interleukin-18-binding protein promotes virulence by reducing gamma interferon production and natural killer and T-cell activity. *J Virol* 77: 9960–9968

79 Esteban DJ, Nuara AA, Buller RM (2004) Interleukin-18 and glycosaminoglycan binding by a protein encoded by *Variola virus*. *J Gen Virol* 85: 1291–1299

80 Alejo A, Ruiz-Arguello MB, Ho Y, Smith VP, Saraiva M, Alcami A (2006) A

chemokine-binding domain in the tumor necrosis factor receptor from variola (smallpox) virus. *Proc Natl Acad Sci USA* 103: 5995–6000
81 Huang J, Huang Q, Zhou X, Shen MM, Yen A, Yu SX, Dong G, Qu K, Huang P, Anderson EM et al (2004) The poxvirus p28 virulence factor is an E3 ubiquitin ligase. *J Biol Chem* 279: 54110–54116
82 Senkevich TG, Wolffe EJ, Buller RM (1995) Ectromelia virus RING finger protein is localized in virus factories and is required for virus replication in macrophages. *J Virol* 69: 4103–4111
83 Brick DJ, Burke RD, Minkley AA, Upton C (2000) Ectromelia virus virulence factor p28 acts upstream of caspase-3 in response to UV light-induced apoptosis. *J Gen Virol* 81: 1087–1097

Poxviruses
ed. by Andrew A. Mercer, Axel Schmidt and Olaf Weber

Genus *Orthopoxvirus: Monkeypox virus*

Sandra Essbauer and Hermann Meyer

Bundeswehr Institute of Microbiology, Neuherbergstr. 11, 80937 München, Germany

Abstract

Monkeypox virus is an orthopoxvirus that is genetically distinct from other members of the genus, including *Variola virus*, *Vaccinia virus*, *Ectromelia virus*, *Camelpox virus*, and *Cowpox virus*. It was first identified as the cause of a pox-like illness in captive monkeys in 1958. In the 1970s, human infections occurred in Central and Western Africa clinically indistinguishable from smallpox. In contrast with *Variola virus*, however, *Monkeypox virus* has a wide range of hosts, which has allowed it to maintain a reservoir in wild animals. Human monkeypox was first recognized outside Africa in 2003 during an outbreak in the US that was traced to monkeypox virus-infected rodents imported from West Africa. Today, monkeypox is regarded as the most important orthopoxvirus infection in human beings since the eradication of smallpox. There is currently no proven treatment for human monkeypox, and its potential as an agent of bioterrorism is discussed.

Monkey monkeypox

In 1958, von Magnus et al. [1] observed two outbreaks of a nonfatal pox-like disease in two shipments of cynomolgus monkeys (*Macaca cynomolgus*) arriving in Copenhagen. Skin eruptions developed between 51 and 62 days after arrival and approximately 25% of the animals developed clinical disease. An orthopoxvirus was isolated on the chorioallantoic membrane producing grayish pocks with a hemorrhagic center after 3-day incubation at 35°C, clearly distinguishable from the larger hemorrhagic pocks of cowpox virus and the opaque white pocks of variola virus. Since the virus isolated differed from variola virus and other known poxviruses, it was named *Monkeypox virus* (MPXV) and given recognition as an own species of the genus *Orthopoxvirus*. This Copenhagen strain is regarded as the MPXV reference strain. In the following 10 years, a total of nine monkeypox outbreaks were observed in captive monkey colonies in the US, the Netherlands, and France and several isolates were recovered [2]. Usually no clinical signs are detected until the rash appears and develops into papules on the trunk, the face, and the palms and soles. The papules become vesicular, and then pustular, before scabs form and fall off 7–10 days after onset of the rash. The severity of signs varied among the several different primate species during an outbreak in the Rotterdam zoo with orangutans being particularly susceptible, dying in the acute viremic stage before skin lesions developed. However, there were no reports of infections in humans handling those infected animals [2].

Human monkeypox 1970–1986

In 1970 it was found that a smallpox-like disease of humans living in tropical rain forest areas in several countries in Western and Central Africa was caused by MPXV [3]. At that time smallpox had just been eliminated from these countries. The discovery of MPXV led to a WHO-initiated intensive investigation of the human disease to address public health importance and to determine whether MPXV might represent a threat to the global smallpox eradication campaign. Early epidemiological data came from an analysis of 47 cases of human monkeypox reported before 1980: the case fatality rate was 17%, a secondary transmission was observed in 9% of the cases, and the secondary attack rate was 3.3%, much lower than the 37–88% observed with smallpox. Monkeypox was not considered a serious health problem at that time because there was no evidence of sustained transmissibility in humans: the longest chain of human-to-human transmission was four serial transmissions. According to a mathematical model, MPXV was not able to maintain itself permanently in the human community, instead it had to rely on frequent introductions from an animal reservoir [4].

An intensive health institution-based surveillance system was established in enzootic foci in the Democratic Republic of Congo (DRC) from 1981 to 1986 by the WHO. Of the 338 cases detected by active surveillance, secondary transmission accounted for 28%, and the case fatality rate was 10%. The highest secondary attack rate (13.9%) occurred in unvaccinated household contacts aged 0–4 years [3].

In the 1980s, studies on human monkeypox showed an incubation period of 10–14 days and an infectious period during the first week of the rash. A characteristic 2-day prodrome with fever and malaise occurs in most patients before development of the rash. Clinically, human monkeypox closely resembles discrete ordinary-type or occasionally modified-type smallpox. No case has been seen that is comparable to flat-type or hemorrhagic-type smallpox. The only feature differentiating human monkeypox from smallpox is lymph node enlargement. About 90% of monkeypox patients develop lymphadenopathy, which can be unilateral or bilateral and occurs in the submandibular, cervical, axillary, or inguinal lymph nodes, or any combination of these. Enlargement occurs early at the time of onset of fever, usually 1–3 days before the rash appears. Lesions develop more or less simultaneously and evolve together at the same time through papules, vesicles, pustules and crusts before resolving and leaving scars. This process takes 2–3 weeks. Severe eruptions can cover the entire body, including the palms and soles. Lesions have been noted on the oral mucous membranes. In patients with a smallpox vaccination scar, the monkeypox rash was milder and no deaths occurred. Chickenpox, a disease caused by the unrelated varicella zoster herpesvirus, became the primary differential diagnostic challenge [4].

Human monkeypox 1996/97

After the end of the active WHO surveillance program in 1986 only 13 cases of human monkeypox were reported until 1995. In 1996/97, however, the largest outbreak ever recorded occurred in the Kasai Oriental region of the DRC [5]. During an initial investigation by the WHO and the Center for Disease Control (CDC), a total of 92 cases were identified and in a follow-up investigation a further 419 cases were reported. Epidemiological data pointed to different results as compared to previous outbreaks: the proportion of cases attributed to secondary transmission was three times higher (78% *versus* 28%) and the mortality was much lower, accounting for 1.5% as compared to 10% in the 1980s. To explain the remarkable rise in secondary cases between the 1970–1986 surveillance data and the 1996/97 outbreak data (28% *versus* 78%), it has been assumed that this was due to a waning immunity after cessation of smallpox vaccination. If this were true, one would assume a higher mortality rate as well, which is not the case. Whether more transmissible and less virulent strains are circulating in the DRC cannot be ruled out. Di Giulio and Eckburg [6] assumed that due to a less specific case definition used in the 1996/97 outbreak, as compared to the 1981–86 active surveillance, a substantial proportion of cases were possibly chickenpox. This is a common disease in the DRC [7], and is characterized by a high rate of secondary transmission in susceptible people (>85%) and a low mortality in children (<0.01%).

Monkeypox in the USA in 2003

Human monkeypox was first recognized outside Africa in 2003 in the USA. As of July 8, 2003, 71 cases of monkeypox have been reported to CDC, 49% of the cases were laboratory confirmed. Among 69 patients for whom data were available, 18 (26%) were hospitalized. Two patients, both children, had serious clinical illness. The median incubation period was 12 days (range: 1–31 days). The aggregate clinical signs and symptoms were similar to those described in outbreaks of monkeypox in Africa. Most patients had a prodrome of fever, headache and sweats before skin lesions and prominent lymphadenopathy developed. In some, a localized lesion was followed by systemic disease. Unique clinical manifestations included focal hemorrhagic necrosis and erythematous flares. Unlike the African outbreaks, the US outbreak resulted in no fatalities and there was no documented human-to-human transmission [8]. The majority of patients were exposed to captive prairie dogs. No patients have been confirmed with their only possible exposure to persons with monkeypox, indicating a lack of secondary transmission. Trace-back investigations have determined that all confirmed human cases of monkeypox were associated with prairie dogs obtained from an animal distributor. These prairie dogs appear to have been infected through contact with African rodents (see below). Before that 2003 US outbreak, human monkeypox had never been reported in the Western hemisphere [8]. This less severe epizootic could be due to higher natural resistance of the US population, a healthier patient population lacking background infections, and/or better supportive care for patients. There is, however, a significant possibility that this variability in pathogenicity is secondary to strain-specific differences in virulence. Recently, three cases of serologically confirmed monkeypox have been reported in preimmune individuals at 13, 29 and 48 years after smallpox vaccination with no recognizable disease symptoms [9]. This shows that cross-protective antiviral immunity against West African monkeypox can potentially be maintained for years.

Reservoir

To understand how human monkeypox is derived from an animal source, initial efforts focused on monkeys: serological surveys of Asian monkeys were negative, but specific antibodies were demonstrated in eight species of monkeys living in Western and Central Africa. However, since MPXV does not cause persistent infections, attention was then directed to terrestrial and arboreal rodents. Several epidemiological studies were conducted in the DRC, and in 1985 attention focused on animals found near villages in which cases of human monkeypox had recently occurred. MPXV-specific antibodies were found in two species of squirrel (*Funisciurus anerythrus*, and *Heliosciurus rufobrachium*) and MPXV was recovered from a diseased squirrel [10]. A subsequent seroprevalence study done as part of the investigation of the 1996/97 outbreak in the DRC showed that 39–50% of *Funisciurus* spp and 50% of *Heliosciurus* spp squirrels were seropositive [5]. In conclusion, conditions that facilitate outbreaks of human monkeypox in Africa are (i) enzootic circulation of MPXV in animals living in agricultural areas and forests surrounding human settlements, (ii) use of poorly cooked meat of wild animals, and (iii) close contact with animals, such as hunting, skinning, and playing with carcasses [7].

Detailed investigations to identify how prairie dogs in the 2003 US outbreak became infected, demonstrated contact of prairie dogs with African rodents. An animal distributor in Texas had imported a shipment of small mammals from Ghana that contained 762 African rodents, including rope squirrels (*Funisciurus* sp.), tree squirrels (*Heliosciurus* sp.), Gambian giant rats (*Cricetomys* sp.), brushtail porcupines (*Atherurus* sp.), dormice (*Graphiurus* sp.), and striped mice (*Hybomys* sp.). CDC laboratory testing of some animals from this shipment confirmed the presence of MPXV by PCR and virus isolation in several rodent species, including one Gambian rat, three dormice, and two rope squirrels. Whether MPXV has already spread to North American rodent populations is unknown, but has substantial implications for both human and animal health. In this respect, it is interesting to note that experimentally infected ground squirrels (*Spermophilus tridecemlineatus*) are able to develop a fulminant illness [11].

Monkeypox virus genome

To address the question whether MPXV and *Variola virus* are closely related, genomic analysis were performed [12]. The central region of the MPXV genome encodes essential enzymes and structural proteins, and is almost identical to that of other orthopoxviruses, including variola virus. However, the end regions of the MPXV genome, which encode virulence and host-range factors, differ substantially [13] like those of the other orthopoxvirus species. Comparative analysis of the genomes of MPXV and variola virus revealed that MPXV is a distinct species, which evolved from an orthopoxvirus ancestor independently of variola virus. Thus, MPXV is not a direct ancestor of *Variola virus* (or *vice versa*), and *Variola virus* cannot be readily "derived" from MPXV.

Whole genome restriction fragment length polymorphism (RFLP) analysis and single gene phylogeny already had suggested the existence of two geographically distinct MPXV clades from Western Africa and the Congo basin (see Fig. 1). Today, this has been confirmed by whole genome sequencing of several MPXV strains and thereby provided clues to understand differences in disease pathology [14, 15]. Open reading frame comparisons indicated that in West African/US MPXV isolates the complement control protein (CCP) is not functional. CCP orthologues, which are also present in variola virus, inhibit the classical and alternate complement pathways and prevent complement-mediated virus neutralization. The lack of virus neutralization might explain why Congo basin MPXVs are more virulent for cynomolgus monkeys as compared to West African/US MPXVs [15], which did not cause any case fatalities during the US 2003 human monkeypox outbreak. Virulence differences are further supported by epidemiological analyses, which showed a similar prevalence of antibodies in non-vaccinated humans in both regions, while >90% of reported cases occurred in the

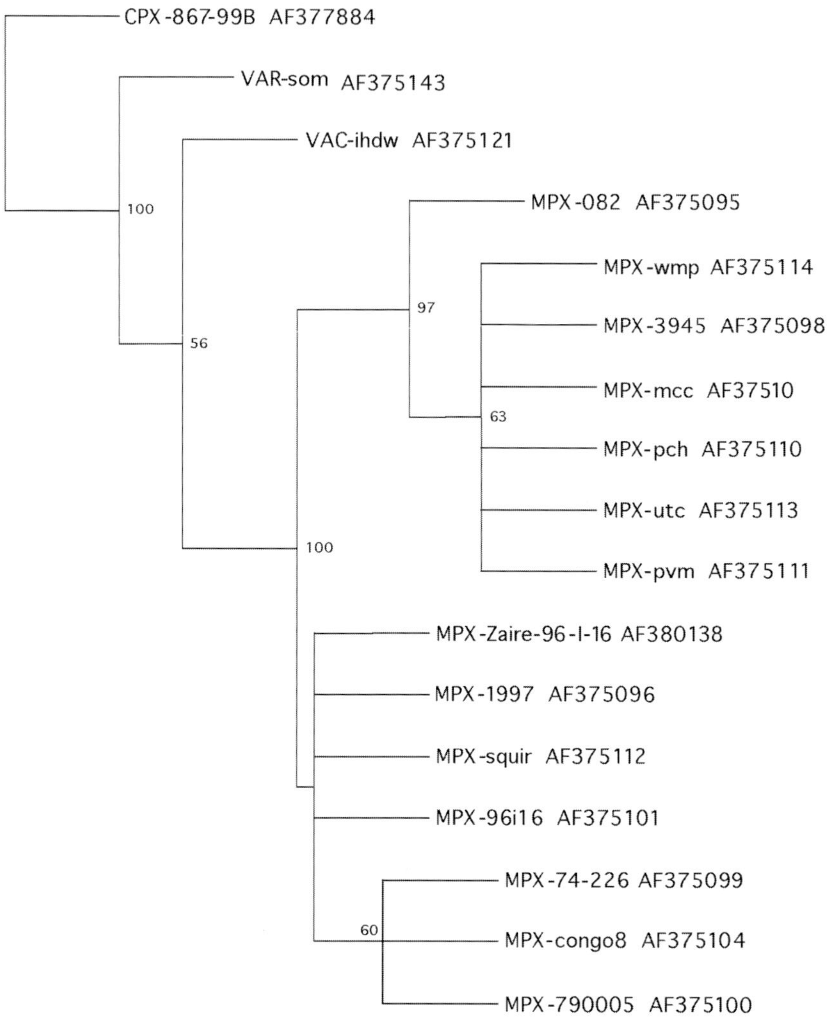

Figure 1. Hemagglutinin gene dendrogram of monkeypox virus isolates. Sequences were compared by means of neighbor-joining methods, and significant bootstrap values for major nodes are shown. Strains of the upper clade originated from Western Africa, whereas strains of the lower clade are from the Congo basin. Accession numbers are given. MPX, monkeypox virus, VAR, variola virus, VAC, vaccinia virus, CPX, cowpox virus

Congo basin and no fatal cases were observed outside of this region [14]. It is noteworthy that the genomic changes described have been reproducibly maintained for over 30 years in isolates from those regions.

Monkeypox virus diagnosis and animal models

Although clinical characteristics might be helpful in differentiating various poxvirus infections from other causes of vesiculopustular rashes, laboratory confirmation is required for definitive diagnosis [16]. Suitable specimens for testing include crusts, vesicle fluids, skin biopsy tissues and blood. A combination of methods, including electron microscopy, virus growth in cell cultures and/or on the chorioallantoic membranes of 12-day-old chicken embryos, as well as DNA amplification assays, are used to identify and differentiate poxviruses. Electron microscopy is a first-line method to rapidly differentiate orthopoxviruses from herpesviruses (causing chickenpox) due to their different morphology; however, it is not possible to specifically differentiate within the genus *Orthopoxvirus* at the species level. MPXV can be easily grown in a variety of established cell culture lines, such as Vero, MA104 and others. PCR protocols to identify and differentiate orthopoxviruses are available based on sequences of the hemagglutinin, the cytokine response modifier B (crmB) or the A-type inclusion (ATI) protein gene [16]. Specificity of the assays is proven by either restriction endonuclease digestion or sequencing of the amplicons. By amplifying sequences of the ATI gene even a differentiation of Western Africa from Congo basin MPXV strains is possible due to different-sized amplicons [14, 17]. Sequences of the hemagglutinin gene have been proven useful for phylogenetic studies. Recently, an orthopoxvirus-specific IgM assay was described and applied to determine acute-phase humoral immunity to MPXV in the 2003 US outbreak [18]. IgM antibody detection allows a broader window for sample collection beyond the rash stage of illness which is of advantage to demonstrate disease retrospectively and/or from remote locations.

The perceived risk of a deliberate use of smallpox and the severe side effects of the currently available smallpox vaccine led the scientific community to search for safer vaccines [19]. A major limitation, however, is the inability to assess efficacy in phase 3 clinical trials in humans. Therefore, several Rhesus macaque models of challenge infection with MPXV have been developed to test new candidate smallpox vaccines, to determine correlates of immunity, and to evaluate the efficacy of antiviral substances [20, 21].

References

1 Von Magnus P, Andersen EK, Petersen BK, Birch-Andersen A (1959) A pox-like disease in cynomolgus monkeys. *Acta Pathol Microbiol Scand* 46: 156

2 Arita I, Gispen R, Kalter SS, Wah LT, Marennikova SS, Netter R, Tagaya I (1972) Outbreaks of monkeypox and serological surveys in non-human primates. *Bull World Health Organ* 46: 625

3 Jezek Z, Marennikova SS, Mutumbo M, Nakano JH, Paluku KM, Szczeniowski

M (1986) Human monkeypox: a study of 2,510 contacts of 214 patients. *J Infect Dis* 154: 551–555

4 Jezek Z, Szczeniowski M, Paluku KM, Mutombo M (1987) Human monkeypox: clinical features of 282 patients. *J Infect Dis* 156: 293–298

5 Hutin YJ, Williams RJ, Malfait P, Pebody R, Loparev VN, Ropp SL, Rodriguez M, Knight JC, Tshioko FK, Khan AS et al (2001) Outbreak of human monkeypox, Democratic Republic of Congo, 1996 to 1997. *Emerg Infect Dis* 7: 434–438

6 Di Giulio DB, Eckburg PB (2004) Human monkeypox: an emerging zoonosis. *Lancet Infect Dis* 4: 15–25

7 Meyer H, Perrichot M, Stemmler M, Emmerich P, Schmitz H, Varaine F, Shungu R, Tshioko F, Formenty P (2002) Outbreaks of disease suspected of being due to human monkeypox virus infection in the Democratic Republic of Congo in 2001. *J Clin Microbiol* 40: 2919–2921

8 Reed KD, Melski JW, Graham MB, Regnery RL, Sotir MJ, Wegner MV, Kazmierczak JJ, Stratman EJ, Li Y, Fairley JA et al (2005) The detection of monkeypox in Humans in the Western Hemisphere. *N Engl J Med* 350: 342–350

9 Hammarlund E, Lewis MW, Carter S, Amanna I, Hansen SG, Strelow LI, Wong SW, Yoshihara P, Hanifin JN, Slifka M (2005) Multiple diagnostic techniques identify previously vaccinated individuals with protective immunity against monkeypox. *Nat Med* 11: 1005–1011

10 Arita I, Jezek Z, Khodakevich I, Ruti K (1985) Human monkeypox: a newly emerged orthopoxvirus zoonosis in the tropical rain forests of Africa. *Am J Trop Med Hyg* 34: 781–789

11 Tesh RB, Watts DM, Sbrana E, Siirin M, Popov VL, Xiao SY (2004) Experimental infection of ground squirrels (*Spermophilus tridecemlineatus*) with monkeypox virus. *Emerg Infect Dis* 10: 1563–1567

12 Douglass N, Dumbell K (1992) Independent evolution of monkeypox and variola viruses. *J Virol* 66: 7565–7567

13 Shchelkunov SN Totmenin AV, Babkin IV, Safronov PF, Ryazankina OI, Petrov NA, Gutorov VV, Uvarova EA, Mikheev MV, Sisler JR et al (2001) Human monkeypox and smallpox viruses: genomic comparison. *FEBS Lett* 509: 66–70

14 Likos AM, Sammons SA, Olson VA, Frace AM, Li Y, Olsen-Rasmussen M, Davidson W, Galloway R, Khristova ML, Reynolds MG et al (2005) A tale of two clades: monkeypox viruses. *J Gen Virol* 86: 2661–2672

15 Chen N, Li G, Liszewski MK, Atkinson JP, Jahrling PB, Feng Z, Schriewer J, Buck C, Wang C, Lefkowitz EJ et al (2005) Virulence differences between monkeypox virus isolates from West Africa and the Congo basin. *Virology* 340: 46–63

16 Damon IK, Esposito JJ (2003) Poxviruses that infect humans. In: PR Murray, EJ Baron, JH Jorgensen, MA Pfaller, MH Yolker (eds): *Manual of clinical microbiology*, 8th edn. ASM Press, Washington DC, 1583–1591

17. Meyer H, Ropp SL, Esposito JJ (1997) Gene for A-type inclusion body protein is useful for a polymerase chain reaction assay to differentiate orthopoxviruses. *J Virol Methods* 64: 217–221

18 Karem KL, Reynolds M, Braden Z, Lou G, Bernard N, Patton J, Damon IK (2005) Characterization of acute-phase humoral immunity to monkeypox: use of immunoglobulin M enzyme-linked immunosorbent assay for detection of monkeypox infection during the 2003 North American outbreak. *Clin Diag Lab Immunol* 12: 867–872

19 Breman JG, Henderson DA (1998) Poxvirus dilemmas: monkeypox, smallpox, and biological bioterrorism. *N Engl J Med* 339: 556–559

20 Earl PL, Americo JL, Wyatt LS, Eller LA, Whitbeck JC, Cohen GH, Eisenberg RJ, Hartmann CJ, Jackson DL, Kulesh DA et al (2004) Immunogenicity of a highly attenuated MVA smallpox vaccine and protection against monkeypox. *Nature* 428: 182–185

21 Zaucha GM, Jahrling PB, Geisbert TW, Swearengen JR, Hensley L (2001) The pathology of experimental aerosolized monkeypox virus infection in cynomolgus monkeys (*Macaca fascicularis*). *Lab Invest* 81: 1581–1600

Poxviruses
ed. by Andrew A. Mercer, Axel Schmidt and Olaf Weber

Genus *Orthopoxvirus: Cowpox virus*

Sandra Essbauer and Hermann Meyer

Bundeswehr Institute of Microbiology, Neuherbergstr. 11, 80937 München, Germany

Abstract

Cowpox virus (CPXV) is distinguished from other orthopoxvirus (OPV) species by producing cytoplasmic A-type inclusion bodies and flattened pocks with a hemorrhagic center on the chorioallantoic membrane. CPXV is endemic to Western Eurasia and naturally infects a broad range of host species including domestic animals, and zoo animals, as well as humans. Infections in humans seem to increase in importance due to a changed epidemiology in the rodent reservoir hosts or in the biotype of the virus. Genetic characterization of CPXV isolates revealed differences which do not correlate with either host species or geographic origin. Phylogenetic analyses suggested a rodent-transmitted CPXV as an ancestor of all other OPV species. So far, only two strains from the UK and Russia are entirely sequenced. Sequence data from other strains isolated in Germany and Scandinavia are needed to better understand differences in virulence and severity of infection.

The history of cowpox virus

Cowpox entered medical history by Edward Jenner's publications "Inquiry" and "Further observations on the Variolae Vaccinae" in 1798/99: he demonstrated the efficacy of cowpox virus ("true cowpox", "variolae vaccinae") scarification to induce a protective immunity against challenge with variola virus (VARV) [1]. The designation cowpox virus (CPXV) refers to its association with pustular lesions on the teats of milking cows. Bovine cowpox was once a sporadic disease, and until the early 1970s was believed to be spread enzootically in cattle only [2, 3]. Zoonotic transmission to humans (milkers) has traditionally occurred *via* contact with infected cows. Beside "true cowpox", Jenner already recognized a second clinical entity, "spurious cowpox", that was transmissible to man but did not induce immunity against smallpox [1]. "Spurious cowpox" is caused by *Pseudocowpox virus*, a virus belonging to the genus *Parapoxvirus*, which occurs frequently and still is an occupational hazard for farmers [4]. In contrast, the epidemiology of CPXV is different: today, it is seen in a broad range of host species, but rarely in cattle. Host species include domestic, zoo and wild animals (Tabs 1 and 2). Zoo animals, in particular elephants, seem to be highly susceptible due to conditions in animal holding and/or individual physical conditions. Since domestic cats ("catpox"), elephants ("elephantpox") and humans ("cowpox-like") are often found infected, the designation "cowpox" is quite misleading [2]. Based on epidemiological data rodents seem to be natural reservoirs of CPXV [2, 3, 5].

Geographic distribution and host range of cowpox virus

First reports of CPXV infections originate from England and Russia [2, 6]. Infections of CPXV or evidence for the presence of CPXV by serological or PCR studies have been reported in countries listed in Table 1. In general, CPXV is endemic to Western Eurasia. Out of 26 outbreaks described in zoo animals between 1960 and 1990, 25 were localized within a 1070-km diameter circle with the center near Magdeburg, Germany, with only a single outbreak in Moscow outside this circle. Table 2 summarizes clinical entities of CPXV infections in animals and humans that have been reported during the last 5 years.

Long-term studies on CPXV infections gave evidence that wild rodents harbor CPXV, although the virus has rarely been isolated. A seasonal variation has been shown [7, 8]. Infections also seem to have an impact on host dynamics [9–11]. Further studies on rodent species as carriers for CPXV are needed to gain information about local reservoirs, the transmission and maintenance of CPXV and the influence of climate, ecological factors and population density.

Cowpox virus infections

The first zoonotic transmission of CPXV from a cat to men was published in 1985 from the Netherlands [12]. Baxby and co-workers [2] summarized 54 human CPXV cases from 1969 to 1993. Human infections are generally mild and self limiting. The virus enters the body via lesions of the skin or mucous membranes and a localized pustular skin infection develops, often on the hands. Scratches or abrasions of the skin caused by a rural, infected cat may determine localization of the lesions elsewhere, e.g., on face, neck or feet (see Tab. 2). The draining lymph nodules become swollen and secondary lesions might occur sporadically. Usually pocks heal after 3–4 weeks, bacterial superinfections may prolong infections (5–8 weeks) [2, 13]. Necrotic conjunctivitis has been reported in some cases [2]. A systemic involvement and/or fatal outcome of human infections has been reported for immunocompromised individuals, e.g., in Darier's disease [14], in atopic patients

[15–17], or is associated with moderate atopic dermatitis [18]. Recent CPXV infections were often, but not exclusively, found in individuals aged <30 years who had never received smallpox vaccination. Young people as well as workers in zoos and circuses [2, 6, 19] may be also at greater risk to acquire an infection because of their close contact with animals. Differential diagnosis has to be made carefully with regards, for example, herpesviruses, cutaneous anthrax and sporothrix [20, 21].

More than 400 cases of CPXV infections in domestic cats have been described in Middle Europe. Clinical findings include multiple, widespread skin lesions (primarily seen on head, oral cavity, neck, forelimb or paws), conjunctivitis or purulent ocular discharge. In cats, infections may be fatal if inner organs such as the lungs are infected (e.g., necrotizing pneumonia [6, 22, 23]), or co-infections/immunodeficiency are present [24]. The outcome of the infection is strongly dependent on the CPXV strain, the route, site and dose of infection as well as the treatment [23, 25]. In cats, an accumulation of CPXV infections occurs in late summer and autumn, which is explained by a higher density of potentially infected rodents [2, 5, 26]. The seroprevalence of CPXV is quite variable, ranging in cats and foxes from 0% to 16% [18, 26–28].

As shown in Tables 1 and 2 several fatal poxvirus infections have been reported in zoo animals within the last few years. Modified vaccinia virus Ankara (MVA) was shown to protect rabbits against a dermal and intradermal challenge infection with CPXV [29]. Therefore, in Germany MVA is authorized for vaccination of zoo animals. Concerning the distribution within the European Union, a special authorization of the German Federal Office for Economy and Export Control exists. From 1999 to 2002, 217 vaccine doses have been distributed to 11 zoos and circuses in Germany, Austria and the Netherlands to immunize elephants, tapirs and rhinoceroses.

Diagnosis of cowpox virus

There are two features that differentiate CPXV from other orthopoxvirus (OPV) species: the presence of large eosinophilic A-type inclusion (ATI) bodies in the cytoplasm and the induction of 2–4-mm flattened, fairly rounded pocks with a red central hemorrhagic area on the chorioallantoic membrane (CAM) of embryonated eggs at 72 h post infection. ATI bodies have been used to retrospectively diagnose CPXV infections in histological sections of dermal specimens [5, 30]. ATI bodies consist of a 160-kDa protein, one of the most abundantly synthesized late proteins, and other factors (e.g., structural protein P4c) that drive the inclusion of mature virions [31]. Classical tools for the diagnosis of CPXV in swabs or bioptates are propagation on appropriate cell cultures and electron microcopy. PCR assays targeting different genes (e.g., hemagglutinin gene [32]; ATI gene [33]; crmB gene [34]), restriction fragment length polymorphism (RFLP)

Table 1. Geographic distribution and host range of CPXV

Geographic origin	Species	Transmission to man	Reference
England	Cats (*Felis sylvestris f. Catus*)	yes	[2, 25]
	Dogs (*Canis lupus familiaris*)	-	[64]
	Cheetahs (*Acinonyx jubatus*)	-	[22]
	Bank voles (*Clethrionomys glareolus*)	-	[7, 8, 65]
	Field voles (*Microtus agrestis*)	-	[7, 8, 65]
	Wood mice (*Apodemus sylvaticus*)	-	[7, 8, 65]
	House mice (*Mus musculus*)	-	[7, 8, 65]
Sweden	Cats (*Felis sylvestris f. catus*)	yes	[2, 55]
Norway	Cats (*Felis sylvestris f. catus*)	yes	[55]
	Lynx (*Lynx lynx*)	-	[66]
	Foxes (*Vulpes vulpes*)	-	[66]
	Bank voles (*C. glareolus*)	-	[67]
	Gray-sided voles (*C. rufocanus*)	-	[67]
	Red-backed voles (*C. rutilus*)	-	[67]
	Wood mice (*A. sylvaticus*)	-	[67]
	Common shrew (*Sorex araneus*)	-	[67]
Finland	Different species	yes	[18]
Denmark	Okapi (*Okapia johnstoni*)	-	[54]
	Cats (*F. sylvestris f. catus*)	yes	[68]
Russia	Cheetahs (*Acinonyx jubatus*)	yes	[6]
	Lions (*Panthera leo*)	-	[6]
	Black panther (*Panthera padus*)	-	[6]
	Ocelot (*Felis pardalis*)	-	[6]
	Jaguar (*Felis onca*)	-	[6]
	Pumas (*Felis concolor*)	-	[6]
	Anteaters (*Myrmecophaga tridactyla*)	-	[6]
	Far eastern cats (*Felis bengalis*)	-	[6]
	Common rat (*Rattus norvegicus*)	yes	[6]
	Root voles (*Microtus oeconomus*)	-	[69]
	House mouse (*M. musculus*)	yes	[70]
Turkmenia	Ground squirrel (*Citellus fulvus*)	-	[70, 71]
	Giant gerbils (*Rhombomys opimus*)	-	[71]
Georgia	Gerbils (*Meriones lybicus*)	-	[72]
Austria	Cats (*F. sylvestris f. catus*)	yes	[72]
	Asian elephants (*Elephas maximus*)	-	[72]
Italy	Cats (*F. sylvestris f. catus*)	-	[73]
Germany	Cats (*F. sylvestris f. catus*)	yes	[36, 53, 74]
	Dogs (*C. lupus familiaris*)	-	[53]
	Horses (*Equus caballus*)	-	[53, 75]
	Cows (*Bos taurus*)	-	[36]
	Asian elephant (*Elephas maximus*)	-	[36, 54, 76, 77]
	African elephant (*Loxodonta africana*)	-	[77]
	Lama (*Lama glama pacos*)	-	[77]
	Black rhinoceros (*Diceros bicornis*)	-	[78][a]
	White rhinoceros (*Ceratotherium s. simum*)	-	[80]
	Beaver (*Castor fibor canadensis*)	-	[35]

Table 1. Geographic distribution and host range of CPXV

Geographic origin	Species	Transmission to man	Reference
Germany	Bearcat (*Aiulurus fulgens*)	-	[35]
	Cats (*F. sylvestris f. catus*)	yes	[36, 53, 74]
	Foxes (*V. vulpes*)	-	[77, 81]
	Wild boar (*Sus scrofa*)	-	[78]
	Stone marten (*Martes martes*)	-	[77]
	Common rat (*R. norvegicus*)	-	[78]
	Bank voles (*C. glareolus*)	-	b
	Field voles (*M. agrestis*)	-	b
	Yellow-necked mice(*Apodemus flavicollis*)	-	b
Belgium	Foxes (*V. vulpes*)	-	[81]
	Bank voles (*C. glareoulus*)	-	[81]
	Wood mice (*A. sylvaticus*)	-	[81]
France	Asian elephants (*E. maximu*)	-	b
	Cats (*F. sylvestris f. catus*)	yes	[2, 14]
The Netherlands	Asian elephants (*E. maximus*)	-	[54]
	Okapis (*Okapia johnstoni*)	yes	[54]
	Cats (*F. sylvestris f. catus*)	-	[12, 23]
	Rats (*R. norvegicus*)	yes	[82]

[a] Also J. Kiessling, personal communication.
[b] S. Essbauer, unpublished data.

and random amplified polymorphic DNA analysis (RAPD [35]) of genomic DNA, Southern blot [36] and dot-blot assays [37] have been used for differentiation of OPVs to the species or strain level. Recently, real-time PCRs have been established (e.g., [38, 39]). Retrospectively, OPV-specific antibodies in sera can be determined by plaque reduction test or with a competition or antigen-capture ELISA [13, 26]. Positive serological findings have to be appraised keeping former smallpox vaccinations in mind.

Evolution of cowpox virus

So far, two CPXV strains have been sequenced completely: CPXV strain Brighton Red (CPXV BR, [40]; 224 501 bp, 235 open reading frames (ORFs), GenBank no: AF482758) originating from the hand of a milker in Great Britain in 1938, and strain GRI-90 isolated in 1990 from a 4-year-old girl in Moscow who had contact with a mole ([41]; 223 666 bp, 214 ORFs, GenBank no: X94355). DNA sequencing demonstrated that CPXVs have the largest genome of the OPV species. The central region of the genome (about 90 genes) is highly conserved in gene content and arrangement, and is similar to that of all other chordopoxviruses (poxviruses of vertebrates)

Table 2. Clinical characteristics of laboratory confirmed cowpox virus infections between 2000 and 2005

Host	Disease	Location	Ref.
Rhinoceros	Lesions on lip, spread to the skin of the whole body and feet	Germany	[a]
Boy (13 years) Cat	Ulceration around anus, buttocks, femur, penis Not given	Denmark	[68]
Man (54 years) Cat (4 weeks) Woman (20 years) Boy (14 years)	Pocks on arms and foreleg Ulcerated nodules at head, *Sporothrix schenkii* co-infection Ulcerative lesions on forearm, head and groin Severe lesions on arms and foreleg	Germany	[13, 83]
Foal (6 days)	Ulcerative lesions in several tissues, streptococcal septicemia, execution	Germany	[75]
Girl	Ulcerations arm, hand, shoulder, neck	Germany	[b]
Elephant	Pocks on body, feet, severe ulcerations; fatal	France	[b]
4 cats	Ulcerative lesions	UK	[30]
Boy (11 years) Cat	Sacral wound lesions Multifocal cutaneous lesions	France	[84]
4-a-old-girl Dog[c]	Severe, generalized eruption Not given	Finland	[9]
Man (26 years) Cat	Ulcer on finger (Veterinarian) Not given	England	[19]
Woman (56 years) Cat	Ulcerative lesions neck No symptoms, refused to eat	Austria	[85]
Woman (36 years) Cat	Ulcer on eye-brow Purulent nodule forepaw	Germany	[21]
Girl (14 years) Rat	Lesions in face Clinically ill	The Netherlands	[b]
Woman (21 years) Cat	Swelling neck Not given	The Netherlands	[86]
Man	Papule on the eye-lid	Germany	[13]
Girl (10 years) Cat[c]	Severe erythematous eruption on ear, hands, feet and back, around anus and vagina Not given	Germany	[13]
Cat (12 weeks)	Multiple red papules on face, head and right hind foot; fatal	Germany	[13]
2 elephants	Several pox viral lesions on knees, fore-foot, carpial joint; fatal	Germany	[13]
Elephant	Stillbirth	Germany	[76]
12-year-old boy Cat[c]	Necrotic ulcers with surrounding ery-thema on upper left arm Not given	Germany	[87]

Table 2 (continued)

Host	Disease	Location	Ref.
Girl (11 years) Cat	Ulcerative nodule neck, blister on leg Not given	Germany	[17]
Girl (9 years) Cat	Left forearm Bad general condition	Germany	[88]
Woman (30 years)	Right submental ulcer	Germany	[88]
Woman (25 years)	Facial lesion	England	[89]
Girl (7 years) Cat	Black crust on back, satellite lesion Not given	England	[89]

[a] Also J. Kiessling, personal communication.
[b] S. Essbauer, unpublished data.
[c] Serologically proven.

[41]. Analysis of the left and right variable terminal DNA regions of CPXV GRI-90 revealed segments that are unique to CPXV DNA [42]. Like other OPVs, about 30–40% of the CPXV genome encodes products that play important roles in virus pathogenesis and host range. Several CPXV ORFs have structural similarity to immunomodulatory and host range function genes/proteins; others mimic functions without having a cellular counterpart, e.g., by interfering with activation cascades (for reviews see [43–46]). Phylogenetic analyses of CPXV Brighton and GRI-90 based on 12 proteins lead to the suggestion that CPXV BR and GRI-90 should be separate OPV species [41, 42].

Evidence for the evolution of OPV from CPXV was gained from the comparison of ORFs, investigation of co-linearity of full-length genomes and also generation of phylogenetic trees. CPXV GRI-90 has the most comprehensive (complete and intact) set of genes compared to other OPV [43, 44, 48]. Further data supporting CPXV as the progenitor for OPV include the observation of sequences formerly described to be VARV-specific in some German CPXV strains [49]. CPXV strains have also been shown to contain a large ORF, which is highly conserved within the genus OPV but was exclusively found as fragmented ORF in VARV and camelpox virus [50].

Cowpox virus heterogeneity

Independent of the host species from which they are derived, CPXVs have quite uniform biological properties and resemble the classic CPXV BR strain. RFLPs generated with *Hind*III, and to lesser extent *Bam*HI, *Xho*I and/or *Sma*I, and construction of physical genome maps are optimal methods for differentiating CPXV strains [31, 51]. Naidoo et al. [52] were the first to confirm that the genomes of CPXVs isolated from cats in England are closely related to those originating from cows and their handlers. Minor differences found in the isolates did not correlate with the geographic origin of the strains. German CPXVs isolated between 1985 and 1991 [36] and in 1998 [53] from cats ("catpox"), humans ("cowpox-like"), elephant ("elephantpox"), dog, horse and cow ("cowpox") were more variable and differed from CPXV BR. In contrast to the UK, in Germany different strains seem to circulate in different regions at a time [33, 36, 53, 54]. RFLP of genomic DNA of CPXV isolates from Sweden and Norway showed also variation of strains dependent on the geographic location [55]. In summary, RFLP studies of German CPXV isolates revealed a higher variation in genotypes than in the UK or Scandinavia, and seem to reflect a geographically independent evolution of these viruses in defined rodent reservoirs. However, as described above, only two sequences from CPXV have been published: the UK strain (CPXV BR) originating over 75 years ago that might due to changes during passages not show the original genetic features, and CPXV GRI from Russia isolated 25 years ago. Knowledge on "actual" circulating strains and from the "center" of CPXV infections, i.e., Germany, or also from Scandinavia, is lacking, but genomic sequencing is currently under investigation. Further genome sequences of such strains will be of evolutionary, epidemiological and taxonomic importance. These may also contribute to clarifying differences in virulence and severity of infections.

Cowpox virus as a model

There are only few experimental animal infection models available for evaluation of antiviral compounds against OPVs. BALB/c mice have been used since 1985 as a model for CPXV studies [56]. Footpad inoculation was established by Miller et al. [57] by investigating the role of the host's complement during the initial response to a CPXV infection. *In vivo* models that may be useful in evaluating antivirals for use in the event of a release of poxviruses by bioterrorists include the intranasal or aerosolic CPXV infection of mice [58]. Aerosolic CPXV induces severe lesions in the lungs; in comparison, intranasally infected mice showed hemorrhagic bronchial, tracheal and nasal lesions [59]. The latter is comparable to the hemorrhagic outcome of VARV infections and, therefore, seems an excellent model for studying the efficacy of antiviral substances. Although several other substances have been tested, the acyclic cytidine analog cidofovir (HPMPC, Vistide, CDV) is the drug of choice for OPV treatment (for review see [59–61]). However, CDV is poorly absorbed in the gut when administered by the oral route, causes localized fibrosis at infection sites and is nephrotoxic. Therefore, the delivery of the drug directly to the respiratory tract is the best prophylactic strategy, and maximizes the tissue concentration at the site of initial viral replication, while minimizing its accumulation in the kidneys [62, 63]. The described investigations with CPXV in lab mice only represent the first step in establishing therapies and also new vaccines against VARV and MPXV. Therefore, for subsequent analysis of therapeutics and especially for vaccine developments, rhesus monkeys have to be used as ultimate challenge models.

References

1 Baxby D (1981) *Jenner's Smallpox Vaccine; the Riddle of Vaccinia Virus and its origin*. Heinemann, London

2 Baxby D, Bennett M, Getty B (1994) Human cowpox 1969–93: a review on 54 cases. *Br J Dermatol* 131: 598–607

3 Baxby D, Bennett M (1997) Cowpox; a re-evaluation of the risks of human cowpox based on new epidemiological information. *Arch Virol* (Suppl) 11: 1–12

4 Buettner M, Rhiza H-J (2002) Parapoxviruses: From the lesion to the viral genome. *J Vet Med B* 49: 7–16

5 Pfeffer M, Pfleghaar S, von Bomhard D, Kaaden O-R, Meyer H (2002) Retrospective investigation of feline cowpox in Germany. *Vet Rec* 150: 50–51

6 Marrenikova SS, Maltseva NN, Korneeva VI, Garanina NM (1977) Outbreak of pox disease among carnivora (felidae) and edentate. *J Infect Dis* 135: 358–366

7 Chantrey J, Meyer H, Baxby D, Begon M, Bown KJ, Hazel SM, Jones T, Montgomery WI, Bennett M (1999) Cowpox: reservoir hosts and geographic range. *Epidemiol Infect* 122: 455–460

8 Hazel SM, Bennett M, Chantrey J, Brown J, Cavanagh R, Jones TR (2000) A longitudinal study of an endemic disease in its wildlife reservoir: cowpox and wild rodents. *Epidemiol Infect* 124: 551–562

9 Feore SM, Bennett M, Chantrey J, Jones T, Baxby D, Begon M (1997) The effect of cowpox virus infections on fecundity in bank voles and wood mice. *Proc Biol Sci* 264: 1457–1461

10 Begon M, Hazel SM, Baxby D, Bown K, Cavanagh R, Chantrey J, Jones T, Bennett M (1999) Transmission dynamics of a zoonotic pathogen within and between wildlife host species. *Proc Biol Sci* 266: 1939–1945

11 Telfer S, Bennett M, Bown K, Cavanagh R, Crespin L, Hazel S, Jones T, Begon M (2002) The effects of cowpox virus on survival in natural rodent populations: increases and decreases. *J Anim Ecol* 71: 558–568

12 Willemse A, Egberink HF (1985) Transmission of cowpox virus infection from domestic cat to man. *Lancet* 1: 1515

13 Essbauer S, Meyer H, Kaaden O-R, Pfeffer M (2002) Recent cases in the German poxvirus consular laboratory. *Rev Med Vet* 153: 635–642

14 Claudy AL, Gaudin OG, Granouillet R (1982) Pox virus infection in Darier's disease. *Clin Exp Dermatol* 7: 261–265

15 Blackford S, Roberts DL, Thomas PD (1993) Cowpox infection causing a

generalized eruption in a patient with atopic dermatitis. *Br J Dermatol* 129: 628–629

16 Czerny C-P, Eis-Hübinger AM, Mayr A, Schneweis KE, Pfeiff P (1991) Animal poxviruses transmitted from cat to man: current event with lethal end. *J Vet Med B* 38: 421–431

17 Wienecke R, Wolff H, Schaller M, Meyer H, Plewig G (2000) Cowpox virus infection in an 11-year-old girl. *J Am Acad Dermatol* 42: 892–894

18 Pelkonen PM, Tarvainen K, Hynninen A, Kallio ER, Henttonen K, Palva A, Vaheri A, Vapalahti O (2003) Cowpox with severe generalized eruption, Finland. *Emerg Infect Dis* 9: 1458–1461

19 Lawn SD, Planche T, Riley P, Holwill S, Silman N, Beweley K, Rice P, Wansbrough-Jones MH (2003) A black necrotic ulcer. *Lancet* 361: 1518

20 Lewis-Jones MS, Baxby D, Cefai C, Hart CA (1993) Cowpox can mimic anthrax. *Br J Dermatol* 129: 625–627

21 Steinborn A, Essbauer S, Marsch WC (2003) [Human cowpox/catpox infection. A potentially unrecognized disease] [Article in German]. *Dtsch Med Wochenschr* 128:607–610

22 Baxby D, Ashton DG, Jones DM, Thomsett LR (1982) An outbreak of cowpox in captive cheetahs: virological and epidemiological studies. *J Hyg* 89: 365–372

23 Hinrichs U, van de Poel PH, van den Ingh TS (1999) Necrotizing pneumonia in a cat caused by an orthopox virus. *J Comp Pathol* 121: 191–196

24 Brown A, Bennett M, Gaskell CJ (1989) Fatal poxvirus infection in association with FIV infection. *Vet Rec* 124: 19–20

25 Bennett M, Gaskell CJ, Gaskell RJ,. Baxby D, Kelly DF (1989) Studies on poxvirus infections in cat. *Arch Virol* 104: 19–33

26 Bennett M, Gaskell CJ, Gaskell RJ,. Baxby D, Gruffyd-Jones TJ (1986) Poxvirus infections in the domestic cat: some clinical and epidemiological investigations. *Vet Rec* 118: 387–390

27 Czerny C-P, Wagner K, Gessler K, Mayr A, Kaaden O-R (1996) A monoclonal blocking ELISA for detection of orthopox virus antibodies in feline sera. *Vet Microbiol* 52: 185–200

28 Tryland M, Sandvik T, Holtet L, Nilsen H, Olsvik O, Traavik T (1998) Antibodies to orthopoxvirus in domestic cats in Norway. *Vet Rec* 143: 105–109

29 Munz E, Linckh S, Renner-Muller IC, Reimann M (1993) [The effectiveness of immunization with vaccinia virus type "MVA" against an infection with cowpox virus type "OPV 85" in rabbits] [Article in German]. *J Vet Med B* 40: 131–140

30 Godfrey DR, Blundell CJ, Essbauer S, Pfeffer M, Shearer DH, Rest JR, Baker JF (2004) Unusual presentations of cowpox infection in cats. *J Small Anim Pract* 45: 202–205

31 Fenner F, Wittek R, Dumbell KR (1989) The pathogenesis, pathology and immunobiology of orthopoxvirus infections. In: *The Orthopoxviruses*. Academic Press, London, 85–141

32 Ropp SI, Jin Q, Knight JC, Masung RF, Esposito JJ (1995) PCR strategy for identification and differentiation of smallpox and other orthopoxviruses. *J Clin Microbiol* 33: 2069–2076

33 Meyer H, Ropp SL, Esposito JJ (1997) Gene for A-type inclusion body protein

is useful for a polymerase chain reaction assay to differentiate orthopoxviruses. *J Virol Methods* 64: 217–221

34 Loparev VN, Massung RF, Esposito JJ, Meyer H (2001) Detection and differentiation of old world orthopoxviruses: restriction fragment length polymorphism of the crmB gene region. *J Clin Microbiol* 39: 94–100

35 Stemmler M, Neubauer H, Meyer H (2001) Comparison of closely related orthopoxvirus isolates by random amplified polymorphic DNA and restriction length polymorphism analysis. *J Vet Med B* 48: 647–654

36 Meyer H, Schay C, Mahnel H, Pfeffer M (1999) Characterization of orthopoxviruses isolated from man and animals in Germany. *Arch Virol* 144: 491–501

37 Meyer H, Osterrieder N, Pfeffer M (1993) Differentiation of species of the genus Orthopoxvirus in a dot blot assay using digoxigenin-labeled DNA-probes. *Vet Microbiol* 34: 333–344

38 Olson VA, Laue T, Laker MT, Babkin IV, Drosten C, Shchelkunov SN, Niedrig M, Damon IK, Meyer H (2004) Real-time PCR system for detection of orthopoxviruses and simultaneous identification of smallpox virus. *J Clin Microbiol* 42: 1940–1946

39 Panning M, Asper M, Kramme S, Schmitz H, Drosten C (2004) Rapid detection and differentiation of human pathogenic orthopox viruses by a fluorescence resonance energy transfer real-time PCR assay. *Clin Chem* 50: 702–708

40 Downie AW (1939) A study of the lesions produced experimentally by cowpox virus. *J Pathol* 48: 361–378

41 Marennikova SS, Gashnikov PV, Zhukova OA, Riabchikova EI, Strel'tsov VV, Riazankina OI, Chekunova EV, Ianova NN, Shchelkunov SN (1996) [The biotype and genetic characteristics of an isolate of the cowpox virus causing infection in a child] [Article in Russian]. *Zh Mikrobiol Epidemiol Immunobiol* 4: 6–10

42 Gubser C, Hue S, Kellam P, Smith GL (2004) Poxvirus genomes: a phylogenetic analysis. *J Gen Virol* 85: 105–117

43 Shchelkunov SN, Safronov PF, Totmenin AV, Petrov NA, Ryazankina OI, Gutorov VV, Kotwal GJ (1998) The genomic sequence analysis of the left and right species-specific terminal region of a cowpox virus strain reveals unique sequences and a cluster of intact ORFs for immunomodulatory and host range proteins. *Virology* 243: 432–460

44 Seet BT, Johnston JB, Brunetti CR, Barrett JW, Everett H, Cameron C, Sypula J, Nazarian SH, Lucas A, McFadden G (2003) Poxviruses and immune evasion. *Annu Rev Immunol* 21: 377–423

45 Johnston JB, McFadden G (2003) Poxvirus immunomodulatory strategies: current perspectives. *J Virol* 77: 6093–6100

46 Bowie AG, Zhan J, Marshall WL (2004) Viral appropiation of apoptotic and NF-kappaB signaling pathways. *J Cell Biochem* 91: 1099–1108

47 Boomker JM, de Leij LF, The TH, Harmsen MC (2005) Viral chemokine-modluatory proteins: tools and targets. *Cytokine Growth Factor Rev* 16: 91–103

48 McLysaght A, Baldi PF, Gaut BS (2003) Extensive gene gain associated with adaptive evolution of poxviruses. *Proc Natl Acad Sci USA* 100: 15655–15660

49 Meyer H, Neubauer H, Pfeffer M (2002) Amplification of ‚variola virus-specific' sequences in German cowpox virus isolates. *J Vet Med B* 49: 17–19

50 Meyer H, Totmenin A, Gavrilova E, Shchelkunov S (2005) Variola and camelpox virus-specific sequences are part of a single large open reading frame identified in two German cowpox virus strains. *Virus Res* 108: 39–43
51 Mackett M, Archard LC (1979) Conservation and variation in orthopoxvirus genome structure. *J Gen Virol* 45: 683–701
52 Naidoo J, Baxby D, Bennett M, Gaskell RM, Gaskell CJ (1992) Characterization of orthopoxviruses isolated from feline infections in Britain. *Arch Virol* 125: 261–272
53 Pfeffer M, Burck G, Meyer H (1999) [Cowpox viruses in Germany: an analysis of 5 cases in 1998] [Article in German]. *Berl Münch Tierärztl Wochenschr* 112: 334–338
54 Pilaski J, Rosen A, Darai G (1986) Comparative analysis of the genomes of orthopoxviruses isolated from elephant, rhinoceros, and okapi by restriction enzymes. *Arch Virol* 88: 135–142
55 Tryland M, Sandvik T, Hansen H, Haukenes G, Holtet L, Bennett M, Mehl R, Moens U, Olsvik O, Traavik T (1998) Characteristics of four cowpox virus isolates from Norway and Sweden. *APMIS* 106: 623–635
56 Buller RML (1985) The BALB/c mouse as a model to study orthopoxviruses. *Curr Top Microbiol Immunol* 122: 148–153
57 Miller CG, Justus DE, Jayaraman S, Kotwal GJ (1995) Severe and prolonged inflammatory response to localized cowpox virus infection in footpads of C5-deficient mice: investigation of the role of host complement in poxvirus pathogenesis. *Cell Immunol* 162: 326–332
58 Quenelle DC, Collins DJ, Wan WB, Beadle JR, Hostetler KY, Kern ER (2004) Oral treatment of cowpox and vaccinia virus infections in mice with ether lipid esters of cidofovir. *Antimicrob Agents Chemother* 48: 404–412
59 Martinez MJ, Bray MP, Huggins JW (2000) A mouse model of aerosol-transmitted orthopoxviral disease: morphology of experimental aerosol-transmitted orthopoxviral disease in a cowpox virus-BALB/c mouse system. *Arch Pathol Lab Med* 124: 362–377
60 de Clercq E (2002) Cidofovir in the treatment of poxvirus infections. *Antiviral Res* 55: 1–13
61 Smee DF, Sidwell RW (2003) A review of compounds exhibiting anti-orthopoxvirus activity in animal models. *Antiviral Res* 57: 41–52
62 Bray M, Martinez M, Kefauver D, West M, Roy C (2002) Treatment of aerosolized cowpox virus infection in mice with aerosolized cidofovir. *Antiviral Res* 54: 129–142
63 Roy CJ, Baker R, Washburn K, Bray M (2003) Aerosolized cidofovir is retained in the respiratory tract and protects mice against intranasal cowpox virus challenge. *Antimicrob Agents Chemother* 47: 2933–2937
64 Smith KC, Bennett M, Garrett DC (1999) Skin lesions caused by orthopoxvirus infection in a dog. *J Small Anim Pract* 40: 495–497
65 Crouch AC, Baxby D, McCracken CM, Gaskell RM, Bennett M (1995) Serological evidence for the reservoir hosts of cowpox virus in British wildlife. *Epidemiol Infect* 115: 185–191
66 Tryland M, Sandvik T, Arnemo JM, Stuve G, Olsvik Ø, Traavik T (1998)

Antibodies against orthopoxviruses in wild carnivores from Fennoscandia. *J Wildl Dis* 34: 443–450

67 Sandvik T, Tryland M, Hansen H, Mehl R, Moens U, Olsvik O, Traavik T (1998) Naturally occurring orthopoxviruses: potential for recombination with vaccine vectors. *J Clin Microbiol* 36: 2542–2547

68 Christensen LS, Nielsen EB, Nowicki J, Anderson J, de Stricker K (2005) Påvisning af kokoppevirus (cowpoxvirus) i. Danmark. *Ugeskr Læger* 167: 1646–1647

69 Lvov SD, Gromashevskyi VL, Marrenikova SS, Bogoyavlenskyi GV, Bajluk FN, Butenko AM, Gushchian E, Shelukhina EM, Thukova OA, Morozova TN (1988) [Poxvirus isolation from Microtus oeconomus Pal. 1776 in Colsky peninsula] [in Russian]. *Vopr Virusol* 1: 92–94

70 Marrenikova SS, Wojnarowska I, Bochanek W, Dziok AF, Sheluckhina EM (1984) [Cowpox in man] [Article in Russian]. *Zh Mikrobiol Epidemiol Immunbiol* 8: 64–69

71 Marennikova SS, Ladnyj ID, Ogorodinikova ZI, Shelukhina EM, Maltseva NN (1978) Identification and study of a poxvirus isolated from wild rodents in Turkmenia. *Arch Virol* 56: 7–14

72 Nowotny N (1994) The domestic cat: a possible transmitter of viruses from rodents to man. *Lancet* 343: 921

73 Canese MG, Lavazza A, Massone A, Galeano F, Boldini M (1997) Feline poxvirus infection. *Schweiz Arch Tierheilkd* 139: 454–457

74 Mahnel H (1991) [Catpox in Germany] [Article in German]. *Tierärztl Prax* 19: 419–422

75 Ellenberger C, Schuppel KF, Mohring M, Reischauer A, Alex M, Czerny CP, Fercho A, Schoon HA (2005) Cowpox virus infection associated with a streptococcal septicaemia in a foal. *J Comp Pathol* 132: 101–105

76 Pilaski J, Roesen-Wolff A (1988) Poxvirus infection in zoo-kept mammals. In: G Darai (ed): *Virus diseases in laboratory and captive animals*. Martinus Nijhoff Publishers, Boston, 83–100

77 Wisser J, Pilaski J, Strauss G, Meyer H, Burck G, Truyen U, Rudolph M, Frolich K (2001) Cowpox virus infection causing stillbirth in an Asian elephant (*Elephas maximus*). *Vet Rec* 149: 244–246

78 Mayr A, Lauer J, Czerny C-P (1995) [New facts on the distribution of orthopox viruses] [Article in German]. *Praktische Tierarzt* 11: 961–967

79 Schaller K, Pilaski J (1979) [Pocks in white rhinoceroses (Ceratotherium s. simum) in Muenster zoo] [Article in German]. *Zool Garten NF* 49: 169–184

80 Mueller T, Henning K, Kramer M, Czerny CP, Meyer H, Ziedler K (1996) Seroprevalence of orthopox virus specific antibodies in red foxes (*Vulpes vulpes*) in the Federal State Brandenburg. *J Wildl Dis* 32: 348–353

81 Boulanger D, Crouch A, Brochier B, Bennett M, Clement J, Gaskell RM, Baxby D, Pastoret PP (1996) Serological survey for orthopoxvirus infection of wild mammals in areas where a recombinant rabies virus is used to vaccinate foxes. *Vet Rec* 138: 247–249

82 Wolfs TF, Wagenaar JA, Niesters HG, Osterhaus AD (2002) Rat-to-human transmission of cowpox infection. *Emerg Infect Dis* 8: 1495–1496

83 Coras B, Essbauer S, Pfeffer M, Meyer H, Schröder J, Stolz W, Landthaler M,

Vogt T (2004) A cowpox microepidemic, transmitted by a domestic cat. *Lancet* 365: 9457

84 Heilbronner C, Harzic M, Ferchal F, Pothier A, Charara O, Beal G, Bellaiche M, Lesca C, Foucaud P (2004) [Cowpox virus infection in a child]. *Arch Pediatr* 11: 335–339

85 Hawranek T, Tritscher M, Muss WH, Jecel J, Nowotny N, Kolodziejek J, Emberger M, Schaeppi H, Hintner H (2003) Feline orthopoxvirus infection transmitted from cat to human. *J Am Acad Dermatol* 49: 513–518

86 Oosterling RJ, Diepersloot RJ (2002) [Diagnostic image (75). A veterinary assistant with a swelling on the neck. Cowpox]. *Ned Tijdschr Geneesk D* 146: 262

87 Schupp P, Pfeffer M, Meyer H, Burck G, Kolmel K, Neumann C (2001) Cowpox virus in a 12-year-old boy: rapid identification by an orthopoxvirus-specific polymerase chain reaction. *Br J Dermatol* 145: 146–150

88 Feuerstein, B, M Jurgens, E Schnetz, Fartasch M, Simon M (2000) [Cowpox/ Catpox. Two clinical cases] [Article in German]. *Hautarzt* 51: 852–856

89 Stewart KJ, Telfers S, Bown KJ, White MI (2000) Cowpox infection: not yet consigned to history. *Br J Plast Surg* 53: 348–350

Poxviruses
ed. by Andrew A. Mercer, Axel Schmidt and Olaf Weber

Genus *Molluscipoxvirus*

Joachim J. Bugert

Senior Lecturer in Virology, Department of Medical Microbiology, Cardiff University School of Medicine, Wales College of Medicine, Heath Park, Cardiff CF14 4XN, UK

Abstract

Molluscum contagiosum (MC) is a common wart-like skin infection mainly seen in children and caused by *Molluscum contagiosum virus* (MCV). The typical poxvirus particle morphology and genome organization of MCV led to its classification as a member of the family *Poxviridae* where it is the sole member of the genus *Molluscipoxvirus*. The genome of MCV type 1 (MCV 1/80) has been completely sequenced (GenBank accession U60315). Of 182 hypothetical MCV open reading frames (>45 amino acids) only 35 have a significant homology to coding sequences of other poxviruses. Unique MCV genes include mc159, an apoptosis inhibitor (vFLIP), mc054, a viral IL-18 binding protein, mc148, a soluble IL-8 antagonist, and mc162, a Hrs (hepatocyte growth factor-regulated tyrosine kinase substrate) binding protein. MCV does not encode an epidermal growth factor (EGF) homolog. MCV shares a number of genes only with para- and avipoxviruses and stands out as phylogenetically distinct from all other poxviruses. This is reflected in a number of unique biological characteristics that set MCV apart from other poxviruses: MCV replication *in vivo* is limited to differentiating keratinocytes of the spineous layer of the human epidermis. MCV induces an enhanced rate of mitosis in keratinocytes, possibly by way of EGF receptor up-regulation, and interferes with the normal epidermal cell differentiation program. The lack of local inflammation gives typical MCV lesions a pearly bland appearance. MC infection can persist in human skin for years. An inflammatory reaction, spontaneous or induced by trauma, frequently leads to the sudden and complete disappearance of MCV lesions. The local, subacute and proliferative nature of the MC infection puts MCV close to a group of animal poxviruses causing slow growing skin tumors. MCV replicates inefficiently in skin xenotranplants to immunodeficient mice. There is currently no cell- or tissue culture system that supports replication of MCV *in vitro*.

Introduction

After the eradication of *Variola virus*, the only remaining poxvirus with a significant prevalence in the human population is *Molluscum contagiosum virus* (MCV), the type member of the genus *Molluscipoxvirus*. MCV causes benign tumors of the skin mainly in children and immunodeficient individu-

Table 1. Summary of the phenotype of MCV

Members of the genus	MCV types 1–4
Host range	Human
Virion morphology (shape, size)	Brick 210_360 nm
Genome size (% GC content)	190 215 bp ± ~100 (63% G+C)
Isolate designation and GenBank accession	MCV type 1; U60315
Major biological features	1. Human host (at present no cell culture system) 2. Epidermal tissue tropism (cellular gene acquisition) 3. Immune evasion (weak inflammatory response) 4. Induces epidermal dedifferentiation 5. Induces epidermal hyperproliferation 6. Induces keratinocyte surface receptor upregulation (EGF and transferrin receptors) 7. Analogies to human papillomaviruses

als. The lesions are limited to the epidermis, can persist for years and show only weak signs of inflammation [1]. MCV lesions have been histopathologically classified as acanthomas: benign hyperproliferative processes confined to the epidermal layers of the skin.

Taxonomy

Based on its poxvirus-like particle morphology, MCV was first reported as an unclassified member of the family *Poxviridae* [2, 3]. It was reclassified as the type member in a separate genus *Molluscipoxvirus* by the International Committee on Taxonomy of Viruses (ICTV) in 1991 [4], recognizing its poxvirus-like genome structure, in particular the inverted terminal repeats, in the absence of significant cross-hybridization to other poxvirus genomes [5, 6]. MCV particle analysis in transmission electron microscopy shows spherical, ellipsoidal, brick-shaped, miniature and incomplete forms of MCV [7] (Tab. 1 and Fig. 1).

History

Thomas Bateman (1778–1821) first used the name 'molluscum contagiosum' to describe dome-shaped flesh colored papules with a central indentation and a diameter of between 2 and 5 mm [8]. In 1841 W. Henderson und Robert Paterson independently observed intracytoplasmic inclusions in the epidermal tissues of molluscum contagiosum (MC) lesions, hence Henderson-Paterson bodies [9, 10]. M. Juliusberg demonstrated in 1905 that the etiological agent of MC cannot be removed by filtration through

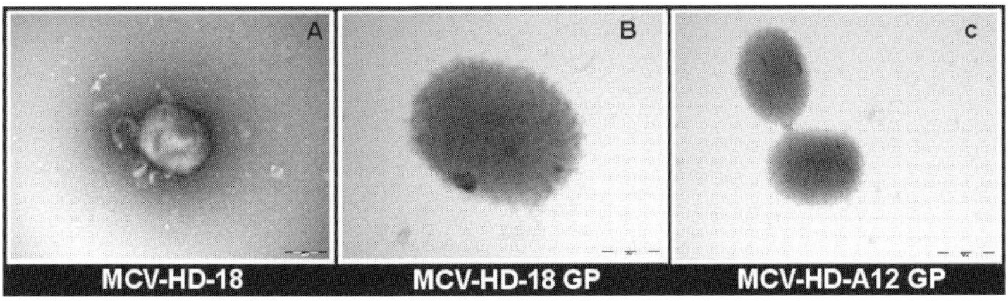

Figure 1. Negative stain of MCV particles, ammonium-molybdate technique. (A) loose membrane fragments in virions (isolate MCV–HD 18) filtered through a 0.45-µm Millipore filter (bar 200 nm). (B) MC virions (isolate MCV–HD 18) after Optiprep® gradient purification (bar 100 nm). (C) MC virions (isolate MCV–HD A12) after Optiprep® gradient purification (bar 100 nm). Electron microscopy: Bugert and Hobot, Cardiff University School of Medicine, 2005.

Chamberland filters, implicating a viral etiology [11]. In 1911 Lipschütz observed 'elementary bodies', essentially a particular matter, inside of Henderson-Paterson bodies [12]. Goodpasture, King und Woodruff recognized similarities between MC elementary bodies and 'Borrel' particles of fowlpox virus in 1927, and concluded that the etiological agent of MC must be a poxvirus [13, 14]. Electron microscopy revealed the dimension of MCV particles as approximately 360 × 210 nm [15, 16].

Disease: clinical aspects, diagnosis and treatment

Clinical aspects of the MC infection

MC is a common infection and could become a public health issue, especially in areas with low sanitary and hygienic standards. The virus is transmitted by smear infection and spreads rapidly among children in day-care centers and kindergartens. Despite the benign and self-limited nature of the infection, one-third of children have symptoms including pruritus, erythema and, occasionally, bacterial superinfection with inflammation and pain. Patients with pruritus spread the virus through scratching [17]. MC frequently occurs around the eyelid, where it is difficult to treat and occasionally causes MC conjunctivitis [18, 19]. Unusual cases of MC include an infant with extensive eruptive MC scattered over the back and buttocks that became inflamed with blackening (possible hemorrhage) and then healed spontaneously [20], or MC associated with papillomatosis (common warts) [21]. MCV presents with an extensive clinical picture in atopic dermatitis [22] and other skin-specific and systemic immune dysfunctions. Spontaneous MCV regression may occur by noninflammatory and traumatic-inflammatory processes [23].

MC in human immunodeficiency virus (HIV) infections used to be very common (up to 30% of HIV-infected individuals in stage 4 clinical disease) before the onset of HAART and cidofovir human cytomegaly virus (HCMV) prophylaxis [24].

Diagnosis of MCV infection

MCV is diagnosed clinically and by the typical histopathology found in sections of lesion biopsies [25]. Molecular diagnostics by *in situ* hybridization and PCR have been described for unclear cases [26–31]. MCV ELISAs have been described for serological surveys [32–34].

Prevention and treatment of MCV infection

MC is best prevented by exposure prophylaxis. Once acquired, MC lesions are generally self limiting, it may take between 6 months and 5 years for lesions to disappear. Patients with immune dysfunction or atopic skin conditions have difficulties clearing lesions. There has been a continued debate about whether MC lesions should be treated or allowed to resolve spontaneously [35]. Therapy is recommended for genital MC to avoid sexual transmission and should begin with gentle skin care and antipruritics to prevent symptoms [17]. Available treatment options are:

1. In-office-curettage (surgical): classical removal of the lesion with a sharp spoon, which leaves occasional scarring. While adults cope well with unanesthetized curettage of lesions, children require local anesthetics or less painful therapeutic options.
2. In-office-cryosurgery: current technique combines lidocaine/prilocaine topical anesthesia with hyperfocal cryotherapy. Most lesions treated regress without leaving scars [36].
3. Novel at-home painless MCV treatment options in extensive cases are ointments containing retinoids, alpha-hydroxy acids and the topical immunomodulators tacrolimus (e.g., 0.1% ointment)/pimecrolimus, imiquimod or podophyllotoxin (0.5% ointment). However, topical immunomodulators may predispose patients to skin infections [22, 37, 38]. Although a variety of such at-home therapies are available, no at-home treatment is as effective as surgical in-office therapy.
   Not-available for topical treatment or outside of the hospital at the present time are:
4. Antivirals specifically active against MCV DNA polymerase, like acyclic nucleoside phosphonates (HPMPC: cidofovir, Vistide; PMEA: adefovir dipivoxil, Hepsera; and PMPA: tenofovir, Viread). These agents are effective *in vivo* against a wide variety of DNA virus infections [39, 39].

There is anecdotal evidence that i.v. and topical cidofovir works against MCV; however, comprehensive clinical studies are lacking [24]. Possible alternative MCV-specific antivirals that are presently not pharmaceutically refined target the viral topoisomerase: lamellarin H [40], coumermycin A1 (50% inhibitory concentration, 32 μM) and cyclic depsipeptide sansalvamideA [41, 42].

All surgical treatments are painful to some degree and carry the risk of leaving scars. Immunomodulators may predispose to bacterial and fungal infections. Specific antivirals are the most expensive treatment option. Further research in large clinical trials is required to increase current knowledge on prevention, optimal treatment, and long-term outcome with this disease.

Epidemiology

MCV molecular epidemiology

First available in the early 1970s was the method known as DNA fingerprinting, which uses bacterial DNA restriction enzymes, to assess genetic variation of viral genome nucleic acids. This method requires access to the viral genome in sufficient quantities to be visualized with ethidium bromide stain on agarose gels. The first purification of MCV DNA suitable for this purpose was reported by Pierie and coworkers [16], who found that MCV can be isolated in large quantities from clinical lesion material. In 1977, Parr and coworkers [43] first observed genetic variations between MCV isolates based on differences in restriction enzyme patterns. Later work in the laboratories of G. Darai and L.C. Archard [44–49] established 2–3 main genetic types, respectively, and a number of subtypes, based on their *Bam*HI viral genomic DNA restriction pattern. Porter and coworkers [47, 48] reported, in two studies of patients seen in London hospitals, a ratio of MCV types 1:2 of about 3:1. Darai and coworkers [45] differentiated MCV types 1, 1 variant (1v), 2, and 2 variant (2v) and went on to characterize 222 MCV isolates from the Crampian region in Scotland. They found that MCV type 1/1v was about 40-fold more common than type 2/2v in this population, and that MCV genotypes did not change over time (up to 3 years) in the same patient, or when passed on in a contact group, e.g., family.

In a study of MCV in Australia, HIV infections were indicated for the first time in the study group. MCV 1 or 1v were found in 59% of lesions obtained from 75 Australian patients, 29% of whom were HIV positive, 32% contained MCV 2 or 2v, 4% contained multiple MCV types, whereas 5% of lesions submitted contained no detectable MCV DNA. The overall ratio of MCV 1/1v to MCV 2/2v was determined to be approximately 1.75:1. MCV type 2 was more frequently detected in general, and specifically in lesions from anogenital areas and immunosuppressed (HIV-positive) patients [29].

A Japanese study looked at genomes of 477 Japanese strains of MCV and classified four *Bam*HI restriction types, including a newly detected type (MCV type 4). The common markers of the variants of MCV-1 were 24-kbp fusion fragments generated by the loss of a *Bam*HI site between the D2 and F fragments of MCV-1p. The variants of MCV-1 were classified into three groups (MCV-1va, MCV-1vb, MCV-1vc), with the variability among them being due to additions and losses of *Bam*HI sites located in the right terminus and around the E and I fragments of MCV-1va. Considerable numbers of *Bam*HI restriction sites were conserved between MCV-2 and 4, indicating a close analogy between them. The prevalence ratios of MCV types [MCV-1 (MCV-1p):MCV-2:MCV-3:MCV-4], was determined to be 436 (0):13:24:4. Thus, the molecular epidemiology of MCV in Japan is characterized by the absence of the European prototype of MCV-1, the exclusive occurrence and abundance of variants of MCV-1, a greater prevalence of MCV-3 over MCV-2, and the presence of MCV-4 [50, 51]. An independent Japanese study of 171 Japanese patients examined whether there were geographic differences in the incidence of MCV types and whether a correlation existed between MCV types and the age, sex, and clinical status of the patients. The ratio of MCV 1 to MCV 2 was 13:1. MCV 1 was commonly detected in children (98%) and adult women (92%). MCV 2 was more frequently isolated from adult men (44%) and from patients with HIV infection (75%) [52]. In a Spanish study of 147 patients, 97 (66%) were children under 10 years, of whom 49% had atopic dermatitis. Atopic patients presented with larger lesions. The MCV 1/MCV 2 ratio was 146:1 [53]. Table 2 presents a summary of the prevalence of MCV genetic types.

MCV seroepidemiology

Using protein preparations from MC lesion biopsies, an early study looked for MCV-specific antibodies [54]. The first comprehensive study comparing 35 HIV-positive MC cases and a random group of 357 persons (ages, 1 week–69 years) was done 1992 in Australia using a virus-coated MCV ELISA format [55]. MCV antibody was identified in 77% of persons with MC lesions: in 17 of 24 HIV-1-negative persons and in 10 of 11 who were HIV-1 positive. No relationship was evident between the serological responses and the number of lesions or the duration of infection. The population survey revealed an overall seropositivity rate of 23%. The lowest antibody prevalence was in children aged 6 months to 2 years (3%), and seropositivity increased with age to reach 39% in persons ≥50 years old, indicating that MC is a very common viral infection [55]. To optimize ELISAs using recombinant MCV antigens, a library of MCV genome fragments was transferred into a cowpox virus expression system and screened with 12 sera from MC patients. Two major antigenic proteins of 70 and 34 kDa were detected by immunoblotting and mapped to the open-reading frames mc133L (70-kDa

Table 2. Prevalence of MCV genetic types

MCV type	England [47] $n=46$	Scotland [45] $n=222$	England [48] $n=93$	Australia [29] $n=75$	Japan [50] $n=477$	Japan [52] $n=171$	Spain [53] $n=147$
Type 1	74%	96% 1p	76%	59% 1p	91% 1v+	92% 1p	99.4% 1p
Type 2	26%	4%	24%	32%	3%	7%	0.6%
Type 3					5% (?1v)		
Type 4					1% (?2v)		

protein: MC133) and mc084L (34-kDa protein: MC084), respectively [56]. This was roughly confirmed in an independent study using protein preparations of the virus-induced lesions, where three immunoreactive proteins of 74/80, 60, and 35 kDa were detected. The 35- and 74/80-kDa proteins turned out to be virus specific, whereas the 60-kDa protein band was composed of a mix of human keratins [53]. MC133L and MC084L were found to be predominantly expressed on the surface of recombinant virus-infected HeLa cells. MC084R is also detectable on the surface of MC virion particles [56]. The same group assessed the seroprevalence of antibodies against MCV in 508 Japanese subjects with or without clinical MCV infection using a recombinant truncated MC133L ELISA. Antibodies to MCV were present in 7 (58%) of 12 patients with MC, 7 (6%) of 108 healthy controls, 7 (9%) of 76 patients with atopic dermatitis, and 7 (18%) of 39 patients with systemic lupus erythematosus, although no clinical MCV infection was observed in the latter three groups. Of 7 HIV-positive patients with MC, 1 (14%) was antibody positive, compared with 5 (2%) of 266 HIV-positive patients without MC [57]. Table 3 summarizes the seroprevalence of MCV in different geographical and clinical populations.

Pathology

MCV pathogenesis

MCV probably enters the epidermis through microlesions. The typical MCV lesion contains conglomerates of hyperplastic epithelial cells organized in follicles and lobes, which all develop into a central indentation towards the surface of the skin. The central indentation is filled with cellular debris and fatty acids, and is extremely rich in elementary viral particles, creating a waxy plug-like structure. This plug gets mobilized and spreads the infection to other areas of surrounding skin or contaminates objects (contagion) in a process similar to holocrine secretion. The whole lesion has the appear-

Table 3. Seroprevalence of MCV in different geographical and clinical populations

Clinical status	Australia [55]	Japan [28, 29]
	$n=392$	$n=508$
MC	77%	58% (12)
Atopic dermatitis	nd	9% (76)
SLE	nd	18% (39)
HIV	91%	2–14% (273)
Overall	23%	6% (108)
Age 6 months–2 years	3%	nd
Age 50+ years	39%	nd

ance of a hair follicle where the hair is replaced by the virus containing plug [58]. The periphery of the MCV lesion is characterized by basaloid epithelial cells with prominent nuclei, large amounts of heterochromatin, slightly basophilic cytoplasm, and increased visibility of membranous structures, which are larger than normal basal keratinocytes. These hyperplastic cells divide faster than normal basal cells, the cytoplasm contains a large number of vacuoles, and they sit on top of an intact basal membrane [59, 60]. The lesion is, therefore, a strictly intraepidermal hyperplastic process (acanthoma). Distinct poxviral factories (inclusion bodies) appear about four cell layers away from the basal membrane in the stratum spinosum [61]. The inclusion bodies grow and push cellular organelles including the cells nucleus to the side. Cells with inclusion bodies no longer show mitoses. The cytoplasm of MCV-producing cells shows keratinization, which is not expected at that stage of keratinocyte differentiation, and indicates dyskeratinization in the sense of abnormal differentiation [62]. MCV lesions are conspicuous for the absence of immune effector cells. There are actually fewer immune cells than in surrounding uninfected skin, e.g., no circulating tissue macrophages, suggesting a local immune evasive effect. MCV-infected cells show increased epidermal growth factor (EGF) receptor and transferrin receptor surface density [63]. MCV might use a vegatative mechanism of replication. Figure 2 shows a summary of the pathogenesis of MC.

MCV tissue and cell tropism

Classical electron microscopy studies [59, 60] indicate that MCV is a virus infecting keratinocytes. Granular cells of MCV-infected epidermis contain filaggrin, a skin-type keratin pair (K1/K10), and trichohyalin, a hyperproliferation-related keratin pair (K6/K16) [62]. More recently, eosinophilic

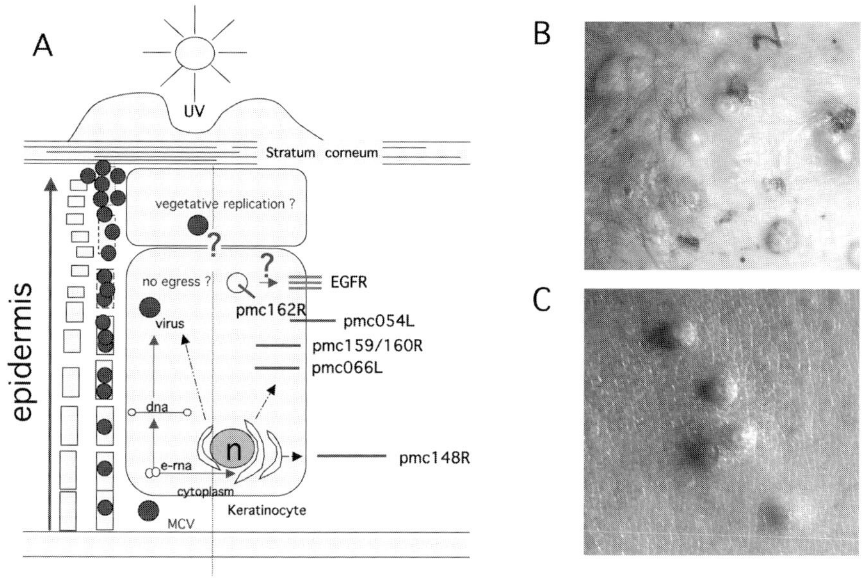

Figure 2. (A) MCV replication in the epidermis. Examples of MCV proteins with known functions: (a) membrane proteins: MC054L-IL-18BP, MC162: Hrs binding protein (possible effect on cell surface receptor regulation), (b) cytoplasmic proteins: MC159/160-FLICE inhibitors, MC066-glutathione peroxidase, (c) secreted proteins: MC148R-chemokine antagonist. Virions are shown as ● circles, cell surface receptors as triplet of lines ≡ (example EGF receptor). (B) Large number of MCV lesions on the forehead of an immunocompromised patient: area 2 of 10 with a diameter of 5 cm each. Individual lesions are between 0.5 and 3 mm in diameter. (C) Distinct group of MCV lesions in an immunocompetent patient. Individual lesions are between 2 mm in diameter. Photography: Turner and Bugert, NIH, Dermatology Service and NIAID, 1995.

intranuclear inclusion bodies, resembling poxviral factories, were described in a melanocytic nevus and confirmed as MCV specific with reverse transcriptase *in situ* PCR [64]. The latter finding has so far not been independently confirmed.

MCV host range

While there is a general consensus that MCV is restricted to the human host, two reports in the more recent literature describe a MCV-like infection in the equine host: Three horses in the Chingola district of Zambia were found to be suffering from a slow progressive skin disease with lesions varying from 4 to 20 mm in diameter in various areas of the body. Microscopically, cytoplasmic inclusions containing many pox virions were found. Attempts at culturing the virus were unsuccessful [65]. There is one report in the literature of 'equine MCV' being closely related to human

MCV by *in situ* hybridization using human MCV hybridization probes [66]. This report has not been followed up by 'equine MCV' sequence information.

Working with MCV – molecular biology

Molecular biological analyses of a virus require an *in vitro* system for faithful amplification of either the virus (cell culture system or animal model) or its genome (PCR-based systems/sequencing). Neither was available for MCV for many years.

Cell culture and animal systems

Abortive cell culture systems

Over the course of many years, a large number of primary cells and cell lines were tried for replication of MCV. MCV does not produce infectious progeny in these cells. Nongenetic reactivation, demonstrated for other chordopoxviruses of different genera, does not work with MCV [16, 67–71]. Only human fibroblasts and keratinocytes turned out to be susceptible for MCV infection and MCV early mRNAs can be isolated from abortively infected cells [72–74].

As early as 1967 Postlethwaite and colleagues [75] at the University of Aberdeen reported cell culture studies with MCV, initially using mouse embryo fibroblasts. At the same time biological assays for interferon (IFN) activity were developed using the same mouse embryo fibroblasts and encephalomyocarditis virus (EMCV) as a readout system [76]. It was found that prior infection of mouse embryo fibroblasts with MCV interfered with the development of EMCV cytopathic effect in a dose-dependent manner. Furthermore, it was observed that MCV does not seem to shut down host protein synthesis and does not, in contrast to vaccinia virus, seem to inhibit the cellular type 1 IFN response.

These observations were confirmed recently for human cell lines. MCV induces IFN-β, but not IFN-α or IL-8, in human MRC5 and HaCaT cells. It induces IL-8 only in A549 epithelial lung cells and human MM6 macrophages, but not in MRC5 or HaCaT cells (Bulek et al., unpublished observation).

MCV lesion core and biopsy material

Currently MCV is isolated from patient specimens. MCV purified from the debris core of MCV lesions or from biopsy material can be used for infection studies, electron microscopy, viral DNA extraction, and analyses of early mRNA synthesized by *in vitro* transcription of permeabilized virions [77].

Foreskin xenograft models

MCV replication was observed in human foreskin grafts to the skin of athymic mice. MCV-infected xenografts developed morphological changes indistinguishable from patient biopsy samples [78]. In an independent approach, infection with MCV type 1 and 2 virions induced similar histological changes in human foreskin fragments transferred to the renal capsule of athymic mice. Cytoplasmic inclusions containing typical poxvirus particles were seen within 2–3 weeks of implantation. Attempts to pass virus from one infected implant to another were not successful. These findings were confirmed by Paslin and coworkers [79, 80].

Even though the xenograft models seem to work *in vivo*, the 'Buller system' is hampered by low efficiency of MCV-infected graft 'take', and a long (146 days) delay before the development of MCV inclusion bodies. Because only one mouse took the infected foreskin graft, there was no attempt to passage the infection. For the 'Fife system', although lesions developed faster, it was found that no infectious progeny were produced.

Genome

There still is no *in vitro* system for replication of MCV. However, beginning in 1985, the DNA- and PCR-based methods allowed an indirect access to the possible biological properties of MCV. Genome cloning and the complete genome sequence revealed similarities and amazing differences between MCV and other poxviruses.

MCV plasmid clone library and previous limited MCV genome sequencing projects

Using DNA fingerprinting with selected enzymes and denaturation/rehybridization studies, the genome of MCV was found to have a very high G+C content of 63%, which differed from vaccinia virus (G+C content of 30%) and resembled more the viruses of the herpesvirus family and parapoxviruses [43, 44]. Purified DNA restriction fragments as well as recombinant plasmid clones derived by either single or double-digestion of genomic DNA from the subtype I of MCV and DNA hybridization were subsequently used for the establishment of the viral genetic map [5, 6, 46, 47, 49, 81] and for limited genome sequencing using Klenow enzyme, ss phage DNA and

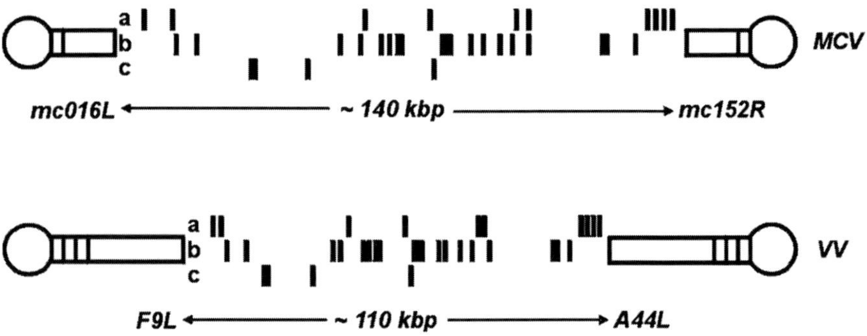

Figure 3. Schematic alignment of the genomes of molluscum contagiosum virus (MCV) and vaccinia virus (VV). The central conserved portion of the MCV genome (mc016L to mc162R: ~140 kbp) corresponds to ~110 kbp of the vaccinia genome between the genes encoding for vaccinia proteins F9L and A44L. The genes encoding amino acid homologs of structural proteins (a), proteins of the DNA expression (b) and of the replication machinery (c) are positionally but not always orientationally conserved between the two poxvirus genomes. Genes with other functions and genes without significant amino acid homology are interspersed.

the radioactive Sanger-ddNTP protocols. Early sequencing studies already revealed that a centrally conserved poxviral gene arrangement [82] was apparently absent in the terminal regions, where neither significant nucleic acid homologies with the vaccinia virus standard genome (Copenhagen), nor in fact any known gene sequences were found [83]. Limited sequencing was carried on until 1996 [6, 44, 83–90] when the complete genome DNA sequence of MCV type 1/80 was determined by fluorescent label sequencing at the LVD, NIAID (NIH, Bethesda, MD) using the overlapping MCV genome fragment library established in the Darai laboratory in Heidelberg. This library was made available to the ATCC in 2004 and is presently prepared for release.

Complete MCV genome sequence and phylogeny

The genome of MCV was found to comprise 190 289 bp (± ~50 bp) of double-stranded DNA with covalently closed ends encoding at least 182 hypothetical genes of 45 amino acids and longer [91, 92]. Most predicted proteins in the central part of the MCV genome show strong homology to structural proteins of other poxviruses, whereas all the proteins encoded at both ends and numerous proteins interspersed in the center of the MCV genome are unique (Fig. 3).

Typical examples of MCV proteins with homologs in other poxvirus genera (avipoxviruses, parapoxviruses) are the p37k major capsid protein homolog [82, 93, 94] and the MCV DNA polymerase [85, 87]. Unique MCV genes can be divided into two functional classes: (1) genes encoding proteins dealing with the host immune system (host-response evasion factors) and (2) genes encoding proteins supporting MCV replication in the host cell or the host tissue (host cell/tissue-modulating factors). MCV-specific host-response evasion factors have been extensively reviewed by several investigators [95, 96] (for review of poxviral homologs of cellular genes see [97]). Typical MCV host cell/tissue-modulating factors are MC066, a selenocysteine-containing glutathione peroxidase that inhibits peroxide- and UV-mediated apoptosis and MC159, a FLICE inhibitor presumably inhibiting apoptosis in MCV-infected keratinocytes. An epidermal growth factor homolog similar to the ones expressed by other poxviruses was not found in the genome of MCV-1. However, Nanney and coworkers observed that MCV-infected basal keratinocytes show an increased density of EGF receptor and transferrin receptor expression, in comparison to uninfected skin [98]. In a phylogenetic analysis of 26 poxvirus genomes, MCV turned out to be the second-most divergent poxvirus genome in the subfamily *Chordopoxvirus*es, after *Avipoxviruses* [99]. MCV seems to have a high degree of homology to crocodile poxvirus, a phylogenetically very old virus (G. Smith, personal communication). The following paragraphs describe the few MCV genes that are well characterized or currently investigated in the author's laboratory.

MCV SLAM homology proteins

MCV genes mc002, mc161 and mc162 were identified by Senkevich and coworkers [91] in the 1996 genome sequencing project and designated a gene family. The genes of this family were predicted to encode a group of MCV proteins with weak N-terminal amino acid homology to each other and to the Ig domain of the human SLAM (signaling lymphocytic activation molecule) protein cd150 [100]. As a first step towards the functional characterization of the MCV SLAM homology family, mRNA transcription in MCV-infected skin tissue and MRC-5 fibroblasts was analyzed by Bugert and coworkers [101] and cDNA expression libraries were established. MCV SLAM homologs MC002 and MC162 contain proline-rich motifs, also known as PY motifs. There is preliminary evidence that these MCV proteins bind to Nedd4-family E3 ubiquitin ligases AIP4 and Nedd4 and that the interaction is mediated by the tyrosine residues of both PY motifs. A PY motif-independent *in vitro* interaction with Hgs/Hrs (hepatocyte growth factor-regulated tyrosine kinase substrate) was confirmed by co-immunoprecipitation by Hgs/Hrs and by co-localization with early endosomal antigen 1 (EEA1) and the transferrin receptor in transfected human epithelial cells. MC162 may be involved in endosomal sorting mechanisms (Melquiot and coworkers, unpublished observation).

MCV IL-18 binding protein(s)

Three MCV hypothetical proteins, MC051L, MC053L, and MC054L, have 20–35% amino acid sequence identities with human IL-18-binding protein (hIL-18BP), a naturally occurring antagonist of the proinflammatory cytokine IL-18.

Of the three, only MC054L binds hIL-18. hIL-18 is a proinflammatory cytokine that activates natural killer cells and is required for a Th1 cell response by inducing synthesis of IFN-γ. Recombinant MC054L is cleaved into two subprotein units by the cellular protease furin. Full-length MC054L, but not the N-terminal IL-18 binding fragment, binds to the cell surface and the extracellular matrix. Full-length MC054 might neutralize locally produced IL-18, whereas the N-terminal fragment is soluble and free to systemically neutralize IL-18 [102–105]. These data have been confirmed and compared to the characteristics of other poxviral IL-18 binding proteins, including those encoded by vaccinia, ectromelia and smallpox viruses [106, 107].

MCV chemokine antagonist

MC148R encodes a competitive CCR8 receptor antagonist without agonistic activity. This MCV protein is probably the best characterized biochemically and in further applications. Initial studies suggested that the protein is secreted [108] and demonstrated a broad range inhibitory activity against diverse β-chemokine receptors [109], as well as inhibitory effects on human hematopoietic progenitor cells [110]. A candidate gene for an MC148 human homolog was then discovered mapping to chromosome 9p13 in humans, where IL-11Ra had been assigned, hence its name, IL-11R α-locus chemokine (ILC). ILC has the highest homology to MC148R among the known human CC chemokines, and is strongly and selectively expressed in the human skin [111]. In an attempt to demonstrate usefulness, MC148 was described to mediate cardiac allograft survival in mice. The same activity was shown for the agonistic viral macrophage-inflammatory protein-1 (vMIP-1) encoded by the human herpesvirus 8 (HHV-8) [112]. Later studies revealed that MC148 is actually a highly selective antagonist for the human, but not the murine, CCR8 receptor [113–115]. This selective binding activity was used to competitively antagonize rescue of thymic lymphoma cells from dexamethosine-induced apoptosis by the agonistic HHV-8-encoded chemokine vMIP-1 [116].

MCV topoisomerase

All poxviruses studied so far encode a type 1B topoisomerase that introduces transient nicks into DNA and thereby relaxes DNA supercoils. The MCV topoisomerase (MC087) was characterized by Y. Hwang. MCV topoisomerase cleaves just 3′ of the sequence 5'-[T/C]CCTT-3'. MCV topoisomerase is sensitive to inhibition by coumermycin A1 (50% inhibitory concentration, 32 μM) and can be selectively inhibited by cyclic depsipeptide sansalvamide A, a natural compound identified from a library of marine extracts and natural products from microorganisms. Chemically related cyclic depsipeptides represent potentially promising alternative MCV antivirals [41, 42, 117–119].

MCV vFLIP proteins

MCV open reading frames mc159 and mc160 encode proteins with death effector domains (DED) that share substantial homology to the DEDs present in the adaptor molecule Fas-associated death domain protein (FADD) and the initiating death protease FADD-like IL-1β-converting enzyme (FLICE ; caspase-8), both cellular regulators of apoptosis. In transfection experiments by two independent laboratories, it was determined that MC159 protein protects cells from Fas- and TNFR1-induced apoptosis [120, 121]. Using a MC159-expressing vaccinia virus depleted of vaccinia anti-apoptotic genes, Shisler and Moss [122] found that MC159 blocked Fas-induced apoptosis. However, binding of FADD and caspase-8 to MCV MC159 v-FLIP seems not to be sufficient to exert anti-apoptotic activity [123, 124]. Recently, Wu and colleagues [125] expressed MC159 in a T cell-specific manner. MC159 protein blocks CD95-induced apoptosis in thymocytes and peripheral T cells, but also impairs post-activation survival of *in vitro*-activated primary T cells, despite normal early activation parameters. In a study analyzing the relationship of MC159L to PKR, it was found that MC159 does not associate with PKR directly, and cannot block PKR-induced phosphorylation of eIF-2α, so the infected cell is predicted to produce IFN-β. However, MC159L was found to inhibit NF-κB activation [126]. Although the MC160 protein associated with FADD and procaspase-8 in co-immunoprecipitation studies, no protection against morphological or biochemical changes associated with Fas-induced apoptosis were discerned and the MC160 protein itself was degraded. Co-expression of MC159, as well as other caspase inhibitors, protected the pmv160 protein from degradation, suggesting a functional relationship between the two viral proteins [122].

Our current knowledge of MCV prompt a series of interesting questions that will form the basis of on-going research with this virus. A selection of these questions are outlined below.

1. MCV host range: only humans?
   Is equine MCV a reality? Biopsy specimens from laboratories reporting this possibility should now be reevaluated to obtain sequence information.

2. Why were there so many more MCV type 2 isolates in the London patient groups in comparison to the Scottish patients (1987–1989 studies in two UK populations)?
   The large discrepancy in MCV type 1:2 ratio between Scottish and London populations in the epidemiological studies by the Darai and the Archard laboratories has never been explained. It is possible that the higher proportion of MCV type 2 is due to unknown HIV infections in the London patient group (HIV testing was sporadic in the late 1980s). Another UK study involving both geographical areas might help to settle the issue.
3. Is MCV-2 a clinically/genetically distinct virus?
   MCV-2 is clearly more often isolated from HIV-positive patients. Does the virus genetically reflect this characteristic? MCV-2 sequence data (60 kb), generated in Heidelberg in 1997 (Lohmüller et al., unpublished observation), were from the centrally conserved core of the genome and showed very little genetic variation. *Bam*HI restriction site variation in the central part of the genome was explained by single-point mutations. Terminal regions of the genome were not sequenced. Nevertheless, it would be interesting to sequence a complete MCV type 2 genome.
4. Is MCV-induced cytokine induction and TLR signaling different to that seen with other poxviruses?
   MCV does not induce a systemic cytokine/immune response. Why then does it encode a protein (MC053) that binds human IL-18? Does IL-18 induce different cytokines in the skin? In contrast to vaccinia virus, MCV has no known inhibitors of TLR signaling (A52R) or IFN induction and release (E3L, K3L). It would be interesting to use MCV as a model for unmodulated poxviral TLR signaling.
5. The fate of MCV in skin equivalents:
   It would be interesting to see whether MCV can replicate in differentiating keratinocyte cultures, like keratinocyte raft cultures, or multicellular epidermal barrier models (skin equivalent). Would MCV replicate there in a vegetative fashion, in analogy to human papillomavirus, where dividing cells receive their share of MCV particles?
6. Is the Hrs-negative cell phenotype induced by MC162 *in vitro* a possible explanation for vacuolizing infection and/or host cell hyperproliferation?
   Does Hrs binding by MC162 cause a redistribution of surface receptors in MCV-infected cells and is MC162 expression responsible for the vacuolization of keratinocytes in the early stages of MCV infection of basal layer keratinocytes ? This can best be answered in a differentiating keratinocyte model.

References

1 Heng MC, Steuer ME, Levy A, McMahon S, Richman M, Allen SG, Blackhart B (1989) Lack of host cellular immune response in eruptive molluscum contagiosum. *Am J Dermatopathol* 11: 248–254
2 Fenner F (1976) Classification and nomenclature of viruses. *Intervirology* 7: 115
3 Matthews REF (1981) The classification and nomenclature of viruses: Summary of results of the meetings of the International Committee on Taxonomy of Viruses in Strasbourg. *Intervirology* 16: 53–60
4 Francki RIB, Fauquet CM, Knudson DL, Brown F (1992) *ICTV: report.* Springer-Verlag, New York, 97
5 Bugert J, Rosen-Wolff A, Darai G (1989) Genomic characterization of Molluscum contagiosum virus type 1: identification of the repetitive DNA sequences in the viral genome. *Virus Genes* 3: 159–173
6 Bugert JJ, Darai G (1991) Stability of molluscum contagiosum virus DNA among 184 patient isolates: evidence for variability of sequences in the terminal inverted repeats. *J Med Virol* 33: 211–217
7 Mihara M (1991) Three-dimensional ultrastructural study of molluscum contagiosum in the skin using scanning-electron microscopy. *Br J Dermatol* 125: 557–560
8 Bateman T (1814) *A practical synopsis of cutaneous diseases*, 3rd edn. Longman Hurst Rees Orme & Brown, London
9 Henderson W (1841) Notice of the molluscum contagiosum. *Edinb Med Surg J* 56: 213–218
10 Paterson R (1841) Causes and observations on the molluscum contagiosum of Bateman with an account of the minute structure of the tumors. *Edinb Med Surg J* 56: 279–288
11 Juliusberg M (1919) Molluscum Contagiosum. *Dtsch Med Wschr* 31: 1598
12 Lipschütz B (1919) Weitere Beiträge zur Kenntnis des Molluscum Contagiosum. *Arch Derm Syph* 107: 387–396
13 Goodpasture EW, King H (1927) A cytologic study of molluscum contagiosum. *Am J Pathol* 3: 385–394
14 Goodpasture EW, Woodruff CE (1931) A comparison of the inclusion bodies of fowlpox and molluscum contagiosum. *Am J Pathol* 7: 1–7
15 Fenner F, Burnett FM (1957) A short description of the poxvirus group (vaccinia and related viruses). *Virology* 4: 305–314
16 Pirie GD, Bishop PM, Burke DC, Postlethwaite R (1971) Some properties of purified molluscum contagiosum virus. *J Gen Virol* 13: 311–320
17 Silverberg N (2003) Pediatric molluscum contagiosum: optimal treatment strategies. *Paediatr Drugs* 5: 505–512
18 Ueyama Y, Osamura Y, Shimamura K, Nishimura M, Machida S, Tamaoki N (1985) Molluscum contagiosum occurring in an epidermal cyst on the eyelid. Light and electron-microscopic studies with literature review. *Acta Pathol Jpn* 35: 193–198
19 Khaskhely NM, Maruno M, Hoshiyama Y, Uezato H, Nonaka S (2000)

Molluscum contagiosum appearing as a solitary lesion on the eyelid. *J Dermatol* 27: 68–70
20 Ogino A, Ishida H (1984) Spontaneous regression of generalized molluscum contagiosum turning black. *Acta Derm Venereol* 64: 83–85
21 Payne D, Yen A, Tyring S (1997) Coinfection of molluscum contagiosum with human papillomavirus. *J Am Acad Dermatol* 36: 641–644
22 Wetzel S, Wollenberg A (2004) Eczema molluscatum in tacrolimus treated atopic dermatitis. *Eur J Dermatol* 14: 73–74
23 Pierard-Franchimont C, Legrain A, Pierard GE (1983) Growth and regression of molluscum contagiosum. *J Am Acad Dermatol* 9: 669–672
24 Meadows KP, Tyring SK, Pavia AT, Rallis TM (1997) Resolution of recalcitrant molluscum contagiosum virus lesions in human immunodeficiency virus-infected patients treated with cidofovir. *Arch Dermatol* 133: 987–990
25 Chan EL, Kingston MA, Carlin EM (2004) The laboratory diagnosis of common genital viral infections. *J Fam Plann Reprod Health Care* 30: 24–25
26 Forghani B, Oshiro LS, Chan CS, Hurst JW, Dennis J, Darai G, Warford AL, Cohen RM (1992) Direct detection of Molluscum contagiosum virus in clinical specimens by *in situ* hybridization using biotinylated probe. *Mol Cell Probes* 6: 67–77
27 Hurst JW, Forghani B, Chan CS, Oshiro L, Darai G (1991) Direct detection of molluscum contagiosum virus in clinical specimens by dot blot hybridization. *J Clin Microbiol* 29: 1959–1962
28 Thompson CH, Biggs IM, Zwart-Steffe RT (1990) Detection of molluscum contagiosum virus DNA by *in situ* hybridization. *Pathology* 22: 181–186
29 Thompson CH, Zwart-Steffe RT, Biggs IM (1990) Molecular epidemiology of Australian isolates of molluscum contagiosum. *J Med Virol* 32: 1–9
30 Thompson CH (1997) Identification and typing of molluscum contagiosum virus in clinical specimens by polymerase chain reaction. *J Med Virol* 53: 205–211
31 Nunez A, Funes JM, Agromayor M, Moratilla M, Varas AJ, Lopez-Estebaranz JL, Esteban M, Martin-Gallardo A (1996) Detection and typing of molluscum contagiosum virus in skin lesions by using a simple lysis method and polymerase chain reaction. *J Med Virol* 50: 342–349
32 Konya J, Thompson CH (1999) Molluscum contagiosum virus: antibody responses in persons with clinical lesions and seroepidemiology in a representative Australian population. *J Infect Dis* 179: 701–704
33 Konya J, Thompson CH, Zwart-Steffe RT (1992) Enzyme-linked immunosorbent assay for measurement of IgG antibody to Molluscum contagiosum virus and investigation of the serological relationship of the molecular types. *J Virol Methods* 40: 183–194
34 Thompson CH (1998) Immunoreactive proteins of molluscum contagiosum virus types 1, 1v, and 2. *J Infect Dis* 178: 1230–1231
35 Tyring SK (2003) Molluscum contagiosum: the importance of early diagnosis and treatment. *Am J Obstet Gynecol* 189 (3 Suppl): S12–S16
36 Bardenstein DS, Elmets C (1995) Hyperfocal cryotherapy of multiple Molluscum contagiosum lesions in patients with the acquired immune deficiency syndrome. *Ophthalmology* 102: 1031–1034

37 Berman B (2002) Imiquimod: a new immune response modifier for the treatment of external genital warts and other diseases in dermatology. Int *J Dermatol* 41 (Suppl 1): 7–11

38 Markos AR (2001) The successful treatment of molluscum contagiosum with podophyllotoxin (0.5%) self-application. *Int J STD AIDS* 12: 833

39 De Clercq E (2003) Potential of acyclic nucleoside phosphonates in the treatment of DNA virus and retrovirus infections. *Expert Rev Anti Infect Ther* 1: 21–43

40 Bailly C (2004) Lamellarins, from A to Z: a family of anticancer marine pyrrole alkaloids. *Curr Med Chem Anticancer Agents* 4: 363–378

41 Hwang Y, Wang B, Bushman FD (1998) Molluscum contagiosum virus topoisomerase: purification, activities, and response to inhibitors. *J Virol* 72: 3401–3406

42 Hwang Y, Rowley D, Rhodes D, Gertsch J, Fenical W, Bushman F (1999) Mechanism of inhibition of a poxvirus topoisomerase by the marine natural product sansalvamide A. *Mol Pharmacol* 55: 1049–1053

43 Parr RP, Burnett JW, Garon CF (1977) Ultrastructural characterization of the Molluscum contagiosum virus genome. *Virology* 81: 247–256

44 Darai G, Reisner H, Scholz J, Schnitzler P, Lorbacher DR (1986) Analysis of the genome of molluscum contagiosum virus by restriction endonuclease analysis and molecular cloning. *J Med Virol* 18: 29–39

45 Scholz J, Rosen-Wolff A, Bugert J, Reisner H, White MI, Darai G, Postlethwaite R (1988) Molecular epidemiology of molluscum contagiosum. *J Infect Dis* 158: 898–900

46 Scholz J, Rosen-Wolff A, Bugert J, Reisner H, White MI, Darai G, Postlethwaite R (1989) Epidemiology of molluscum contagiosum using genetic analysis of the viral DNA. *J Med Virol* 27: 87–90

47 Porter CD, Muhlemann MF, Cream JJ, Archard LC (1987) Molluscum contagiosum: characterization of viral DNA and clinical features. *Epidemiol Infect* 99: 563–567

48 Porter CD, Blake NW, Archard LC, Muhlemann MF, Rosedale N, Cream JJ (1989) Molluscum contagiosum virus types in genital and non-genital lesions. *Br J Dermatol* 120: 37–41

49 Porter CD, Archard LC (1992) Characterisation by restriction mapping of three subtypes of molluscum contagiosum virus. *J Med Virol* 38: 1–6

50 Nakamura J, Muraki Y, Yamada M, Hatano Y, Nii S (1995) Analysis of molluscum contagiosum virus genomes isolated in Japan. *J Med Virol* 46: 339–348

51 Nakamura J, Arao Y, Yoshida M, Yamada M, Nii S (1992) Molecular epidemiological study of molluscum contagiosum virus in two urban areas of western Japan by the in-gel endonuclease digestion method. *Arch Virol* 125: 339–345

52 Yamashita H, Uemura T, Kawashima M (1996) Molecular epidemiologic analysis of Japanese patients with molluscum contagiosum. *Int J Dermatol* 35: 99–105

53 Agromayor M, Ortiz P, Lopez-Estebaranz JL, Gonzalez-Nicolas J, Esteban M, Martin-Gallardo A (2002) Molecular epidemiology of molluscum contagiosum virus and analysis of the host-serum antibody response in Spanish HIV-negative patients. *J Med Virol* 66: 151–158

54 Shirodaria PV, Matthews RS, Samuel M (1979) Virus-specific and anticellular antibodies in molluscum contagiosum. *Br J Dermatol* 101: 133–140
55 Thompson CH, Zwart-Steffe RT, Donovan B (1992) Clinical and molecular aspects of molluscum contagiosum infection in HIV-1 positive patients. *Int J STD AIDS* 3: 101–106
56 Watanabe T, Morikawa S, Suzuki K, Miyamura T, Tamaki K, Ueda Y (1998) Two major antigenic polypeptides of molluscum contagiosum virus. *J Infect Dis* 177: 284–292
57 Watanabe T, Nakamura K, Wakugawa M, Kato A, Nagai Y, Shioda T et al (2000) Antibodies to molluscum contagiosum virus in the general population and susceptible patients. *Arch Dermatol* 136: 1518–1522
58 Reed RJ, Parkinson RP (1977) The histogenesis of molluscum contagiosum. *Am J Surg Pathol* 1: 161–166
59 Vreeswijk J, Leene W, Kalsbeek GL (1977) Early host cell-Molluscum contagiosum virus interactions. *J Invest Dermatol* 69: 249–256
60 Vreeswijk J, Leene W, Kalsbeek GL (1976) Early interactions of the virus Molluscum contagiosum with its host cell. Virus-induced alterations in the basal and suprabasal layers of the epidermis. *J Ultrastruct Res* 54: 37–52
61 Shelley WB, Burmeister V (1986) Demonstration of a unique viral structure: the molluscum viral colony sac. *Br J Dermatol* 115: 557–562
62 Manabe M, Yaguchi H, Butt KI, O'Guin WM, Sun TT, Ogawa H (1996) Expression of keratohyalin-trichohyalin hybrid granules in molluscum contagiosum. *Int J Dermatol* 35: 106–108
63 Viac J, Chardonnet Y (1990) Immunocompetent cells and epithelial cell modifications in molluscum contagiosum. *J Cutan Pathol* 17: 202–205
64 Hahm GK, McMahon JT, Nuovo GJ, Pellegrini AE, Vadmal MS (2002) Eosinophilic intranuclear inclusion bodies in a melanocytic nevus. *Cutis* 69: 223–226
65 Lange L, Marett S, Maree C, Gerdes T (1991) Molluscum contagiosum in three horses. *J S Afr Vet Assoc* 62: 68–71
66 Thompson CH, Yager JA, Van Rensburg IB (1998) Close relationship between equine and human molluscum contagiosum virus demonstrated by *in situ* hybridisation. *Res Vet Sci* 64: 157–161
67 Bugert JJ, Melquiot N, Kehm R (2001) Molluscum contagiosum virus expresses late genes in primary human fibroblasts but does not produce infectious progeny. *Virus Genes* 22: 27–33
68 Brown T, Butler P, Postlethwaite R (1973) Non-genetic reactivation studies with the virus of Molluscum contagiosum. *J Gen Virol* 19: 417–421
69 Postlethwaite R, Lee YS (1970) Sedimentable and non-sedimentable interfering components in mouse embryo cultures treated with molluscum contagiosum virus. *J Gen Virol* 6: 117–125
70 Robinson HJ Jr, Prose PH, Friedman-Kien AE, Neistein S, Vilcek J (1969) The molluscum contagiosum virus in chick embryo cell cultures: an electron microscopic study. *J Invest Dermatol* 52: 51–56
71 Shand JH, Gibson P, Gregory DW, Cooper RJ, Keir HM, Postlethwaite R (1976) Molluscum contagiosum – a defective poxvirus? *J Gen Virol* 33: 281–295

72 Melquiot NV, Bugert JJ (2004) Preparation and use of molluscum contagiosum virus from human tissue biopsy specimens. *Methods Mol Biol* 269: 371–384
73 McFadden G, Pace WE, Purres J, Dales S (1979) Biogenesis of poxviruses: transitory expression of Molluscum contagiosum early functions. *Virology* 94: 297–313
74 Bugert JJ, Lohmuller C, Darai G (1999) Characterization of early gene transcripts of molluscum contagiosum virus. *Virology* 257: 119–129
75 Postlethwaite R, Watt JA, Hodgkiss W (1967) The virus of molluscum contagiosum and its adsorption to mouse embryo cells in culture. *J Gen Virol* 1: 269–280
76 Postlethwaite R (1968) Analysis of molluscum-induced interference in mouse embryo cells: growth of encephalomyocarditis virus and dose-response relationships in molluscum-inhibited cultures. *J Gen Virol* 2: 167–175
77 Melquiot NV, Bugert JJ (2004) Preparation and use of molluscum contagiosum virus from human tissue biopsy specimens. *Methods Mol Biol* 269: 371–384
78 Buller RM, Burnett J, Chen W, Kreider J (1995) Replication of molluscum contagiosum virus. *Virology* 213: 655–659
79 Fife KH, Whitfeld M, Faust H, Goheen MP, Bryan J, Brown DR (1996) Growth of molluscum contagiosum virus in a human foreskin xenograft model. *Virology* 226: 95–101
80 Paslin D, Krowka J, Forghani B (1997) Molluscum contagiosum virus grows in human skin xenografts. *Arch Dermatol Res* 289: 486–488
81 Porter CD, Archard LC (1987) Characterization and physical mapping of Molluscum contagiosum virus DNA and location of a sequence capable of encoding a conserved domain of epidermal growth factor. *J Gen Virol* 68: 673–682
82 Blake NW, Porter CD, Archard LC (1991) Characterization of a molluscum contagiosum virus homolog of the vaccinia virus p37K major envelope antigen. *J Virol* 65: 3583–3589
83 Bugert JJ, Raab K, Rosen-Wolff A, Janssen W, Darai G (1993) Determination of the position of the boundaries of the terminal repetitive sequences within the genome of molluscum contagiosum virus type 1 by DNA nucleotide sequence analysis. *Virology* 192: 391–396
84 Hadasch RP, Bugert JJ, Janssen W, Darai G (1993) Characterization of the genome of molluscum contagiosum virus type 1 between the genome coordinates 0. 045 and 0. 075 by DNA nucleotide sequence analysis of a 5. 6-kb HindIII/MluI DNA fragment. *Intervirology* 36: 32–43
85 Sonntag KC, Darai G (1996) Strategy for identifying the gene encoding the DNA polymerase of molluscum contagiosum virus type 1. *Virus Genes* 13: 31–44
86 Sonntag KC, Clauer U, Bugert JJ, Schnitzler P, Darai G (1995) Identification and properties of the genes encoding the poly(A) polymerase and a small (22 kDa) and the largest subunit (147 kDa) of the DNA-dependent RNA polymerase of molluscum contagiosum virus. *Virology* 210: 471–478
87 Sonntag KC, Darai G (1995) Evolution of viral DNA-dependent RNA polymerases. *Virus Genes* 11: 271–284
88 Moratilla M, Agromayor M, Nunez A, Funes JM, Varas AJ, Lopez-Estebaranz

JL, Esteban M, Martin-Gallardo A (1997) A random DNA sequencing, computer-based approach for the generation of a gene map of molluscum contagiosum virus. *Virus Genes* 14: 73–80
89 Martin-Gallardo A, Moratilla M, Funes JM, Agromayor M, Nunez A, Varas AJ, Collado M, Valencia A, Lopez-Estebaranz JL, Esteban M (1996) Sequence analysis of a Molluscum contagiosum virus DNA region which includes the gene encoding protein kinase 2 and other genes with unique organization. *Virus Genes* 13: 19–29
90 Douglass NJ, Blake NW, Cream JJ, Soteriou BA, Zhang HY, Theodoridou A Archard LC (1996) Similarity in genome organization between Molluscum contagiosum virus (MCV) and vaccinia virus (VV): identification of MCV homologues of the VV genes for protein kinase 2, structural protein VP8, RNA polymerase 35 kDa subunit and 3beta-hydroxysteroid dehydrogenase. *J Gen Virol* 77: 3113–3120
91 Senkevich TG, Bugert JJ, Sisler JR, Koonin EV, Darai G, Moss B (1996) Genome sequence of a human tumorigenic poxvirus: prediction of specific host response-evasion genes. *Science* 273: 813–816
92 Senkevich TG, Koonin EV, Bugert JJ, Darai G, Moss B (1997) The genome of molluscum contagiosum virus: analysis and comparison with other poxviruses. *Virology* 233: 19–42
93 Sullivan JT, Mercer AA, Fleming SB, Robinson AJ (1994) Identification and characterization of an orf virus homologue of the vaccinia virus gene encoding the major envelope antigen p37K. *Virology* 202: 968–973
94 Calvert JG, Ogawa R, Yanagida N, Nazerian K (1992) Identification and functional analysis of the fowlpox virus homolog of the vaccinia virus p37K major envelope antigen gene. *Virology* 191: 783–792
95 Moss B, Shisler JL, Xiang Y, Senkevich TG (2000) Immune-defense molecules of molluscum contagiosum virus, a human poxvirus. *Trends Microbiol* 8: 473–477
96 McFadden G (1998) Even viruses can learn to cope with stress. *Science* 279: 40–41
97 Bugert JJ, Darai G (2000) Poxvirus homologues of cellular genes. *Virus Genes* 21: 111–133
98 Nanney LB, Ellis DL, Levine J, King LE (1992) Epidermal growth factor receptors in idiopathic and virally induced skin diseases. *Am J Pathol* 140: 915–925
99 Gubser C, Hue S, Kellam P, Smith GL (2004) Poxvirus genomes: a phylogenetic analysis. *J Gen Virol* 85: 105–117
100 Sidorenko SP, Clark EA (2003) The dual-function CD150 receptor subfamily: the viral attraction. *Nat Immunol* 4: 19–24
101 Bugert JJ, Melquiot NV, Darai G (2000) Mapping of mRNA transcripts in the genome of molluscum contagiosum virus: transcriptional analysis of the viral slam gene family. *Virus Genes* 21: 189–192
102 Xiang Y, Moss B (2003) Molluscum contagiosum virus interleukin-18 (IL-18) binding protein is secreted as a full-length form that binds cell surface glycosaminoglycans through the C-terminal tail and a furin-cleaved form with only the IL-18 binding domain. *J Virol* 77: 2623–2630

103 Xiang Y, Moss B (2001) Correspondence of the functional epitopes of poxvirus and human interleukin-18-binding proteins. *J Virol* 75: 9947–9954

104 Xiang Y, Moss B (1999) IL-18 binding and inhibition of interferon gamma induction by human poxvirus-encoded proteins. *Proc Natl Acad Sci USA* 96: 11537–11542

105 Xiang Y, Moss B (1999) Identification of human and mouse homologs of the MC51L-53L-54L family of secreted glycoproteins encoded by the Molluscum contagiosum poxvirus. *Virology* 257: 297–302

106 Smith VP, Bryant NA, Alcami A (2000) Ectromelia, vaccinia and cowpox viruses encode secreted interleukin-18-binding proteins. *J Gen Virol* 81: 1223–1230

107 Esteban DJ, Nuara AA, Buller RM (2004) Interleukin-18 and glycosaminoglycan binding by a protein encoded by *Variola virus*. *J Gen Virol* 85: 1291–1299

108 Bugert JJ, Lohmuller C, Damon I, Moss B, Darai G (1998) Chemokine homolog of molluscum contagiosum virus: sequence conservation and expression. *Virology* 242: 51–59

109 Damon I, Murphy PM, Moss B (1998) Broad spectrum chemokine antagonistic activity of a human poxvirus chemokine homolog. *Proc Natl Acad Sci USA* 95: 6403–6407

110 Krathwohl MD, Hromas R, Brown DR, Broxmeyer HE, Fife KH (1997) Functional characterization of the C---C chemokine-like molecules encoded by molluscum contagiosum virus types 1 and 2. *Proc Natl Acad Sci USA* 94: 9875–9880

111 Ishikawa-Mochizuki I, Kitaura M, Baba M, Nakayama T, Izawa D, Imai T, Yamada H, Hieshima K, Suzuki R, Nomiyama H et al (1999) Molecular cloning of a novel CC chemokine, interleukin-11 receptor alpha-locus chemokine (ILC), which is located on chromosome 9p13 and a potential homologue of a CC chemokine encoded by molluscum contagiosum virus. *FEBS Lett* 460: 544–548

112 DeBruyne LA, Li K, Bishop DK, Bromberg JS (2000) Gene transfer of virally encoded chemokine antagonists vMIP-II and MC148 prolongs cardiac allograft survival and inhibits donor-specific immunity. *Gene Ther* 7: 575–582

113 Luttichau HR, Gerstoft J, Schwartz TW (2001) MC148 encoded by human molluscum contagiosum poxvirus is an antagonist for human but not murine CCR8. *J Leukoc Biol* 70: 277–282

114 Luttichau HR, Lewis IC, Gerstoft J, Schwartz TW (2001) The herpesvirus 8-encoded chemokine vMIP-II, but not the poxvirus-encoded chemokine MC148, inhibits the CCR10 receptor. *Eur J Immunol* 31: 1217–1220

115 Luttichau HR, Stine J, Boesen TP, Johnsen AH, Chantry D, Gerstoft J, Schwartz TW (2000) A highly selective CC chemokine receptor (CCR)8 antagonist encoded by the poxvirus molluscum contagiosum. *J Exp Med* 191: 171–180

116 Spinetti G, Bernardini G, Camarda G, Mangoni A, Santoni A, Capogrossi MC, Napolitano M (2003) The chemokine receptor CCR8 mediates rescue from dexamethasone-induced apoptosis via an ERK-dependent pathway. *J Leukoc Biol* 73: 201–207

117 Hwang Y, Rhodes D, Bushman F (2000) Rapid microtiter assays for poxvirus topoisomerase, mammalian type IB topoisomerase and HIV-1 integrase: application to inhibitor isolation. *Nucleic Acids Res* 28: 4884–4892

118 Hwang Y, Park M, Fischer WH, Burgin A Jr, Bushman F (1999) DNA contacts by protein domains of the molluscum contagiosum virus type-1B topoisomerase. *Virology* 262: 479–491
119 Hwang Y, Burgin A Jr, Bushman F (1999) DNA contacts stimulate catalysis by a poxvirus topoisomerase. *J Biol Chem* 274: 9160–9168
120 Hu S, Vincenz C, Buller M, Dixit VM (1997) A novel family of viral death effector domain-containing molecules that inhibit both CD-95- and tumor necrosis factor receptor-1-induced apoptosis. *J Biol Chem* 272: 9621–9624
121 Bertin J, Armstrong RC, Ottilie S, Martin DA, Wang Y, Banks S, Wang GH, Senkevich TG, Alnemri ES, Moss B et al (1997) Death effector domain-containing herpesvirus and poxvirus proteins inhibit both Fas- and TNFR1-induced apoptosis. *Proc Natl Acad Sci USA* 94: 1172–1176
122 Shisler JL, Moss B (2001) Molluscum contagiosum virus inhibitors of apoptosis: The MC159 v-FLIP protein blocks Fas-induced activation of procaspases and degradation of the related MC160 protein. *Virology* 282: 14–25
123 Garvey T, Bertin J, Siegel R, Lenardo M, Cohen J (2002) The death effector domains (DEDs) of the molluscum contagiosum virus MC159 v-FLIP protein are not functionally interchangeable with each other or with the DEDs of caspase-8. *Virology* 300: 217–225
124 Garvey TL, Bertin J, Siegel RM, Wang GH, Lenardo MJ, Cohen JI (2002) Binding of FADD and caspase-8 to molluscum contagiosum virus MC159 v-FLIP is not sufficient for its antiapoptotic function. *J Virol* 76: 697–706
125 Wu Z, Roberts M, Porter M, Walker F, Wherry EJ, Kelly J, Gadina M, Silva EM, DosReis GA, Lopes MF et al (2004) Viral FLIP impairs survival of activated T cells and generation of $CD8^+$ T cell memory. *J Immunol* 172: 6313–6323
126 Gil J, Rullas J, Alcami J, Esteban M (2001) MC159L protein from the poxvirus molluscum contagiosum virus inhibits NF-kappaB activation and apoptosis induced by PKR. *J Gen Virol* 82: 3027–3034

Poxviruses
ed. by Andrew A. Mercer, Axel Schmidt and Olaf Weber

Genus *Yatapoxvirus*

Geoffrey L. Smith

Department of Virology, Faculty of Medicine, Imperial College London, St. Mary's Campus, Norfolk Place, London W2 1PG, UK

Abstract

*Yatapoxvirus*es are a small group of *Chordopoxvirus*es that infect humans and primates. There are two viruses in this genus, *Yaba monkey tumour virus* (YMTV) and *Tanapox virus* (TANV), hence the name Yatapox. A third virus called *Yaba-like disease virus* (YLDV) is very closely related to TANV so that YLDV and TANV are considered strains of the same species. TANV and YMTV infect primates in equatorial Africa and these infections may be transmitted to man by biting insects as zoonoses. Notable feature of yatapoxviruses are their slow growth in cell culture and the ability of YMTV to induce tumours (histiocytomas) in primates. Here the properties of the *Yatapoxvirus* genus are described.

Introduction

Taxonomically the *Yatapoxvirus* genus lies within the *Chordopoxvirinae* subfamily of the *Poxviridae*. Three yatapoxviruses have been described: *Yaba monkey tumour virus* (YMTV), *Tanapox virus* (TANV) and *Yaba-like disease virus* (YLDV), although the latter two viruses are considered strains of the same species. Like other poxviruses, yatapoxviruses are large, complex viruses that replicate in the cell cytoplasm, encode many enzymes for transcription and replication, and have double stranded DNA genomes of greater than 134 kb. TANV, YMTV and YLDV were all isolated form primates and serological studies indicate that yatapoxvirus infections are frequent in primates across equatorial Africa. However, it is uncertain if primates are the natural, or only, reservoir of these viruses. *Yatapoxvirus*es can infect man as zoonoses and this is not uncommon adjacent to the rivers such as the Tana River Basin in Kenya and the Zaire River in Zaire.

Discovery of yatapoxviruses

Yaba monkey tumour virus (YMTV)

In 1957 Bearcroft and Jamieson working in Yaba, Lagos, Nigeria identified a cutaneous tumour on an rhesus monkey (*Mucaca mulatta*) and shortly thereafter found similar tumours on other imported rhesus monkeys that were housed in the same animal colony in Africa [1]. The clustered incidence of the tumours suggested an infective agent was responsible and subsequently Andrewes and co-workers identified the causative agent as a poxvirus [2, 3]. This virus became known as *Yaba monkey tumour virus* (YMTV) after its origin and ability to induce tumours in primates. The tumours induced by YMTV in Asiatic monkeys are benign histiocytomas that resolve spontaneously in 1–2 months [4-6]. Electron microscopy confirmed that the virus responsible was similar to other poxviruses, such as *Vaccinia virus* (VACV) [7, 8]. However, no antigenic relationship to VACV, *Monkeypox virus* (MPXV) and *Orf virus* could be established, and animals infected previously with VACV or MPXV remained susceptible to YMTV challenge [3, 7, 9, 10]. Similarly, although sera from YMTV-infected animals recognized cells infected with YMTV, these sera did not recognize cells infected with the orthopoxviruses VACV or MPXV, and serum from animals infected with VACV or MPXV did not recognize YMTV-infected cells. Accidental infection of humans, who had been vaccinated against smallpox, by a needle stick and deliberate infection of volunteers induced skin lesions, demonstrating that YMTV could infect man and such infections were not prevented by prior smallpox vaccination [11–13].

Yaba-like disease virus (YLDV)

In 1966 there were outbreaks of poxvirus infections in three primate colonies in USA (Brookes Air Force Base in Texas, the Oregon Regional Primate Center and the National Center for Primate Biology, Davis, California). Notably, each infection derived from primates housed together by a single importer. For a review, see [14]. During the Texas outbreak a virus was isolated from skin lesions of an infected rhesus monkey [15]. Analysis of the structure and antigenic properties of this virus confirmed that it was a poxvirus and was related to YMTV [15, 16]. However, it was distinct from YMTV by two criteria: first, serum from YMYV-infected animals neutralized YMTV 10-fold more efficiently than the new virus; second, although both viruses induced cytopathic effect (CPE) slowly in cell culture, the new virus did not induce mini-tumours characteristic of YMTV [16]. Therefore, it seemed to represent a new virus species. Indistinguishable viruses were isolated from rhesus monkeys in other primate centres (Oregon Regional Primate Center and the National Center for Primate Biology, Davis,

California) [14, 17]. The virus from Oregon was called *1211 agent* [18], the virus from Texas was called *Yaba-related* (Y-R) *virus* [16] and the virus from California was termed *Yaba-like disease virus* (YLDV) [19]. All these very likely represent the same species.

Tanapox virus (TANV)

Tanapox virus (TANV) was isolated in the Tana River basin, Kenya from members of the Wapakomo tribe who suffered an epidemic of a febrile illness in 1957 and 1962 [20]. Both epidemics were linked to periods of extensive flooding so that the population was morooned together with wild and domestic animals in cramped conditions on islands surrounded by flood water. During these periods large numbers of mosquitoes were present and it was estimated that humans received up to 600 bites per hour. Consequently, it was thought that infection was transmitted mechanically from animals (possibly primates) to man by insect bite. Infected patients developed a fever and one or two vesicular lesions that resembled pocks but which regressed without pustulation [20]. The causative agent was a poxvirus and was called TANV after its geographical origin. TANV is distinct from YMTV. However, its biological and antigenic properties, and the disease it induced in humans, were indistinguishable from those of the three viruses isolated from primate colonies in USA in 1966 [21]. Thus TANV and YLDV are strains of the same virus. However, analysis of virus DNA showed that there are small differences in the pattern of restriction sites in the genomes of YLDV and TANV [22], and comparison of 23.2 kb of DNA from near each terminus of the virus genomes showed they differed in 1.4% of nucleotides [23].

Epidemiology

The natural host(s) of yatapoxviruses remains uncertain. It was noted originally that although Asiatic monkeys (*Mucaca mulatta*, *Mucaca irus* and *Mucaca speciosa*) were susceptible to YMTV, African monkeys (*Cercopithecus aethiops*, *Cercopithecus mona* and *Cercopithecus fuliginosus*) from both West and central Africa appeared immune to YMTV-induced tumours. To test if this resistance was due to genetic factors or to prior exposure to YMTV or related viruses that rendered adults immunologically resistant, African monkeys born in captivity in USA were compared with African or Asian monkeys for their sensitivity to experimental infection by YMTV. The development of YMTV-induced lesions in the African animals born in USA confirmed that these species were susceptible and suggested that the resistance in Africa might be due to prior exposure to this or a related virus [24]. In turn, this suggested that infections in African monkeys might be widespread.

Subsequent serological studies investigated how widespread infections with YMTV or TANV were in African green monkeys (*Cercopithecus aethiops* $n=55$) and Asiatic cynomolgus (*Macaca iris*, $n=166$), rhesus (*Mucaca mulatta*, $n=14$) and bonnet (*Mucaca radiata*, $n=83$) monkeys [25]. The African green monkeys were all captured in Uganda, the bonnet and rhesus monkeys were from India and the cynomolgus monkeys were from Cambodia, Vietnam, Philippines, Indonesia and Malaya. In Asiatic cynomolgus, bonnet and rhesus monkeys the incidence of antibodies to YMTV was 19.9, 8.4 and 0%, respectively. But in African green monkeys the incidence was much higher at 76.4% [25]. In contrast, antibody to TANV (agent 1211) was not detected in the Asiatic monkeys and only 5.5% of African green monkeys were seropositive. These data suggest that the African green monkey is a natural host for YMTV, or is very frequently infected from another source. Asiatic monkeys were also infected by YMTV, but less frequently. The host for TANV could not be deduced from this investigation, although it was clear that African green monkeys could be infected infrequently.

Downie and España, 1972, proposed that the natural host for TANV may be African monkeys in which it caused an inapparent disease [21]. However, under the unusual conditions caused by flooding in which man and animals are close together and there were large numbers of mosquitoes, the virus was transmitted mechanically by insect bite to man as a zoonosis. Similarly, it was proposed that infection of African green monkeys by YMTV was asymptomatic, but that when these primates were housed with rhesus monkeys the virus was transmitted and histiocytomas developed in the rhesus animals. The principle of a virus causing asymptomatic infection in its natural host but significant disease in another host is well known in virology. The ability of *Myxoma virus* to induce myxomatosis in the European rabbit, but not to cause disease in its natural host, the South American rabbit, is a good example with another poxvirus.

Infections in humans in certain geographical areas were also common. A serological survey of humans in the Tana River valley in 1971 showed that 16.3% of the population had antibodies to TANV. The presence of antibodies in children born after the last recorded outbreak of TANV, in 1962, demonstrated that the virus remained in the area and infections were ongoing [26]. It was suggested that the route of transmission might be *via* mosquito bites because the incidence and distribution of antibodies to *West Nile virus* (a flavivirus that is transmitted by mosquito bite) in the same sera showed a very similar pattern. Another study in a more extended region along the Tana River in 1976, found 9.2% of the population contained neutralizing antibody to TANV [27]. A similar study in Zaire reported 264 laboratory confirmed TANV infections between 1979 and 1983. Most cases occurred near to the Zaire River and 50% were in children <15 years old [28].

Travellers to equatorial Africa have been infected with TANV and sometimes the infection is apparent only after the traveler returns home

[29–31]. The infection can be diagnosed by polymerase chain reaction (PCR) [31, 32].

Disease and pathogenesis

YMTV and TANV differ in the disease they cause despite having a similar host range and being immunologically related. The lesion formed by YMTV in either primates or humans is proliferative and involves mesodermal cells. In their comparison of infections caused by YMTV and TANV, Downie and España (1973) reported that YMTV infection induced tumour-like masses of polyglonal mononuclear cells [33]. Subsequently, the lesion became infiltrated by lymphocytes and polymorphonuclear leukocytes [3]. Eosinophilic inclusion bodies were present in infected cells. In contrast, TANV infection was restricted to the epidermis and there was a swelling and hypertrophy of the epidermal layer [28, 33].

A direct comparison of infection of rhesus monkeys by TANV and YMTV showed that these viruses induce quite different lesions [33]. Intradermal infection of rhesus monkeys with TANV induced lesions that appeared in 3–4 days, reached a maximum size (1.5 cm) in one or two weeks and then regressed. In contrast, YMTV-induced lesions appeared more slowly and were apparent as nodules after 7–10 days. These continued to grow and became raised tumours peaking in size (4–5 cm diameter) after 3–6 weeks and then slowly regressed in 2–3 months.

TANV infections in man usually occur as isolated lesions on exposed skin, consistent with the proposed transmission by insect bite. Following an incubation period of 5–7 days, the patient develops fever and headache, sometimes with backache and prostration. There is usually only a single lesion, and only very seldom more than 2, a feature distinguishing TANV infection from other poxvirus diseases, such as smallpox and monkeypox. The lesion starts as a papule and grows into a raised, umbilicated vesicle that does not become pustular [20]. Histological examination of biopsy material showed pronounced dermal hyperplasia and cytoplasmic eosinophilic inclusions, typical of poxvirus infection [20]. Lesions regress eventually, usually within 4-6 weeks. The disease progression in animal handlers infected with YLDV was indistinguishable and occurred mostly on the hands or forearms and often at sites of injury.

Virus structure

Electron microscopy of cells infected with YLDV revealed typical poxvirus particles with dimensions of 220 to 310 nm long by 125 to175 nm wide [16]. These virions had an electron dense core that was often dumbbell shaped and was surrounded by an electron dense layer and membrane. These are equivalent to intracellular mature virus (IMV) particles of VACV. An analysis of YMTV-infected cells reported essentially the same virion structure [34]. The outer surface of YMTV contains thread-like tubules, but these are irregular [34] and not organized in a criss-cross pattern as seen on the surface of *Orf virus* [35]. Like VACV, yatapoxviruses produce several types of infectious virion. In addition to IMV, there are intracellular enveloped virus (IEV) particles that contain additional membranes. These are produced by wrapping IMV with intracellular cisternae [16, 22, 34, 36] and are separable from IMV by CsCl density gradient centrifugation [22, 36]. Virus released from cells by exocytosis has an additional lipid membrane compared to IMV [22, 36].

Genome structure and phylogenetic relationships

The genome of YMTV was cloned and restriction enzyme maps were established in the mid 1980s [37, 38]. The YMTV genome mass was calculated to be 95.0×10^6 Daltons and, like other poxviruses, contained terminal hairpins [37]. A comparison of YMTV, YLDV and TANV showed that the genomes of YLDV and TANV were very similar, but distinguishable, whereas the genome of YMTV was more divergent [22]. Sequencing of the YLDV [23] and YMTV [39] genomes confirmed that these are quite distinct and share only 78% nucleotide identity.

The YLDV genome (strain Davis) is 144.6 kb (excluding the terminal hairpins), encodes 151 genes of 60 or more codons, is 73% A+T and contains inverted terminal repeats of 1.88 kb [23]. In contrast, the YMTV genome is 134.7 kb, encodes 140 genes and is 70% A+T [39]. YLDV encodes all the genes found in YMTV. As with other poxviruses, the central region encodes the genes for replication and structural proteins, while the terminal regions contain non-essential genes for host range, virulence and immune modulation (see below). Less sequence is available for TANV, but the sequence of 23.2 kb from the left and right terminal regions of TANV showed it shared 98.6% nucleotide identity with the corresponding region of YLDV [23].

Phylogenetic comparisons showed that the *Yatapoxvirus* genus is distinct from other *Chordopoxvirus* genera and is more closely related to the *Capripoxvirus*, *Suipoxvirus* and *Leporipoxvirus* genera than to the *Orthopoxvirus* genus [23, 39, 40]. The genomes of yatapoxviruses are smaller than most chordopoxviruses at between 135 and 146 kb.

Replication cycle

The development of tissue culture systems to replicate YMTV and other yatapoxviruses enabled a more detailed characterization of these viruses

[41, 42]. YMTV replication is limited to several monkey kidney cell lines [43, 44]. Like other poxviruses, the majority of the YMTV infectivity remained intracellular and infected cells developed cytoplasmic, eosinophilic, inclusion bodies [16]. Similar observations were made for TANV and YLDV [22, 36, 45]. The development of quantitative replication systems for these viruses also enabled the titration of neutralizing antibodies from infected animals or man [42]. Compared to other poxviruses, yatapoxviruses grow slowly with plaques or foci taking more than a week to be clearly visible. In susceptible cell lines, such as BSC-1, TANV produces CPE more quickly than YMTV and the lesions are different. TANV induces focal lesions and the cells appear granular before rounding up. In contrast, YMTV produced small foci of heaped cells [33], alterations to the surface of monkey kidney cells [46] and development of cytoplasmic lipid vacuoles [47].

The ability of YMTV to induce histiocytomas in primates and foci of heaped cells in cell culture prompted a search for the regions of the genome responsible for this transforming property. UV-inactivated YMTV induced cell transformation and several fragments of virus DNA of 3.9, 4.8 and 5.1 kbp were detected in transformed cells [48]. These cells also expressed YMTV proteins of 160, 140, 107 and 74 kDa.

Virus specific enzymes

A study of the enzymes present in purified YMTV virions showed that, like VACV, YMTV packaged an RNA polymerase, acidic DNAase, nucleotide phosphohydrolase (NTPase) and neutral DNAase [49]. Moreover, infection by YMTV complemented a host-dependent conditional lethal mutant of VACV and restored plaque formation by this virus, suggesting the existence of a transcription system in YMTV compatible with that of VACV [50]. The sequencing of the YLDV and YMTV genomes [23, 39] confirmed that yatapoxviruses contain the enzymes for transcription and DNA replication that are present in other poxviruses, such as VACV. Both YMTV [51] and YLDV [23] encode a thymidine kinase.

DNA replication

Virus DNA synthesis occurs in the cytoplasm and starts between 3–9 h post infection (p.i.), peaks at about 18 h and continues for 2–3 days p.i., depending on the multiplicity of infection and the cell line used [52, 53]. Virus DNA was seen in the cytoplasm by autoradiography and histochemical analysis [6, 53, 54] or by incorporation of the acid-insoluble radioactive thymidine [52]. The latter study showed that virus DNA became resistant to DNAase as virus morphogenesis progressed and this was maximal at 4 day p.i. [52].

Host DNA synthesis in the nucleus was inhibited when B type inclusions appeared in the cytoplasm [6].

Morphogenesis

The morphogenesis of YMTV in monkey kidney cells was studied by electron microscopy by several groups [8, 34, 55]. These analyses revealed a series of events similar to those described by Dales and co-workers for VACV [56]. The first structures seen were arcs (or crescents) that grew by addition of micelles to form immature virions. Before the virus membrane was sealed, electron dense material containing the virus DNA was packaged inside the virus particle [34]. Thereafter, the core condensed to form electron dense infectious virions that are equivalent to IMV of VACV. During this condensation, additional structures were seen within the virion, including a rectangular-shaped core, prior to the appearance of the dumbbell-shaped core characteristic of the IMV particle [34]. As noted above under virus structure, additional enveloped forms of virus are produced that are equivalent to VACV IEV and extracellular enveloped virus (EEV), which is released by exocytosis [22, 36]. With YLDV the extracellular virus represented only 3% of total infectivity at 3 day p.i. when maximum intracellular titres had been produced [36].

Cell-to-cell spread

A notable feature of yatapoxviruses is their slow replication in cell culture so that plaques formed by TANV and YLDV take about 10 days to form. With VACV the spread of virus from cell to cell is aided by polymerization of thick actin bundles beneath enveloped virions on the cell surface. VACV mutants that are deficient in actin polymerization form small plaques; for review see [57]. In addition, the VACV protein A36 is essential for actin polymerization and a recognizable orthologue is not encoded by the YLDV genome [23]. It was surprising, therefore, to find that YLDV-infected cells do form actin tails beneath enveloped virus at the cell surface [36]. Nonetheless, these are not sufficient to enable rapid cell-to-cell spread of virus. The absence of a recognizable A36-like protein suggests that at least one other YLDV protein is needed for the polymerization of actin. One of the glycoproteins present on the outer envelope of the EEV form of VACV is called B5. This protein is needed for virus morphogenesis [58, 59] and entry of VACV EEV [60]. A related protein, Y144, is encoded by YLDV in the region of the YLDV genome corresponding to that of VACV *B5R* [23], and this is also present in YLDV EEV particles [36]. However, the Y144 protein was unable to complement for loss of VACV B5 and so is functionally distinct [36].

Immune modulation

Like other chordopoxviruses, yatapoxviruses express several immunomodulators. The first one reported was a 38-kDa protein that was secreted from TANV-infected cells early during infection and that bound human interleukin (IL)-2, IL-5 and interferon (IFN)-γ [61]. The supernatant of TANV-infected cells also contained a TNF-α inhibitor [62] that was purified on a TNF-α affinity column and found to be a 45-kDa glycoprotein. Amino acid sequencing and computational analysis mapped the protein to the *2L* gene [63]. The 2L protein did not bind IL-2, IL-5 or IFN-γ and so is distinct from the factor identified by Essani et al. 1994 [63]. Proteins related to 2L are expressed by all yatapoxviruses. Notably, TANV 2L bound and inhibited human but not mouse TNF-α consistent with the primate host range of this virus.

The genome sequence of YLDV predicted several other immunomodulators [23]. These include proteins related to chemokine receptors, a type I IFN-binding protein, an IL-10 family member, an IL-18 binding protein and intracellular inhibitors of apoptosis and IFN-induced antiviral proteins. Several of these have been characterised. Genes *7L* and *145R* encode transmembrane glycoproteins related to the chemokine receptor 8 (CCR8). The Y7 protein binds chemokine CCL1 (originally called I-309) [64] and affected virus virulence when expressed by recombinant VACV [65]. YLDV protein Y134 is related to IL-19, IL-20 and IL-24, all members of the IL-10 family of cytokines. The protein is secreted from cells as a monomeric glycoprotein and stimulated signal transduction from class II cytokine receptors IL-20Ralpha/IL-20Rbeta (IL-20R type1) and IL-22R/IL-20Rbeta (IL-20R type 2). A VACV recombinant expressing Y134 had a reduced virulence compared to control viruses [66]. Lastly, an intracellular protein, Y34, that is related to the VACV dsRNA-binding protein E3, has been characterised and the N-terminal domain has been expressed and crystallized complexed to Z DNA [67].

Use as a recombinant vector

The slow replication cycle of *Yatapoxvirus*es suggested that these viruses would continue to express antigens for a prolonged period of time and, therefore, they might be useful recombinant vaccines or vectors for cancer gene therapy [68]. An additional advantage of recombinant yatapoxviruses is that the human population is mostly immunologically naïve against these viruses, whereas many humans were vaccinated with VACV against smallpox.

Future research topics

The yatapoxviruses remain a poorly characterized group of chordopoxviruses that have some interesting and unusual properties that should be investigated further. These include the reason for the slow rate of virus replication, the mechanism by which YMTV induces transformation of histiocytes resulting in formation of histiocytomas in primates, and the novel immune evasion strategies of these viruses.

References

1 Bearcroft WG, Jamieson MF (1958) An outbreak of subcutaneous tumors in rhesus monkeys. *Nature* 182: 195–196
2 Andrewes CH, Allison AC, Armstrong JA, Bearcroft WG, Niven JSF, Pereira HG (1959) A virus disease of monkeys causing large superficial growths. *Acta Unio internat contra cancrum* 15
3 Niven JSF, Armstrong JA, Andrewes CH, Pereira HG, Valentine RC (1961) Subcutaneous growths in monkeys produced by a poxvirus. *J Pathol Bacteriol* 81: 1–14
4 Feltz ET (1961) *Proc Amer Assoc Cancer Res* 3
5 Sproul EE, Metzgar RS, Grace JT Jr (1963) The pathogenesis of Yaba virus-induced histiocytomas in primates. *Cancer Res* 23: 671–675
6 Kato S, Tsuru K, Miyamoto H (1965) Autoradiographic studies on the Yaba monkey tumor virus and host cell interaction. *Biken J* 8: 45–53
7 Owens G, Metzgar R, Grace JT, Jr. (1964) Ultrastructure and Related Immunologic Characteristics of the Yaba Virus. *J Surg Res* 26: 297–305
8 De Harven E, Yohn DS (1966) The fine structure of the Yaba monkey tumor poxvirus. *Cancer Res* 26: 995–1008
9 Ambrus CM, Feltz ET, Grace JT Jr, Owens G (1963) A virus induced tumor in primates. *Natl Cancer Inst Monogr* 10: 447–458
10 Behbehani AM, Bolano CR, Kamitsuka PS, Wenner HA (1968) Yaba tumor virus. I. Studies on pathogenesis and immunity. *Proc Soc Exp Biol Med* 129: 556–561
11 Grace JT Jr, Mirand EA, Millian SJ, Metzgar RS (1962) Experimental studies of human tumors. *Fed Proc* 21: 32–36
12 Grace JT, Jr., Mirand EA (1963) Human susceptibility to a human tumor virus. *Ann NY Acad Sci* 108: 1123
13 Grace JT Jr, Mirand EA (1965) Yaba virus infection in humans. *Exp Med Surg* 23: 213–216
14 Espana C (1971) Review of some outbreaks of viral disease in captive nonhuman primates. *Lab Anim Sci* 21: 1023–1031
15 Casey HW, Woodruff JM, Butcher WI (1967) Electron microscopy of a benign epidermal pox disease of rhesus monkeys. *Am J Pathol* 51: 431–446
16 Crandell RA, Casey HW, Brumlow WB (1969) Studies of a newly recognized poxvirus of monkeys. *J Infect Dis* 119: 80–88
17 Hall AS, McNulty WP (1967) A contagious pox disease in monkeys. *J Am Vet Med Assoc* 151: 833–838
18 Nicholas AH, McNulty WP (1968) *In vitro* characteristics of a poxvirus isolated from rhesus monkeys. *Nature* 217: 745–746
19 Hull RN (1968) The simian viruses. In S Gard, C Hallauer, KF Meyer (eds):

Virology Monographs. Springer-Verlag, Vienna, Volume 2, *Die Virusforschung in Einzeldarstellungen*, pp. 1–66

20 Downie AW, Taylor-Robinson CH, Caunt AE, Nelson GS, Manson-Bahr PE, Matthews TC (1971) Tanapox: a new disease caused by a poxvirus. *Br Med J* 1: 363–368

21 Downie AW, Espana C (1972) Comparison of Tanapox virus and Yaba-like viruses causing epidemic disease in monkeys. *J Hyg (Lond)* 70: 23–32

22 Knight JC, Novembre FJ, Brown DR, Goldsmith CS, Esposito JJ (1989) Studies on Tanapox virus. *Virology* 172: 116–124

23 Lee HJ, Essani K, Smith GL (2001) The genome sequence of Yaba-like disease virus, a yatapoxvirus. *Virology* 281: 170–192

24 Ambrus JL, Strandstrom HV (1966) Susceptibility of Old World monkeys to Yaba virus. *Nature* 211: 876

25 Tsuchiya Y, Tagaya I (1971) Sero-epidemiological survey on Yaba and 1211 virus infections among several species of monkeys. *J Hyg (Lond)* 69: 445–451

26 Manson-Bahr PE, Downie AW (1973) Persistence of tanapox in Tana River valley. *Br Med J* 2: 151–153

27 Axford JS, Downie AW (1979) Tanapox. A serological survey of the lower Tana River Valley. *J Hyg (Lond)* 83: 273–276

28 Jezek Z, Arita I, Szczeniowski M, Paluku KM, Ruti K, Nakano JH (1985) Human tanapox in Zaire: clinical and epidemiological observations on cases confirmed by laboratory studies. *Bull World Health Organ* 63: 1027–1035

29 Croitoru AG, Birge MB, Rudikoff D, Tan MH, Phelps RG (2002) Tanapox virus infection. *Skinmed* 1: 156–157

30 Dhar AD, Werchniak AE, Li Y, Brennick JB, Goldsmith CS, Kline R, Damon I, Klaus SN (2004) Tanapox infection in a college student. *N Engl J Med* 350: 361–366

31 Stich A, Meyer H, Kohler B, Fleischer K (2002) Tanapox: first report in a European traveller and identification by PCR. *Trans R Soc Trop Med Hyg* 96: 178–179

32 Zimmermann P, Thordsen I, Frangoulidis D, Meyer H (2005) Real-time PCR assay for the detection of tanapox virus and yaba-like disease virus. *J Virol Methods* 130: 149–153

33 Downie AW, Espana C (1973) A comparative study of Tanapox and Yaba viruses. *J Gen Virol* 19: 37–49

34 Rouhandeh H, Vafai A, Kilpatrick D (1984) The morphogenesis of Yaba monkey tumor virus in a cynomolgus monkey kidney cell line. *J Ultrastruct Res* 86: 100–105

35 Nagington J, Newton AA, Horne RW (1964) The structure of Orf virus. *Virology* 23: 461–472

36 Law M, Hollinshead M, Lee HJ, Smith GL (2004) Yaba-like disease virus protein Y144R, a member of the complement control protein family, is present on enveloped virions that are associated with virus-induced actin tails. *J Gen Virol* 85: 1279–1290

37 Kilpatrick D, Rouhandeh H (1987) The analysis of Yaba monkey tumor virus DNA. *Virus Res* 7: 151–157

38 Kilpatrick DR, Rouhandeh H (1985) Cloning and physical mapping of Yaba monkey tumor virus DNA. *Virology* 143: 399–406
39 Brunetti CR, Amano H, Ueda Y, Qin J, Miyamura T, Suzuki T, Li X, Barrett JW, McFadden G (2003) Complete genomic sequence and comparative analysis of the tumorigenic poxvirus Yaba monkey tumor virus. *J Virol* 77: 13335–13347
40 Gubser C, Hue S, Kellam P, Smith GL (2004) Poxvirus genomes: a phylogenetic analysis. *J Gen Virol* 85: 105–117
41 Feltz ET (1964) *In vitro* culture of Yaba virus-induced tumour from monkeys. *Nature* 202: 625–626
42 Yohn DS, Grace JT Jr, Haendiges VA (1964) A quantitative cell culture assay for Yaba tumour virus. *Nature* 202: 881–883
43 Tsuchiya Y, Tagaya I, Tsuruhara T (1969) Titration and extensive serial passages of Yaba virus *in vitro*. *Jpn J Microbiol* 13: 103–117
44 Olsen RG, Yohn DS (1970) Immunodiffusion analysis of Yaba poxvirus structural and associated antigens. *J Virol* 5: 212–220
45 Mediratta S, Essani K (1999) The replication cycle of tanapox virus in owl monkey kidney cells. *Can J Microbiol* 45: 92–96
46 Rouhandeh H, Richards JC (1980) Surface membrane redistribution and stabilization of concanavalin A-specific receptors following Yaba tumor poxvirus infection. *Biochim Biophys Acta* 600: 301–312
47 Rouhandeh H, Kilpatrick D, Vafai A (1982) The molecular biology of Yaba tumour pox virus: analysis of lipids, proteins and DNA. *J Gen Virol* 62: 207–218
48 Rouhandeh H, Vafai A (1982) A novel cell transformation with DNA-containing cytoplasmic Yaba tumor poxvirus. *Virology* 120: 77–92
49 Schwartz J, Dales S (1971) Biogenesis of poxviruses: identification of four enzyme activities within purified Yaba tumor virus. *Virology* 45: 797–801
50 Tsuchiya Y, Tagaya I (1979) Plaque formation by a host range mutant of vaccinia virus in non-permissive cells co-infected with Yaba virus. *J Gen Virol* 43: 193–202
51 Amano H, Ueda Y, Miyamura T (1995) Identification and characterization of the thymidine kinase gene of Yaba virus. *J Gen Virol* 76: 1109–1115
52 Rouhandeh H, Rouhandeh ML (1973) Nucleic acid synthesis in cytoplasm of Yaba monkey tumor virus-infected cells. *J Virol* 12: 1407–1413
53 Yohn DS, Marmol FR, Olsen RG (1970) Growth kinetics of Yaba tumor poxvirus after *in vitro* adaptation to cercopithecus kidney cells. *J Virol* 5: 205–211
54 Yohn DS, Haendiges VA, Grace JT Jr (1966) Yaba tumor poxvirus synthesis *in vitro*. I. Cytopathological, histochemical, and immunofluorescent studies. *J Bacteriol* 91: 1977–1985
55 Tsuruhara T (1971) Immature particle formation of Yaba poxvirus studied by electron microscopy. *J Natl Cancer Inst* 47: 549–554
56 Dales S, Mosbach EH (1968) Vaccinia as a model for membrane biogenesis. *Virology* 35: 564–583
57 Smith GL, Vanderplasschen A, Law M (2002) The formation and function of extracellular enveloped vaccinia virus. *J Gen Virol* 83: 2915–2931
58 Engelstad M, Smith GL (1993) The vaccinia virus 42-kDa envelope protein is

required for the envelopment and egress of extracellular virus and for virus virulence. *Virology* 194: 627–637

59 Wolffe EJ, Isaacs SN, Moss B (1993) Deletion of the vaccinia virus B5R gene encoding a 42-kilodalton membrane glycoprotein inhibits extracellular virus envelope formation and dissemination. *J Virol* 67: 4732–4741

60 Law M, Carter GC, Roberts KL, Hollinshead M, Smith GL (2006) Ligand-induced and nonfusogenic dissolution of a viral membrane. *Proc Natl Acad Sci USA* 103: 5989–5994

61 Essani K, Chalasani S, Eversole R, Beuving L, Birmingham L (1994) Multiple anti-cytokine activities secreted from tanapox virus-infected cells. *Microb Pathog* 17: 347–353

62 Paulose M, Bennett BL, Manning AM, Essani K (1998) Selective inhibition of TNF-alpha induced cell adhesion molecule gene expression by tanapox virus. *Microb Pathog* 25: 33–41

63 Brunetti CR, Paulose-Murphy M, Singh R, Qin J, Barrett JW, Tardivel A, Schneider P, Essani K, McFadden G (2003) A secreted high-affinity inhibitor of human TNF from Tanapox virus. *Proc Natl Acad Sci USA* 100: 4831–4836

64 Najarro P, Lee HJ, Fox J, Pease J, Smith GL (2003) Yaba-like disease virus protein 7L is a cell-surface receptor for chemokine CCL1. *J Gen Virol* 84: 3325–3336

65 Najarro P, Gubser C, Hollinshead M, Fox J, Pease J, Smith GL (2006) Yaba-like disease virus chemokine receptor 7L, a CCR8 orthologue. *J Gen Virol* 87: 809–816

66 Bartlett NW, Dumoutier L, Renauld JC, Kotenko SV, McVey CE, Lee HJ, Smith GL (2004) A new member of the interleukin 10-related cytokine family encoded by a poxvirus. *J Gen Virol* 85: 1401–1412

67 Ha SC, Lokanath NK, Van Quyen D, Wu CA, Lowenhaupt K, Rich A, Kim YG, Kim KK (2004) A poxvirus protein forms a complex with left-handed Z-DNA: crystal structure of a Yatapoxvirus Zalpha bound to DNA. *Proc Natl Acad Sci USA* 101: 14367–14372

68 Hu Y, Lee J, McCart JA, Xu H, Moss B, Alexander HR, Bartlett DL (2001) Yaba-like disease virus: an alternative replicating poxvirus vector for cancer gene therapy. *J Virol* 75: 10300–10308

Poxviruses
ed. by Andrew A. Mercer, Axel Schmidt and Olaf Weber

Genus *Parapoxvirus*

Stephen B. Fleming and Andrew A. Mercer

Department of Microbiology, University of Otago, PO Box 56, 700 Cumberland Street, Dunedin, New Zealand

Abstract

Highly contagious pustular skin infections of sheep, goats and cattle that were unwittingly transmitted to humans from close contact with infected animals, have been the scourge of shepherds, herdsmen and dairy farmers for centuries. In more recent times we recognise that these proliferative pustular lesions are likely to be caused by a group of zoonotic viruses that are classified as parapoxviruses. In addition to infecting the above ungulates, parapoxviruses have more recently been isolated from seals, camels, red deer and reindeer and most have been shown to infect man. The parapoxviruses have one of the smallest genomes of the poxvirus family (140 kb) yet share over 70% of their genes with the most virulent members. Like other poxviruses, the central core of the genomes encode factors for virus transcription and replication, and structural proteins, whereas the terminal regions encode accessory factors that give the parapoxvirus group many of its unique features. Several genes of parapoxviruses are unique to this genus and encode factors that target inflammation, the innate immune responses and the development of acquired immunity. These factors include a homologue of mammalian interleukin (IL)-10, a chemokine binding protein and a granulocyte-macrophage colony stimulating factor /IL-2 binding protein. The ability of this group to reinfect their hosts, even though a cell-mediated memory response is induced during primary infection, may be related to their epitheliotropic niche and the immunomodulators they produce. In this highly localised environment, the secreted immunomodulators only interfere with the local immune response and thus do not compromise the host's immune system. The discovery of a vascular endothelial growth factor-like gene may explain the highly vascular nature of parapoxvirus lesions. There are many genes of parapoxviruses which do not encode polypeptides with significant matches with protein sequences in public databases, separating this genus from most other mammalian poxviruses. These genes appear to be involved in inhibiting apoptosis, manipulating cell cycle progression and degradation of cellular proteins that may be involved in the stress response, thus allowing the virus to subvert intracellular antiviral mechanisms and enhance the availability of cellular molecules required for replication. Parapoxviruses in common with *Molluscum contagiosum virus* lack a number of genes that are highly conserved in other poxviruses, including factors for nucleotide metabolism, serine protease inhibitors and kelch-like proteins. It is apparent that parapoxviruses have evolved a unique repertoire of genes that have allowed adaptation to the highly specialised environment of the epidermis.

Taxonomy

The classification of the parapoxviruses has evolved slowly and there has been much confusion over the nomenclature used [1]. Members of the genus of the *Chordopoxvirus* subfamily that we now call the parapoxviruses, although having long been recognised as causing poxvirus-like disease, were not classified as poxviruses until 1956 [2]. At this time the members were few and included pustular dermatitis of sheep and goats and milkers nodes. In 1964, three viruses we now recognise as parapoxviruses,were listed as Group II poxviruses in "Viruses of Vertebrates" by Andrews 1964 [3]. Here the diseases of orf (synonyms: contagious pustular dermatitis, contagious ecthyma of sheep, sore mouth, scabby mouth, contagious pustular stomatitis; infectious labial dermatitis), milkers nodes (synonyms: pseudocowpox, paravaccinia), and stomatitis papulosa (of cattle) were included. The viruses associated with these diseases had a similar morphology and the "ball of yarn" appearance was described. The classification of the above as a distinct group within the poxviruses was described by the International Committee on Nomenclature of Viruses in 1971 but in addition to bovine papular dermatitis virus, milkers nodes and orf, the group also included chamois contagious ecthyma virus [4]. In 1976, the International Committee on Taxonomy of Viruses (ICTV) introduced the scheme of genera within families of viruses and here the subgroup became the *Parapoxvirus* genus within the family *Poxviridae* [5]. The genus was described as viruses of ungulates that infect man and *Orf virus* (ORFV) was chosen as the type species. The ICTV classification of the parapoxvirus genus now includes ORFV (syn. contagious pustular dermatitis virus and contagious ecthyma virus), *Bovine papular stomatitis virus* (BPSV) [syn bovine papular (pustular) stomatitis virus], *Pseudocowpox virus* (PCPV) (syn milker's nodule virus, paravaccinia virus) and the more recent member, *Parapoxvirus of red deer in New Zealand* (PVNZ) [6]. Tentative species of the genus include seal parapoxvirus, parapoxvirus of camels (contagious ecthyma of camels or Ausdyk disease), and chamois contagious ecthyma virus. A poxvirus able to cause fatal disease in red squirrels was initially considered a possible parapoxvirus, largely on the basis of its virion morphology. More recent DNA sequence data indicate that this virus is not a parapoxvirus and it remains an unclassified poxvirus [7].

Features that have proven useful in classifying viruses as parapoxviruses include the distinctive virion morphology when viewed by electron microscopy, the high G+C content of the genome and host range. However, each of these features have now been associated with poxviruses that are not parapoxviruses and further analysis, particularly DNA sequence, will be required to support the inclusion of additional viruses in the genus.

History of parapoxviruses

The history of the parapoxviruses has been reviewed by Robinson and Lyttle [1] and is covered here only briefly. Contagious pustular dermatitis or ORFV was first described in 1787, although shepherds have long recognised scabby disease of sheep [8]. However, it was another 100 years before the contagious nature of ORFV was recognised [9] and the susceptibility of humans to infection was reported [10]. In 1923, it was reported that the disease could be transmitted between sheep, by an agent that was smaller than most bacteria and could be included in the group of "filterable" viruses [11]. Aynaud also demonstrated that ORFV could be distinguished from *Vaccinia virus* (VACV) in that it did not cross-protect and he described the natural disease, its histological appearance, the susceptibility of the virus to solvents and chemicals, the development and duration of immunity, the lack of protection afforded by passive transfer of serum and the development of a vaccine which was live unattenuated ORFV. Today the vaccine against ORFV is still live unattenuated ORFV but it is commonly propagated in cell culture.

Although the disease we now know as pseudocowpox was present in cattle for a long time prior to the 1930s, it could not be readily distinguished from cowpox. In a review of the early literature Bonnevie [12] recognised that some smallpox vaccinations called "vaccine rouge" produced forms of lesions different from that caused by true cowpox and that vaccination material from these lesions did not protect from cowpox. Such infections were called false cowpox, paravaccine, milkers warts and milkers nodules and did not protect against smallpox. Lipschutz referred to the disease in humans as paravaccinia and along with others could distinguish the agent of milkers nodules from that causing cowpox by the application of the Pauls test, which involved the inoculation of the infectious material onto the cornea of rabbits [13]. Unlike cowpox, milkers nodules did not produce a lesion. In 1963, the virus was isolated in cell cultures from teat lesions in cattle and from milkers nodules and the virions were shown by electron microscopy to resemble those of ORFV and BPSV.

The early literature describing the disease caused by BPSV was reviewed by Griesemer and Cole [14], while the more recent literature has been reviewed by Robinson and Lyttle [1]. The disease was first described in Belgium in 1884 and given the name "la stomatite papillaire ou papillomateuse" (papular or papillomatous stomatitis) [15]. The definitive characterisation of bovine papular stomatitis was performed by Plowright and Ferris [16] and Griesemer and Cole [17] who reported the isolation of the virus from cell culture and the reproduction of the disease in calves. The first report of transmission of bovine papular stomatitis to humans was that of Carson and Kerr [18].

Reports of parapoxvirus diseases in camels [19–24], seals [25–33], red deer [34, 35], and reindeer [36–38] have only appeared since the late 1960s;

however, these diseases have probably been in existence for as long as the parapoxviruses described above.

Epidemiology

ORFV, BPSV, and PCPV are ubiquitous in sheep-producing and cattle-producing countries worldwide [1, 39]. Reports of parapoxviruses of camels and seals have increased in recent years suggesting a wider distribution than previously thought. It is believed that the spread and maintenance of the infections in each species is related to the resistant nature of the virions in the environment and the short-lived immunity to reinfection [1].

ORFV primarily infects animals less than 1 year old, affecting lambs and kids shortly after birth and at 3–4 months [40, 41]. Adults may also be affected and outbreaks have been observed at all times of the year. The incidence in a flock may reach 90%, but mortality is usually low. Spread in a flock is rapid and occurs by contact with affected animals or shed scabs [41, 42]. Lambs may spread the virus to the udder and teats of the ewe while suckling [40]. The virus may survive in chronically infected animals [40, 43, 44].

Recently, the prevalence of parapoxvirus infections of Japanese serows (*Capricornis crispus*) and Japanese deer (*Cervus nippon centralis*) was reported [45]. The serological survey suggested that parapoxviruses of Japanese serows is widespread in Japan. Characterisation of the DNA of isolates circulating in Japanese serows suggests that they are likely to be ORFV [46].

The parapoxvirus disease of camels called Ausdk or camel contagious ecthyma was first described in the Soviet Union in 1972 [19]. The disease has since been recorded in Mongolia [20, 21], Somalia [47], Kenya [22] and Libya [23]. In the Turkans district of Kenya outbreaks were only detected in camel calves (*Camelus dromedaries*) [48]. Mortality among camel calves is one of the most serious problems faced by camel herdsmen. Evidence suggests that parapoxvirus of camels is ORFV. Cases of contagious ecthyma of sheep occurring in camels have been reported [24] and more recently serological analysis of infected camels in Libya suggest that these infections are also caused by ORFV [23].

Parapoxvirus of reindeer (*Rangifer tarandus tarandus*) has been reported in Finland and Norway. A severe outbreak occurred in Finland during the winter of 1992–93 when approximately 400 reindeer died and 2800 showed clinical signs of disease [36]. Sporadic outbreaks have been reported since [38]. More recently, parapoxvirus infections of reindeer have been reported in semi-domesticated reindeer in Norway [37]. It has been shown that the parapoxvirus infections in Norway were likely caused by ORFV [49]. Genomic comparisons of one standard ORFV strain NZ2 ($ORFV_{NZ2}$) and the reindeer isolates, employing restriction fragment length polymorphism, random amplified polymorphic DNA analysis and partial DNA sequencing of specific genes demonstrated high similarity between the reindeer viruses and known ORFV strains. It has been suggested that the virus may have been transferred from sheep and goats to reindeer *via* people, equipment and common use of pastures and corrals. Analysis of the viruses recovered from reindeer in Finland suggest that one disease outbreak was caused by ORFV and another by PCPV [38].

PVNZ is clearly distinct from the other recognised species of parapoxviruses. Curiously, it has only ever been reported in New Zealand [34, 35] even though red deer in New Zealand are derived from animals introduced from Europe in the 19th century and the country has no indigenous ungulate species. These observations suggest that PVNZ is probably present in other countries. The recent determination of the genome sequence of deerpox virus confirmed that it is likely to represent a new genus, and that it is clearly not a parapoxvirus and is distinct from PVNZ [50].

It is now evident that infections of seal species and other pinnipeds by parapox-like viruses are widespread. The first report appeared in 1969 and described the infection of Californian sea lions (*Zaophus californianus*) [26]. Since this time infections attributed to parapoxviruses have been reported in South American sea lions (*Otaria bryonia*) [25], harbour seals (*Phoca vitulina*) in the German North sea [27, 28], Northern fur seals (*Callorhinus ursinus*) [29], grey seals (*Halichoerus grypus*) around the coast of Cornwall [30] and other parts of the world [31, 32] and the Weddell seal (*Leptonychotes weddellii*) in Queen Maud Land Antarctica [33]. Early reports were generally confined to observations of the histopathology of the lesions and electron microscopy of the virus particles. More recent reports have included *in situ* hybridisation with parapoxvirus-specific DNA probes and sequence analysis of PCR products. The emerging picture is that the viruses infecting pinnipeds are likely to form one or more new species within the *Parapoxvirus* genus, although the separation between pinnipeds and the currently recognized hosts for parapoxviruses (ungulates) introduces a note of caution.

Pathogenesis

In general the pathology of parapoxvirus infection of mammals is confined to the epithelium and oral mucosa. The virus usually infects through abrasions and breaks to the skin, and the clinical pathology observed at sites of infection is typically the formation of pustules and scabs [1, 17, 22, 26, 34, 39, 42]. There is little evidence that parapoxviruses can spread systemically [1].

Parapoxvirus lesions evolve through the stages of macule, papule, vesicle, pustule, scab and resolution. The infection begins as reddening and swelling around the sites of inoculation and small vesicles develop within 24 h. The lesions take on a pustular appearance as they develop. The pustular nature of the lesions is due to a large infiltration of polymorphonucleocytes. Adjacent lesions may coalesce as the disease progresses eventually forming a scab. Underlying the scabby lesions, the dermis becomes oedematous and proliferative, which gives a granulomatous appearance to the lesion. The lifting and cracking of scabs can result in the discharge of blood. Usually the resolution of the lesions takes up to 4–6 weeks, but there have been cases of persistent infection of ORFV in East Friesian sheep in New Zealand in which large tumour-like growths have developed (unpublished observation) and a report of a severe long-lasting contagious ecthyma in a goat's kid that lasted for 6 months [51].

In ORFV-infected sheep and goats, the lesions most often form around the muzzle and buccal cavity [1, 52]. ORFV lesions are normally benign; however, more serious complications can arise with secondary infections by bacteria or fungi. ORFV infections often cause a debilitating disease in young lambs or kids affecting the animals ability to feed. The lesions of PCPV are normally found on the teats of cattle and spread to mouths of calves [1]. With red deer (*Cervus elaphus*) lesions usually occur around the muzzle and face and multifocal scabby lesions on the velvet of stags have been recorded [34]. Parapoxvirus infections of fawns can be more serious and in addition to encrustations around the face and mouth, lesions covering 60–90% of the body have been seen [34]. Studies in infected Finnish reindeer (*R. tarandus tarandus*) have noted erosions, papules, pustules and ulcers in the mouth [36, 38]. In harbour seals (*P. vitulina*) lesions of the skin and mucosa of the oral cavity have been reported [28] and in infections of grey seals (*H. grypus*) cutaneous pocks have progressed to involve extensive regions of the skin [53]. An elevated skin lesion of 3 cm in diameter has been observed in the Weddell seal consisting of partly fresh and partly necrotic tissue and proliferative papilloma-like structures [33].

The histopathological features of natural and experimental infections of ORFV [1, 54–56], PCPV [57] and BPSV [14, 17] have been described and many of the features are common to all three viruses. Parapoxvirus infections are markedly proliferative. The infected epidermis is characterised by vacuolation and swelling of keratinocytes in the stratum spinosum, reticular degeneration, marked epidermal proliferation, intra-epidermal microabscesses and accumulation of scale-crust. Intracytoplasmic eosinophilic inclusion bodies may be visible in ballooning keratinocytes 72 h after infection. Epidermal proliferation leads to markedly elongated rete pegs. Neutrophils migrate into areas of reticular degeneration and form microabscesses that subsequently rupture on the surface. A thick layer of scale crust is built up, composed of hyperkeratosis, proteinaceous fluid, degenerating neutrophils, cellular debris and bacteria. Dermal lesions include oedema, marked capillary dilation and infiltration of inflammatory cells. Papillomatous growths that consist of pseudoepitheliomatous hyperplasia and granuloma formation often develop in natural ORFV infections and may become extensive [40].

Many, perhaps all, parapoxviruses can infect humans. Infections of humans have been reported for ORFV, BPSV and PCPV [1], as well as unclassified parapoxviruses isolated from reindeer [36] and seals [32].

Human infection by PVNZ has yet to be reported. Milkers nodules and ORFV infections of humans have been noted for centuries. The virus often infects the hands of people coming in close contact with infected animals. ORFV lesions are relatively common in people working in the sheep industry; however, recently it has been reported that ORFV infections coincided with the Islamic practice "feast of sacrifice" in which sheep are manipulated for slaughter with bare hands [58]. Unlike the lesions of animals they remain localised as foci of infection. The progression of the disease caused by ORFV from infection to resolution has been divided into six stages [1, 59]. A maculopapular stage (days 1–7), which is characterised by vacuolisation of the cells of the upper epidermis; a target stage (days 7–14) macroscopically having a red centre surrounded by a white ring of maculopapular stage cells, which is further surrounded by a red halo of inflammation; an acute stage (days 14–21) where the epidermis has disappeared, and in some areas hair follicles are dilated and full of pycnotic cells; a regenerative stage (days 21–28) where the epithelium is regenerating; a papilloma stage (days 28–35) characterised by a raised epidermal lesion with finger-like projections of epidermis extending down into the dermis; and a regressive phase (after 35 days) in which the skin returns to its normal thickness and appearance, often without scarring. The appearance of milkers' nodules are similar, with lesions beginning as reddish purple, raised nodules turning bullous or pustular, and surrounded by a red halo of inflammation. The lesions resolve in 5–6 weeks [60]. Parapoxvirus infections reported in handlers of reindeer and musk-oxen in Norway are markedly granulomatous and, unlike orf and milkers nodules, may take many months to heal [61]. More serious complications of orf in humans are large highly vascularised tumour-like lesions of the skin. These tumour-like lesions have been noted in immunocompromised people [62, 63], but have also been seen in people with apparently normal immune systems. ORFV infections can cause complications such as erythema multiforme reactions and in these cases individuals present with rashes on the backs of hands, legs and ankles [64–67]. Cases of severe forms of erythema multiforma, known as Stevens-Johnson syndrome, have been reported and involve rashes on mucous membranes and skin [68]. In immune-impaired individuals severe progressive disease can develop and cases have been reported presenting with multiple lesions [69]. The apparently successful use of cidofovir to treat a giant non-resolving ORFV lesion in an immunocompromised patient has been reported [70]. Immunity against ORFV is short lived and both animals and humans are susceptible to reinfection.

Virion structure

The virions of parapoxviruses have a characteristic ovoid structure and this unique morphology has formed the basis for their inclusion as a separate group in the poxvirus family [1]. Electron microscopy of ORFV reveals a virion with a long axis of approximately 260 nm and a short axis of 160 nm [71–75]. Negatively stained preparations of parapoxviruses appear in two forms. In the capsular form where the stain has penetrated the virion, a finely crenelate membrane appears to surround an inner amorphous core, whereas virions that are impervious to the stain reveal a regular array of tubule-like structures arranged in a criss-cross manner along the length of the particle [73, 76]. Where the virus has been propagated in cell culture, virions that appear in the medium are surrounded by a membranous structure 9–18 nm thick. It has been suggested that this membrane, by analogy to VACV, has been derived from the Golgi. The criss-cross pattern seen by electron microscopy is apparently due to superimposed images of the tubule-like structure as it winds its way in a spiral around the viral particle much like a ball of wool. More recently, the surface ultrastructure of ORFV has been described using ultra high resolution scanning electron microscopy where spirally arranged protrusions are visible on the surface of the virion [77].

Few studies have been performed to characterise the polypeptides that make up the virion particles of the parapoxviruses. Preliminary characterisation of ORFV virion polypeptides [78] showed that up to 35 polypeptides could be resolved by polyacrylamide gel electrophoresis. Analysis of ORFV virion polypeptides solubilized by treatment with NP-40 and 2-mercaptoethanol showed that 13 of 35 polypeptide bands distinguishable in whole virion preparations, were found in supernatant fractions after detergent treatment. There appeared to be considerable enrichment for a polypeptide of 38.5 kDa. There were varying degrees of enrichment for the other 12 polypeptides. The major band in virus preparations was 64.5 kDa and was thought to be a major core polypeptide. Others have detected about 30-40 structural proteins of ORFV [79–81]. Studies on PCPV have shown that up to 40 polypeptides can be resolved by SDS-PAGE [82].

Monoclonal antibodies raised against ORFV particles have helped to identify the proteins that make up the virion structure. The majority of these antibodies have reacted with proteins of 65, 39 or 22 kDa [83, 84]. The gene encoding the immunodominant 39-kDa protein is a homologue of the VACV gene H3L gene [83–85]. VAC H3L encodes an immunodominant virion membrane protein of 35 kDa [86] that is a member of the C-terminal anchor proteins [87] and has a role in virus maturation [88] and intracellular mature virus (IMV) adsorption to mammalian cells [89]. There is strong evidence that a polypeptide of about 40 kDa is the major component of the surface tubule [78–80, 82, 90].

DNA analysis of parapoxvirus genomes has revealed further homologues of VACV structural proteins. VACV has two infectious forms; IMV that are particles that have an outer membrane derived from the intermediate compartment, and extracellular enveloped virus (EEV), which are IMV particles that have an outer membrane derived from the trans-Golgi network (reviewed in [91]). Viral encoded proteins that have been incorporated into these membranes of VACV have been identified. ORFV and BPSV have homologues of the IMV-associated proteins as well as homologues of several of the EEV-associated proteins (see below). The discovery of such homologues in conjunction with the morphology of the virus suggests that the structure and morphogenesis of the parapoxviruses and VACV may be similar.

Immune response to parapoxviruses

Most of our knowledge of immunity to parapoxviruses comes from studies with ORFV. The current ORFV vaccine is live unattenuated virus that elicits protective immunity for approximately 6–8 months [92]. In view of the deficiencies of the current vaccine, an in-depth understanding of the protective immune response against ORFV has been undertaken by several laboratories.

Although the current evidence strongly suggests that cell-mediated immunity is likely to play a major role in conferring protective immunity against ORFV infection, the role of antibody in protection is less clear. Understanding the mechanisms of protective immunity to ORFV is complicated by the fact that immunity is short lived, whether it is induced by natural or experimental infection. Although there is general agreement that ORFV is able to reinfect its host, albeit the lesions are smaller and resolve sooner, there has been much debate over the role of humoral immunity in preventing or reducing the severity of lesions during reinfection. There are a number of reports that suggest that antibody is not important in protection or recovery. Early studies reported by Aynaud in 1923 showed that serum from immune animals was not protective [11] and many years later it was shown that colostrum passed onto lambs from their immune dams did not confer protection [93–95]. Others have shown that there was no relationship between antibody titre and severity of lesions. In experiments carried out by McKeever et al. [80], it was observed that lambs that were seropositive were not protected from infection. Some investigators dispute the lack of importance of antibody. Lloyd [41] showed a strong correlation between IgG2 and the resolution of lesions subsequent to challenge, suggesting that a specific isotype was important in defence against ORFV infection. Lloyd suggested that the involvement of IgG2 in the immune response might explain observations by Buddle and Pulford [93] that colostral antibody failed to protect lambs from ORFV infection since IgG1 but not IgG2 is selectively transported in milk of ruminants.

Other approaches to examine the inflammatory and immune responses to ORFV infection have involved histology of infected tissue where the cell types that infiltrate into lesions have been analysed [55, 56, 96–99]. These studies showed that neutrophils accumulated in a biphasic manner with an initial influx at 24 h, followed by a second phase at 4 days post-infection, which coincided with the appearance of viral antigen in the epidermis [55, 96]. An influx of basophils also coincided with the appearance of antigen. A dense mass of MHC class II$^+$ dendritic cells (DC) developed in the necrotising dermis adjacent to infected hair follicles and under infected degenerating epidermis [56]. The MHC class II$^+$ cells accumulating in the dermis were shown to be CD1$^-$ cells (acetylcholine esterase negative) that could be further subdivided based on Factor XIII expression [98]. These cells appear to form a barrier to invasion and may be involved in the immune response or wound repair [56, 98]. There was no evidence of epidermal Langerhans cell (CD1$^+$, acetylcholine esterase positive) involvement in the response [56]. In addition, different classes of T cells also accumulated including CD4$^+$, CD8$^+$ and T19/WC$^+$ cells [97]. Anderson et al. [99] showed that CD4$^+$ cells and DC accumulated to greater numbers than other cell types over the first 8 days. CD4$^+$ cells concentrated in the papillary dermis. CD8$^+$ cells were seen throughout the dermis and occasionally in the epidermis proximal to virus-infected epithelium. Studies of CD8$^+$ T cells in ORFV lesions have suggested that, although these cells are recruited to the site of virus infection, they become trapped underneath the ORFV lesion and are unable to gain access to virus-infected cells [100]. In spite of the presence of activated cytolytic CD8$^+$ T cells, the virus was able to replicate for several days. B cells were generally restricted to the reticular dermis underlying the virus-infected epithelium. T19$^+$ cells were distributed throughout the dermis and occasionally in the epidermis.

The dynamics of the local immune response to ORFV infection has been studied by examining the cells and soluble mediators in afferent and efferent lymph draining from the site of infection. These studies have involved cannulating the afferent and efferent lymph ducts of prefemoral or popliteal lymph nodes draining an infection site in the hind flank of sheep [92, 101–105]. Acquired immunity to pathogens that infect skin is initiated in the peripheral lymph nodes. Antigen is carried to lymph nodes by antigen-presenting cells (APC) *via* the afferent lymphatic ducts. Antibody and cytotoxic T cells produced by the lymph nodes leave *via* the efferent lymph ducts and migrate to the infected site. In addition lymphocytes migrating from blood to the site of infection, cycle through the lymph node by passive movement and become activated during this process. Studies in sheep have shown that the local immune response to ORFV in reinfected animals was a biphasic lymph cell response involving CD4$^+$ T cells, CD8$^+$ T cells, B cells and DC (reviewed in [92]). The studies showed that CD4$^+$ T cells were the most numerous lymphocyte subset in afferent lymph and peaked on days 4 and 12 post infection in reinfected sheep [104]. A similar pattern was also seen in the production of granulocyte-macrophage colony stimulating factor (GM-CSF), interleukin-1 (IL-1), IL-8, IL-2 and interferon-γ (IFN-γ) in lymph cells cultured from afferent lymph collected at various times post infection. The study also showed that reinfected animals produce a strong memory response when given inactivated ORFV, which is essentially a delayed-type hypersensitivity response as shown by Buddle and Pulford [93]. Cytokine analysis of ORFV-infected tissue has also shown that the immune response to ORFV is predominantly a Th1 response [99]. Cells expressing tumour necrosis factor-α (TNF-α) included epidermal cells, vascular endothelium and uncharacterised cells that had lymphocyte morphology. The numbers of these cells increased more rapidly in skin after reinfection. Cells expressing IFN-γ mRNA were only detected after reinfection and these cells had lymphocyte morphology.

The components of the immune response that are important in protection from ORFV have been studied by immunosuppressing animals with the drug cyclosporin-A prior to infection [106], and more recently by the depletion of specific lymphocyte subtypes [107]. Cyclosporin-A caused severe ORFV lesions to develop and was associated with the inhibition of IFN-γ and IL-2. The lymphocyte depletion studies revealed that $CD4^+$ T cells and antibody to a lesser extent are important for clearance of ORFV. The depletion of $CD4^+$ cells was associated with virus persistence and correlated with previous studies showing that $CD4^+$ T cells were the predominant T cells in skin and draining lymph node [108]. Although there was no correlation between $CD8^+$ T cell depletion and size and resolution of ORFV lesions in this study, the role of $CD8^+$ T cells cannot be excluded, since not all $CD8^+$ T cells were depleted. The study suggested that the function of $CD4^+$ T cells as helper cells for antibody could be important because of the correlation seen between antibody titres and lesion size.

The conclusion from these studies is that sheep produce a normal antiviral immune and inflammatory response to ORFV in spite of the fact that ORFV is able to repeatedly reinfect sheep and replicate over a short period of time. Furthermore, a memory response is indicated by a delayed-type hypersensitivity reaction to ORFV antigen in previously exposed animals. The discovery of immune modulators encoded by ORFV (see below) [109–114] may explain how ORFV is able to avoid, at least temporarily, the effects of host immunity. The accumulating evidence suggests that the immune evasion strategies of the parapoxviruses are similar across the genus ([115] and unpublished data).

Molecular biology

Genome

The first reports on the molecular analysis of parapoxviruses showed that the genome of BPSV comprised linear double-stranded (ds)DNA of approximately 135 kbp with cross-linked ends [116]. Also at this time the nucleotide composition of the DNAs of BPSV, ORFV and PCPV were determined and the genomes of these viruses were found to be unusually G+C rich compared with other poxviruses, approximately 63% [117]. Restriction endonuclease cleavage analyses of their genomes showed marked variability, although DNA/DNA hybridisation revealed strong inter-species homology between regions within the central core of the genomes, suggesting that, although there were sequence differences, their genomes were genetically conserved. There was a lack of cross-hybridisation between the terminal fragments of the parapoxviral genomes, suggesting significant differences in these areas [118, 119]. The genomic studies generally supported the classification of the above as separate species of parapoxviruses, which hitherto had been based on host range and pathology.

Over the last two decades, most studies on the genetic structure of the parapoxviruses were carried out with ORFV [39, 52, 120–124]. Detailed restriction endonuclease cleavage maps were produced for 16 New Zealand isolates and the complete genome of ORFV strain NZ2 was cloned [125–127]. Sequencing of selected regions across the $ORFV_{NZ2}$ genome revealed homologues of VACV genes. These included a dUTPase [128], homologues of VACV H4L (RNA polymerase-associated protein RAP94), H5R (35-kDa virion envelope antigen) [123] H6R (topoisomerase) [129] and the 14K fusion protein [130]. The distribution of these genes suggested that ORFV and VACV were colinear [123]. Further "spot sequencing" over the entire genome identified further homologues of VACV and supported the notion that many genes in ORFV conserved the order, orientation and spacing of genes seen in VACV [124]. Sequencing of the terminal regions identified genes that did not have counterparts in VACV and were likely to be involved in pathogenesis and virulence. These included a vascular endothelial growth factor (VEGF) [112], a homologue of IL-10 [110], a chemokine binding protein (CBP) [131] and a GM-CSF/IL-2 inhibitory factor (GIF) [109] at the right end of the genome. Moreover, there were a number of open reading frames that did not show matches with protein sequences in public databases, some of which had ankyrin repeats [132] and some of which appeared to be homologues of VACV genes with no known function. In addition, early and late promoter sequences were identified by transcriptional mapping [123, 133–136]. The early transcriptional termination motif, TTTTTNT, discovered in VACV, is conserved in ORFV [133, 137]. Furthermore, it was shown with VACV recombinants in which multi-gene ORFV fragments were inserted, that early ORFV genes were faithfully transcribed, demonstrating the conservation of transcriptional regulation between ORFV and orthopoxviruses [134, 135]. In addition, the inverted terminal repeat (ITR) of the $ORFV_{NZ2}$ genome was described [112].

Only recently have the genomes of ORFV (three strains) and BPSV (strain BV-AR02) [115] been fully sequenced (see Tab. 1). The genome sequences have provided further insights into the unique characteristics of the parapoxviruses and have allowed comparisons to be made within the genus and with members of the *Chordopoxviridae* subfamily.

Table 1. Species within the genus parapoxvirus

Members of the genus	Host range	Virion morphology	Genome size	GenBank accession no.
Orf virus	Sheep, goats, Japanese serow, camels, humans	Ovoid 260–160 nm	138 kbp 64% G+C	OV-NZ2, DQ184476, OV-IA82, AY386263, OV-SA00, AY386264
Bovine papular stomatitis virus	Cattle, humans	Ovoid 260–160 nm	134 kbp	BV-AR02, AY386265
Pseudocowpox virus	Cattle, humans	Ovoid 260–160 nm		
Parapoxvirus of red deer in NZ	Red deer	Ovoid 260–160 nm		
Sealpox virus (tentative)	Seal sp, humans	Ovoid 260–160 nm		
Ausdyk virus (tentative)	Camels	Ovoid		
Parapoxvirus of reindeer (tentative)	Reindeer, humans	Ovoid		
Chamois contagious ecthyma virus (tentative)	Chamois	Ovoid		

Our analysis of the ORFV genome sequences predicts 132 genes in the 138-kbp genome [138], whereas BPSV lacks one ORFV gene of unknown function but has two additional ankyrin F-box genes, giving a total of 133 genes [115, 139]. Sequences of only single genes of PCPV and PVNZ have been published; however, comparisons of these sequences and of as-yet unpublished partial genome sequences from this laboratory have confirmed the identity of ORFV, BPSV, PCPV and PVNZ as separate species within the *Parapoxvirus* genus [28, 38, 140]. Phylogenetic analyses of these sequences have, surprisingly, indicated a closer relationship between PCPV and ORFV rather than between PCPV and the other bovine parapoxvirus, BPSV.

The central core of ORFV and BPSV genomes contains homologues of VACV genes involved in replication and transcription of the genome as well as genes encoding proteins associated with structure and morphogenesis, including homologues of proteins that are incorporated into the membrane of the IMV and EEV (Fig. 1). The central region of the ORFV and BPSV genomes lack two genes (VACV D9R, a putative nucleoside triphosphate pyrophosphohydrolase, and VACV F15R, unknown function) present in all other chordopoxviruses, indicating that the minimum essential chordopoxvirus genome is 88 genes [141, 142].

The terminal regions of the parapoxvirus genomes comprising approximately 20% of the genome show substantial variation from that seen in

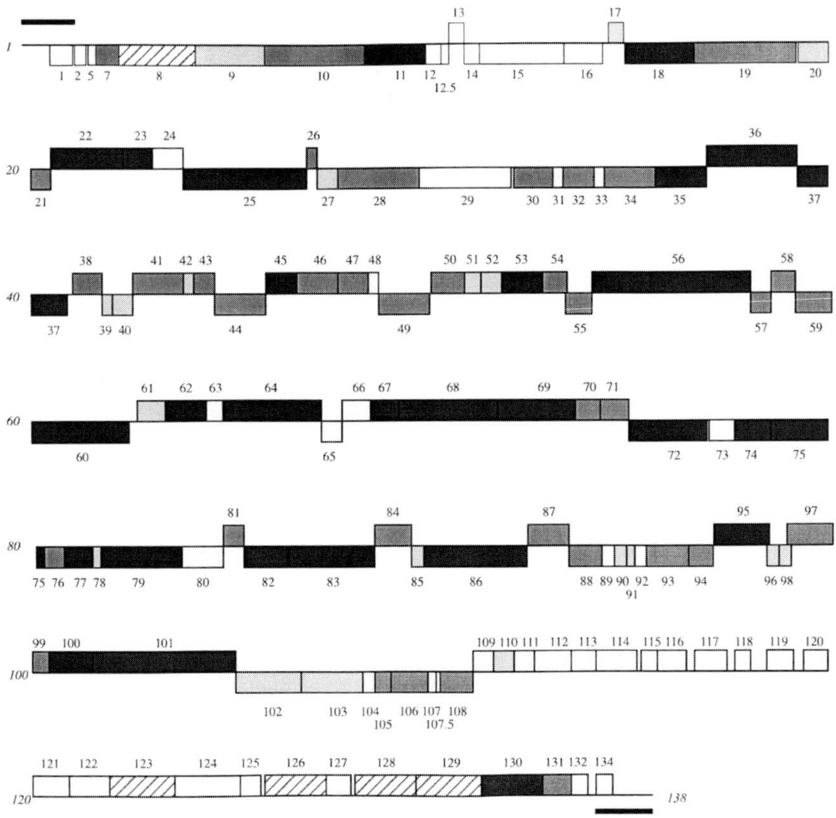

Figure 1. ORFV NZ2 genetic map. The assigned open reading frames of ORFV are shown as boxes on a line representing the genome. Boxes above the line represent open reading frames transcribed rightward and those below the line are transcribed leftward. Each line except the last corresponds to 20 kb as indicated by the numbers in italics at the left of each line. The boxes are shaded to indicate the approximate BLASTP bit score with the orthologous gene in VACV (Copenhagen). The four shades of grey from darkest to lightest correspond to bit scores of greater than 300, 100–300, 55–99 and 34–54, respectively. The speckled boxes represent scores of less than 34. White boxes are those ORFV genes for which no significant BLASTP match with a VACV protein was detected. White boxes with cross-hatching represent genes encoding ankyrin repeat proteins (see text). Figure from [138].

other poxviruses (Fig. 1). For example the ORFV genome includes 31 genes that lack clear matches in VACV, and 17 that have no significant homology with genes from all other poxvirus genera. Many of these are located in a 25-kbp region at the right terminus and are likely to encode factors that are involved in pathogenesis and virulence. Sequence analysis of approximately 25 kbp of the PCPV and PVNZ genomes has revealed the presence of this extended genus-specific region in these two other species (unpublished).

Comparisons of predicted protein sequences of the three fully sequenced ORFV isolates revealed a degree of inter-isolate sequence variation that is uncommon among chordopoxviruses. For instance, amongst the 20 most variant genes, the average predicted amino acid sequence identity was only 80% [138]. Most of these genes are not seen in other poxviruses and have unknown functions. However, two of the most variant proteins are orthologs of envelope glycoproteins present in all mammalian poxviruses (VACV A33R and A34R). A33R has been shown to be a target of neutralizing antibody, leading to the suggestion that inter-isolate variation might represent "escape mutants" and be linked to the ability of ORFV to reinfect previously infected animals [138]. It has also been proposed that some of the inter-isolate variation seen in these ORFV proteins might be associated with host-specific requirements for infection of different species, such as sheep and goat [115]. A homologue of the transcription factor VLTF-4 that shows little variability in capripoxviruses, *Sheeppox virus* and *Goatpox virus* is highly variable in ORFV and BPSV, suggesting that it may play a role in host range [115]. Both ORFV and BPSV encode proteins that are apparent homologues of orthopoxvirus proteins involved in the formation of A-type inclusions.

Parapoxviruses, in common with *Molluscum contagiosum virus* (MOCV), lack some genes that are highly conserved in other chordopoxviruses and that are likely involved in nucleotide metabolism, including ribonucleotide reductase, thymidine kinase, guanylate kinase, thymidylate kinase and a putative ribonucleotide reductase cofactor. Parapoxviruses also lack a Ser/Thr protein kinase and the serine protease inhibitor and the kelch-like gene families found in all other chordopoxviruses except MOCV [115]. These genes are known to affect host responses including inflammation, apoptosis, complement activation and coagulation and are associated with virulence. The absence of these genes may, at least in the case of parapoxviruses, be compensated for by an alternative set of genus-specific genes involved in host manipulation. Phylogenetic analysis suggests that parapoxviruses and MOCV, although clearly divergent from one another, share a separation from the other genera of mammalian poxviruses.

The full genomes of three ORFV isolates and one BPSV isolate have been shown to share an average nucleotide composition of 64% G+C. However, points of marked deviation from this average were observed in near-terminal regions in such a distinctive and uniform pattern as to form a signature [138]. In contrast, representatives of other poxvirus genera, including the high G+C of MOCV, display more uniform G+C contents across their genomes. In some cases the parapoxviral regions of uniform deviation in G+C content coincide with regions that show significant inter-isolate sequence variation. These results suggest a selective pressure to maintain unusually low regions of G+C content in specific regions of the parapoxvirus genome, independent of coding potential.

The ORFV genome is subject to rearrangement of terminal sequences when the virus is passaged in cell culture [143]. Similar rearrangements have been reported in other poxviruses [144–147]. Such terminal rearrangements have occurred in the highly passaged and attenuated strain of $ORFV_{D1701}$, that has given rise to a considerably enlarged ITR compared with low passage field isolates of ORFV [39, 148]. This has resulted in the duplication of some genes and the loss of others. We have observed spontaneous terminal transposition-deletion variants of $ORFV_{NZ2}$ that emerged during serial passage in bovine testis cells. Characterisation of one of the variants revealed that 6.6 kb of DNA at the left end of the genome had been replaced by 19.3 kb from the right end. The transposition resulted in the deletion at the left end of 3.3 kb encoding three genes and the terminal sequence of a fourth [143].

Virulence genes

IL-10

The discovery of an IL-10-like gene in a poxvirus was first reported in ORFV [110]. Since then, IL-10-like genes have been found in other parapoxviruses including BPSV [115] and PVNZ (unpublished) and yatapoxviruses (*Yaba-like disease virus* (YLDV)) [149] and capripoxviruses (*Lumpy skin disease virus*, *Goatpox virus* and *Sheeppox virus*) [150]. Mammalian IL-10 is a multifunctional cytokine that has suppressive effects on inflammation, anti-viral responses and T helper type 1 (Th1) effector function [151]. The inhibition of a Th1 response occurs indirectly through antigen-presenting macrophages and DC. In addition, IL-10 has co-stimulatory functions and is a costimulator of T lymphocytes associated with Th2 responses, mast cells and B cells.

$ORFV_{NZ2}$-IL-10 is 186 amino acid peptide with a molecular mass of 21.7 kDa and BPSV-IL-10 has 185 amino acids making the parapoxvirus IL-10s slightly larger than their mammalian counterparts. The gene is expressed early and is flanked by typical poxvirus early transcriptional sequences [110]. The homologies of the predicted polypeptide sequences of $ORFV_{NZ2}$-IL-10 with IL-10s of mammals and herpesviruses are: ovine 80%, bovine 75%, human 67% mouse 64%, Epstein-Barr virus (EBV) 63% and equine herpesvirus 2 67%. The homology of BPSV with bovine IL-10 is 75%. It is clear from sequence alignments of both ORFV-IL-10 and BPSV-IL-10, that they most closely resemble their natural host. The amino acid sequence identity of the parapoxvirus IL-10 with mammalian IL-10 is highest over the C-terminal two thirds of the polypeptide, although the relatedness at the nucleotide level is less apparent and reflects differences in codon usage and the high G+C content of the parapoxvirus genomes in general. Curiously, the N-terminal region of the parapoxviral IL-10 contains little similarity to mammalian or herpesvirus IL-10s [110].

The close similarity between the IL-10s of herpesviruses and their hosts suggested there were selective pressures for the viral IL-10 to resemble their eukaryotic counterparts, which is also apparent with the parapoxviruses. However, the discovery of IL-10-like genes in members of two other poxvirus genera (*Yatapoxvirus* and *Capripoxvirus*) and in the herpesvirus, cytomegalovirus (CMV) [152, 153], which are only approximately 20% identical to mammalian IL-10, would seem to refute this notion, although few studies have been performed on the functional characterisation of these IL-10 variants. It is possible that some of the viral IL-10s may have evolved from captured host gene(s) other than IL-10 but which are structurally similar to mammalian IL-10. It has recently been shown that YLDV-IL-10 is functionally more similar to IL-24 than IL-10 [154].

The functional characterisation of parapoxvirus IL-10 has thus far been carried out with ORFV-IL-10. These studies have revealed that it appears to have all the activities of mammalian IL-10. Using murine, ovine and human cells ORFV-IL-10 has been shown to inhibit the production of TNF-α and IL-8 by LPS-activated macrophages and PMA/calcium ionophore-activated keratinocytes, and IFN-γ and GM-CSF from Con A-activated peripheral blood lymphocytes [122, 155]. In addition, ORFV-IL-10 costimulates mast cells and thymocyte proliferation [110, 122, 155]. It is active on APC and has been shown to inhibit maturation and antigen presentation of murine bone marrow-derived DC [156] and human blood-derived monocyte DC (Chan, Baird, Mercer, Fleming, unpublished). These activities suggest that the parapoxviral IL-10 will have a role in suppressing inflammation and the development of the innate responses and acquired immunity.

Studies on viral IL-10-like molecules have provided insights into structure - function aspects of cellular IL-10. The active form of mammalian IL-10 is a homodimer. The three-dimensional structure of human IL-10 [157–159] and its interaction with its receptor at the molecular level has been determined [160]. It has been shown that a total of 27 amino acids of IL-10 contact the binding interface of the IL-10 receptor. These amino acids are located within both the near N-terminal and the C-terminal regions of IL-10. Examination of ORFV-IL-10 reveals that it conserves 11 of the 16 N-terminal amino acids of human IL-10 that make contact with the receptor and 10 of the 11 C-terminal residues. Although ORFV-IL-10 and EBV-IL-10 resemble their host counterparts only ORFV-IL-10 has all the functional activities of mammalian IL-10, whereas EBV-IL-10 has only a subset of activities, having evolved a more immunosuppressive form [161–164]. It was originally thought that EBV IL-10 lacked immunostimulatory activities because of differences at the N terminus, which had been suggested to contain the immunostimulatory domain; however, studies on ORFV-IL-10 showed that it was also different within this region, although it costimulated thymocytes and mast cells [122, 155]. The concept that IL-10 has multiple domains is no longer accepted and it is believed that essentially two regions bind to the receptor, one region at the near N terminus and the other at the C terminus [165]. It is intriguing that ORFV has not evolved a more immunosuppressive form of this virokine, like EBV IL-10. This may suggest that mutations of the ORFV-IL-10 to a potentially more immunosuppressive form may compromise the coexistence of host and virus.

Chemokine binding protein

In common with orthopoxviruses and leporipoxviruses, the parapoxviruses encode a CBP [111, 115, 131, 166, 167]. Chemokines are a large family of molecules that recruit and activate immune cells at sites of inflammation and infection [168, 169]. Thus far, a CBP has been found in ORFV, BPSV, PVNZ (unpublished). The most well characterised of these is the CBP of $ORFV_{NZ2}$, which is a protein of 286 amino acids with a predicted molecular mass of 31.2 kDa [111]. $ORFV_{NZ2}$-CBP shows surprisingly low similarity to CBPs of orthopoxviruses or leporipoxviruses with only approximately 16% amino acid identity. The parapoxvirus CBPs are more similar to ORFV-GIF at the polypeptide level than to other poxvirus proteins (approximately 20% identical at the amino acid level). This suggests that the *Parapoxvirus*, *Orthopoxvirus* and *Leporipoxvirus* genera share a common ancestral gene that became modified during the course of evolution to create different binding specificities [111]. The orthopoxvirus and leporipoxvirus CBPs share a high level of identity and many of the highly conserved regions of sequence within these CBPs are not apparent in the parapoxvirus CBPs. In addition, only six of the eight cysteine residues present in other poxvirus CBPs are found in parapoxvirus CBPs. The viral CBPs, including those found in the herpesvirus group, bear no sequence or structural homology to any known G-protein coupled receptors or mammalian proteins.

The ORFV-CBP has been shown to have a unique binding profile amongst the poxvirus CBPs with the most significant difference being that in addition to binding a number of CC inflammatory chemokines, it also binds the C chemokine lymphotactin that the other poxviruses do not bind [111]. To date, it has been shown that the ORFV-CBP binds the CC chemokines eotaxin, MCP-3, MCP-1, MIP-1b and MIP-1a and I309 and lymphotactin with high affinity. In common with the other poxvirus CBPs, ORFV-CBP does not bind the homeostatic chemokines MDC or TARC.

The binding site of ORFV-CBP to human MCP-1 has been examined at the molecular level using single amino acid mutants of MCP-1. The studies revealed that ORFV-CBP binds to residues that are critical for the interaction of MCP-1 with CCR2b (MCP-1 receptor) and demonstrates that ORFV-CBP occludes the receptor binding site of the chemokine in a similar manner to other poxvirus CBP [111]. The findings suggest that viral CBPs are likely to act as competitive inhibitors *in vivo*. In addition, it has been shown that ORFV-CBP inhibits chemokine-induced signalling in a dose-dependent manner in a calcium flux assay [111].

The binding activities of ORFV-CBP suggest that it blocks the recruitment of monocytes, macrophages, DC, natural killer (NK) cells and T cells to sites of infection. ORFV-CBP does not bind the homeostatic chemokines such as monocyte-derived or thymus- and activation-regulated chemokines, suggesting the importance of inhibiting the inflammatory CC-chemokines rather than the homeostatic CC-chemokines. In addition, lymphotactin has been implicated in the chemotaxis of T cells, neutrophils and B cells that express the lymphotactin receptor XCR1 [111]. Furthermore, the binding spectrum of ORFV-CBP suggests that in addition to inhibiting chemokine-induced chemotaxis, it has evolved to target Th1 antiviral responses. MIP-1α, MIP-1β, RANTES and lymphotactin can function in concert with IFN-γ as Th1 cytokines that can coactivate macrophages and promote NK cells and $CD8^+$ T cells in driving Th1 responses [111].

GM-CSF/IL-2 inhibitory factor

The GM-CSF/IL-2 inhibitory factor (GIF) discovered in ORFV has not been reported in any virus other than the parapoxviruses [109, 170]. GIF was originally identified as an activity produced from primary ovine skin keratinocytes infected with ORFV. Although GM-CSF was up-regulated at the transcriptional level, the secreted protein could not be detected in ORFV-infected cell culture supernatants, whereas the inflammatory cytokines IL-1β and TNF-α were detected. GIF is highly conserved within ORFV strains. ORFV strains orf 11 and MRI scab are predicted to encode proteins with 98% identity to $ORFV_{NZ2}$ GIF. Homologues of GIF have more recently been identified in BPSV [115] and PVNZ (unpublished). GIF has sequence similarities with poxvirus CBPs (see above), suggesting extensive divergence from a poxvirus ancestral gene. GIF has 32% amino acid similarity with the VACV A41L protein but that protein does not bind GM-CSF, IL-2 or a range of chemokines and, while it appears to be involved in reducing the migration of inflammatory cells, its function has not been fully defined [171].

GIF exists in solution as either a dimer or a tetramer and both forms are functionally active. It has been shown to bind ovine GM-CSF and ovine IL-2 with high affinity with Kd of 369 pM and 1.04 nM, respectively; however, it does not bind the human equivalents of these molecules, highlighting the adaptation of ORFV to its ovine host [109]. In biological assays, GIF has been shown to inhibit the haemopoietic activity of GM-CSF in a soft-agar bone marrow cell colony assay and ovine IL-2 in a T cell proliferation assay [109]. Furthermore, the activity has been detected in cannulated afferent lymph from ORFV-infected sheep, in which the highest GIF activity detected corresponded to the time of maximum growth of the virus [109]. Sequence comparisons of IL-2 and GM-CSF have not revealed a potential binding domain shared by these cytokines. The only common feature is that they are members of the short-chain, four-α-helical bundle family of cytokines that also includes IL-4; however, GIF does not bind IL-4 [109].

Vascular endothelial growth factor

A gene encoding a polypeptide with homology to mammalian VEGF has been identified in ORFV, [112, 172–174], BPSV [115], PCPV [175], and PVNZ (unpublished data). The viral VEGF is thought to explain the extensive proliferation of vascular endothelial cells, dilation of blood vessels and dermal swelling seen in parapoxvirus lesions. Indeed, reports from as early as 1890 use terms such as "readily bleed" in describing ORFV lesions [9]. VEGF-like factors are not encoded by any other poxviruses and the only other occurrence of a potential viral VEGF is in two closely related iridoviruses of fish [176, 177].

Members of the mammalian VEGF family are major regulators of the formation of new blood vessels during embryogenesis and angiogenesis. The family currently comprises VEGF-A, placental growth factor (PlGF), VEGF-B, VEGF-C and VEGF-D [178]. These factors mediate endothelial cell proliferation, vascular permeability, angiogenesis and lymphangiogenesis *via* the tyrosine kinase receptors VEGFR-1 (Flt-1), VEGFR-2 (KDR/Flk1), and VEGFR-3 (Flt-4) [179]. In general VEGFR-1 plays a role in haematopoietic cell differentiation and migration, VEGFR-2 is involved in vascular endothelial cell mitogenesis, and VEGFR-3 is involved in the regulation of lymphangiogenesis.

The viral VEGFs bind and induce autophosphorylation of VEGFR-2 but do not bind VEGFR-3 and show little recognition of VEGFR-1 [172–174]. This receptor binding spectrum differs from that of all mammalian VEGF family members and the viral VEGFs have been classified as a new subgroup of the family, called VEGF-E [172]. The ORFV and PCPV VEGF have been shown to share a disulphide-linked homodimeric structure with mammalian VEGF, to be mitogenic for endothelial cells and to induce vascular permeability.

Variants of VEGF-E were revealed during the genetic analysis of different strains of ORFV. $ORFV_{NZ2}$ encodes a polypeptide of 14.7 kDa, whereas the $ORFV_{NZ7}$ encodes a polypeptide of 16 kDa. Both forms of VEGF-E show low amino acid sequence identity to mammalian VEGF with $ORFV_{NZ2}$ VEGF-E showing 35% and ORFVNZ7 25% identity to human VEGF-A. Intriguingly, these two viral VEGFs are only 41% identical to each other. The VEGF of PCPV shows 27% amino acid identity to human VEGF-A and 41% and 61% amino acid identity to VEGF encoded by ORFV strains NZ2 and NZ7, respectively [175]. Similar levels of sequence relatedness are observed for the VEGF of BPSV [115] and PVNZ (unpublished).

The sequence disparity of the NZ2 and NZ7 VEGFs has been examined further by sequence analysis of 21 ORFV isolates [180]. It was found that most carried the NZ2-like version but their amino acid sequences varied by up to 31%. Despite the sequence variations, structural predictions for the viral VEGFs were similar to the structure determined for VEGF-A. In addition, the viral VEGFs are all equally active mitogens, stimulating proliferation of human endothelial cells *in vitro* and dermal vascularisation of sheep *in vivo* with potencies equivalent to VEGF-A [181]. It has been suggested that the extensive sequence divergence seen in at least the ORFV VEGF may have been generated primarily by selection against VEGFR-1 binding and its associated recruitment and activation of cells involved in antiviral responses [181].

A recombinant ORFV, in which the VEGF gene was deleted, has been used to assess the contribution of this gene to the vascular responses in infected sheep. The striking proliferation of blood vessels within the dermis underlying the site of infection was absent in sheep infected with the VEGF deletion mutant; however, viral replication in the early stages was not impaired but appeared reduced later in infection [182]. Epidermal hyperplasia is a feature of the response to ORFV infection and this feature was also reduced in infections with the VEGF deletion mutant. The epidermal and vascular responses seen in ORFV lesions are reminiscent of a sustained wound healing response and extravagantly proliferative ORFV lesions have been reported in immunocompromised individuals. Expression of a viral VEGF might assist in maintaining a regenerative response and thereby support extended viral growth. Parapoxviruses do not encode the epidermal growth factor seen in several other poxviruses and which has been associated with localised cellular proliferation.

Another possible role for the viral VEGF relates to the extensive scab formation seen in ORFV lesions. Scab shed from ORFV lesions contains substantial amounts of infectious virus and the scab provides protection from environmental inactivation. In this way the virus remains available to infect naïve animals as much as a year after being shed. The viral VEGF is able to induce vascular permeability and would seem to contribute to scab formation since lesions induced by VEGF-deleted ORFV have essentially no scab [182].

IFN-resistance gene

ORFV is resistant to type 1 and type 2 IFN. A homologue of the VACV IFN resistance factor E3L has been described for ORFV [113, 114] and homologues have since been discovered in BPSV [115]. The E3L gene product inhibits IFN-mediated down-regulation of protein synthesis by binding dsRNA thus preventing the activation of the dsRNA-dependent IFN inducible protein kinase (PKR) [183]. During the antiviral response, PKR phosphorylates itself and the translation initiation factor eIF2-2, thus blocking protein translation and viral replication. The ORFV E3L homologue (ORFV 020) is 31% identical and 57% similar to VACV E3L at the protein level and is expressed early [113]. A predicted dsRNA binding motif is present in ORFV 020 and it has been shown to bind specifically to dsRNA and to competitively inhibit the activation (phosphorylation) of the ovine dsRNA-dependent PKR gene. In addition, cell lysates from ORFV-infected cells diminished PKR phosphorylation, which was also observed in the presence of cytosine arabinoside, indicating that the inhibitory activity is encoded by an early gene [114]. Further, transient expression of ORFV 020 protected Semliki forest virus from the inhibitory effects of IFN-α.

The predicted protein sequence of the BPSV E3L homologue (BPSV-020) is 53% identical to the ORFV protein and it includes a predicted dsRNA binding motif. Both BPSV and ORFV 020 proteins have evidence of a N-terminal Z-DNA binding domain that, in the case of VACV E3L, has been linked to pathogenicity in mouse infection models [184].

Anti-apoptosis

Recently the VACV IFN resistance factor, the E3L protein, has been shown to have anti-apoptotic properties and it has been suggested that these functions are linked to its N-terminal Z-DNA binding domain acting as a transcriptional transactivator of a range of cellular genes [185]. Inspection of the ORFV and BPSV genomes reveals that the VACV E3L homologues are the only parapoxvirus proteins with clear links to the inhibitors of apoptosis identified in other poxviruses. Despite this, investigations in this laboratory have revealed that ORFV is a potent inhibitor of apoptosis and we have identified a mitochondrial-targeted ORFV protein that blocks UV-induced apoptosis and which shows some similarities to Bcl-2 family members (unpublished). Related proteins are present in each of BPSV, PCPV and PVNZ.

Ankyrin repeat, F-box-like proteins

In common with all other chordopoxviruses except MOCV, parapoxviruses encode several proteins carrying the ankyrin repeat motif. This motif is named after the cytoskeleton protein, ankyrin, which contains 24 copies of the motif. The motif is recognised as a mediator of protein-protein interactions. ORFV encodes five such proteins and BPSV seven. Each of the ORFV genes can be paired with a corresponding gene in BPSV, but the direct relationships between the parapoxvirus proteins and other chordopoxvirus ankyrin repeat genes are less clear. In fact, any one of the parapoxvirus ankyrin repeat proteins shows more similarity to all of the other parapoxvirus ankyrin repeat proteins than to any of the ankyrin repeat proteins in other poxviruses. However, all five ORFV and seven BPSV ankyrin repeat proteins carry the C-terminal F-box-like domain present in most poxviral ankyrin repeat proteins and this has led to the suggestion that these proteins may function within the ubiquitin–proteasome system by acting as recognition subunits of cellular ubiquitin ligase complexes [139]. The proteins targeted by the viral ankyrin-F-box proteins might be involved in modulating cellular stress responses or cell cycle regulation [186, 187].

Parapoxviruses and immune evasion

It has become apparent over the last decade that parapoxviruses, like other poxviruses, encode an arsenal of weapons that allows this group to temporarily suppress the host's defences and thus create a window of opportunity in which to replicate. The immunomodulators that have been discovered thus far suggest that this group has the capability to target inflammatory processes, the innate responses such as apoptosis, NK cell activity and antiviral effects of IFN, and the development of adaptive immunity. Although these targets are common to almost all of the poxviruses, the virulence factors encoded by the parapoxviruses in many cases are unique.

As described above, parapoxviruses replicate exclusively within the epidermis and in the case of ORFV within keratinocytes. The skin is the largest organ of the body and has evolved a highly specialised defence system to respond rapidly to invading organisms. Keratinocytes are the principle immune cell within the epidermis and act as proinflammatory signal transducers responding to non-specific stimuli by secreting inflammatory cytokines, chemotactic factors and adhesion molecules into the extracellular fluid of the epidermal compartment [188]. In the initial phase of non-specific cutaneous inflammation, keratinocytes release IL-1β and TNF-α. IL-1β and TNF-α activate dermal vascular endothelium, which up-regulates the expression of adhesion molecules involved in the recruitment of leukocytes to the endothelium. In conjunction with chemokines, these cytokines direct the migration of leukocytes from the circulatory system into the epidermis. TNF-α is down-regulated in activated keratinocytes by cellular IL-10 [189], suggesting that the production of proinflammatory cytokines produced by these cells may be the main targets of viral IL-10 during the early stages of cutaneous inflammation. There is no evidence that parapoxviruses produce receptor-like homologues of IL-1β or TNF-α to sequester these cytokines. Furthermore, there is no evidence at this time to suggest that parapoxviruses produce factors other than IL-10 that disrupt the induction of the proinflammatory signalling cascade in virus infected cells. Poxviruses in general have developed multiple strategies to minimize the deleterious effects of proinflammatory cytokines but few encode a viral IL-10. It is likely that parapoxvirus factors will be discovered in the future that specifically target pathways that lead to the induction of proinflammatory cytokines in virus-infected cells. In addition, the production of proinflammatory cytokines secreted by immigrating macrophages and $CD8^+$ cells are likely to be blocked by viral IL-10.

Apoptosis can be induced by a variety of extracellular inducers including TNF, FAS, IFN, NK cells and cytotoxic T lymphocytes (CTL), as well as agents such as UV light, serum growth factor deprivation and hypoxia and within the cell by macromolecular synthesis such as viral dsRNA. Thus far the parapoxviruses have only been shown to encode one factor that directly inhibits apoptosis and evidence suggests that it acts *via* the mitochondria by inhibiting the release of cytochrome c (unpublished). There is no evidence that parapoxviruses produce factors that bind caspases and factors that disrupt the cellular death effector domains of the TNF or FAS receptor mechanisms common to other poxviruses [190–193]. Furthermore, serpins have not been found, such as CrmA that protects cells from perforin-dependent apoptosis induced by CTL and NK cells [194, 195].

The activities of poxvirus anti-apoptotic proteins are closely interrelated with strategies that target intracellular elements in the IFN response pathway, including the PKR and 2',5' oligoadenylate synthetase [196, 197]. Both of these enzymes are activated by dsRNA. In addition, dsRNA is known to initiate cascades that inhibit protein synthesis and induce apoptosis by activating caspase-8 [198]. As described above, it has been established that ORFV produces a homologue of VAC E3L that binds dsRNA and blocks PKR activation. It has not been established, however, that it blocks other elements in the IFN response pathway that have been reported for VAC E3L, such as inhibiting the induction of IFN-α/β [199], reducing adenosine deaminase editing activity and mediating virus host range [200].

The binding activities of ORFV-CBP (inflammatory CC chemokines and lymphotactin) [111] suggest that parapoxviruses have the capability to establish a blockade to prevent the recruitment of inflammatory cells to the site of infection, in particular monocytes, NK cells, T cells and DC. In addition, the ability of ORFV-CBP to bind lymphotactin suggests that lymphocytes, B cells, DC and NK cells are of particular significance in the immune response to parapoxviruses. Although lymphotactin is also a chemotactic factor for neutrophils, the heavy infiltration of polymorphs into ORFV lesions suggests that these cells are being recruited to the site of infection predominantly by the CXC chemokines to which CBP does not bind. It has recently been reported that $CD8^+$ cytotoxic T cell infiltration into tumours is enhanced by transgene expression of lymphotactin by $CD8^+$ T cells [201]. In light of this observation, it is interesting to note that activated $CD8^+$ cells appear to become trapped under ORFV lesions [100], suggesting that the specificity of CBP for lymphotactin may provide an explanation for this observation.

The discovery of a secreted ORFV GM-CSF/IL-2 binding protein signals the importance of these cytokines in the immune response to parapoxviruses. GM-CSF is produced by a variety of cell types including T cells and keratinocytes [109] and stimulates the recruitment and/or activation of neutrophils, monocytes and eosinophils in tissues [202]. In addition, GM-CSF is involved in the maturation of DC. IL-2 stimulates T cell and NK cell activation and proliferation. It also stimulates the proliferation of activated B cells and may play a role in the survival of cytotoxic T cells at the site of the infection. It is tempting to speculate that $CD8^+$ cytotoxic T cells are a major target of ORFV immunomodulators and that their proliferation, migration, activation and survival are affected by these factors. In addition, GIF could also be interfering with the maturation of DC as discussed below.

IFN-γ is associated with Th1 anti-viral immune responses and all poxviruses have evolved mechanisms to limit its actions [196]. IFN-γ is produced by $CD4^+$, $CD8^+$ and NK cells and has various effects on cells. It stimulates the production of IgG2a synthesis in B cells, inhibits Th2 cell growth, activates MHC class I and class II in macrophages and activates NK cells. Most poxviruses sequester extracellular IFN-γ by producing soluble IFN-γ receptor-like proteins [197]. There is no evidence that parapoxviruses encode such factors. However, parapoxviruses have the potential to suppress the production of IFN-γ since this cytokine is inhibited in NK cells, $CD4^+$ Th1 cells and $CD8^+$ cells by IL-10. In addition to their role in inflammation, TNF-α and IFN-γ are involved in the antiviral innate responses and specific early immune responses. IFN-γ acts synergistically to enhance antiviral cytotoxic activity of TNF-α and the anti-viral activities of IFN-α and IFN-β.

A further point of intervention by parapoxviruses could involve APC, which could be of particular significance during reinfection and persistent infections. It is apparent that the host produces a memory response to ORFV [93, 104], inferring that ORFV has the capability to replicate, albeit temporarily, in the immune host. The question is how ORFV is able to subvert the reactivation of memory T cells during reinfection. The evidence suggests that dermal DC or blood-derived DC are involved in initiating the immune response to ORFV, since Langerhans cells do not appear to play a role [56]. In the normal course of events DC are recruited to the site of infection, capture antigen, mature and migrate to the lymph node in response to constitutive chemokines where they present antigen to naïve T cells or memory T cells. APC other than DC may be involved during reinfection. Parapoxviruses have the potential to disrupt this process at multiple points. It is possible that the viral secreted immunomodulators GIF, IL-10, CBP, and VEGF work in concert to inhibit this process. DC have been observed to accumulate at the site of infection in ORFV-infected animals [56] and it has been observed that there is a reduction in DC trafficking from the epidermis to the lymph node at a point when ORFV replication is maximal, suggesting intervention by viral immunomodulators [92]. Although GIF and viral IL-10 have the potential to disrupt antigen presentation and activation of $CD4^+$ and $CD8^+$ T cells in the lymph node, we have no evidence that the viral cytokines are carried into the lymph node by passive movement. If this is the case, viral IL-10 could potentially block the development of the acquired immune response and may have effects on the development of immune memory, such as the induction of tolerogenic T cells. The IL-2 binding properties of GIF could block clonal expansion of $CD8^+$ cells and the sequestering of lymphotactin could all impact on the development of a Th1 response [131]. It has also been reported that ORFV induces apoptosis in APC *via* the CD95 pathway in a mouse model [203] and CMV-IL-10 has been shown to increase apoptosis associated with DC maturation [204]. This may be a further mechanism that the parapoxviruses exploit to reduce or delay the development of the acquired immune response. It is also possible that parapoxviral IL-10 could skew the immune response towards a Th2 response during the early phase of infection, as proposed for CMV *via* viral IL-10 [204] and that may also involve the induction of immunological tolerance. Such a response might explain persistent parapoxvirus infections.

In conclusion, the accumulated evidence suggests that the parapoxviruses have evolved mechanisms to temporarily delay viral clearance by a Th1 immune response. It is possible that this strategy is only successful where virus replication is localised and restricted to specific tissues, such as the skin epithelium. The short range effects of the secreted viral immunomodulators in this instance are unlikely to compromise the general integrity of the host's immune system such as might occur with a more generalised infection.

Parapoxviruses in immunotherapy and recombinant vaccines

Although ORFV encodes potential immune-evasion factors, the attenuated strain D1701 possesses a variety of immunostimulatory properties [205–209]. Moreover, the massive accumulation of DC that occurs around the lesion in the natural host [98] is thought to indicate some chemoattractive activities. These properties lead to the development of the so-called 'paraimmunity inducer' licensed as immunomodulator Baypamun® [203, 205, 206]. Recent studies with inactivated $ORFV_{D1701}$ have shown that it induces a complex autoregulatory cytokine response that involves the up-regulation of IL-12, IL-18, IFN-γ and other Th1 cytokines and their subsequent down-regulation that is accompanied by the induction of IL-4 [210]. The powerful immune enhancing effect of D1701 may have application in immunotherapy. ORFV has been shown to mediate anti-viral activity and is effective in mice infected with herpes simplex virus type 1, in a guinea pig model of recurrent genital herpes disease and in a transgenic mouse model of human HBV replication, without any signs of inflammation or other side effects [210].

The potential and development of parapoxviruses as recombinant vaccines in permissive and non-permissive hosts has been described [1, 211–215]. The use of parapoxviruses in permissive hosts may have advantages over other recombinant viral vaccines since parapoxviruses only cause localised skin lesions that resolve within weeks and they do not cause systemic infection [1]. In addition, ORFV represents a promising candidate as a novel vaccine vector due to its immunomodulating properties even in non-permissive hosts [211]. Recombinant parapoxvirus vectors have been shown to induce protective immunity against the lethal alphaherpes virus of swine and pseudorabies virus in a non-permissive mouse model [215]. $ORFV_{D1701}$

recombinants have been produced that express the glycoproteins gC and gD of pseudorabies virus. The study demonstrated the potential of the parapoxvirus recombinant vector vaccines to efficiently prime both protective humoral and cell-mediated immune mechanisms in a non-permissive host species for the virus. In a further study, intramuscular injection of recombinant $ORFV_{D1701}$ expressing the nucleoprotein p40 of Borna disease virus was shown to protect rats against Borna disease virus infection of the brain [211]. The results of investigations thus far suggest that recombinant parapoxviruses have exciting potential as new vaccine vector.

References

1 Robinson AJ, Lyttle DJ (1992) Parapoxviruses: their biology and potential as recombinant vaccines. In: M Binns, GL Smith (eds): *Recombinant poxviruses*. CRC Press, Boca Raton, 285–327

2 Downie AW, Dumbell KR (1956) Poxviruses. *Annu Rev* Microbiol 10: 237–252

3 Andrewes C, Pereira (eds) (1964) *Viruses of vertebrates*. Baillière, Tindall, Cassell, London

4 Wildy P (1971) Classification and nomenclature of viruses. First report of the International Committee on Nomenclature of Viruses. *Monogr Virol* 5: 28; cited in [1]

5 Fenner F (1976) Classification and nomenclature of viruses. Second report of the International Committee on Taxonomy of Viruses. *Intervirology* 7: 1–115

6 Fauquet CM, Mayo, MA, Maniloff J, Desselberger U, Ball LA (eds) (2005) *Virus Taxonomy. Eighth report of the International committee on Taxonomy of viruses*. Academic Press, Elservier, London, 117–133

7 Thomas K, Tompkins DM, Sainsbury AW, Wood A, Dalziel R, Nettleton PF, McInnes CJ (2003) A novel poxvirus lethal to red squirrels (*Sciurus vulgaris*). *J Gen Virol* 84: 3337–3341

8 Steeb (1787) Von der Schaf-Raude (Grind); cited in: H. Nürnberg: Über den ansteckenden Maulgrind der Schafe und Ziegen. Dr. med. vet. thesis, Friedrich-Wilhelms-Universität, Berlin

9 Walley T (1890) Contagious dermatitis: "orf" in sheep. *J Comp Pathol Ther* 3: 357–360

10 Hansen (1879) Tidsskr Vet 9: 298; cited in: Hodgson-Jones IS (1951) Orf in London. *Br Med J* 1: 795

11 Aynaud M (1923) La stomatite pustuleuse contagieuse des ovins (chancre du mouton. *Ann Inst Pasteur (Paris)* 36: 498–527

12 Bonnevie P (1937) Milker's warts: infection from "false cowpox" with a paravaccinia virus. *Br J Dermatol* 49: 165; cited in: M Binns, GL Smith (eds): *Recombinant poxviruses*. CRC Press, Boca Raton

13 Lipschutz B (1932) Paravaccine, Julius Springer, Berlin; cited in: M Binns, GL Smith (eds): *Recombinant poxviruses*. CRC Press, Boca Raton

14 Griesemer RA, Cole CR (1960) Bovine papular stomatitis. I. Recognition in the United States. *J Am Vet Med Assoc* 137: 404–410

15 Degive A (1884) Une affection-type ou maladie inedite – la stomatite papillaire

ou papillomateuse – observee sur quatre genesis. *Ann Med Vet* 33: 369; cited in: M Binns, GL Smith (eds): *Recombinant poxviruses*. CRC Press, Boca Raton
16 Plowright WR, Ferris RD (1959) Papular stomatitis of cattle. II. Reproduction of the disease with culture-passaged virus. *Vet Rec* 71: 828; cited in: M Binns, GL Smith (eds): *Recombinant poxviruses*. CRC Press, Boca Raton
17 Griesemer RA, Cole CR (1961) Bovine papular stomatitis. II. The experimentally produced disease. *Am J Vet Res* 22: 473–481
18 Carson CA, Kerr KM (1967) Bovine papular stomatitis with apparent transmission to man. *J Am Vet Med Assoc* 151:183–187
19 Rosliakov AA (1972) Comparative ultrastructure of viruses of camel pox, pox-like disease of camels (AUZDUK) and contagious ecthyma of sheep. *Voprosi Virusol* 17: 26–30
20 Dashtseren T, Solovyev BV, Varejka F, Khokhoo A (1984) Camel contagious ecthyma (Pustular Dermatitis). *Acta Virol* 28:128–133
21 Jezek Z, Kriz B, Rothbauer V (1983) Camelpox and its risk to the human population. *J Hyg Epidemiol Microbiol Immunol* 27: 29–42
22 Munz E, Schillinger D, Reimann M, Mahnel H (1986) Electron microscopical diagnosis of Ecthyma contagiosum in camels (*Camelus dromedarius*). First report of the disease in Kenya. *Zentralbl Veterinarmed B* 33: 73–77
23 Azwai SM, Carter SD, Woldehiwet Z (1995) Immune responses of the camel (*Camelus dromedarius*) to contagious ecthyma (*Orf*) virus infection. *Vet Microbiol* 47: 119–131
24 Hartung J (1980) Contagious ecthyma of sheep (cases in man, dog, alpaca and camel). *Tieraerztl Prax* 8: 435–438
25 Wilson TM, Poglayen-Neuwall I (1971) Pox in South American sea lions (Otaria byronia). *Can J Comp Med* 35: 174–177
26 Wilson T, Cheville N, Karstad L (1969) Seal pox. *Bull Wild Dis Assoc* 5: 412–418
27 Wilson TM, Dykes RW, Tsai KS (1972) Pox in young, captive harbor seals. *J Am Vet Med Assoc* 161: 611–617
28 Becher P, Konig M, Muller G, Siebert U, Thiel HJ (2002) Characterization of sealpox virus, a separate member of the parapoxviruses. *Arch Virol* 147: 1133–1140
29 Hadlow WJ, Cheville NF, Jellison WL (1980) Occurence of pox in northern fur seal on the Pribilof Islands in 1951. *J Wildl Dis* 16: 305 312
30 Simpson VR, Stuart NC, Stack MJ, Ross HA, Head JC (1994) Parapox infection in grey seals (*Halichoerus grypus*) in Cornwall. *Vet Rec* 134: 292–296
31 Osterhaus AD, Broeders HW, Visser IK, Teppema JS, Vedder EJ (1990) Isolation of an orthopoxvirus from pox-like lesions of a grey seal (*Halichoerus grypus*). *Vet Rec* 127: 91–92
32 Hicks BD, Worthy GA (1987) Sealpox in captive grey seals (*Halichoerus grypus*) and their handlers. *J Wildl Dis* 23: 1–6
33 Tryland M, Klein J, Nordoy ES, Blix AS (2005) Isolation and partial characterization of a parapoxvirus isolated from a skin lesion of a Weddell seal. *Virus Res* 108: 83–87
34 Horner GW, Robinson AJ, Hunter R, Cox BT, Smith R (1987) Parapoxvirus infections in New Zealand farmed red deer. *NZ Vet J* 35: 41–45

35 Robinson AJ, Mercer AA (1995) Parapoxvirus of red deer: evidence for its inclusion as a new member in the genus parapoxvirus. *Virology* 208: 812–815
36 Buttner M, von Einem C, McInnes C, Oksanen A (1995) Clinical findings and diagnosis of a severe parapoxvirus epidemic in Finnish reindeer. *Tierarztl Prax* 23: 614–618
37 Tryland M, Josefsen TD, Oksanen A, Aschfalk A (2001) Parapoxvirus infection in Norwegian semi-domesticated reindeer (*Rangifer tarandus tarandus*). *Vet Rec* 149, 394–395
38 Tikkanen MK, McInnes CJ, Mercer AA, Buttner M, Tuimala J, Hirvela-Koski V, Neuvonen E, Huovilainen (2004) Recent isolates of parapoxvirus of Finnish reindeer (*Rangifer tarandus tarandus*) are closely related to bovine pseudocowpox virus. *J Gen Virol* 85: 1413–1418
39 Buttner M, Rziha HJ (2002) Parapoxviruses: from the lesion to the viral genome. *J Vet Med B Infect Dis Vet Public Health* 49: 7–16
40 Reid HW (1991) Orf. In: WB Martin, ID Aitken (eds) *Diseases of sheep*. Blackwell, London, 265–269
41 Lloyd JB (1996) A study of the immune response of sheep to orf virus. *Ph.D thesis*, Department of Veterinary Pathology, University of Sydney, Sydney
42 Blood DC, Radostits OM, Henderson JA, Arundel JH, Gay CC (1983) *Veterinary medicine: a textbook of the diseases of cattle, sheep, goats and horses.* Bailliere Tindall, London, 945–946
43 Greig A, Linklater KA, Clark WA (1984) Persistent orf in a ram. *Vet Rec* 115: 149
44 McKeever DJ (1984) Persistent orf. *Vet Rec* 115: 334–335
45 Inoshima Y, Yamamoto Y, Takahashi T, Shino M, Katsumi A, Shimizu S, Sentsui H (2001) Serological survey of parapoxvirus infection in wild ruminants in Japan in 1996–99. *Epidemiol Infect* 126: 153–156
46 Inoshima Y, Murakami K, Wu D, Sentsui H (2002) Characterization of parapoxviruses circulating among wild Japanese serows (*Capricornis crispus*). *Microbiol Immunol* 46: 583–587
47 Maollin AS, Zessin KH (1988) Outbreak of camel contagious ecthyma in central Somalia. *Trop Anim Health Prod* 20: 185
48 Gitao CG (1994) Outbreaks of contagious ecthyma in camels (*Camelus dromedarius*) in the Turkana district of Kenya. *Rev Sci Tech* 13: 939–945
49 Klein J, Tryland M (2005) Characterisation of parapoxviruses isolated from Norwegian semi-domesticated reindeer (*Rangifer tarandus tarandus*). *Virol J* 2: 79
50 Afonso CL, Delhon G, Tulman ER, Lu Z, Zsak A, Becerra VM, Zsak L, Kutish GF, Rock DL (2005) Genome of deerpox virus. *J Virol* 79: 966–977
51 Abu Elzein EM, Housawi FM (1997) Severe long-lasting contagious ecthyma infection in a goat's kid. *Zentralbl Veterinarmed B* 44: 561–564
52 Haig DM, Mercer AA (1998) Ovine diseases. Orf. *Vet Res* 29:311–326
53 Nettleton PF, Munro R, Pow I, Gilray J, Gray EW, Reid HW (1995) Isolation of a parapoxvirus from a grey seal (*Halichoerus grypus*). *Vet Rec* 137: 562–564
54 McKeever DJ, Jenkinson DM, Hutchison G, Reid HW (1988) Studies of the pathogenesis of orf virus infection in sheep. *J Comp Pathol* 99: 317–328
55 Jenkinson DM, McEwan PE, Onwuka SK, Moss VA, Elder HY, Hutchison G,

Reid HW (1990) The polymorphonuclear and mast cell responses in ovine skin infected with orf virus. *Vet Dermatol* 1: 71–77
56 Jenkinson DM, Hutchison G, Onwuka SK, Reid HW (1991) Changes in the MHC class II dendritic cell population of ovine skin in response to orf virus infection. *Vet Dermatol* 2: 1–9
57 Groves RW, Wilson-Jones E, MacDonald DM (1991) Human orf and milkers' nodule: a clinicopathologic study. *J Am Acad Dermatol* 25: 706–711
58 Ghislain PD, Dinet Y, Delescluse J (2001) Orf in urban surroundings and religious practices: a study over a 3-year period. *Ann Dermatol Venereol* 128: 889–892
59 Leavell UW, McNamara J, Muelling RJ, Landrum F (1965) Ecthyma contagiosum virus (orf). *South Med J* 58: 239–243
60 Becker FT (1940) Milkers nodules. *JAMA* 115: 2140–2144
61 Falk ES (1978) Parapoxvirus infections of reindeer and musk ox associated with unusual human infections. *Br J Dermatol* 99: 647–654
62 Savage J, Black MM (1972) "Giant orf" of a finger in a patient with lymphoma. *Proc R Soc Med* 64: 766–768
63 Tan ST, Blake GB, Chambers S (1991) Recurrent orf in an immunocompromised host. *Br J Plastic Surg* 44: 465–467
64 Agger WA, Webster SB (1983) Human orf infection complicated by erythema multiformae. *Cutis* 31: 334–338
65 Blakemore F, Abdussalam M, Goldsmith WN (1948) A case of orf (contagious pustular dermatitis): identification of the virus. *Br J Dermatol* 60: 404–409
66 Fastier LB (1957) Human infections with the virus of ovine contagious pustular dermatitis. *NZ Med J* 56: 121–123
67 Mourtada I, Le Tourneur M, Chevrant-Breton J, Le Gall F (2000) Human orf and erythema multiforme. *Ann Dermatol Venereol* 127: 397–399
68 Erickson GA, Carbrey EA, Gustafson GA (1975) Generalised contagious ecthyma in a sheep rancher: diagnostic considerations. *J Am Vet Med Assoc* 166: 262–263
69 Sanchez RL, Hebert A, Lucia H, Swedo J (1985) Orf. A case report with histologic, electron microscopic, and immunoperoxidase studies. *Arch Pathol Lab Med* 109: 166–170
70 Geerinck K, Lukito G, Snoeck R, De Vos R, De Clercq E, Vanrenterghem Y, Degreef H, Maes B. (2001) A case of human orf in an immunocompromised patient treated successfully with cidofovir cream. *J Med Virol* 64: 543–549
71 Abdussalam M, Cosslett VE (1957) Contagious pustular dermatitis. *J Comp Pathol* 67:145–156
72 Reczko E (1957) Electronenmikroskopische untersuchungen am virus der stomatitis papulosa. *Zentralbl Bakteriol Abt Orig B* 169: 425–453
73 Nagington J, Horne RW (1962) Morphological studies of orf and vaccinia viruses. *Virology* 16: 248–260
74 Nagington J, Newton AA, Horne RW (1964) The structure of orf virus. *Virology* 23: 461–472
75 Peters D, Muller G, Buttner D (1964) The fine structure of paravaccinia viruses. *Virology* 23: 609–611

76 Mitchiner MB (1969) The envelope of vaccinia and orf viruses: an electron-cytochemical investigation. *J Gen Virol* 5: 211–220

77 Hiramatsu Y, Uno F, Yoshida M, Hatano Y, Nii S (1999) Poxvirus virions: their surface ultrastructure and interaction with the surface membrane of host cells. *J Electron Microsc (Tokyo)* 48: 937–946

78 Ballasu TC, Robinson AJ (1987) Orf virus replication in bovine testis cells: kinetics of viral DNA, polypeptide, and infectious virus production and analysis of virion polypeptides. *Arch Virol* 97: 267–281

79 Buddle BM, Dellers RW, Schurig GG (1984) Heterogeneity of contagious ecthyma virus isolates. *Am J Vet Res* 45: 75–79

80 McKeever DJ, Reid HW, Inglis NF, Herring AJ (1987) A qualitative and quantitative assessment of the humoral antibody response of the sheep to orf virus infection. *Vet Microbiol* 15: 229–241

81 Rosenbusch RF, Reed DE (1983) Reaction of convalescent bovine antisera with strain-specific antigens of parapoxviruses. *Am J Vet Res* 44: 875–878

82 Thomas V, Flores L, Holowczak JA (1980) Biochemical and electron microscopic studies of the replication and composition of milker's node virus. *J Virol* 34: 244–255

83 Housawi FM, Roberts GM, Gilray JA, Pow I, Reid HW, Nettleton PF, Sumption KJ, Hibma MH, Mercer AA (1998) The reactivity of monoclonal antibodies against orf virus with other parapoxviruses and the identification of a 39 kDa immunodominant protein. *Arch Virol* 143: 2289–2303

84 Czerny CP, Waldmann R, Scheubeck T (1997) Identification of three distinct antigenic sites in parapoxviruses. *Arch Virol* 142: 807–821

85 Scagliarini A, Ciulli S, Battilani M, Jacoboni I, Montesi F, Casadio R, Prosperi S (2002) Characterisation of immunodominant protein encoded by the F1L gene of orf virus strains isolated in Italy. *Arch Virol* 147: 1989–1995

86 Zinoviev VV, Tchikaev NA, Chertov O, Malygin EG (1994) Identification of the gene encoding vaccinia virus immunodominant protein p35. *Gene* 147: 209–214

87 da Fonseca FG, Wolffe EJ, Weisberg A, Moss B (2000) Characterization of the vaccinia virus H3L envelope protein: topology and posttranslational membrane insertion via the C-terminal hydrophobic tail. *J Virol* 74: 7508–7517

88 da Fonseca FG, Wolffe EJ, Weisberg A, Moss B (2000) Effects of deletion or stringent repression of the H3L envelope gene on vaccinia virus replication. *J Virol* 74: 7518–7528

89 Lin CL, Chung CS, Heine HG, Chang W (2000) Vaccinia virus envelope H3L protein binds to cell surface heparan sulfate and is important for intracellular mature virion morphogenesis and virus infection *in vitro* and *in vivo*. *J Virol* 74: 3353–3365

90 Yirrell DL, Vestey JP, Norval M (1994) Immune responses of patients to orf virus infection. *Br J Dermatol* 130: 438–443

91 Smith GL, Vanderplasschen A (1998) Extracellular enveloped vaccinia virus. In: L Enjuanes, SG Siddell, W Spaan (eds): *Coronaviruses and Arteriviruses*. Plenum Press, London, 395–414

92 Haig DM, McInnes CJ (2002) Immunity and counter-immunity during infection with the parapoxvirus orf virus. *Virus Res* 88: 3–16

93 Buddle BM, Pulford HD (1984) Effect of passively-acquired antibodies and vaccination of the immune response to contagious ecthyma virus. *Vet Microbiol* 9: 515–522
94 Robinson AJ, Mercer AA (1988) Orf virus and vaccinia virus do not cross-protect sheep. *Arch Virol* 101: 255–259
95 Mercer AA, Yirrell DL, Reid HW, Robinson AJ (1994) Lack of cross-protection between vaccinia virus and orf virus in hysterectomy-procured, barrier maintained lambs. *Vet Microbiol* 41: 373–382
96 Jenkinson D, McEwan PE, Onwuka SK, Moss VA, Elder HY, Hutchison G, Reid H W (1990) The pathological changes and polymorphonuclear and mast cell responses in the skin of specific pathogen-free lambs following primary and secondary challenge with orf virus. *Vet Dermatol* 1: 139–150
97 Jenkinson DM, Hutchison G, Reid HW (1992) The B and T cell responses to orf virus infection of ovine skin. *Vet Dermatol* 3: 57–64
98 Lear A, Hutchison G, Reid HW, Norval M, Haig DM (1996) Phenotypic characterisation of the dendritic cells accumulating in ovine dermis following primary and secondary orf virus infections. *Eur J Dermatol* 6: 135–140
99 Anderson IE, Reid HW, Nettleton PF, McInnes CJ, Haig DM (2001) Detection of cellular cytokine mRNA expression during orf virus infection in sheep: differential interferon-gamma mRNA expression by cells in primary versus reinfection skin lesions. *Vet Immunol Immunopathol* 83: 161–176
100 Haig DM, Hutchinson G, Thomson J, Yirrell D, Reid HW (1996) Cytolytic activity and associated serine protease expression by skin and afferent lymph CD8+ T cells during orf virus reinfection. *J Gen Virol* 77: 953–961
101 Yirrell DL, Reid HW, Norval M, Entrican G, Miller HR (1991) Response of efferent lymph and popliteal lymph node to epidermal infection of sheep with orf virus. *Vet Immunol Immunopathol* 28: 219–235
102 Yirrell DL, Reid HW, Norval M, Miller HR (1991) Qualitative and quantitative changes in ovine afferent lymph draining the site of epidermal orf virus infection *Vet Dermatol* 2: 133–141
103 Haig DM, Entrican G, Yirrell DL, Deane D, Millar HR, Norval M, Reid HW (1992) Differential appearance of interferon and colony stimulating activity in afferent versus efferent lymph following orf virus infection in sheep. *Vet Dermatol* 3: 221–229
104 Haig D, Deane D, Percival A, Myatt N, Thomson J, Inglis L, Rothel J, Heng-Fong S, Wood P, Miller HR, Reid HW (1996) The cytokine response of afferent lymph following orf virus reinfection of sheep. *Vet Dermatol* 7: 11–20
105 Haig DM, Hopkins J, Miller HR (1999) Local immune responses in afferent and efferent lymph. *Immunology* 96: 155–163
106 Haig DM, McInnes CJ, Hutchison G, Seow HF, Reid HW (1996) Cyclosporin A abrogates the acquired immunity to cutaneous reinfection with the parapoxvirus orf virus. *Immunology* 89: 524–531
107 Lloyd JB, Gill HS, Haig DM, Husband AJ (2000) *In vivo* T-cell subset depletion suggests that $CD4^+$ T-cells and a humoral immune response are important for the elimination of orf virus from the skin of sheep. *Vet Immunol Immunopathol* 74: 249–262
108 Haig DM, Deane DL, Myatt N, Thomson J, Entrican G, Rothel J, Reid HW

(1996) The activation status of ovine CD45R+ and CD45R− efferent lymph T cells after orf virus reinfection. *J Comp Pathol* 115: 163–174
109 Deane D, McInnes CJ, Percival A, Wood A, Thomson J, Lear A, Gilray J, Fleming S, Mercer A, Haig D (2000) Orf virus encodes a novel secreted protein inhibitor of granulocyte-macrophage colony-stimulating factor and interleukin-2. *J Virol* 74: 1313–1320
110 Fleming SB, McCaughan CA, Andrews AE, Nash AD, Mercer AA (1997) A homologue of interleukin-10 is encoded by the poxvirus orf virus. *J Virol* 71: 4857–4861
111 Seet BT, McCaughan CA, Handel TM, Mercer AA, Brunetti C, McFadden G, Fleming SB (2003) Analysis of an orf virus chemokine-binding protein: Shifting ligand specificities among a family of poxvirus viroceptors. *Proc Natl Acad Sci USA* 100: 15137–15142
112 Lyttle DJ, Fraser KM, Fleming SB, Mercer AA, Robinson AJ (1994) Homologs of vascular endothelial growth factor are encoded by the poxvirus orf virus. *J Virol* 68: 84–92
113 McInnes CJ, Wood AR, Mercer AA (1998) Orf virus encodes a homolog of the vaccinia virus interferon-resistance gene E3L. *Virus Genes* 17: 107–115
114 Haig DM, McInnes CJ, Thomson J, Wood A, Bunyan K, Mercer A (1998) The orf virus OV20.0L gene product is involved in interferon resistance and inhibits an interferon-inducible, double-stranded RNA-dependent kinase. *Immunology* 93: 335–340
115 Delhon G, Tulman ER, Afonso CL, Lu Z, de la Concha-Bermejillo A, Lehmkuhl HD, Piccone ME, Kutish GF, Rock DL (2004) Genomes of the parapoxviruses ORF virus and bovine papular stomatitis virus. *J Virol* 78:168–177
116 Menna A, Wittek R, Bachmann PA, Mayer A, Wyler R (1979) Physical characterisation of a stomatitis papulosa virus genome: a cleavage map for the restriction endonucleases HindIII and EcoRI. *Arch Virol* 59: 145–156
117 Wittek R, Kuenzle CC, Wyler R (1979) High G+C content in parapoxvirus DNA. *J Gen Virol* 43: 231–234
118 Wittek R, Herlyn M, Schumperli D, Bachmann PA, Mayr A, Wyler R (1980) Genetic and antigenic heterogeneity of different parapoxvirus strains. *Intervirology* 13: 33–41
119 Gassmann U, Wyler R, Wittek R (1985) Analysis of parapoxvirus genomes. *Arch Virol* 83: 17–31
120 Wood AR, McInnes CJ (2003) Transcript mapping of the ‚early' genes of Orf virus. *J Gen Virol* 84: 2993–2998
121 McInnes CJ, Wood AR, Nettleton PE, Gilray JA (2001) Genomic comparison of an avirulent strain of Orf virus with that of a virulent wild type isolate reveals that the Orf virus G2L gene is non-essential for replication. *Virus Genes* 22: 141–150
122 Haig DM, Thomson J, McInnes CJ, Deane DL, Anderson IE, McCaughan CA, Imlach W, Mercer AA, Howard CJ, Fleming SB (2002) A comparison of the anti-inflammatory and immunostimulatory activities of orf virus and ovine interleukin-10. *Virus Res* 90: 303–316
123 Fleming SB, Blok J, Fraser KM, Mercer AA, Robinson AJ (1993) Conservation

of gene structure and arrangement between vaccinia virus and orf virus. *Virology* 195: 175–184

124 Mercer AA, Lyttle DJ, Whelan EM, Fleming SB, Sullivan JT (1995) The establishment of a genetic map of orf virus reveals a pattern of genomic organization that is highly conserved among divergent poxviruses. *Virology* 212: 698–704

125 Robinson AJ, Ellis G, Ballasu T (1982) The genome of orf virus: restriction endonuclease analysis of viral DNA isolated from lesions of orf virus in sheep. *Arch Virol* 71: 43–55

126 Robinson AJ, Barns G, Fraser K, Carpenter E, Mercer AA (1987) Conservation and variation in orf virus genomes. *Virology* 157: 13–23

127 Mercer AA, Fraser K, Barns G, Robinson AJ (1987) The structure and cloning of orf virus DNA. *Virology* 157: 1–12

128 Mercer AA, Fraser KM, Stockwell PA, Robinson AJ (1989) A homologue of retroviral pseudoproteases in the parapoxvirus orf virus. *Virology* 172: 665–668

129 Klemperer N, Lyttle D J, Tauzin D, Traktman P, Robinson AJ (1995) Identification and characterization of the orf virus type I topoisomerase. *Virology* 206, 203–215

130 Naase M, Nicholson BH, Fraser KM, Mercer AA, Robinson AJ (1991) An orf virus sequence showing homology to the 14K ‚fusion' protein of vaccinia virus. *J Gen Virol* 72: 1177–1181

131 Seet BT, McFadden G (2002) Viral chemokine-binding proteins. *J Leukoc Biol* 72: 24–34

132 Sullivan JT, Fraser KM, Fleming SB, Robinson AJ, Mercer AA (1995) Sequence and transcriptional analysis of an orf virus gene encoding ankyrin-like repeat sequences. *Virus Genes* 93: 277–282

133 Fleming SB, Fraser KM, Mercer AA, Robinson AJ (1991) Vaccinia virus-like early transcriptional control sequences flank an early gene in orf virus. *Gene* 97: 207–212

134 Fleming SB, Mercer AA, Fraser KM, Lyttle DJ, Robinson AJ (1992) *In vivo* recognition of orf virus early transcriptional promoters in a vaccina virus recombinant. *Virology* 187: 464–471

135 Vos JC, Mercer AA, Fleming SB, Robinson AJ (1992) *In vitro* recognition of an orf virus early promoter in a vaccinia virus extract. *Arch Virol* 123: 223–228

136 Sullivan JT, Fleming SB, Robinson AJ, Mercer AA (1995) Sequence and transcriptional analysis of a near-terminal region of the orf virus genome. *Virus Genes* 11: 21–29

137 Sullivan JT, Mercer AA, Fleming SB, Robinson AJ (1994) Identification and characterization of an orf virus homologue of the vaccinia virus gene encoding the major envelope antigen p37K. *Virology* 202: 968–973

138 Mercer AA, Ueda N, Friederichs SM, Hofmann K, Fraser KM, Bateman T, Fleming SB (2006) Comparative analysis of genome sequences of three isolates of Orf virus reveals unexpected sequence variation. *Virus Res* 116: 146–158

139 Mercer AA, Fleming SB, Ueda N (2005) F-Box-Like domains are present in most poxvirus ankyrin repeat proteins. *Virus Genes* 31: 127–133

140 Inoshima Y, Murakami K, Yokoyama T, Sentsui H (2001) Genetic heteroge-

neity among parapoxviruses isolated from sheep, cattle and Japanese serows (*Capricornis crispus*). *J Gen Virol* 82: 1215–1220
141 Upton C, Slack S, Hunter AL, Ehlers A, Roper RL (2003) Poxvirus orthologous clusters: toward defining the minimum essential poxvirus genome. *J Virol* 77: 590–600
142 Gubser C, Hue S, Kella P, Smith GL (2004) Poxvirus genomes: a phylogenetic analysis. *J Gen Virol* 85: 105–117
143 Fleming SB, Lyttle DJ, Sullivan JT, Mercer AA, Robinson AJ (1995) Genomic analysis of a transposition-deletion variant of orf virus reveals a 3.3 kbp region of non-essential DNA. *J Gen Virol* 76: 2969–2978
144 Esposito JJ, Cabradilla CD, Nakano JH, Obijeski JF (1981) Intragenomic sequence transposition in monkeypox virus. *Virology* 109: 231–243
145 Pickup DJ, Ink BS, Parsons BL, Hu W, Joklik WK (1984) Spontaneous deletions and duplications of sequences in the genome of cowpox virus. *Proc Natl Acad Sci USA* 81: 6817–6821
146 Moyer RW, Rothe CT (1980) The white pock mutants of rabbit poxvirus. I. Spontaneous host range mutants contain deletions. *Virology* 102: 119–132
147 Kotwal GJ, Moss B (1988) Analysis of a large cluster of nonessential genes deleted from a vaccinia virus terminal transposition mutant. *Virology* 167: 524–537
148 Cottone R, Buttner M, Bauer B, Henkel M, Hettich E, Rziha HJ (1998) Analysis of genomic rearrangement and subsequent gene deletion of the attenuated Orf virus strain D1701. *Virus Res* 56: 53–67
149 Lee HJ, Essani K, Smith GL (2001) The genome sequence of Yaba-like disease virus, a yatapoxvirus. *Virology* 281: 170–192
150 Tulman ER, Afonso CL, Lu Z, Zsak L, Kutish GF, Rock DL (2001) Genome of lumpy skin disease virus. *J Virol* 75: 7122–7130
151 Moore KW, De Waal Malefyte R, Coffman R, O'Garra A (2001) Interleukin-10 and interleukin-10 receptor. *Annu Rev Immunol* 19: 683–704
152 Kotenko SV, Saccani S, Izotova LS, Mirochnitchenko OV, Pestka S (2000) Human cytomegalovirus harbors its own unique IL-10 homolog (cmvIL-10). *Proc Natl Acad Sci USA* 97: 1695–1700
153 Lockridge KM, Zhou SS, Kravitz RH, Johnson JL, Sawai ET, Blewett EL, Barry PA (2000) Primate cytomegaloviruses encode and express an IL-10-like protein. *Virology* 268: 272–280
154 Bartlett NW, Dumoutier L, Renauld JC, Kotenko SV, McVey CE, Lee HJ, Smith GL (2004) A new member of the interleukin 10-related cytokine family encoded by a poxvirus. *J Gen Virol* 85: 1401–1412
155 Imlach W, McCaughan CA, Mercer AA, Haig D, Fleming SB (2002) Orf virus-encoded interleukin-10 stimulates the proliferation of murine mast cells and inhibits cytokine synthesis in murine peritoneal macrophages. *J Gen Virol* 83: 1049–1058
156 Lateef Z, Fleming SB, Halliday G, Faulkner L, Mercer A, Baird M (2003) Orf virus-encoded interleukin-10 inhibits maturation, antigen presentation and migration of murine dendritic cells. *J Gen Virol* 84: 1101–1109
157 Zdanov A, Schalk-Hihi C, Gustchina A, Tsang M, Weatherbee J, Wlodawer A

(1995) Crystal structure of interleukin-10 reveals the functional dimer with an unexpected topological similarity to interferon gamma. *Structure* 3: 591–601
158 Zdanov A, Schalk-Hihi C, Wlodawer A (1996) Crystal structure of human interleukin-10 at 1.6 Å resolution and a model of a complex with its soluble receptor. *Protein Sci* 5: 1955–1962
159 Walter MR, Nagabhushan TL (1995) Crystal structure of interleukin 10 reveals an interferon gamma-like fold. *Biochemistry* 34: 12118–12125
160 Josephson K, Logsdon NJ, Walter MR (2001) Crystal structure of the IL-10/IL-10R1 complex reveals a shared receptor binding site. *Immunity* 15: 35–46
161 MacNeil IA, Suda T, Moore KW, Mosmann TR, Zlotnik A (1990) IL-10, a novel growth cofactor for mature and immature T cells. *J Immunol* 145: 4167–4173
162 Go NF, Castle BE, Barrett R, Kastelein R, Dang W, Mosmann TR, Moore KW, Howard M (1990) Interleukin 10, a novel B cell stimulatory factor: unresponsiveness of X chromosome-linked immunodeficiency B cells. *J Exp Med* 172: 1625–1631
163 Vieira P, de Waal-Malefyt R, Dang MN, Johnson KE, Kastelein R, Fiorentino DF, deVries JE, Roncarolo MG, Mosmann TR, Moore KW (1991) Isolation and expression of human cytokine synthesis inhibitory factor cDNA clones: homology to Epstein-Barr virus open reading frame BCRFI. *Proc Natl Acad Sci USA* 88: 1172–1176
164 Suzuki T, Tahara H, Narula S, Moore KW, Robbins PD, Lotze MT (1995) Viral interleukin 10 (IL-10), the human herpes virus 4 cellular IL-10 homologue, induces local anergy to allogeneic and syngeneic tumors. *J Exp Med* 182: 477–486
165 Fickenscher H, Hor S, Kupers H, Knappe A, Wittmann S, Sticht H (2002) The interleukin-10 family of cytokines. *Trends Immunol* 23: 89–96
166 Smith C, Smith T, Smolak P, Friend D, Hagen H, Gerhart M, Park L, Pickup D, Torrance D, Mohler K et al (1997) Poxvirus genomes encode a secreted, soluble protein that preferentially inhibits beta chemokine activity yet lacks sequence homology to known chemokine receptors. *Virology* 236: 316–327
167 Graham KA, Lalani AS, Macen JL, Ness TL, Barry M, Liu LY, Lucas A, Clark-Lewis I, Moyer RW, McFadden G (1997) The T1/35kDa family of poxvirus-secreted proteins bind chemokines and modulate leukocyte influx into virus-infected tissues. *Virology* 229: 12–24
168 Rossi D, Zlotnik A (2000) The biology of chemokines and their receptors. *Annu Rev Immunol* 18: 217–242
169 Murphy PM, Baggiolini M, Charo IF, Hebert CA, Horuk R, Matsushima K, Miller LH, Oppenheim JJ, Power CA (2000) International union of pharmacology. XXII. Nomenclature for chemokine receptors. *Pharmacol Rev* 52: 145–176
170 McInnes CJ, Deane D, Haig D, Percival A, Thomson J, Wood AR (2005) Glycosylation, disulfide bond formation, and the presence of a WSXWS-like motif in the orf virus GIF protein are critical for maintaining the integrity of Binding to ovine granulocyte-macrophage colony-stimulating factor and interleukin-2. *J Virol* 79: 11205–11213
171 Ng A, Tscharke DC, Reading PC, Smith GL (2001) The vaccinia virus A41L

protein is a soluble 30 kDa glycoprotein that affects virus virulence. *J Gen Virol* 82: 2095–2105
172 Ogawa S, Oku A, Sawano A, Yamaguchi S, Yazaki Y, Shibuya M (1998) A novel type of vascular endothelial growth factor, VEGF-E (NZ-7 VEGF), preferentially utilizes KDR/Flk-1 receptor and carries a potent mitotic activity without heparin- binding domain. *J Biol Chem* 273: 31273–31282
173 Meyer M, Clauss M, Lepple-Wienhues A, Waltenberger J, Augustin HG, Ziche M, Lanz C, Buttner M, Rziha HJ, Dehio C (1999) A novel vascular endothelial growth factor encoded by Orf virus, VEGF-E, mediates angiogenesis via signalling through VEGFR-2 (KDR) but not VEGFR-1 (Flt-1) receptor tyrosine kinase. *EMBO J* 18: 363–374
174 Wise LM, Veikkola T, Mercer AA, Savory LJ, Fleming SB, Caesar C, Vitali A, Makinen T, Alitalo K, Stacker SA (1999) Vascular endothelial growth factor (VEGF)-like protein from orf virus NZ2 binds to VEGFR2 and neuropilin-1. *Proc Natl Acad Sci USA* 96: 3071–3076
175 Ueda N, Wise LM, Stacker SA, Fleming SB, Mercer AA (2003) Pseudocowpox virus encodes a homolog of vascular endothelial growth factor. *Virology* 305: 298–309
176 He JG, Deng M, Weng SP, Li Z, Zhou SY, Long QX, Wang XZ, Chan SM (2001) Complete genome analysis of the mandarin fish infectious spleen and kidney necrosis iridovirus. *Virology* 291: 126–139
177 Lu L, Zhou SY, Chen C, Weng SP, Chan S M, He JG (2005) Complete genome sequence analysis of an iridovirus isolated from the orange-spotted grouper, *Epinephelus coioides*. *Virology* 339: 81–100
178 Ferrara N, Gerber HP, LeCouter J (2003) The biology of VEGF and its receptors. *Nat Med* 9: 669–676
179 Stacker SA, Achen MG (1999) The vascular endothelial growth factor family: signalling for vascular development. *Growth Factors* 17: 1–11
180 Mercer AA, Wise LM, Scagliarini A, McInnes CJ, Buttner M, Rziha HJ, McCaughan C A, Fleming SB, Ueda N, Nettleton PF (2002) Vascular endothelial growth factors encoded by Orf virus show surprising sequence variation but have a conserved, functionally relevant structure. *J Gen Virol* 83: 2845–2855
181 Wise LM, Ueda N, Dryden NH, Fleming SB, Caesar C, Roufail S, Achen MG, Stacker SA, Mercer AA (2003) Viral vascular endothelial growth factors vary extensively in amino acid sequence, receptor-binding specificities, and the ability to induce vascular permeability yet are uniformly active mitogens. *J Biol Chem* 278: 38004–38014
182 Savory LJ, Stacker SA, Fleming SB, Niven BE, Mercer AA (2000) Viral vascular endothelial growth factor plays a critical role in orf virus infection. *J Virol* 74: 10699–10706
183 Chang HW, Watson JC, Jacobs BL (1992) The E3L gene of vaccinia virus encodes an inhibitor of the interferon-induced, double-stranded RNA-dependent protein kinase. *Proc Natl Acad Sci USA* 89: 4825–4829
184 Vijaysri S, Talasela L, Mercer AA, McInnes CJ, Jacobs BL, Langland JO (2003) The Orf virus E3L homologue is able to complement deletion of the vaccinia virus E3L gene *in vitro* but not *in vivo*. *Virology* 314: 305–314
185 Kwon JA, Rich A (2005) Biological function of the vaccinia virus Z-DNA-bind-

ing protein E3L: Gene transactivation and antiapoptotic activity in HeLa cells. *Proc Natl Acad Sci USA* 102: 12759–12764
186 Camus-Bouclainville C, Fiette L, Bouchiha S, Pignolet B, Counor D, Filipe C, Gelfi J, Messud-Petit F (2004) A virulence factor of myxoma virus colocalizes with NF-kappaB in the nucleus and interferes with inflammation. *J Virol* 78: 2510–2516
187 Johnston JB, Wang G, Barrett JW, Nazarian SH, Colwill K, Moran M, McFadden G (2005) Myxoma virus M-T5 protects infected cells from the stress of cell cycle arrest through its interaction with host cell cullin-1. *J Virol* 79: 10750–10763
188 Bos JD, Kapsenberg ML (1993) The skin immune system: progress in cutaneous biology. *Immunol Today* 14: 75–78
189 Becherel PA, LeGoff L, Frances C, Chosidow O, Guillosson JJ, Debre P, Mossalayi MD, Arock M (1997) Induction of IL-10 synthesis by human keratinocytes through CD23 ligation: a cyclic adenosine 3',5'-monophosphate-dependent mechanism. *J Immunol* 159: 5761–5765
190 Garvey TL, Bertin J, Siegel RM, Wang GH, Lenardo J, Cohen JI (2002) Binding of FADD and caspase-8 to molluscum contagiosum virus MC159 v-FLIP is not sufficient for its antiapoptotic function. *J Virol* 76: 697–706
191 Garvey T, Bertin J, Siegel R, Lenardo M, Cohen J (2002) The death effector domains (DEDs) of the molluscum contagiosum virus MC159 v-FLIP protein are not functionally interchangeable with each other or with the DEDs of caspase-8. *Virology* 300: 217–225
192 Shisler JL, Moss B (2001) Molluscum contagiosum virus inhibitors of apoptosis: The MC159 v-FLIP protein blocks Fas-induced activation of procaspases and degradation of the related MC160 protein. *Virology* 282: 14–25
193 Thome M, Schneider P, Hofmann K, Fickenscher H, Meinl E, Neipel F, Mattmann C, Burns K, Bodmer J, Schroter M et al (1997) Viral FLICE-inhibitory proteins (FLIPs) prevent apoptosis induced by death receptors. *Nature* 386: 517–521
194 Quan LT, Caputo A, Bleackley RC, Pickup DJ, Salvesen GS (1995) Granzyme B is inhibited by the cowpox virus serpin cytokine response modifier A. *J Biol Chem* 270: 10377–10379
195 Ray CA, Black RA, Kronheim SR, Greenstreet TA, Sleath PR, Salvesen GS, Pickup DJ (1992) Viral inhibition of inflammation: cowpox virus encodes an inhibitor of the interleukin-1 beta converting enzyme. *Cell* 69: 597–604
196 Sen GC (2001) Viruses and interferons. *Annu Rev Microbiol* 55: 255–281
197 Johnston JB, McFadden G (2003) Poxvirus immunomodulatory strategies: current perspectives. *J Virol* 77: 6093–6100
198 Gil J, Esteban M (2000) Induction of apoptosis by the dsRNA-dependent protein kinase (PKR): mechanism of action. *Apoptosis* 5: 107–114
199 Xiang Y, Condit RC, Vijaysri S, Jacobs B, Williams BR, Silverman RH (2002) Blockade of interferon induction and action by the E3L double-stranded RNA binding proteins of vaccinia virus. *J Virol* 76: 5251–5259
200 Langland JO, Jacobs BL (2002) The role of the PKR-inhibitory genes, E3L and K3L, in determining vaccinia virus host range. *Virology* 299: 133–141
201 Huang H, Bi XG, Yuan JY, Xu SL, Guo XL, Xiang J (2005) Combined CD4+

Th1 effect and lymphotactin transgene expression enhance $CD8^+$ Tc1 tumor localization and therapy. *Gene Ther* 12: 999–1010
202 McNiece I (1997) Interleukin-3 and the colony-stimulating factors. In: DG Remick, JS Friedland (eds): *Cytokines in health and disease*, 2nd edn. Marcel Dekker, Ann Arbor, 41–43
203 Kruse N, Weber O (2001) Selective induction of apoptosis in antigen-presenting cells in mice by Parapoxvirus ovis. *J Virol* 75: 4699–4704
204 Chang WL, Baumgarth N, Yu D, Barry PA (2004) Human cytomegalovirus-encoded interleukin-10 homolog inhibits maturation of dendritic cells and alters their functionality. *J Virol* 78: 8720–8731
205 Buttner M (1993) Principles of paramunization. Option and limits in veterinary medicine. *Comp Immunol Microbiol Infect Dis* 16: 1–10
206 Fachinger V, Schlapp T, Saalmuller A (2000) Evidence for a parapox ovis virus-associated superantigen. *Eur J Immunol* 30: 2962–2971
207 Fachinger V, Schlapp T, Strube W, Schmeer N, Saalmuller A (2000) Poxvirus-induced immunostimulating effects on porcine leukocytes. *J Virol* 74: 7943–7951
208 Forster R, Wolf G, Mayr A (1994) Highly attenuated poxviruses induce functional priming of neutrophils *in vitro*. *Arch Virol* 136: 219–226
209 Mayr A, Buttner M, Wolf G, Meyer H, Czerny C (1989) Experimental detection of the paraspecific effects of purified and inactivated poxviruses. *Zentralbl Veterinarmed B* 36: 81–99
210 Weber O, Siegling A, Friebe A, Limmer A, Schlapp T, Knolle P, Mercer A, Schaller H, Volk HD (2003) Inactivated parapoxvirus ovis (Orf virus) has antiviral activity against hepatitis B virus and herpes simplex virus. *J Gen Virol* 84: 1843–1852
211 Henkel M, Planz O, Fischer T, Stitz L, Rziha HJ (2005) Prevention of virus persistence and protection against immunopathology after Borna disease virus infection of the brain by a novel Orf virus recombinant. *J Virol* 79: 314–325
212 Rziha H, Henkel M, Cottone R, Bauer B, Auge U, Gotz F, Pfaff E, Rottgen M, Dehio C, Buttner M (2000) Generation of recombinant parapoxviruses: non-essential genes suitable for insertion and expression of foreign genes. *J Biotechnol* 83: 137–145
213 Rziha HJ, Henkel M, Cottone R, Meyer M, Dehio C, Buttner M (1999) Parapoxviruses: potential alternative vectors for directing the immune response in permissive and non-permissive hosts. *J Biotechnol* 73: 235–242
214 Marsland BJ, Tisdall DJ, Heath DD, Mercer AA (2003) Construction of a recombinant orf virus that expresses an Echinococcus granulosus vaccine antigen from a novel genomic insertion site. *Arch Virol* 148: 555–562
215 Fischer T, Planz O, Stitz L, Rziha HJ (2003) Novel recombinant parapoxvirus vectors induce protective humoral and cellular immunity against lethal herpesvirus challenge infection in mice. *J Virol* 77: 9312–9323

Poxviruses
ed. by Andrew A. Mercer, Axel Schmidt and Olaf Weber

Genus *Capripoxvirus*

Adama Diallo[1] and Gerrit J. Viljoen[2]

[1]Animal Production Unit, FAO/IAEA Agriculture and Biotechnology Laboratory, International Atomic Energy Agency, Wagrammerstrasse 5, P.O. Box 100, 1400 Vienna, Austria; [2]Animal Production and Health Section, FAO/IAEA Joint Division, International Atomic Energy Agency (AIEA), Wagrammerstrasse 5, P.O. Box 100, 1400 Vienna, Austria

Abstract

The *Capripoxvirus* genus is composed of three closely related viruses: *Goatpox virus* (GTPV), *Sheeppox virus* (SPPV) and *Lumpy skin disease virus* (LSDV). The natural hosts from which these were isolated include goats, sheep and cattle, respectively, although domestic buffaloes are also susceptible to LSDV. Cross protection can be induced by all three viruses. Unfortunately, serological distinction between these viruses is not possible. Previous classification was based only on animal host origins, but today differentiation is possible using genomic DNA restriction digestion patterns or comparisons of gene sequences. Although most strains grow readily in goat, sheep or cattle, their pathogenicities may differ according to the animal origin. The diseases they cause are characterized by fever, papules, and nodular and sometimes pustular lesions on the skin. The nodules can be also found in internal organs, particularly the lungs. They induce immune depression in infected hosts, thereby favoring secondary bacterial infections with an associated increase in the mortality rate. A high morbidity is, however, usually observed with economic implications in the case of lumpy skin disease, such as loss of milk production in cows, infertility in bulls following orchitis and damage caused to hides. *Capripoxvirus* diseases are of a transboundary nature and are on the World Organization for Animal Health (OIE: *Office International des Epizooties*) list of important animal diseases that need to be notified. The geographical distributions of these three viruses differ: whereas sheeppox and goatpox viruses are endemic to Asia, the Middle East and Africa south of the equator, LSDV is mainly confined to sub-Saharan Africa. These differences in geographical distribution may be an indication that GTPV and SPPV evolved separately from LSDV.

Viruses of the Capripoxvirus genus

The *Capripoxvirus* genus, one of the eight members of the subfamily *Chordopoxvirinae*, is composed of three important pathogens that infect only ungulates, i.e., *Lumpy skin disease virus* (LSDV), *Goatpox virus* (GTPV) and *Sheeppox virus* (SPPV), which are isolated from cattle, goat and sheep, respectively. Early and separate electron microscopic observations of these viruses indicated that size distinctions could be made [1–5]. Kitching and Smale [6], however, did not find significant size differences between intact capripoxviruses. All virions have an ovoid shape with an average size of 294 × 273 nm. Since they can not be differentiated by morphology or by serology, capripoxviruses were mainly classified according to the animal origin.

Their genomes consist of double-stranded DNA of about 150 kb with terminal repeated sequences at each end [7]. Early molecular studies of these genomes indicated the usefulness of restriction endonuclease analysis for the comparative study of capripoxvirus strains [8, 9]. Although the patterns of fragments generated by the digestion of their genomic DNA with *Hind*III are similar, suggesting a close relationship between viruses within the genus, they do have some specific and marked differences that can be related to animal origin. The Kenya sheeppox isolate KS1 is an exception as it was subsequently proven to be an LSDV [8]. By *Hind*III digestion of viral DNA, Kitching et al. [9] have shown that cattle field isolates of capripoxvirus have been very stable over a period of 30 years in Sub-Saharan Africa. The full genome sequences for some strains of all three capripoxviruses are now available [10–12]. They are about 151 kbp long and contain 156 putative genes. Comparison of these sequences with those of other chordopoxviruses has shown a high degree of co-linearity and amino acid identity in the central region of the genome, except for some gene inversions in fowlpoxviruses and insertions in both *Molluscum contagiosum virus* and fowlpoxviruses [13]. Within this poxvirus subfamily, the genomes of capripoxviruses have the highest A-T content, 73–75%, while that of *Molluscum contagiosum virus* is only 36% [13]. The first gene sequence comparisons indicated the close relationship between capripoxviruses and leporipoxviruses within the *Poxvirus* family [10, 14, 15]. A recent phylogenetic analysis has shown that capripoxviruses form an important cluster with the *Suipoxvirus*, *Leporipoxvirus* and *Yatapoxvirus* genera and that within this group, *Capripoxvirus* and *Suipoxvirus* are the closest and seem to have evolved from a common ancestor [13]. The genome sequence data now available have also confirmed the high similarity between the three viruses of the *Capripoxvirus* genus as they share 96–97% nucleotide identity [11]. The main differences between LSDV on the one hand and SPPV and GTPV genomes on the other are located in the terminal regions of the genomes, known to contain genes that are possibly involved in viral virulence and in determining host range of poxviruses [16]. Nine LSDV genes in this region with likely virulence and host range functions are in fact disrupted in the GTPV and SPPV genomes [10, 11]. Genetic differences in these regions between virulent and attenuated strains of different capripoxviruses have also been identified [11, 12]. A thorough investigation of these regions might help in developing more effective vaccines. A recent study to help elucidate the relationships between SPPV and its host has shown that the virus has the capacity to inhibit local macrophage function soon after inoculation. At a later stage, however, splenic macrophage activity as well as lymphocytic responsiveness is enhanced [17]. The SPPV proteins involved in these immunomodulatory mechanisms have not yet been identified.

History and epidemiology of capripoxvirus infections

Based on the fact that LSDV genes are absent or fragmented in SPPV and GTPV genomes, Tulman et al. [11] suggested that the latter viruses are derived from an LSDV-like ancestor that became adapted to sheep and/or goats. If this is true, then lumpy skin disease (LSD) or LSD-like diseases were ignored for many centuries, as the first report of disease dates back only to 1929 in Zambia [18]. After many attempts to isolate the causative agent, a poxvirus was eventually isolated from bovine skin lesions and identified as causing true LSD in cattle [5, 19, 20]. The first isolate was obtained in South Africa and known as the Neethling isolate, or LSDV type-Neethling [19, 21]. From its original focus in Zambia, LSD then spread steadily to almost all sub-Saharan countries by the end of the 1970s [22]. It was later also identified in Egypt in May 1988 [23, 24]. It still remains a cattle disease restricted primarily to the African continent, with the exception of cases reported in Madagascar in 1954 [22] and two others in 1989 in dairy cattle in Israel and in Arabian oryx in Saudi Arabia [25, 26].

In contrast to LSD, sheeppox is a very old disease with many cases already reported in the first century A.D. [27]. In 1902, Borrel identified the causative agent as a virus, which was first cultivated *in vitro* in 1933 by Bridre [28, 29]. It is not clear if the history of goatpox is similar to that of sheeppox [27]. Most cases of goatpox, however, were reported in 1884 in North Africa and Spain, and in Italy in 1898, although one case had already been reported by Hansen in Norway in 1879 (cited in [27]). Sheeppox and goatpox are more widely distributed than LSD. The endemic areas of the former diseases extend from China to Afghanistan, Turkey, the Middle East and all African countries north of the Equator. During the 1990s, occasional sheeppox outbreaks were reported mainly in Bulgaria and Greece. Three epidemiological patterns of capripoxvirus infections are found in Africa: in the region between the southern Sahara and northern equatorial areas, all three diseases coexist; in contrast, southern Africa has only LSD and northern Africa, with the exception of Egypt, only sheeppox. The epidemiological distribution, and in particular, the limitation of the spread of sheep- and goatpox south of Kenya, remains unknown.

Epidemiology of capripoxvirus infections appears complex. As far as small ruminants are concerned, there are many reported field outbreaks affecting either sheep or goats, while other reports indicate the involvement of both species [30–36]. The host specificity of capripoxvirus strains is in fact not limited to either goats or sheep, and the apparent conflicting reports on sheeppox/goatpox outbreaks may rather reflect the differing degrees of virulence between species, with goat isolates giving less severe disease in sheep and vice versa [9, 35–37]. Thus, goatpox and sheeppox outbreaks may be caused by separate viruses according to their relative virulence for goats or sheep. In the case of LSDV, only one association with sheeppox was reported in Kenya. The capripoxvirus strain KS 0240, also named KS1, was isolated from a sheep in Kenya but was shown to be a LSDV according to genome mapping and sequencing data analysis [8, 11, 38]. Neither sheeppox nor goatpox has been reported in sheep or in goats in South Africa where LSD is endemic, and this might indicate that LSDV cannot cause serious disease in these species. This is strengthened by experimental findings that inoculation of different LSDV strains into sheep and goats only induced a single granulomatous reaction at the site of inoculation [9]. The initial cases of LSD in Egypt affected both cattle and domestic buffaloes, although the latter seemed to be less susceptible [23]. In wildlife, only one report mentioned the natural infection of an Arabian oryx (*Oryx leucoryx*) in Saudi Arabia [26]. Earlier, susceptibility of wildlife to LSDV was demonstrated by both experimental infection [39] and serological surveys, which revealed the presence of capripoxvirus antibodies in some animals (Davies et al., 1981 as cited in [26, 40]). While Davies was suggesting wild buffaloes as possible reservoir for LSDV, Hedger and Hamblin [40] considered the role of wildlife as negligible in its epidemiology due to the low prevalence of serological positive samples.

The mode of LSDV transmission has not yet been clearly established. Following an investigation, it was concluded that the in-contact mode of infection is extremely inefficient and that inoculation of the virus is required to establish infection [41]. During these experiments, the intravenous route was the most effective means of inducing generalized lesions. These results in addition to the observation that LSD is prevalent mainly in wet seasons and during times when insects are abundant, strongly suggest a major role for biting arthropods in mechanical transmission of the causal agent between animals. Under experimental conditions, the mosquito *Aedes aegypti* has been shown to transmit LSDV from infected to susceptible animals. Trials using several other biting insects were unsuccessful [42]. Successful transmission of capripoxviruses to sheep or goats by *Stomoxys calcitrans* has also been reported [43, 44]. It seems that capripoxviruses can propagate between sheep and goats by aerosol, requiring close contact between animals, with those that have developed severe clinical disease with multiple external lesions being a potent source of infectious virus [33–36, 45]. The persistence of the virus in scab material might also constitute an important factor in the maintenance of the disease in the field [34].

Clinical signs and lesions

Lumpy skin disease

Infected cattle develop clinical signs after an incubation period of 4–14 days and in some cases up to 4 weeks after viral contact. Initially, a fever of about 40–41°C occurs, lasting for up to 2 weeks in some cases. At the same time, the affected animal may show depression, salivation and ocular and

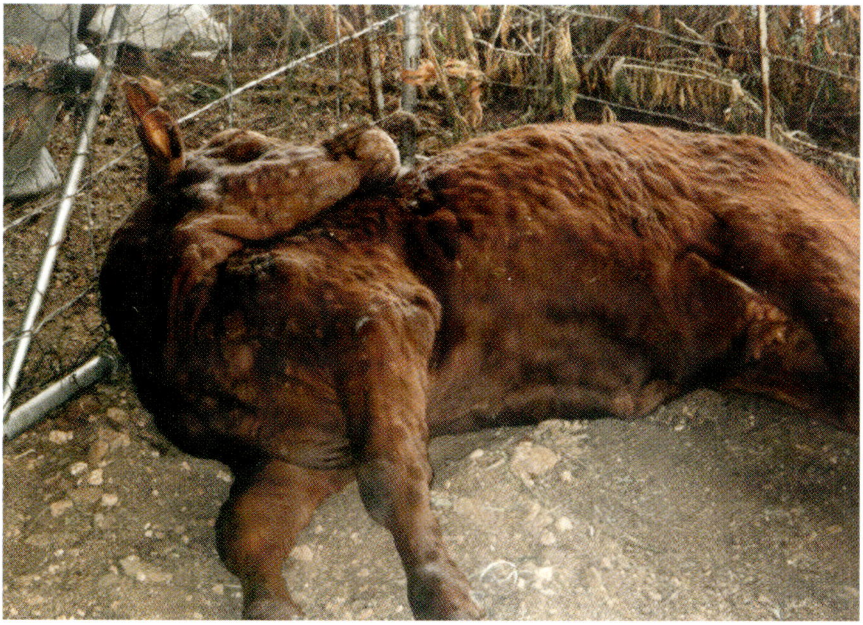

Figure 1. Young calf showing undisrupted lumps due to lumpy skin disease virus infection (Courtesy of D. Wallace, Onderstepoort Veterinary Institute, South Africa).

nasal discharges. The superficial lymph nodes are usually enlarged. Skin lesions appear 4–10 days after the onset of the disease consisting initially of erythematous raised foci and surrounding hair with a star-like appearance. These lesions then rapidly give rise to well-circumscribed nodules that are at first mainly limited to the head and around the eyes, the neck and on the perineum. They then spread to the sides and even to the entire body surface, including the ventral surfaces in severe cases (see Fig. 1). They may sometimes also be found on mucosal surfaces such as in the nostrils. The nodules are circular with a diameter between 0.5 and 5 cm; they are also firm and painless and involve both the skin and subcutaneous tissues. The number of nodules ranges from a few to several hundred, with some fusing to form large plaques. They contain a clear serous and sometimes purulent exudate. Some nodules persist for months and some become dry and hard, forming dark scabs within 3 weeks. They then detach leaving ulcers that eventually heal within few weeks. In bulls, the genitalia can also be affected and can give rise to an orchitis with temporary or permanent infertility. In cows, the formation of nodules on the udders and teats are followed by secondary bacterial infections causing mastitis. Microscopic lesions include ballooning degeneration of cells in the epidermis, eosinophilic intracytoplasmic inclusion bodies, vasculitis and perivascular fibroplasia.

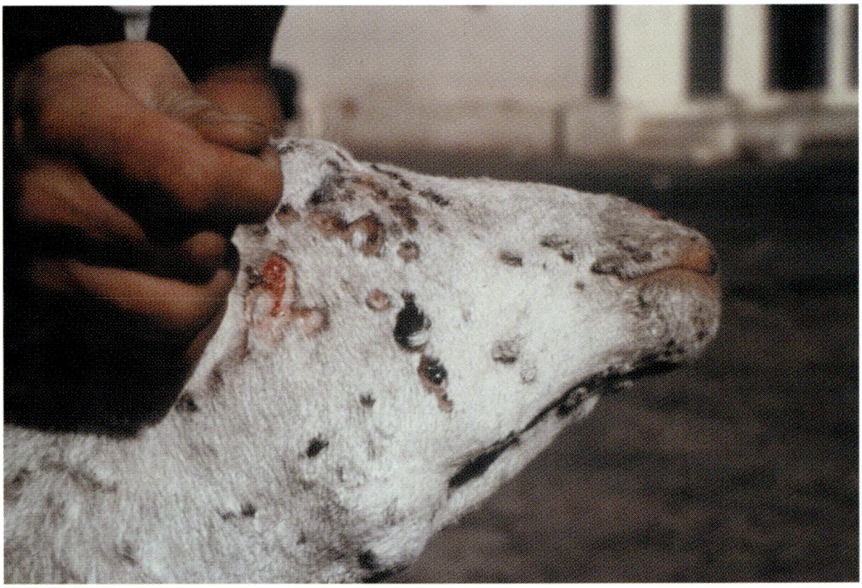

Figure 2. Goat at the stage of pustule and scab lesions of capripox disease (Prof. J. Chantal, National Veterinary School of Toulouse, France).

Sheeppox and goatpox

Clinically, it is not possible to distinguish the diseases caused by SPPV and GTPV. They are therefore described as an entity. The clinical signs seen are very variable, depending not only on individual host susceptibility but also on the virus strain. As indicated previously, the same virus can have different pathogenicities in goats and in sheep. The incubation period is approximately 6–12 days but can be as long as 3 weeks, or shorter than 4 days under experimental conditions. The first clinical sign is a rise in rectal temperature to 40°C and above. In peracute cases, death can occur prior to the development of skin lesions. In acute cases, which are most commonly seen, skin lesions appear 2–5 days after the onset of the disease. These consist of maculae or small circumscribed hyperemic areas that are only obvious on unpigmented regions of the skin. A day later, they develop into papules or hard swellings of 0.5–1 cm or even 3 cm in diameter. These lesions may cover the whole body or they may be restricted to hairless/wool-less areas such as the face groin, axilla and perineum. These lesions can also be seen in the nose, eye, mammary glands, vulva, prepuce and mouth, making feeding painful with the latter. During this phase of papule eruptions, ocular and nasal discharges occur. They are initially serous but become mucopurulent and can make breathing difficult. The rectal temperature of the affected animal, which is high at the beginning

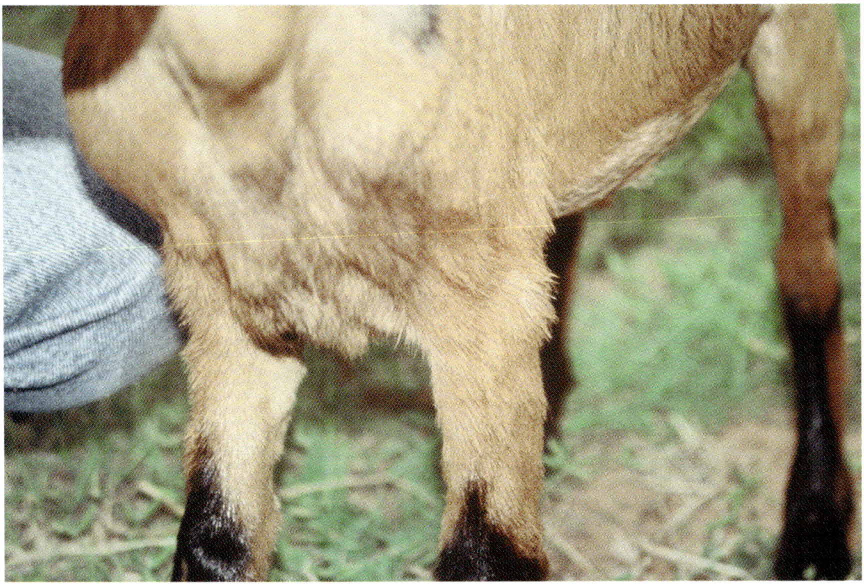

Figure 3. Goat showing the "stone pox" form, large circumscribed nodules, of capripox disease (photo A. Diallo).

of the disease drops gradually to normal. The superficial lymph nodes are enlarged. If death does not occur at this stage, the papules evolve to form pustules and scabs following the necrosis of tissues in about 10 days (see Fig. 2). The scabs persist for about 6 weeks and eventually detach from the skin. In some cases, these papules evolve quickly into firm, circumscribed nodules known as "stone pox", each with variable diameters that can be as large as 5 cm (see Fig. 3). These are located mainly on the head, neck, back, the legs, the tail and sometime genital organs of the animal. This form of sheeppox/goatpox, which is seen mainly in goats in sub-Saharan countries, is not found in north Africa [27]. Following necrosis, the nodules detach and leave ulcerative lesions that form scars in about 3 weeks. The nodules may also first retract and form crusts and then scars.

The majority of fatalities occur during the acute phase of the disease at the time of bronchopneumonia following secondary bacterial infection. Young animals are mostly affected, with a mortality rate varying between 50% and 70% [33, 34]. Most adults, however, survive with a mortality rate of about 1%. The post-mortem examination confirms the presence of enlarged and oedematous lymph nodes. Mucous membranes have necrotic lesions. In most cases, multiple nodular lesions are seen in the lungs (see Fig. 4). Papules are also found in the different digestive organs, kidneys and liver.

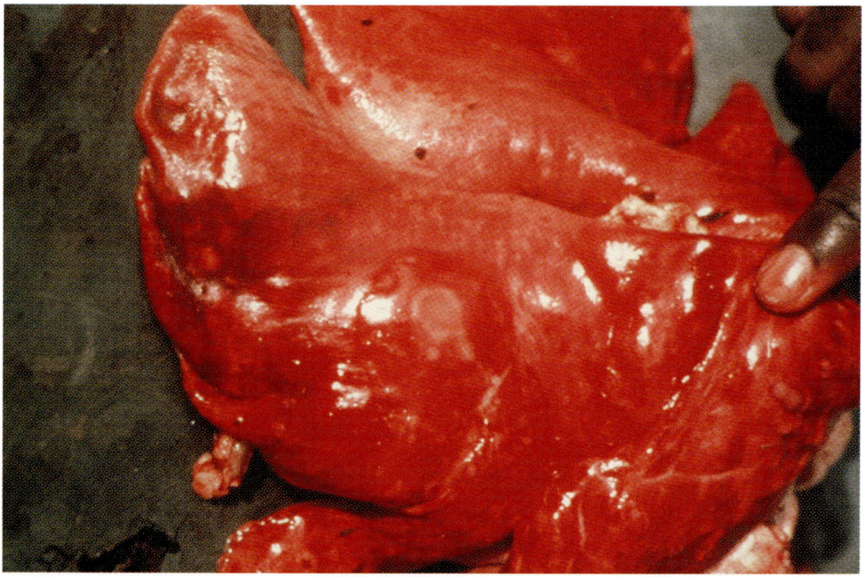

Figure 4. Nodular lesions in the lung from a goat which was infected with capripoxvirus (Prof. J. Chantal, National Veterinary School of Toulouse, France).

Diagnosis

In endemic areas, the diagnosis of different capripoxvirus diseases is easily based on clinical signs. Such clinical diagnoses should nevertheless be considered as presumptive until laboratory confirmation occurs. Differential diagnoses include: (a) in the case of LSD, pseudo-LSD caused by the Allerton virus, a bovine herpesvirus type 2 or bovine herpes mammillitis virus [20, 31, 46–49], and (b) in the case of sheeppox/goatpox, contagious pustular dermatis (Orf) because of the presence of labial crusts, or peste des petits ruminants (PPR) because of purulent oculonasal discharges and bronchopneumonia, although no pustules nor nodules are seen in the latter.

The different laboratory techniques available for diagnosis of capripoxviruses are well reviewed in the Manual of Diagnostic Tests and Vaccines for Terrestrial Animals published by the World Organization for Animal Health, the OIE Manual [50]. The most rapid test for the identification of capripoxviruses is electron microscopy of skin, lymph nodes or lung biopsy samples. In the case of bovine infections, the structure of the capripoxvirus virion (see Fig. 5) is sufficiently different from the herpesvirus to allow for the differentiation between LSD from pseudo-LSD. In the case of small ruminants, the main differential diagnosis needed is between sheeppox and contagious pustular dermatis caused by a parapoxvirus, which is an oval-

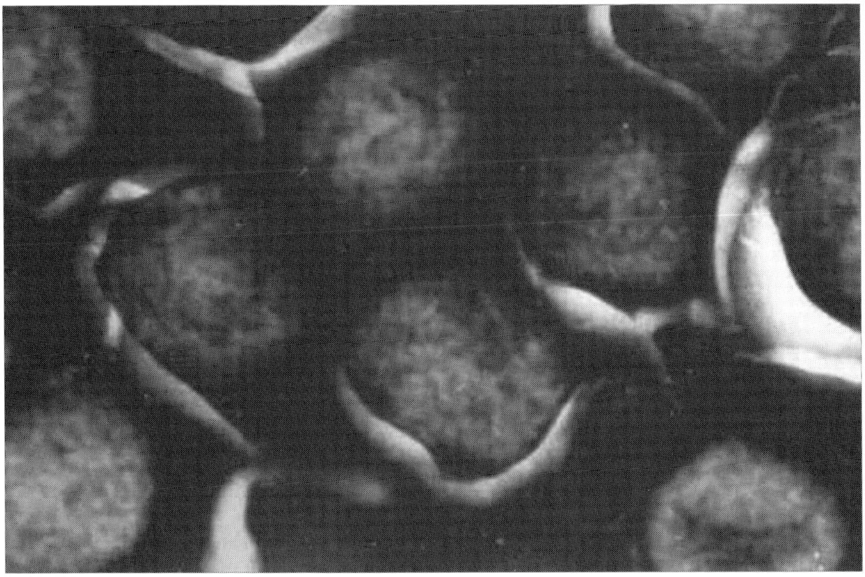

Figure 5. Electron photomicrograph of clustered lumpy skin disease virus particles (×75 000) (Courtesy of L.M. Stannard, University of Cape Town, South Africa).

shaped virus and is also smaller than capripoxviruses. The agar immunodiffusion test (AGID) to detect capripoxvirus antigen in biopsy material is a simple test, which gives results within 48–72 h. A counter immunoelectrophoresis format has also been developed that needs only 45 min to complete [51]. This test is unfortunately not specific and gives cross-reactions with parapoxviruses that share common precipitating antigens with capripoxvirus [52]. A sandwich ELISA for the detection of the capripoxvirus antigen has been developed [53]. It is based on the use of anti-capripoxvirus rabbit serum to capture virus from the test material, and a detection guinea pig antibody against the capripoxvirus protein p32, a major viral protein common to all three capripoxviruses but not shared with parapoxviruses. The most sensitive test for the detection of capripoxviruses is the detection of nucleic acids using PCR [54–56]. Sequencing the amplified DNA products generated by this test allows a rapid identification of the virus strain. As for any other disease, the gold standard test for capripoxvirus detection is pathogen isolation, followed by other means of identification. For virus isolation, the recommended cells are primary or secondary culture lamb testis or kidney cells. As an alternative, bovine cells can also be used. The cytopathic effect (cpe) of the virus on the cells can be seen in 1 week, although this can be up to 2–3 weeks, with several blind passages needed. For antibody detection, the virus neutralization test is presently the most widely used assay. The test serum is either titrated against a constant titer of virus, or virus is titrated against a constant dilution of the serum. In the latter case, the result is expressed as a neutralization index. Other tests such as immunofluorescence or Western blot have been described for the detection of anti-capripoxvirus antibodies [57, 58]. The most promising serological test for capripoxvirus detection is ELISA. The indirect format uses p32, a major capripoxvirus protein [59, 60]. Since immunity to capripoxviruses is mostly cell mediated, serological response of animals to these viruses is sometimes very weak, thus leading to false-negative results. In these cases, animals can still resist challenge with virulent virus.

Control

LSD, sheeppox and goatpox are important veterinary diseases that can impact negatively on international animal trade. In countries previously regarded as free of these diseases, an accidental introduction is dealt with using an eradication programme. In endemic areas, the disease is controlled by vaccination campaigns. Although the three viruses of the genus are sufficiently closely related to provide cross protection [61, 62], attenuated live vaccines were developed independently in different laboratories for use in cattle, or sheep or goats (for review and list of vaccines, see [63]). In South Africa, the control of LSD is ensured by the use of an attenuated vaccine developed more than 40 years ago from a South African field isolate of LSDV. It was attenuated by serial passage in the chorioallantoic membranes of embryonated chicken eggs [21, 64]. Cattle inoculated with this attenuated virus only developed mild local reactions and produced antibodies that persisted upwards of 3 years and were protective against virulent challenge [65]. Not all cattle produce circulating antibodies, but all are still resistant to challenge demonstrating the protective role of cell-mediated immunity. This vaccine is now produced in cell culture. For sheeppox, one of the vaccines that has been widely used is the SPPV Rumania strain. It has been attenuated by serial passages in lamb kidney cell culture by Ramyar and Hessami [66]. One of the goatpox live vaccines is the Mysore strain, which was attenuated on goat testis cells. The Kenyan 0240 vaccine, also named KS1 (for Kenyan Sheep 1), is derived from a virus isolated from a sheep in Kenya and attenuated in lamb testis cell [52]. Genomic DNA analysis of this strain has shown it to be LSDV, even though it had been isolated from a sheep [8, 10]. This vaccine is recommended for the control of capripoxviruses in both sheep and goats but not in cattle because it does seem to have residual pathogenicity for this species [50, 67].

It is claimed that live attenuated capripoxvirus vaccines induce protective immunity for at least 3 years if not lifelong [45, 50]. This characteristic, in addition to the fact that capripoxviruses are host-range restricted to cattle, sheep, goat and some buffalos, makes live attenuated strains excellent candidates for the development of recombinant multiple valence vaccines for use in ruminants, or as non-replicative vaccines in other hosts. A number of recombinant vaccines using the KS1 isolate as the vector have been developed. Recombinants expressing either the fusion or hemagglutinin gene of rinderpest virus were used successfully to protect cattle against both rinderpest and LSD [68–72]. Similarly, recombinant viruses containing the H and F genes of the peste des petits ruminants virus (PPRV) inserted into the genome of KS1 vaccine proved to be excellent dual vaccines that could protect animals against both PPR and goatpox [73, 74]. However, in the case of KS1 recombinants expressing the major core structural protein (VP7) of bluetongue virus (BTV), only partial protection was induced in sheep against a virulent heterotypic BTV challenge [75]. As with the KS1 strain, the southern African vaccine strain of LSDV (Neethling) has also been used as a vector to express different foreign proteins such as the glycoproteins of rabies, bovine ephemeral fever and Rift Valley fever viruses [76, 77]. Although the recombinant LSDV-rabies G protein virus replicates to maturity only in permissive cells, it induces protective immunity in both rabbits and mice [78].

References

1 Abdussalam M (1957) Elementary bodies of sheep pox. *Am J Vet Res* 18: 614

2 Cohen J, Berehi A, Ribero M, Vincent, M (1971) Étude en microscopie électronique de la morphogénèse du virus de la clavelée (variole ovine) en culture de tissu. *Ann Inst Pasteur* 121: 569–577

3 Ghaboussi B (1978) Morphology and physical characteristics of and goat pox viruses. *Arch Inst Razi* 30: 107–115

4 Tantawi HH, Falluji MM (1979) Laboratory characteristics of four strains of goat pox virus. *Acta Virol* 23: 455–460

5 Munz EK, Owen NC (1966) Electron microscopic studies on Lumpy Skin Disease virus type "Neethling". *Onderstepoort J Vet Res* 33: 3–8

6 Kitching RP, Smale C (1986) Comparison of the external dimensions of capripoxvirus isolates. *Res Vet Sci* 41: 425–427

7 Gershon PD, Black DN (1987) Physical characterization of the genome of a cattle isolate of Capripoxvirus. *Virology* 160: 473–476

8 Black DN, Hammond JM, Kitching RP (1986) Genomic relationship between Capripoxviruses. *Virus Res* 5: 277–292

9 Kitching RP, Bhat PP, Black DN (1989) The characterisation of African strains of Capripoxvirus. *Epidemiol Infect* 102: 335–343

10 Tulman ER, Afonso CL, Lu Z, Zsak L, Kutish GF, Rock DL (2001) Genome of Lumpy Skin Disease Virus. *J Virol* 75: 7122–7130

11 Tulman ER, Afonso CL, Lu Z, Zsak L, Sur J-H, Sandybaev NT, Kerembekova UZ, Zaitsev GF, Kutish GF, Rock DL (2002) The genomes of sheepoox and goatpox viruses. *J Virol* 76: 6054–6061

12 Kara PD, Afonso CL, Wallace DB, Kutish GF, Abolnik C, Lu Z, Vreede FT, Taljaard LCF, Zsak A, Viljoen GJ, Rock DL (2003) Comparative sequence

analysis of the South African vaccine strain and two virulent field isolates of lumpy skin disease virus. *Arch Virol* 148: 1335–1356
13 Gubser C, Hue S, Kellam P, Smith GL (2004) Poxvirus genomes: a phylogenetic analysis. *J Gen Virol* 85:105–117
14 Gershon PD, Black DN (1989) The nucleotide sequence around the Capripoxvirus thymidine kinase gene reveals a gene shared specifically with Leporipoxvirus. *J Gen Virol* 70: 525–533
15 Gershon PD, Black DN (1989) A capripoxvirus pseudogene whose only intact homologs are in other poxvirus genomes. *Virology* 172: 350–354
16 Johnston JB, McFadden G (2003) Poxvirus immunomodulatory strategies: current perspectives. *J Virol* 77: 6093–6100
17 Abu-EL-Saad AA, Abdel-Moneim AS (2005) Modulation of macrophage functions by sheeppox virus provides clues to understand interaction of the virus with host immune system. *Virol J* 2005 2:22
18 Coetzer JAW (2004) Lumpy Skin Disease. In: JAW Coetzer, RC Tustin (eds): *Infectious Diseases of Livestock*, 2nd edn. Oxford University Press, Cape Town, 1268–1276
19 Alexander RA, Plowright W, Haig DA (1957) Cytopathogenic agents associated with Lumpy-skin Disease of Cattle. *Bull Epiz Dis Afr* 5: 489–492
20 Haig DA (1957) Lumpy skin disease. *Bull Epiz Dis Afr* 5: 421–430
21 Weiss KE (1963) Lumpy skin disease. Emerging diseases of animals. *FAO Agric Studies* 61: 179–201
22 Ordner G, Lefèvre PC (eds) (1987) *La dermatose nodulaire contagieuse des bovins*. Collection Etudes et Synthèse de l'IEMVT, Paris
23 Ali AA, Esmat M, Attia H, Selim A, Abdel-Hamid YM (1990) Clinical and pathological studies on Lumpy Skin Disease in Egypt. *Vet Rec* 127: 549–550
24 Hafez MAM, Tawfik AM, Maysa Shaker HM, El-Danaf NA (1992) Clinical and pathological studies on Lumpy Skin Disease firstly recorded in Egypt. *Bull Anim Prod Afr* 40: 225–233
25 Yeruham I, Nir O, Braverman Y, Davidson M, Grinstein H, Haymovitch M, Zamir O (1995) Spread of lumpy skin disease in Israeli dairy herds. *Vet Rec* 137: 91–93
26 Greth A, Gourreau JM, Vassart M, Nguyen-Ba-Vy, Wyers M, Lefevre PC (1992) Capripoxvirus Disease in an Arabian Oryx (Oryx leucoryx) from Saudi Arabia. *J Wild Dis* 28: 295–300
27 Lefèvre PC (ed) (1983) *La variole ovine (clavelée) et la variole caprine*. Collection Etudes et Synthèse de l'IEMVT, Paris
28 Borrel A (1902) *Expérience sur la filtration du virus claveleux*. CR Séanc Soc Biol Paris 54: 59–61
29 Bidre J (1935) Essais de culture *in vitro* du virus de la clavelée. Premiers résultats positifs. *CR Séanc Soc Biol Paris* 119: 502–503
30 Burdin ML, Prydie J (1959) Observations on the first outbreak of lumpy skin disease in Kenya. *Bull Epiz Dis Afr* 7: 21–26
31 Capstick PB (1959) Lumpy Skin Disease – experimental infection. *Bull Epiz Dis Afr* 7: 51–62
32 Davies FG (1976) Characteristics of a virus causing a pox disease in sheep

and goats in Kenya, with observations on the epidemiology and control. *J Hyg* (Camb) 76: 163–171

33 Garner MG, Sawarkar SD, Brett EK, Edwards JR, Kulkarni VB, Boyle DB, Singh SN (2000) The extent and impact of sheep pox and goat pox in the state of Maharashtra, India. *Trop Anim Health Prod* 32: 205–223

34 Hailat N, Al-Rawashdeh O, Lafi S, Al-Bateineh Z (1994) An outbreak of sheep pox associated with unusual winter conditions in Jordan. *Trop Anim Health Prod* 26: 79–80

35 Mondal B, Hosamani M, Dutta TK, Senthilkumar VS, Rathore R, Singh RK (2004) An outbreak of sheep pox on a sheep breeding farm in Jammu, India. *Rev Sci Tech Off Int Epiz* 23: 943–949

36 Kitching RP, Taylor WP (1985) Clinical and antigenic relationship between isolates of sheep and goat poxviruses. *Trop Anim Health Prod* 17: 64–74

37 Bidgeh K, Ganda K, Diguimbaye C (1990) Variole caprine au Tchad: étude du pouvoir pathogène du virus chez les ovins et les caprins. *Rev Elev Méd Vét Pays Trop* 44: 33–36

38 Kitching RP, Hammond JM, Taylor WP (1987) A single vaccine for the control of Capripox infection in sheep and goats. *Res Vet Sci* 42: 53–60

39 Young E, Basson PA, Weiss KE (1970) Experimental infection of game animals with Lumpy Skin Disease virus (prototype strain Neethling). *Onderstepoort J Vet Res* 37: 79–88

40 Hedger RS, Hamblin C (1983) Neutralising antibodies to Lumpy Skin Disease in African Wildlife. *Comp Immun Microbiol Infect Dis* 6: 209–213

41 Carn VM, Kitching RP (1995) An investigation of possible routes of transmission of lumpy skin disease virus (Neethling). *Epidemiol Infect* 114: 219–226

42 Chihota CM, Rennie LF, Kitching RP, Mellor PS (2003) Attempted mechanical transmission of lumpy skin disease virus by biting insects. *Med Vet Entomol* 17: 294–300

43 Kitching RP, Mellor PS. (1986) Insect transmission of Capripoxvirus. *Res Vet Sci* 40: 255–258

44 Mellor PS, Kitching RP, Wilkinson PJ (1987) Mechanical transmission of capripox virus and African swine fever virus by *Stomoxys calcitrans. Res Vet Sci* 43:109–112

45 Kitching RP (2004) Sheepox and goatpox. In: JAW Coetzer, RC Tustin (eds): *Infectious Diseases of Livestock*, 2nd edn. Oxford University Press, Cape Town, 1277–1281

46 Burdin ML (1959) The use of histopathological examinations of skin material for the diagnosis of lumpy skin disease in Kenya. *Bull Epiz Dis Afr* 7: 27–36

47 Prydie J, Coackley W (1959) Lumpy skin disease – tissue culture studies. *Bull Epiz Dis Afr* 7: 37–50

48 Davies FG, Krauss H, Lund J, Taylor M (1971) The laboratory diagnosis of lumpy skin disease virus. *Res Vet Sci* 12: 123–127

49 Woods JA, Herring JA, Nettleton PF, Kreuger N, Scott FMM, Reid, HW (1996) Isolation of bovine herpesvirus-2 (BHV-2) from a case of pseudo-lumpy skin disease in the United Kingdom. *Vet Rec* 138: 113–114

50 OIE (2004) *Manual of Diagnostic Tests and Vaccines for Terrestrial Animals*, 5th edn. Office Internationale des Epizooties, Paris

51 Sharma B, Negi BS, Pandey AB, Bandyopadhyay Shankar H, Yadav MP (1988) Detection of goat pox antigen and antibody by the counter immunoelectrophoresis test. *Trop Anim Health Prod* 20: 109–113

52 Kitching RP, Hammond JM, Black DN (1986) Studies on the major common precipitating antigen of Capripoxvirus. *J Gen Virol* 67: 139–148

53 Carn VM (1995) An antigen trapping ELISA for the detection of capripoxvirus in tissue culture supernatant and biopsy samples. *J Virol Methods* 51: 95–102

54 Ireland DC, Binepal YS (1998) Improved detection of capripoxvirus in biopsy samples by PCR. *J Virol Methods* 74: 1–7

55 Mangana-Vougiouka O, Markoulatos P, Koptopoulos G, Nomikou K, Bakandritsos N, Papadopoulos O (1999) Sheep poxvirus identification by PCR in cell cultures. *J Virol Methods* 77: 75–79

56 Markoulatos P, Mangana-Vougiouka O, Koptopoulos G, Nomikou K, Papadopoulos O (2000) Detection of sheep poxvirus in skin biopsy samples by a multiplex polymerase chain reaction. *J Virol Methods* 84: 161–167

57 Davies FG, Otema C (1978) The antibody response in sheep infected with a Kenyan sheep and goat pox virus. *J Comp Pathol* 88: 205–210

58 Chand P, Kitching RP, Black DN (1994) Western blot analysis of virus-specific antibody responses for capripox and contagious pustular dermatitis viral infections in sheep. *Epidemiol Infect* 113: 377–385

59 Carn VM, Kitching RP, Hammond JM, Chand P (1994) Use of a recombinant antigen in an indirect ELISA for detecting bovine antibody to capripoxvirus. *J Virol Methods* 49: 285–294

60 Heine HG, Stevens MP, Foord AJ, Boyle DB (1999) A capripoxvirus detection PCR and antibody ELISA based on the major antigen P32, the homolog of the vaccinia virus H3L gene. *J Immunol Methods* 227: 187–196

61 Capstick PB, Coakley W (1961) Protection of cattle against lumpy skin disease. I. Trials with a vaccine against Neethling type infection. *Res Vet Sci* 2: 362–368

62 Kitching RP (1986) Passive protection of sheep against Capripoxvirus. *Res Vet Sci* 41: 247–250

63 Carn VM (1993) Control of Capripoxvirus infections. *Vaccine* 11: 1275–1279

64 Van Rooyen PJ, Munz EK, Weiss KE (1969) The optimal conditions for the multiplication of Neethling-type LSDV in embryonated eggs. *Onderstepoort J Vet Res* 36: 165–174

65 Weiss KE (1968) Lumpy Skin Disease virus. *Virol Monogr* 3: 111–131

66 Ramyar H, Hessami M (1968) Development of an attenuated live virus vaccine against sheep pox. *Arch Inst Razi* 20: 77–80

67 Yeruham I, Perl S, Nyska A, Abraham A, Davidson M, Haymovitch M, Zamir O, Grinstein H(1994) Adverse reactions in cattle to a capripox vaccine. *Vet Rec* 135: 330–332

68 Romero CH, Barrett T, Evans SA, Kitching RP, Gershon PD, Bostock C, Black DN (1993) Single Capripoxvirus recombinant vaccine for the protection of cattle against Rinderpest and Lumpy skin disease. *Vaccine* 11: 737–742

69 Romero CH, Barrett T, Kitching RP, Carn VM, Black DN (1994) Protection of cattle against rinderpest and lumpy skin disease with a recombinant capripoxvirus expressing the fusion protein gene of rinderpest virus. *Vet Rec* 135:152–154

70 Romero CH, Barrett T, Chamberlain RW, Kitching RP, Fleming M, Black DN

(1994) Recombinant capripoxvirus expressing the hemagglutinin protein gene of rinderpest virus: protection of cattle against rinderpest and lumpy skin disease viruses. *Virology* 204: 425–429

71 Ngichabe CK, Wamwayi HM, Barrett T, Ndungu EK, Black DN, Bostock CJ (1997) Trial of a capripoxvirus-rinderpest recombinant vaccine in African cattle. *Epidemiol Infect* 118: 63–70

72 Ngichabe CK, Wamwayi HM, Ndungu EK, Mirangi PK, Bostock CJ, Black DN, Barrett T (2002) Long term immunity in African cattle vaccinated with a recombinant capripox-rinderpest virus vaccine. *Epidemiol Infect* 128: 343–349

73 Diallo A, Minet C, Berhe G, Le Goff C, Black DN, Fleming M, Barrett T, Grillet C, Libeau G (2002) Goat immune response to capripox vaccine expressing the hemagglutinin protein of peste des petits ruminants. *Ann NY Acad Sci* 969: 88–91

74 Berhe G, Minet C, Le Goff C, Barrett T, Ngangnou A, Grillet C, Libeau G, Fleming M, Black DN, Diallo A (2003) Development of a dual recombinant vaccine to protect small ruminants against peste-des-petits-ruminants virus and capripoxvirus infection. *J Virol* 77: 1571–1577

75 Wade-Evans AM, Romero CH, Mellor P, Takamatsu H, Anderson J, Thevasagayam J, Fleming MJ, Mertens PPC, Black DN (1996) Expression of the major core structural protein (VP7) of bluetongue virus, by a recombinant capripoxvirus, provides partial protection of sheep against a virulent heterotypic bluetongue virus challenge. *Virology* 220: 227–231

76 Aspden K, van Dijk AA, Bingham J, Cox D, Passmore J-A, Williamson A-L (2002) Immunogenicity of a recombinant lumpy skin disease virus (Neethling vaccine strain) expressing the rabies virus glycoprotein in cattle. *Vaccine* 20: 2693–2701

77 Wallace DB, Viljoen GJ (2005) Immune responses to recombinants of the South African vaccine strain of lumpy skin disease virus generated by using thymidine kinase gene insertion. *Vaccine* 23: 3061–3067

78 Aspden K, Passmore J-A, Tiedt F, Williamson A-L (2003) Evaluation of lumpy skin disease virus, a capripoxvirus, as a replication-deficient vaccine vector. *J Gen Virol* 84: 1985–1996

This virus is of primary interest to veterinarians and wildlife managers, and most reports deal with the diagnosis of infected *Sciurus* spp. squirrels. Little fundamental virology has been conducted on SQFV. FIBV was described in 1959 in the European hare (*Lepus europaeus*) and its biology resembles RFV most closely. FIBV is the only leporipoxvirus to arise naturally outside of the Americas. African hares (*Lepus capensis*) in Kenya have been reported with small dermal lesions, for which gross and histopathological analysis suggest that the tumors most closely resemble RFV/SFV [18]. Therefore, the range of FIBV may be extended to include lagomorphs of Africa.

Epidemiology, disease, pathology

Epidemiology

The *Sylvilagus* rabbit species in the Americas have co-evolved in association with several fibroma-like poxviruses [4]. For example, *S. floridanus* of eastern North America is the sole natural host to RFV/SFV. *S. bachmani* of south-western North, and Central America is frequently infected by the California strain of MYXV and *S. braziliensis* is host to the South American strain of MYXV. SQFV and FIBV have traditionally only been reported in North America and Europe, respectively, but there have been reports of a poxvirus fibroma with similarities to RFV/SFV and FIBV found in African hares in Kenya [18]. Whether African hares represent the expansion of FIBV into Africa or a new endemic fibroma virus restricted to the African continent will have to be determined. It would not be surprising to learn that other geographic ranges that support lagomorphs have also established enzootic members of the leporipoxvirus genus.

Infection by leporipoxviruses follows seasonal cycles that correlate well with arthropod vector populations in the wild and breeding cycles of the host. The best information on these cycles is derived from studies carried out in Australia over the past 50 years to monitor MYXV spread in populations of wild rabbits following the release of MYXV in the early 1950s [4, 19–21]. An unanticipated observation following the initial release of MYXV was the relatively rapid attenuation of MYXV in the wild and the simultaneous development of resistance in wild rabbit populations [22–24]. As the virulence of MYXV decreased, infected rabbits lived longer and this allowed more blood meals by mosquitoes and the transmission of the attenuated virus to more hosts [22].

Tissue tropism

The primary vector of transmission of leporipoxviruses is the mosquito, although other biting arthropod vectors like fleas can also transmit the disease and the flea is thought to be the main vector for the transmission of MYXV in Britain [4]. In their natural hosts, leporipoxviruses are introduced into the dermal layer by arthropod vectors, and virus replication initially occurs in the epidermis and sub-dermal regions. The virus does not usually progress to secondary sites in their natural or evolutionary hosts. The exception to this is MYXV infection of *Oryctolagus cuniculus*, where the virus can propagate efficiently in lymphocytes and migrate *via* infected leukocytes through lymphatic channels to establish secondary sites of infection. MYXV transmission from rabbit to rabbit is primarily by mosquitoes, but fleas, black flies, ticks and mites have also been implicated. Many of these biting insects follow seasonal cycles and there has been a correlation between time of year and occurrence of disease. Because of the history of myxoma virus use as a biocontrol agent, much investigation has gone into the confirmation of the strict species tropism of this virus [4]. Numerous animal species, including man, have been tested for susceptibility to MYXV. Injections of selected human volunteers done in Australia during the 1950s confirmed that MYXV was unable to replicate or cause a disease in humans [25]. However, recently the barrier to MYXV infection of primary murine and human fibroblasts has been breached experimentally. In these cases, either blockage of the antiviral state by neutralization of interferon responses [26] or infection of primary tissue before the anti-viral state could be established [27] demonstrated that MYXV could productively infect primary cells from species that are normally resistant to infection. In fact, many human cancer cells are both interferon resistant and fully permissive for MYXV [28].

Disease

Infection of the natural evolutionary host, by each of the four prototype members of the leporipoxviruses, are characterized by the production of skin lesions and tumors. These cutaneous tumors are clinically and histologically similar. Infection of *Sylvilagus* species by RFV/SFV results in tumors that resolve over several months. In contrast, *Oryctolagus* species infected by RFV/SFV can recover in a few weeks (Tab. 2). The fibromas are rarely accompanied by other symptoms, such as fevers or appetite loss, unless the rabbit host is immunocompromised. Infection of *Sylvilagus* species of the Americas with South American MYXV produces cutaneous fibromas in healthy individuals, but immunocompromised rabbits and the very young can be particularly susceptible. *Leporipoxvirus*es from the Americas do not easily cross species barriers. For example, RFV/SFV, which robustly infects *S. floridanus*, only infects *S. bachmani* or *S. braziliensis* poorly *via* the invertebrate vector route [4].

In contrast, infection of *O. cuniculus* with South American MYXV results in lethal myxomatosis [4]. This devastating systemic infection produces numerous tumors on the skin, ears, face and genital regions of the infected animals.

The primary tumor is often large, protuberant and purple/black. Numerous secondary lesions develop over the body within 6–8 days post infection. As the disease progresses, and the immune defenses are breached, the natural micro-flora and -fauna overwhelm the animal, leading to purulent discharge from the nose and eyes. Breathing becomes difficult as the head swells and the congestion develops from progressive bacterial infestation. Myxomatosis is nearly 100% lethal in *O. cuniculus*, and acts to override the immune response within the first days of infection, resulting in the establishment of supervening Gram-negative bacteria infection in the respiratory tract. Infected animals often survive no more than 1–2 weeks before succumbing to the disease. In contrast, infection of the same rabbit species with Californian MYXV causes a more rapid disease with only mild external features; however, the infected animal often dies within the first week of infection. Because California myxomatosis is often associated with decreased survival times, reduced production of lesions, tremors and convulsions, it has been suggested that the Californian strain of myxoma virus is neurovirulent [4, 12].

Pathology

Leporipoxviruses cause proliferative fibromas in *Sylvilagus* rabbits, gray squirrels and hares. Following infection, an acute inflammatory reaction occurs with infiltration of mononuclear and polymorphonuclear cells and proliferation of fibroblast-like cells of uncertain origin. The fibromas consist of pleomorphic cells imbedded in a matrix of intracellular fibrils of collagen. Unlike the transformed cells induced by many other DNA viruses, the cells from poxviral tumors are not immortalized and cannot be propagated independently. Instead, the tumor cells appear to require factors produced during a viral infection to maintain their hyperproliferative state. The speed with which immune cells clear the viral infection and reverse the hyperproliferation can range from 1–2 weeks up to 6 months, depending on both the virus and host.

The principal difference between the benign fibroma syndrome caused by leporipoxviruses in their evolutionary hosts, and the devastating disease caused by MYXV in *Oryctolagus* rabbits, is that the latter virus efficiently propagates in host lymphocytes and migratory leukocytes, and is able to circumvent the cell-mediated immune response to the viral infection (see the next section on the molecular biology of leporipoxvirus immune evasion). MYXV readily migrates to secondary sites within infected immune cells of susceptible rabbits and concomitant cellular proliferation can be detected in the reticulum cells of lymph nodes and spleen as well as the conjunctival and pulmonary alveolar epithelium [4].

Although there are four accepted members of the leporipoxviruses, there is only extensive genetic and pathology information for MYXV and RFV/SFV. MRV has been characterized as a natural recombinant between

RFV/SFV (Boerlage strain) and MYXV (strain unknown) in which a small portion of the RFV/SFV terminal DNA [between S005 (partial), S006, S007 and S 008] have been swapped into the ITRs of MYXV producing duplicated copies of a fusion between M005 [3, 16]. The pathogenesis of MRV is thought to be closely related to MYXV.

Molecular biology: genomics and immune evasion

Genomics

Poxviruses are double-stranded DNA viruses that have a large coding capacity. It is this feature that allows the poxviridae to acquire the diverse genes that allow the virus to evade the host immune system [29]. Many of these immune evasion strategies appear to be derived from host cellular genes that have been co-opted by the virus and re-deployed to act for virus protection [30]. MYXV and RFV/SFV of the leporipoxviruses were among the earliest poxvirus genomes to be completely sequenced [5, 7]. MYXV has a somewhat larger genome and encodes 171 contiguous genes *versus* the 165 encoded by RFV/SFV. The members of the leporipoxviruses have among the longest ITRs in the poxviridae. MYXV encodes 12 ORFs within the 11.5-kb ITR, while RFV/SFV encodes 11 ORFs in a slightly longer ITR of 12.4 kb [5, 7]. In addition, the genetic information is highly conserved between the two genomes with the genetic identity ranging from 87% in the central conserved core to about 70% in the termini. There are 9 genes from MYXV that are either fragmented (6 ORFs), truncated (2 ORFs) or missing (1 ORF) in RFV/SFV [5]. A peculiar feature noted for RFV/SFV was the duplication of the eIF2α homolog (S008.2L/R) and the partial duplication of a kelch repeat protein (S009L/S155R) [7]. In contrast, MYXV contains only a single copy of the eIF2α homolog (M156R) [5]. The structure of M156R has been determined, and it is similar to the structure determined for the vaccinia homolog, K3L [31]. Biochemical analysis has demonstrated that M156R can compete with eIF2α for phosphorylation by the protein kinase PKR [31]. MYXV possesses a single copy of the S009 gene, called M009L; however, it was noted that S155R was likely a pseudogene [7].

Following the sequencing of the RFV/SFV and MYXV genomes, several novel leporipoxvirus genes were noted for which no other poxvirus homologs had been identified [7]. In the intervening years, however, many of these novel leporipoxvirus genes have turned out to be shared amongst other members from other poxviral genera (Tab. 3).

Although MYXV evolved in association with the *Sylvilagus* rabbits of the Americas, it is best known for the disease it produces upon infection of *O. cuniculus*. Because myxomatosis produces such a distinct disease phenotype, any alteration to the virulence of the virus can be readily measured. This dramatic biological interaction between the host and virus, in coordi-

Table 3. Novel leporipoxvirus genes[a]

Leporipoxvirus gene	Domain	Homolog	Predicted function	Ref.
S013L/M013L	Pyrin	YLDV 18L; TPV 18L; DPV83GP024; SPV014	anti-inflammatory	[87]
S017L/ M017L		Novel	Unknown	
S023R/M023R	Renamed S023.5L/ M023.5L	YMTV 028.5L, YLDV 028.5L, SPV026.5, LSDV028.5, VVF14L, MC022.1L		[79]
S119R/M119R		Novel	Unknown	
S125R/M125R		LSDV126; SPV126; SPPV121; DpV83gp136	EEV glycoprotein	
S127L/M127L	Photolyase; FAD binding	Avipoxviruses; Entomopoxviruses	Photolyase	[69]
S130R/M130R		LSDV129; SPPV124; MPVI6L; SPV126; VARV K6L; CMLV073		
S138L/M138L	Glyco transferase	DpV83gp150	Sialyltransferase	[80–82]
S141R/M141R	IgG-like	LSDV138, YMTV141; YLDV141; SPPV131	Viral CD200	[57]

[a]Update of Table 4 from [7].

nation with the use of targeted gene knockout viruses, has allowed for the identification and characterization of the function of numerous MYXV virulence genes that mediate immune evasion, host range and disease pathogenesis [32] (Tab. 4).

Immune evasion

When MYXV first made the species leap into the related, but distinct, European rabbit in 1896, the infection immediately manifested as a new pathogenic syndrome referred to as myxomatosis [4, 9]. This drastic change in the pathogenic phenotype in the infected host emphasizes the unpredictable consequences when viruses cross host-species boundaries. However, because of this very dramatic change in disease presentation, researchers have been able to study how specific MYXV genes contribute to its impressive virulence in *Oryctolagus* [33]. While many of the immune evasion strategies described for MYXV are shared by other poxviruses [29], and a general overview is presented in other chapters within this volume, here we

Table 4. Virulence genes of the leporipoxviruses

Protein	Gene	Description of action	Ref.
M-T1	M001L/R	Chemokine binding protein; specific to CC chemokines	[45]
M-T2	M002L/R	TNF receptor homolog; inhibitor of apoptosis	[39, 40]
M-T4	M004L/R	ER-localized inhibitor of apoptosis in rabbit T lymphocytes	[68]
M-T5	M005L/R	Binds cullin1; alters cell cycle progression; inhibitor of apoptosis in rabbit T lymphocytes; Necessary for infection of some human tumor cell lines	[28, 65, 66]
M-T7	M007L/R	Interferon-γ binding protein; binds chemokines through GAG domains	[43, 44, 83]
Serp 1	M008.1L/R	Serpin; blocks inflammation in experimental animals models	[47, 48, 55, 84]
MGF	M010L	EGF-like growth factor	[46, 85]
M11L	M011L	Blocks apoptosis in rabbit T lymphocytes; inhibits apoptosis in human cells by binding to Bak	[62, 63, 85, 86]
M13L	M013L	Blocks inflammosome within infected cells	[87]
CD47-like	M128L	Down-regulation of macrophages	[56]
SOD	M131R, S131R	Up-regulation of SOD to inhibit Fas-induced apoptosis and promote cell proliferation; protection of the virion	[71] [72] [70]
α-2,3 sialyl-transferase	M138L	Mild virulence factor; may be necessary for sialylation during infection	[80]
OX-2 homolog	M141R	Down-regulation of macrophage and T cell activation	[57]
Zinc ring finger	S143R	Inhibits apoptosis	[88]
Myxoma nuclear factor	M150R	Blocks NF-κB induced inflammation	[61]
Serp2	M151R	Serpin; ICE inhibitor	[59]
Serp3	M152R	Serpin;	[60]
M153/MV-LAP	M153R	Down-regulation of MHC class I, CD94 and CD4	[37, 38]
eIF2α homolog	M156R	Interferon resistance	[31]

briefly summarize only the key distinctive features of the strategies used by the leporipoxviruses.

Leporipoxvirus immunomodulation strategies (Tab. 4) can be subdivided into three broad categories: virostealth, viromimicry and virotransduction [33, 34]. A naive mammalian host is dependent on rapid identification and clearance of virus-infected cells by the innate immune system. For example,

MYXV infection results in the down-regulation of surface molecules that normally signal abnormalities in the cells. MYXV has been shown to down-regulate major histocompatibility complex (MHC) class I and CD4, two sentinel molecules that signal during an innate immune response [35, 36]. The MYXV gene M153R was identified as being critical for the degradation of these two surface markers, as well as CD95 [37, 38]. M153R was shown to be E3 ubiquitin ligase that induced rapid internalization and lysosomal degradation of surface CD4 molecules [38].

The remarkable diversity of the leporipoxvirus-encoded immune evasion genes was first suggested with the identification of a TNF-R homolog that was identified in RFV/SFV and MYXV [39, 40]. The TNF-R mimic from MYXV, designated M-T2, inhibited TNF in a species-specific manner, and also had a secondary property of inhibiting apoptosis in rabbit T lymphocytes [41, 42]. This discovery of dual function by a viral immunomodulator was followed closely by the identification of a viral mimic of the IFN-γ receptor from myxoma virus [43]. Such host-related modulators that were virally encoded but nevertheless resembled host receptors were termed "viroceptors" [29]. TNF and IFN-γ viroceptors have been identified in most poxvirus members and the viroceptor family now includes inhibitors of IFN-α/β as well [29, 34]. In addition to exploiting receptor mimics, poxviruses encode viral mimics of cellular cytokines or cytokine binding proteins or "virokines" [29]. The leporipoxviruses express several virokines such as two types of chemokine binding proteins (CBP) termed CBP-I and -II. CBP-I, or the low-affinity binder, is also the MYXV IFN-γ-viroceptor (M-T7) and represents another example of the dual anti-host properties of some of the viral regulators [44]. The type II CBP is represented by the M-T1 from MYXV [45]. The leporipoxviruses express other virokines as well, such as the myxoma growth factor (MGF), the related SFV growth factor (SGF), and Serp-1. MGF is a virulence factor that appears to promote cell proliferation of both infected and surrounding uninfected cells, thereby improving the cellular environment for virus replication [46]. Serp1 from MYXV is a secreted serpin that acts as a virulence factor for MYXV, whereas the Serp1 gene is fragmented in RFV/SFV [7] and is not expressed. Analysis indicates that Serp1 alters the inflammatory response during an infection [47, 48], and it was this observation that led to the discovery of the use of Serp1 as an anti-inflammatory agent, and suggested a clinical use to alleviate allograft vasculopathy [49, 50], rheumatoid arthritis [51] and injury vasculopathy [52–54]. The use of such viral proteins as anti-inflammatory reagents has been recently reviewed [55].

Two distinct MYXV virulence factors have been shown to down-regulate macrophages during infection. M128L, a cell surface CD47 homolog, is required for full pathogenesis and blocks activation of monocytes and macrophage cells during infection [56]. M141R, a viral CD200 homolog, blocks activation of macrophages in infected lesions and draining lymph nodes and this then down-regulates T lymphocyte activation during infection [57].

Inhibitors of apoptosis

Apoptosis has evolved as an innate cellular defense mechanism against tissue damage or infection. In response to this host strategy, many viruses have evolved or acquired genes that encode regulators that allow the virus to either avoid host cell detection or block cellular signals from triggering apoptosis [58]. The leporipoxviruses encode numerous molecules that act on different aspects of the apoptosis pathways. M151R and M152R encode intracellular serpins denoted as Serp2 and Serp3, respectively. Both are virulence factors, with Serp2 acting to inhibit interleukin-1β-converting enzyme and thus blocking inflammation [59], and Serp3 also involved in virulence [60]. M150R, or the myxoma nuclear factor (MNF), co-localizes with NF-κB in the nucleus and interferes with the NF-κB-induced pro-inflammatory pathway [61].

Another MYXV regulator with an important function is the anti-apoptosis molecule M11L [42]. M11L is targeted to the mitochondria where it interacts with the peripheral benzodiazepine receptor, which controls the inner membrane potential of the mitochondria [62, 63]. By controlling mitochondria membrane integrity, M11L can prevent mitochondria-dependent apoptosis of infected cells. Recently, M11L has been shown to bind to the pro-apoptotic molecule Bak and block caspase-dependent apoptosis [64].

The M-T5 gene of MYXV has been defined as a host range gene because deletion of the gene resulted in rapid shutdown of host and viral protein synthesis, and premature viral abort following infection of rabbit T lymphocytes [65]. This phenomenon was not observed following infection of rabbit fibroblast cells with the same M-T5 knockout virus. Infection of rabbits with the vMyxT5KO resulted in 100% recovery with an almost complete absence of secondary lesions and little edema. Recently, it has been demonstrated that M-T5 binds to cellular cullin-1 and can drive the infected cells through G2/M phase of the cell cycle [66]. Also, M-T5 has been demonstrated to be necessary for MYXV infection of some human cancer cells [28]. In addition to cytoplasmic proteins that are directed to blocking apoptosis, MYXV encodes an ER-retained protein, M-T4, that inhibits apoptosis in rabbit T lymphocytes [67, 68]. The genomes of the leporipoxviruses also encode catalytically active photolyases that act to repair light-dependent DNA damage [69]. This enzyme is found only in the leporipoxviruses, the *Avipoxvirus*es and the entomopoxviruses. Finally, tumorigenic leporipoxviruses encode catalytically inactive homologs of Cu,Zn superoxide dismutase that modulate intracellular redox status to stimulate cell proliferation and inhibit apoptosis [70–72].

The profound virulence of MYXV in the European rabbit led to its exploitation in the early 1950s as a biocontrol agent in Australia. Although initially there was a tremendous reduction in rabbit populations, this strategy of inter-species biological warfare did not prove to be a long-term solution. Not only did resistant rabbits soon emerge and repopulate the infected areas, but the dominant field strains of the virus became progressively attenuated [4, 19–24, 73].

Vaccine strategies

MYXV is an effective vector for antigen presentation in rabbits [74] and cats [75]. Authorities in Australia have experimented with the use of the recombinant MYXV as a delivery system in immunocontraceptive strategies with limited success [76, 77]. Currently, gene knockouts of MYXV are being tested as vaccines for rabbits to protect against myxomatosis. Also, the use of MYXV as an oncolytic virus platform is being investigated [78].

References

1 McFadden G (1999) Poxviruses (Poxviridae): Leporipoxviruses and Suipoxviruses. In: RG Webster, A Granoff (eds): *Encyclopedia of Virology*, 2nd edn. Academic Press, New York, 1381–1388
2 Strayer DS, Cabirac G, Sell S, Leibowitz JL (1983) Malignant rabbit fibroma virus: Observations on the culture and histopathologic characteristics of a new virus-induced rabbit tumor. *J Natl Cancer Inst* 71: 91–104
3 Upton C, Macen JL, Maranchuk RA, DeLange AM, McFadden G (1988) Tumorigenic poxviruses: Fine analysis of the recombination junctions in malignant rabbit fibroma virus, a recombinant between Shope fibroma virus and myxoma virus. *Virology* 166: 229–239
4 Fenner F, Ratcliffe FN (1965) *Myxomatosis*. University Press, Cambridge
5 Cameron C, Hota-Mitchell S, Chen L, Barrett J, Cao J-X, Macaulay C, Willer D, Evans D, McFadden G (1999) The complete DNA sequence of myxoma virus. *Virology* 264: 298–318
6 Labudovic A, Perkins H, van Leeuwen B, Kerr P (2004) Sequence mapping of the Californian MSW strain of Myxoma virus. *Arch Virol* 149: 553–570
7 Willer D, McFadden G, Evans DH (1999) The complete genome sequence of Shope (rabbit) fibroma virus. *Virology* 264: 319–343
8 Moss B (2001) Poxviridae: The viruses and their replication. In: DM Knipe, PM Howley (eds): *Fields Virology*. Lippincott Williams & Wilkins, Philadelphia, 2849–2883
9 Sanarelli G (1898) Das myxomatogene Virus. Beitrag zum Stadium der Krankheitserrege ausser halb des Sichtbaren. *Zentralbl Bakteriol (Abt 1)* 23: 865
10 Aragão HB (1927) Myxoma dos coelhos. *Mem Inst Oswaldo Cruz* 20: 225–247
11 Kessel JF, Prouty CC, Meyer JW (1931) Occurrence of infectious myxomatosis in Southern California. *Proc Soc Exp Biol NY* 28: 413
12 Ladudovic A, Perkins H, van Leeuwen B, Kerr P (2004) Sequence mapping of the Californian MSW strain of Myxoma virus. *Arch Virol* 149: 553–570

13 McFadden G (ed) (1994) *Myxoma, rabbit fibroma, squirrel fibroma and swinepox viruses*. Sanders, San Diego, 1153–1160
14 Angulo E, Cooke B (2002) First synthesize new viruses then regulate their release? The case of the wild rabbit. *Mol Ecol* 11: 2703–2709
15 Shope RE (1932) A filterable virus causing a tumor-like condition in rabbits and its relationship to virus myxomatosum. *J Exp Med* 56: 803–822
16 Block W, Upton C, McFadden G (1985) Tumorigenic poxviruses: Genomic organization of malignant rabbit virus, a recombinant between Shope fibroma virus and myxoma virus. *Virology* 140: 113–124
17 Kilham L, Herman CM, Fisher ER (1953) Naturally occurring fibromas of grey squirrels related to Shope's rabbit fibroma. *Proc Soc Exp Biol NY* 82: 298
18 Karstad L, Thorsen J, Davies G, Kaminjolo JS (1977) Poxvirus fibromas on African hares. *J Wildl Dis* 13: 245–247
19 Merchant JC, Kerr PJ, Simms NG, Robinson AJ (2003) Monitoring the spread of myxoma virus in rabbit *Oryctolagus cuniculus* populations on the southern tablelands of New South Wales, Australia. I. Natural occurrence of myxomatosis. *Epidemiol Infect* 130: 113–121
20 Kerr PJ, Merchant JC, Silvers L, Hood GM, Robinson AJ (2003) Monitoring the spread of myxoma virus in rabbit *Oryctolagus cuniculus* populations on the southern tablelands of New South Wales, Australia. II. Selection of a strain of virus for release. *Epidemiol Infect* 130: 123–133
21 Merchant JC, Kerr PJ, Simms NG, Hood GM, Pech RP, Robinson AJ (2003) Monitoring the spread of myxoma virus in rabbit *Oryctolagus cuniculus* populations on the southern tablelands of New South Wales, Australia. III. Release, persistence and rate of spread of an identifiable strain of myxoma virus. *Epidemiol Infect* 130: 135–147
22 Kerr PJ, Best SM (1998) Myxoma virus in rabbits. *Rev Sci Tech* 17: 256–268
23 Best SM, Kerr PJ (2000) Coevolution of host and virus: the pathogenesis of virulent and attenuated strains of myxoma virus in resistant and susceptible European rabbits. *Virology* 267: 36–48
24 Best SM, Collins SV, Kerr PJ (2000) Coevolution of host and virus: cellular localization of virus in myxoma virus infection of resistant and susceptible European rabbits. *Virology* 277: 76–91
25 Burnet M (1968) *Changing Patterns: An atypical autobiography*. Heinemann, Melbourne
26 Wang F, Ma Y, Barrett JW, Gao X, Loh J, Barton E, Virgin HW, McFadden G (2004) Disruption of Erk-dependent type I interferon induction breaks the myxoma virus species barrier. *Nat Immunol* 5: 1266–1274
27 Johnston JB, Nazarian SH, Natale R, McFadden G (2005) Myxoma virus infection of primary human fibroblasts varies with cellular age and is regulated by host interferon responses. *Virology* 332: 235–248
28 Sypula J, Wang F, Ma Y, Bell J, McFadden G (2004) Myxoma virus tropism in human tumor cells. *Gene Ther Mol Biol* 8: 103–114
29 Seet BT, Johnston JB, Brunetti CR, Barrett JW, Everett H, Cameron C, Sypula J, Nazarian SH, Lucas A, McFadden G (2003) Poxviruses and immune evasion. *Annu Rev Immunol* 21: 377–423

30 Bugert JJ, Darai G (2000) Poxvirus homologues of cellular genes. *Virus Genes* 21: 111–133
31 Ramelot TA, Cort JR, Yee AA, Liu F, Goshe MB, Edwards AM, Smith RD, Arrowsmith CH, Dever Te, Kennedy MA (2002) Myxoma virus immunomodulatory protein M156R is a structural mimic of eukaryotic translation initiation factor eIF2α. *J Mol Biol* 322: 943–954
32 Johnston JB, McFadden G (2004) Technical knockout: understanding poxvirus pathogenesis by selectively deleting viral immunomodulatory genes. *Cell Microbiol* 9: 695–705
33 Nash P, Barrett J, Cao J-X, Hota-Mitchell S, Lalani AS, Everett H, Xu X-M, Robichaud J, Hnatiuk S, Ainslie C, Seet BT, McFadden G (1999) Immunomodulation by viruses: The myxoma virus story. *Immunol Rev* 168: 103–120
34 Johnston JB, McFadden G (2003) Poxvirus immunomodulatory strategies: current perspectives. *J Virol* 77: 6093–6100
35 Boshkov LK, Macen JL, McFadden G (1992) Virus-induced loss of class I major histocompatibility antigens from the surface of cells infected with myxoma virus and malignant rabbit fibroma virus. *J Immunol* 148: 881–887
36 Barry M, Lee SF, Boshkov L, McFadden G (1995) Myxoma virus induces extensive CD4 downregulation and dissociation of $p56^{lck}$ in infected rabbit $CD4^+$ T lymphocytes. *J Virol* 69: 5243–5251
37 Guerin J-L, Gelfi J, Bouillier S, Delverdier M, Bellanger F-A, Bertagnoli S, Drexler I, Sutter G, Messud-Petit F (2002) Myxoma virus leukemia-associated protein is responsible for major histocompatibility complex class I and Fas-CD95 down-regulation and defines scrapins, a new group of surface cellular receptor abductor proteins. *J Virol* 76: 2912–2923
38 Mansouri M, Bartee E, Gouveia K, Nerenberg BTH, Barrett J, Thomas L, Thomas G, McFadden G, Freu K (2003) The PHD/LAP-domain protein M153R of myxoma virus is a ubiquitin ligase that induces the rapid internalization and lysosomal destruction of CD4. *J Virol* 77: 1427–1440
39 Smith CA, Davis T, Wignall JM, Din WS, Farrah T, Upton C, McFadden G, Goodwin RG (1991) T2 open reading frame from Shope fibroma virus encodes a soluble form of the TNF receptor. *Biochem Biophys Res Commun* 176: 335–342
40 Upton C, Macen JL, Schreiber M, McFadden G (1991) Myxoma virus expresses a secreted protein with homology to the tumor necrosis factor receptor gene family that contributes to viral virulence. *Virology* 184: 370–382
41 Schreiber M, Sedger L, McFadden G (1997) Distinct domains of M-T2, the myxoma virus TNF receptor homolog, mediate extracellular TNF binding and intracellular apoptosis inhibition. *J Virol* 71: 2171–2181
42 Macen JL, Graham KA, Lee SF, Schreiber M, Boshkov LK, McFadden G (1996) Expression of the myxoma virus tumor necrosis factor receptor homologue (T2) and M11L genes is required to prevent virus-induced apoptosis in infected rabbit T lymphocytes. *Virology* 218: 232–237
43 Upton C, Mossman K, McFadden G (1992) Encoding of a homolog of the interferon-γ receptor by myxoma virus. *Science* 258: 1369–1372
44 Lalani AS, Graham K, Mossman K, Rajarathnam K, Clark-Lewis I, Kelvin D,

McFadden G (1997) The purified myxoma virus gamma interferon receptor homolog, M-T7, interacts with the heparin binding domains of chemokines. *J Virol* 71: 4356–4363

45 Graham KA, Lalani AS, Macen JL, Ness TL, Barry M, Liu L-Y, Lucas A, Clark-Lewis I, Moyer RW, McFadden G (1997) The T1/35kDa family of poxvirus secreted proteins bind chemokines and modulate leukocyte influx into virus infected tissues. *Virology* 229: 12–24

46 Opgenorth A, Strayer D, Upton C, McFadden G (1992) Deletion of the growth factor gene related to EGF and TGF α reduces virulence of malignant rabbit fibroma virus. *Virology* 186: 175–191

47 Macen JL, Upton C, Nation N, McFadden G (1993) SERP-1, a serine proteinase inhibitor encoded by myxoma virus, is a secreted glycoprotein that interferes with inflammation. *Virology* 195: 348–363

48 Upton C, Macen JL, Wishart DS, McFadden G (1990) Myxoma virus and malignant rabbit fibroma virus encode a serpin-like protein important for virus virulence. *Virology* 179: 618–631

49 Miller L, Dai E, Nash P, Liu L, Icton C, Klironomous D, Fan L, Nation PN, Zhong R, McFadden G, Lucas A (2000) Inhibition of transplant vasculopathy in a rat aortic model after infusion of an anti-inflammatory viral serpin. *Circulation* 101: 1598–1605

50 Hausen B, Boeke K, Berry GJ, Morris RE (2001) Viral serine proteinase inhibitor (Serp-1) effectively decreases the incidence of graft vasculopathy in heterotopic heart allografts. *Transplantation* 72: 364–368

51 Maksymowych WP, Nation N, Nash PD, Macen J, Lucas A, McFadden G, Russell AS (1996) Amelioration of antigen-induced arthritis in rabbits treated with a secreted viral serine proteinase inhibitor. *J Rheumatol* 23: 878–882

52 Dai E, Guan H, Liu L, Little S, McFadden G, Vaziri S, Cao H, Ivanova IA, Bocksch L, Lucas A (2003) Serp-1, a viral anti-inflammatory serpin, regulates cellular serine proteinase and serpin responses to vascular injury. *J Biol Chem* 278: 18563–18571

53 Lucas A, Liu L, Macen J, Nash P, Dai E, Stewart M, Graham K, Etches W, Boshkov L, Nation PN, Humen D, Hobman ML, McFadden G (1996) Virus-encoded serine proteinase inhibitor SERP-1 inhibits atherosclerotic plaque development after balloon angioplasty. *Circulation* 94: 2890–2900

54 Lucas A, Dai E, Liu L, Guan H, Nash P, McFadden G, Miller I (2000) Transplant vasculopathy: viral anti-inflammatory serpin regulation of atherogenesis. *J Heart Lung Transplant* 19: 1029–1038

55 Lucas A, McFadden G (2004) Secreted immunomodulatory viral proteins as novel biotherapeutics. *J Immunol* 173: 4765–4774

56 Cameron CM, Barrett JW, Mann M, Lucas A, McFadden G (2005) Myxoma virus M128L is expressed as a cell surface CD47-like virulence factor that contributes to the downregulation of macrophage activation *in vivo*. *Virology* 337: 55–67

57 Cameron CM, Barrett JW, Liu L, Lucas AR, McFadden G (2005) Myxoma virus M141R expresses a viral CD200 (vOX-2) that is responsible for down-regulation of macrophage and T-cell activation *in vivo*. *J Virol* 79: 6052–6067

58 Barry M, Wasilenko ST, Stewart TL, Taylor JM (2004) Apoptosis regulator genes encoded by poxviruses. *Prog Mol Subcell Biol* 36: 19–37
59 Messud-Petit F, Gelfi J, Delverdier M, Amardeilh M-F, Py R, Sutter G, Bertagnoli S (1998) SERP-2, an inhibitor of the interleukin-1β-converting enzyme, is critical in the pathobiology of myxoma virus. *J Virol* 72: 7830–7839
60 Guerin JL, Gelfi J, Camus C, Delverdier M, Whisstock JC, Amardeihl MF, Py R, Bertagnoli S, Messud-Petit F (2001) Characterization and functional analysis of Serp3: a novel myxoma virus-encoded serpin involved in virulence. *J Gen Virol* 85: 1407–1417
61 Camus-Bouclainville C, Fiette L, Bouchiha S, Pignolet B, Counor D, Filipe C, Gelfi J, Messud-Petît F (2004) A virulence factor of myxoma virus colocalizes with NF-kB in the nucleus and interferes with inflammation. *J Virol* 78: 2510–2516
62 Everett H, Barry M, Lee SF, Sun XJ, Graham K, Stone J, Bleackley RC, McFadden G (2000) M11L: A novel mitochondria-localized protein of myxoma virus that blocks apoptosis in infected leukocytes. *J Exp Med* 191: 1487–1498
63 Everett H, Barry M, Sun X, Lee SF, Frantz C, Berthiaume LG, McFadden G, Bleackley RC (2002) The myxoma poxvirus protein, M11L, prevents apoptosis by direct interaction with the mitochondrial permeability transition pore. *J Exp Med* 196: 1127–1139
64 Wang G, Barrett JW, Nazarian SH, Everett H, Gao X, Bleackley C, Colwill K, Moran MF, McFadden G (2004) Myxoma virus M11L prevents apoptosis through constitutive interaction with Bak. *J Virol* 78: 7097–7111
65 Mossman K, Lee SF, Barry M, Boshkov L, McFadden G (1996) Disruption of M-T5, a novel myxoma virus gene member of the poxvirus host range superfamily, results in dramatic attenuation of myxomatosis in infected European rabbits. *J Virol* 70: 4394–4410
66 Johnston JB, Wang G, Barrett JW, Nazarian SH, Colwill K, Moran M, McFadden G (2005) Myxoma virus M-T5 protects infected cells from the stress of cell cycle arrest through its interaction with host cell cullin-1. *J Virol* 79: 10750–10763
67 Hnatiuk S, Barry M, Zeng W, Liu LY, Lucas A, Percy D, McFadden G (1999) Role of the C-terminal RDEL motif of the myxoma virus M-T4 protein in terms of apoptosis regulation and viral pathogenesis. *Virology* 263: 290–306
68 Barry M, Hnatiuk S, Mossman K, Lee S-F, Boshkov L, McFadden G (1997) The myxoma virus M-T4 gene encodes a novel RDEL-containing protein that is retained within the endoplasmic reticulum and is important for the productive infection of lymphocytes. *Virology* 239: 360–377
69 Bennett CJ, Webb M, Willer DO, Evans DH (2003) Genetic and phylogenetic characterization of the type II cyclobutane pyrimidine dimer photolyases encoded by Leporipoxviruses. *Virology* 315: 10–19
70 Teoh ML, Turner PV, Evans DH (2005) tumorigenic poxviruses up-regulate intracellular superoxide to inhibit apoptosis and promote cell proliferation. *J Virol* 79: 5799–57811
71 Cao JX, Teoh ML, Moon M, McFadden G, Evans D (2002) Leporipoxvirus CnZn superoxide dismutase homologs inhibit cellular superoxide dismutase but are not essential for virus replication or virulence. *J Virol* 296: 125–135
72 Teoh ML, Walasek PJ, Evans DH (2003) Leporipoxvirus Cu,Zn-superoxide dis-

mutase (SOD) homologs are catalytically inert decoy proteins that bind copper chaperone for SOD. *J Biol Chem* 278: 33175–33184
73 Saint KM, French N, Kerr P (2001) Genetic variation in Australian isolates of myxoma virus: an evolutionary and epidemiological study. *Arch Virol* 146: 1105–1123
74 Kerr PJ, Jackson RJ (1995) Myxoma virus as a vaccine vector for rabbits: Antibody levels to influenza virus haemagglutinin presented by a recombinant myxoma virus. *Vaccine* 13: 1722–1726
75 McCabe VJ, Tarpey I, Spibey N (2002) Vaccination of cats with an attenuated recombinant myxoma virus expressing feline calicivirus capsid protein. *Vaccine* 20: 2454–2462
76 Kerr PJ, Jackson RJ, Robinson AJ, Swan J, Silvers L, French N, Clarke H, Hall DF, Holland MK (1999) Infertility in female rabbits (*Oryctolagus cuniculus*) alloimmunized with the rabbit zona pellucida protein ZPB either as a purified recombinant protein or expressed by recombinant myxoma virus. *Biol Reprod* 61: 606–613
77 Kerr PJ, Twigg LE, Silvers L, Lowe TJ, Forrester RI (1998) Serological monitoring of the epidemiology of myxoma virus to assess the effects of imposed fertility control of female rabbits on myxomatosis. *Wildlife Res* 25: 123–131
78 Lun XQ, Yang WQ, Alain T, Shi ZS, Muzik HM, Barrett JW, McFadden G, Bell J, Hamilton MG, Senger DL, Forsyth PA (2005) Myxoma virus is a novel oncolytic virus with significant anti-tumor activity against experimental human gliomas. *Cancer Res* 65: 9982–9990
79 Brunetti CR, Li X, Barrett J, Amano H, Yoshiaki U, Miyamura T, Suzuki T, McFadden G (2003) The complete genome sequence and comparative analysis of the tumorigenic poxvirus Yaba monkey tumor virus. *J Virol* 77: 13335–13347
80 Jackson RJ, Hall DF, Kerr PJ (1999) Myxoma virus encodes an alpha 2,3-sialytransferase that enhances virulence. *J Virol* 73: 2376–2384
81 Nash P, Barry M, Seet BT, Veugelers K, Hota S, Heger J, Hodgkinson C, Graham K, Jackson RJ, McFadden G (2000) Post-translational modification of the myxoma virus anti-inflammatory serpin, SERP-1 by a virally encoded sialyltransferase. *Biochem J* 347: 375–382
82 Sujino K, Jackson RJ, Chan NWC, Tsuji S, Palcic MM (2000) A novel viral alpha 2,3-sialyltransferase (v-ST3Gal I): transfer of sialic acid to fucosylated acceptors. *Glycobiology* 10: 313–320
83 Mossman K, Nation P, Macen J, Garbutt M, Lucas A, McFadden G (1996) Myxoma virus M-T7, a secreted homolog of the interferon-γ receptor, is a critical virulence factor for the development of myxomatosis in European rabbits. *Virology* 215: 17–30
84 Nash P, Whitty A, Handwerker J, Macen J, McFadden G (1998) Inhibitory specificity of the anti-inflammatory myxoma virus serpin, SERP-1. *J Biol Chem* 273: 20982–20991
85 Opgenorth A, Graham K, Nation N, Strayer D, McFadden G (1992) Deletion analysis of two tandemly arranged virulence genes in myxoma virus, M11L and myxoma growth factor. *J Virol* 66: 4720–4731
86 Wang G, Barrett JW, Nazarian SH, Everett H, Gao X, Bleackley C, Colwill

K, Moran MF, McFadden G (2004) Myxoma virus M11L prevents apoptosis through constitutive interaction with Bak. *J Virol* 78: 7097–7111

87 Johnston JB, Barrett JW, Nazarian SN, Goodwin M, Ricuttio D, Wang G, McFadden G (2005) A poxvirus-encoded pyrin domain protein interacts with ASC-1 to inhibit host inflammatory and apoptotic responses to infection. Immunity 23: 587–598

88 Brick DJ, Burke RD, Schiff L, Upton C (1998) Shope fibroma virus Ring finger protein N1r binds DNA and inhibits apoptosis. *Virology* 249: 42–51

Poxviruses
ed. by Andrew A. Mercer, Axel Schmidt and Olaf Weber

Genus *Suipoxvirus*

Gustavo A. Delhon[1,3], Edan R. Tulman[2], Claudio L. Afonso[4], and Daniel L. Rock[1]

[1]*University of Illinois, Department of Pathobiology, College of Veterinary Medicine, 2522 VMBSB, 2001 S. Lincoln Ave, Urbana, IL 61802, USA;* [2]*Center of Excellence for Vaccine Research, University of Connecticut, Storrs, CT 06269, USA;* [3]*Area of Virology, School of Veterinary Science, University of Buenos Aires, 1427 Buenos Aires, Argentina;* [4]*Southeast Poultry Research Laboratory, Agricultural Research Service, United States Department of Agriculture, Athens, GA 30605, USA*

Abstract

Swinepox virus (SWPV) has been classified as the sole member of the genus *Suipoxvirus* in the subfamily *Chordopoxvirinae*. Swine represent the only known host of SWPV; in adult animals the virus usually causes a mild, self-limiting disease. Infection occurs *via* skin abrasions, and the virus replicates in epidermal keratinocytes of the stratum spinosum. Tissues other than the skin are rarely affected. SWPV infection induces protective immunity.

The complete genomic sequence of SWPV (strain 17077–99) is known. The genome contains a central coding region and two identical inverted terminal repeat regions. Four of 150 putative genes seem unique for this virus. A number of SWPV proteins are likely involved in the disruption or modulation of host immune responses as indicated by their similarity to other viral immunomodulators and by the presence of predicted sequences. The distinct nature of the SWPV virulence and host range gene complement suggests that it contributes to SWPV host specificity. Due to its restricted host range, use of SWPV as a vaccine expression vector has been proposed.

Taxonomy

Based on virus antigenic properties and host range [1–4], and cross-protection and DNA cross-hybridization data [1–3, 5], SWPV has been classified as the sole member of the genus *Suipoxvirus* in the subfamily *Chordopoxvirinae* [6]. Phylogenetic and genomic analyses support this classification, indicating that SWPV is most closely related to members of the genera *Capripoxvirus* and *Leporipoxvirus* [7, 8] (Fig. 1).

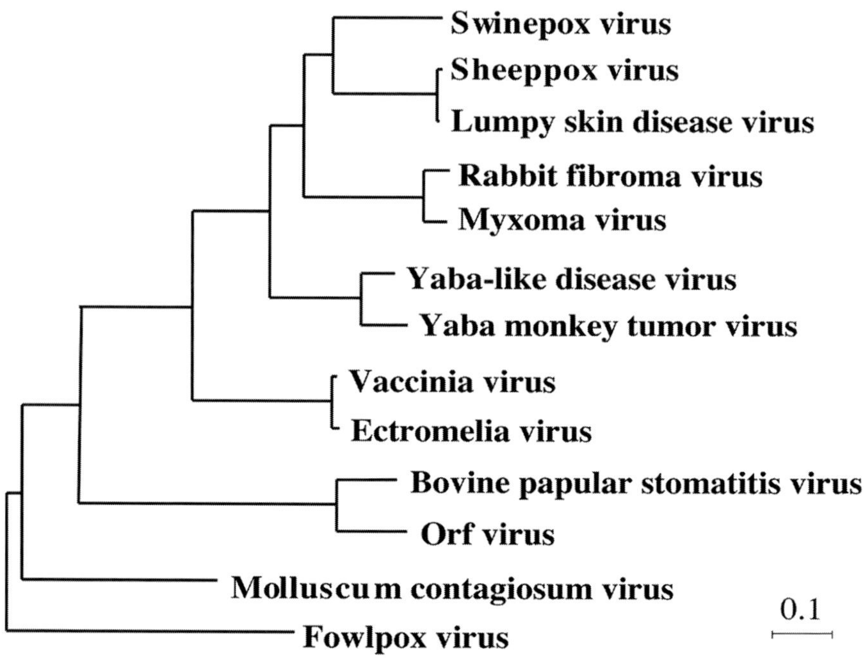

Figure 1. Phylogenetic relationship of swinepox virus to currently classified chordopoxvirus genera using aligned, concatenated datasets of conserved protein sequences and maximum likelihood analysis to produce the tree. Bar represents estimated changes per residue.

History

SWP was first reported in Europe in 1842, and later in Africa and America [9, 10]. Poenaru [11] reproduced the disease by infecting healthy pigs with blood and papulae contents from pigs exhibiting clinical SWP, and demonstrated that the disease was caused by a filterable agent. The identity of the primary causative agent remained elusive, as both a pig-specific poxvirus and *Vaccinia virus* (VACV) were found to induce pox-like disease in swine [1, 5, 12–14]. In the early 1960s, SWPV was first cultured in primary porcine cells and distinguished from VACV based on its immunological and host range properties [1, 2, 4, 5, 15]. The complete SWPV genomic sequence was obtained in 2002 [7].

Epidemiology

Swine represent the only known host of SWPV. Unlike VACV, SWPV fails to experimentally infect or adapt to several mammalian and avian species

[1, 5], with only a single report of productive SWPV infection following intradermal inoculation of rabbits [4]. This restricted host range suggests that swine represent the reservoir of SWPV in nature. SWP is present world-wide with limited serological survey data from Europe indicating that 8–19% of swine serum samples contained anti-SWPV antibodies [2, 16]. Young swine are most often affected, as adult swine rarely present with clinical disease [10, 15]. Morbidity rates can be high (up to 100%), but mortality is generally negligible (less than 5%) [2].

Natural transmission of SWP is not well understood but is often associated with poor sanitation. SWP has been associated with louse (*Haematopinus suis*) infestation. Lice are able to mechanically transmit SWPV and are thought to affect the extent and distribution of cutaneous lesions, which often occur in less keratinized abdominal and inguinal regions [5, 13, 15]. However, SWP without evidence of louse involvement has been described, suggesting the role for other insect vectors or the possibility of horizontal transmission [1, 2, 16, 17]. Vertical SWPV transmission is indicated by sporadic cases of congenital infection resulting in stillborn fetuses with generalized lesions [7, 16, 18].

Disease

SWP is an acute disease characterized by typical poxviral eruptive dermatitis. Animals up to 3 months of age are the most susceptible to clinical disease, while adults usually develop a mild, self-limiting form of the disease. Multiple cutaneous lesions are commonly found on the flanks, belly, inner side of the legs, ears, and, less frequently, on the face of affected animals [1, 2, 10, 17, 19, 20]. Lesions can also be found on the teats of sows and on the face, lips, and tongue of suckling pigs [20]. In congenital infections, lesions are observed over the entire body and in the oral cavity [16, 18]. When virus transmission is associated with mechanical vectors, the distribution of lesions tends to reflect preferred vector feeding areas.

The incubation period is thought to be 4–14 days under field conditions [2, 10] and 3–5 days after intradermal or intravenous virus inoculation [1, 21], although longer periods have been described [5]. Initial lesions are round, flat, pale maculae of 3–5 mm in diameter that over 2 days progress to papulae that are 1–2 mm in height, 1–2 cm in diameter, and occasionally confluent. Appearance of papulae may be accompanied by a slight and transient increase in body temperature and loss of appetite [15, 21]. A true vesicle stage is absent or transient [4, 18, 21, 22]. The lesions usually become umbilicated and shrink about a week after appearing, and they are replaced by crusts, which are ultimately shed, leaving discolored spots [21]. Complete recovery is observed 15–30 days post exposure, but it may be delayed if secondary bacterial infection occurs [1, 2, 10, 23].

Pathology

The most conspicuous histological change caused by SWPV infection is hydropic degeneration of stratum spinosum keratinocytes [1, 10, 16, 18, 20–22, 24, 25]. Hyperplasia of epidermal cells is not as marked as in poxviral infections of other mammals, an observation that might be related to the lack of a SWPV-encoded homologue of the poxviral epidermal growth factor-like gene [1, 7, 10]. The cytoplasm of the infected cell is brightened and enlarged, contains eosinophilic inclusion bodies resembling poxviral type B inclusion bodies [25], and reacts strongly with antibodies against viral antigens [26]. Hydropic degeneration and inclusion bodies are also observed in the outer root sheaths of the hair follicles [21, 22]. The nucleus of affected cells exhibits margination of chromatin and a large, central "vacuole" resembling the nuclear clearing observed in sheeppox virus-infected keratinocytes [10, 21, 22, 24, 25, 27]. No significant fluid accumulation is observed between keratinocytes. Apical keratinocytes undergo necrosis at later stages of infection. Leukocyte infiltration is observed in the underlying dermis and, to a lesser degree, the affected epidermis, with few viral antigen-containing dermal macrophages [26]. When involved, the inguinal lymph nodes present edema, hyperemia, hyperplasia, and few virus antigen-containing cells which may contain infectious virus [21, 24].

Ultrastructurally, infected cells exhibit a marked decrease in keratin precursors (tonofilaments) and loss of intercellular interdigitations characteristic of the stratum spinosum [24, 25]. Individual inclusion bodies consist of electron-dense central cores surrounded by lamellar bodies and maturing viral particles (viroplasm) [19, 24, 25, 28, 29]. The large, well defined nuclear "vacuole" can be more accurately described as a region of low electron density, which lacks a surrounding membrane and contains cross-striated fibrils similar to those observed in the cytoplasm.

Pathogenesis

SWPV may enter the host through pre-existing skin abrasions and preferentially replicates in epidermal keratinocytes of the stratum spinosum [22]. Although mature viral particles have been observed in epidermal basal cells [25] and viral antigen has been detected in dermal macrophages [26], there is no direct evidence that these cell types support virus replication *in vivo*. With the exception of moderate changes in superficial lymph nodes, including edema, hyperemia, and hyperplasia, tissues other than the skin are rarely affected. Infectious virus can be readily isolated from the skin of infected animals as early as 3 days post intradermal inoculation, but can be isolated from regional lymph nodes only when skin lesions are severe [21]. A viremic stage has been suggested to account for virus spread from the primary to secondary sites of replication in the skin and for congenital infection; however, virus has not been isolated from blood of infected animals [5, 16, 18, 21].

Functional studies on SWPV pathogenesis are lacking. The complement of virus genes with putative roles in virulence and host range suggests that modulation of host immune responses and inhibition of apoptosis likely play a role in pathogenesis [7, 30, 31].

Convalescent swine are resistant to SWPV challenge, indicating that infection induces protective immunity [1, 2, 5, 15, 32]. However, the immune mechanisms associated with protection are not known. SWPV neutralizing activity is present in swine sera as early as 7 days post infection; however, low neutralizing titers, delayed kinetics of antibody response, and lack of neutralizing antibodies at 50 days post infection have been reported [5, 15, 22, 33]. Suckling pigs may also be protected by maternal antibody [13], although high neonatal mortality rates have been observed [20]. Decreased mitogen and SWPV-induced proliferative responses have been observed in peripheral blood mononuclear cells from experimentally infected swine [33].

Genome

The complete nucleotide sequence of the SWPV genome was obtained from the 17077-99 strain, which was isolated during an outbreak of SWP in Nebraska (GenBank accession no. AF410153, [7]). The 146,454-base pair (bp), A+T-rich SWPV genome (Tab. 1) is organized with a central unique coding region representing 95% of the genome, and two identical inverted terminal repeat (ITR) regions. SWPV contains 150 putative genes (SPV001-SPV150), 4 of which (SPV018, SPV019, SPV020, and SPV026) have no poxvirus homologues. A conserved central core of 106 genes (SPV021 to SPV125) is largely collinear with genomes of other mammalian poxviruses, and contains homologues of the many genes elucidated in VACV (between F9L to A38L) to be involved in basic poxviral replicative functions, including viral transcription, DNA replication, and virion assembly and maturation [7]. Terminal genomic regions contain genes that likely function in modulation or evasion of host immune responses, modulation or inhibition of host cell apoptosis, or in aspects of cell or tissue tropism [7, 30]. Many potential SWPV host range genes are homologues to genes present in other poxviruses. However, SWPV does contain a unique complement of these genes which likely are important in specifying its restricted host range.

A number of SWPV proteins are potentially secreted or membrane bound and are likely involved in the disruption or modulation of host immune responses, as indicated by similarity to other viral immunomodulators and by the presence of predicted signal peptide or transmembrane sequences (Tab. 2) [7, 30]. Potentially secreted immunomodulators include homologues of IFN-γ receptor (SPV008), IFN-α/β binding protein

Table 1. General characteristics of swinepox virus

Members of the genus	Swinepox virus (SWPV)
Host range	Pig
Virion morphology	Brick-shaped; 320 × 240 nm
Genome size and G+C content	146 kbp; 27.5% G+C

(SPV132), IL-18 binding protein (SPV011), and a novel tanapoxvirus MHC-like TNF-α binding protein (SPV003/SPV148) [34]. Potentially membrane-bound immunomodulators encoded by SWPV include homologues of cellular seven-transmembrane G-protein-coupled CC chemokine receptors (SPV005 and SPV146), CD47 (SPV125), and a MARCH family ubiquitin ligase [30, 35, 36]. SPV005, although truncated, and SPV146 are similar to cellular and viral CC chemokine receptor homologues, including yaba-like disease virus 7L, which is expressed on the surface of virus-infected cells and capable of activating extracellular signal-regulated kinases (ERK1/2) upon binding chemokines [37]. SPV009 contains an LAP/PHD/RING-CH domain similar to cellular and viral MARCH family membrane-bound ubiquitin ligases capable of down-regulating expression of host immuno-regulatory cell surface glycoproteins, including MHC class I, Fas-CD95 and CD4, by M153R, a MARCH ligase and virulence factor of myxoma virus [35, 38, 39].

Several SWPV proteins may have intracellular host range or immune evasion functions (Tab. 2). These include homologues of VACV double-stranded RNA-dependent protein kinase inhibitors (SPV010 and SPV032), which confer resistance to the antiviral effects of IFN and influence virus host range [40]. Poxviral serine proteinase inhibitors (serpins) are known to perform anti-inflammatory roles, and the single serpin encoded in SWPV (SPV145) is similar to LSDV149, YLDV 149R and MYXV M151R [30]. Notably, SPV001, SPV007, SPV133, SPV135 and SPV150 are similar to the poxviral gene family which includes VACV A52R (Family 5, [41]). Although the function of most of these genes is not known, the VACV A52R virulence factor and other VACV proteins with sequence similarity to A52R are able to down-regulate host cell IL-1R/Toll-like receptor (TLR) superfamily signaling mechanisms important for induction of innate immune and inflammatory responses [42–44].

SWPV encodes homologues of several other poxviral proteins known to affect virus virulence, virus growth in specific cell types, and/or apoptotic responses. These include homologues of MYXV M011L apoptosis regulator protein (SPV012), VACV A14.5L virulence protein (SPV103), and VACV C7L host range protein (SPV064), a SWPV protein encoded at the same centrally located locus as homologues in *Leporipoxvirus*, *Yatapoxvirus* and *Capripoxvirus* [7, 45–47]. SPV138 encodes a protein similar to the orthopox-

Table 2. Swinepox virus ORFs with predicted host range and immunomodulatory functions [7]

ORF [a]	Genome position	Length[b]	Predicted structure and/or function[c]
SPV001	736 – 287	150	A52R family protein
SPV003	2452 – 1433	340	MHC-likeTNF binding protein,TM
SPV005	3630 – 2824	269	Chemokine receptor-like protein, TM
SPV006	5285 – 3696	530	Kelch-like protein
SPV007	6038 – 5331	236	A52R family protein
SPV008	6885 – 6064	274	IFN-γ-receptor, SP
SPV009	7385 – 6921	155	LAP/PHD-fingerprotein, TM
SPV010	7705 – 7448	86	elF2γ-1ike PKR inhibitor
SPV011	8146 – 7745	134	IL-18 binding protein, SP
SPV012	8672 – 8172	167	Apoptosis regulator, TM
SPV015	11205 – 9604	534	Kelch-like protein
SPV032	25909 – 25379	177	PKR inhibitor, host range
SPV064	56225 – 56779	185	Host range protein
SPV103	98184 – 98026	53	Virulence factor, TM
SPV125	116661 – 115783	293	CD47-like protein, SP, TM
SPV132	126727 – 127758	344	IFN-α/ß binding protein, SP
SPV133	127790 – 128326	179	A52R family protein
SPV135	129411 – 129974	188	A52R family protein
SPV136	129994 – 131715	574	Kelch-like protein,TM
SPV138	132666 – 133403	246	N1R/p28-like host range protein
SPV141	135128 – 137032	635	Ankyrin repeat protein
SPV142	137100 – 138554	485	Ankyrin repeat protein, TM
SPV143	138662 – 139951	430	Ankyrin repeat protein
SPV144	140003 – 141481	493	Ankyrin repeat protein
SPV145	141494 – 142453	320	Serpin
SPV146	142522 – 143631	370	Chemokine receptor-like protein, TM
SPV148	144003 – 145022	340	MHC-like TNF binding protein, TM
SPV150	145719 – 146168	150	A52R family protein

[a]Swinepox virus ORF number.
[b]Length of ORFs in codons.
[c]Function was deduced from the degree of similarity to known genes and from Prosite signatures. TM, transmembrane; SP, N-terminal signal peptide.

virus p28, an E3 ubiquitin ligase required for ectromelia virus replication in macrophages *in vitro* and virulence *in vivo*, and to homologues encoded by members of the genera *Capripoxvirus*, *Leporipoxvirus*, and *Yatapoxvirus* [48–50]. SWPV also encodes four proteins containing ankyrin-repeat motifs

(SPV141 to SPV144), motifs encoded by most chordopoxviruses in multigene families. Poxviral genes encoding ankyrin-repeats have been associated with host range functions, inhibition of virally induced apoptosis, virulence, and virus/host interaction, and have been suggested to comprise specific gene complements that affect viral host range [51–57]. Similarly, SPV006, SPV015 and SPV136 encode homologues of poxvirus kelch-like proteins. Mutations in pox kelch-like proteins have been associated with altered host range *in vitro*, immunopathology *in vivo*, or viral attenuation [58–60]. The distinct nature of the SWPV multigene family gene complement suggests that it contributes to SWPV host specificity.

Other proteins encoded in terminal regions of the SWPV genome and potentially mediating virus/host interactions include homologues of poxvirus proteins resembling cellular enzymes, including SPV128 (hydroxysteroid dehydrogenase), a gene absent in both capripoxviruses and leporipoxviruses, and SPV129 (superoxide dismutase), SPV130 (DNA ligase) and SPV140 (tyrosine protein kinase) [7]. SWPV encodes a unique complement of enzymes likely involved in nucleotide metabolism, including a ribonucleotide reductase large subunit absent in capripoxviruses, leporipoxviruses, and yatapoxviruses. SWPV also encodes a homologue of the variola virus (strain Bangladesh) B22R (SPV131, 1959 amino acids), a putative membrane protein of unknown function.

Notably absent in SWPV are homologues of genes present in closely related viruses and known to affect virus/host interaction. These include homologues of VACV F1L and myxoma virus M-T4 anti-apoptotic proteins, VACV C23L 35-kDa CC chemokine inhibitor, viral IL-1 and TNF receptors, viral epidermal growth factor-like proteins, and viral homologues of cellular CD200/Ox-2. Also absent in SWPV, similar to capripoxviruses, leporipoxviruses, and yatapoxviruses, are homologues of genes located at the VACV A26L locus and involved in formation of insoluble A-type inclusion bodies [7].

Molecular biology

Studies on the molecular biology of SWPV are limited, with only a few reports addressing characterization and expression of selected viral genes [61–63]. The SWPV homologue of VACV F13L protein P37 (SPV025) has been characterized as a component of the extracellular enveloped virus particle; however, it was unable to functionally complement F13L in VACV replication [62]. Despite sequence differences between SPV010 and VACV K3L-encoded eIF2a-like proteins, both act as pseudosubstrate inhibitors of PKR [61]. Kinetic studies of SWPV replication in swine cells *in vitro* have shown considerable delay in DNA accumulation, RNA transcription, and protein expression relative to VACV, with detectable levels taking at least twice as long to accumulate [3]. In general, SWPV replicates poorly upon initial isolation in swine cell cultures, requiring multiple passages before inducing a cytopathic effect (CPE) [15, 16, 21, 22, 32]. Although SWPV has been reported not to induce CPE and/or replicate in bovine, rabbit, and feline cell cultures [15, 32, 64] and replicate preferentially in cultured cells of swine origin, limited replication in cultures of non-swine cells has been reported [65, 66].

Due to its restricted host range, use of SWPV as a vaccine expression vector has been proposed [67, 68]. Genetically engineered SWPV vectors expressing pseudorabies virus (PrV) and classical swine fever virus antigens have been constructed and in the case of PrV shown to induce immune responses in pigs [66, 69]. SWPV is able to express antigens in non-swine cells and may represent a safe host range-restricted vaccine vector for non-swine species [64, 65]. Cellular immune costimulatory molecules have also been expressed in recombinant SWPV as adjuvants for experimental SWPV-based vaccines [70].

References

1 Schwarte LH, Biester HE (1941) Pox in swine. *Am J Vet Res* 2: 136–140
2 de Boer GF (1975) Swinepox, virus isolation, experimental infections and the differentiation from vaccinia virus infections. *Arch Virol* 49: 141–150
3 Massung RF, Moyer RW (1991) The molecular biology of swinepox virus. II. The infectious cycle. *Virology* 180: 355–364
4 Datt NS (1964) Comparative studies of pigpox and vaccinia viruses. I. Host range pathogenicity. *J Comp Pathol* 74: 62–69
5 Shope RE (1940) Swine pox. *Arch Ges Virusforsch* 1: 457–467
6 Moyer RW, Arif B, Black DN, Boyle DB, Buller RM, Dumbell KR, Esposito JJ, McFadden G, Moss B, Mercer AA et al (2000) Family Poxviridae. In: MHV van Regenmortel, CM Fauquet, DHL Bishop, EB Carstens, MK Estes, SM Lemon, J Maniloff, MA Mayo, DJ McGeoch, CR Pringle, RB Wickner (eds) *Virus taxonomy*. Academic Press, New York
7 Afonso CL, Tulman ER, Lu Z, Zsak L, Osorio FA, Balinsky C, Kutish GF, Rock DL (2002) The genome of swinepox virus. *J Virol* 76: 783–790
8 Schnitzlein WM, Tripathy DN (1991) Identification and nucleotide sequence of the thymidine kinase gene of swinepox virus. *Virology* 18: 727–732
9 Spinola M (1842) Krankheiten der Schweine. Ed A Hieschwald, Berlin, p204
10 McNutt SH, Murray C, Purwin P (1929) Swine pox. *Am Vet Med Assoc* 74: 752–761
11 Poenaru J (1913) Recherches sur le virus filtrant dans la variole des porcelets. *Bull Soc Cent Med Vet* 67: 148
12 Akazawa S, Matsumura J (1937) *Rep Govt Inst Vet Res (Fusan)* X: p8
13 Manninger R, Csontos J, Salyi J (1940) Über die ätiologie des pockenartigen Ausschlages der Ferkel. *Arch Tierheilkunde* 75: 159–179
14 Blakemore F, Abdussalam M (1956) Morphology of the elementary bodies and cell inclusions in swine pox. *J Comp Pathol* 66: 373–377

15 Kasza L, Bohl EH, Jones DO (1960) Isolation and cultivation of swine pox virus in primary cell cultures of swine origin. *Am J Vet Res* 21: 269–273
16 Paton DJ, Brown IH, Fitton J, Wrathall AE (1990) Congenital pig pox: A case report. *Vet Rec* 127: 204
17 Jubb TF, Ellis TM, Peet RL, Parkinson J (1992) Swinepox in pigs in northern Western Australia. *Aust Vet J* 69: 99
18 Borst GH, Kimman TG, Gielkens AL, van der Kamp JS (1990) Four sporadic cases of congenital swinepox. *Vet Rec* 127: 61–63
19 Kim JCS, Luong LC (1975) Ultrastructure of swine pox. *Vet Med Small Anim Clin* 70: 1043–1045
20 Olufemi BE, Ayoade GO, Ikede BO, Akpavie SO, Nwufoh KJ (1981) Swine pox in Nigeria. *Vet Rec* 109: 278–280
21 Kasza L, Griesemer RA (1962) Experimental Swine Pox. *Am J Vet Res* 23: 443–450
22 Meyer RC, Conroy JD (1972) Experimental swinepox in gnotobiotic piglets. *Res Vet Sci* 13: 334–338
23 Miller RC, Olson LD (1980) Experimental induction of cutaneous streptococcal abscesses in swine as a sequela to swinepox. *Am J Vet Res* 41: 341–347
24 Cheville NF (1966) The cytopathology of swine pox in the skin of swine. *Am J Pathol* 49: 339–352
25 Teppema JS, De Boer GF (1975) Ultrastructural aspects of experimental swinepox with special reference to inclusion bodies. *Arch Virol* 49: 151–163
26 Cheville NF (1966) Immunofluorescent and morphologic studies on swinepox. *Pathol Vet* 3: 556–564
27 Plowright W, Ferris RD (1958) The growth and cytopathogenicity of sheep-pox virus in tissue cultures. *Br J Exp Pathol* 39: 424–435
28 Conroy JD, Meyer RC (1971) Electron Microscopy of swinepox virus in germfree pigs and in cell culture. *Am J Vet Res* 32: 2021–2032
29 Smid B, Valicek L, Mensik J (1973) Replication of swinepox virus in the skin of naturally infected pigs. Electron microscopic study. *Zentralbl Veterinarmed B* 20: 603–612
30 Massung RF, Jayarama V, Moyer RW (1993) DNA sequence analysis of conserved and unique regions of swinepox virus: identification of genetic elements supporting phenotypic observations including a novel G protein-coupled receptor homologue. *Virology* 197: 511–528
31 Kawagishi-Kobayashi M, Cao C, Lu J, Ozato K, Dever TE (2000) Pseudosubstrate inhibition of protein kinase PKR by swine pox virus C8L gene product. *Virology* 276: 424–434
32 Garg SK, Meyer RC (1972) Adaptation of swinepox virus to an established cell line. *Appl Microbiol* 23: 180–182
33 Williams PP, Hall MR, McFarland MD (1989) Immunological responses of cross-bred and in-bred miniature pigs to swine poxvirus. *Vet Immunol Immunopathol* 23: 149–159
34 Brunetti CR, Paulose-Murphy M, Singh R, Qin J, Barrett JW, Tardivel A, Schneider P, Essani K, McFadden G (2003) A secreted high-affinity inhibitor of human TNF from Tanapox virus. *Proc Natl Acad Sci USA* 100: 4831–4836
35 Bartee E, Mansouri M, Hovey Nerenberg BT, Gouveia K, Fruh K (2004)

Downregulation of major histocompatibility complex class I by human ubiquitin ligases related to viral immune evasion proteins. *J Virol* 78: 1109–1120

36 Sanderson CM, Parkinson JE, Hollinshead M, Smith GL (1996) Overexpression of the vaccinia virus A38L integral membrane protein promotes Ca^{2+} influx into infected cells. *J Virol* 70: 905–914

37 Najarro P, Lee HJ, Fox J, Pease J, Smith GL (2003) Yaba-like disease virus protein 7L is a cell-surface receptor for chemokine CCL1. *J Gen Virol* 84: 3325–3336

38 Guerin JL, Gelfi J, Boullier S, Delverdier M, Bellanger FA, Bertagnoli S, Drexler I, Sutter G, Messud-Petit F (2002) Myxoma virus leukemia-associated protein is responsible for major histocompatibility complex class I and Fas-CD95 down-regulation and defines scrapins, a new group of surface cellular receptor abductor proteins. *J Virol* 76: 2912–2923

39 Mansouri M, Bartee E, Gouveia K, Hovey Nerenberg BT, Barrett J, Thomas L, Thomas G, McFadden G, Fruh K (2003) The PHD/LAP-domain protein M153R of myxomavirus is a ubiquitin ligase that induces the rapid internalization and lysosomal destruction of CD4. *J Virol* 77: 1427–1440

40 Langland JO, Jacobs BL (2002) The role of the PKR-inhibitory genes, E3L and K3L, in determining vaccinia virus host range. *Virology* 299: 133–141

41 Smith GL, Chan YS, Howard ST (1991) Nucleotide sequence of 42 kbp of vaccinia virus strain WR from near the right inverted terminal repeat. *J Gen Virol* 72: 1349–1376

42 Bowie AG, Haga IR (2005) The role of toll-like receptors in the host response to viruses. *Mol Immunol* 42: 859–867

43 Stack J, Haga IR, Schroder M, Barlett NW, Maloney G, Reading PC, Fitzgerald KA, Smith GL, Bowie AG (2005) Vaccinia virus protein A46R targets multiple toll-like-interleukin-1 receptor adaptors and contributes to virulence. *J Exp Med* 201: 1007–1018

44 DiPerna G, Stack J, Bowie AG, Boyd A, Kotwal G, Zhang Z, Arvikar S, Latz E, Fitzgerald KA, Marshalll WL (2004) Poxvirus protein N1L targets the I-κB kinase complex, inhibits signaling to NF-κB by the tumor necrosis factor superfamily of receptors, and inhibits NF-κB and IRF3 signaling by Toll-like receptors. *J Biol Chem* 279: 36570–36578

45 Everett H, Barry M, Lee SF, Sun X, Graham K, Stone J, Bleackley RC, McFadden G (2000) M11L: a novel mitochondria-localized protein of myxoma virus that blocks apoptosis of infected leukocytes. *J Exp Med* 191: 1487–1498

46 Perkus ME, Goebel SJ, Davis SW, Johnson GP, Limbach K, Norton EK, Paoletti E (1990) Vaccinia virus host range genes. *Virology* 179: 276–286

47 Betakova T, Wolffe E, Moss B (2000) The vaccinia virus A14.5L gene encodes a hydrophobic 53-amino-acid virion membrane protein that enhances virulence in mice and is conserved among vertebrate poxviruses. *J Virol* 74: 4085–4092

48 Senkevich TG, Koonin EV, Buller RM (1994) A poxvirus protein with a RING zinc finger motif is of crucial importance for virulence. *Virology* 198: 118–128

49 Senkevich TG, Wolffe EJ, Buller RM (1995) Ectromelia virus RING finger protein is localized in virus factories and is required for virus replication in macrophages. *J Virol* 69: 4103–4111

50 Nerenberg BT, Taylor J, Bartee E, Gouveia K, Barry M, Fruh K (2005) The

poxviral RING protein p28 is a ubiquitin ligase that targets ubiquitin to viral replication factories. *J Virol* 79: 597–601

51 Gillard S, Spehner D, Drillien R, Kirn A (1986) Localization and sequence of a vaccinia virus gene required for multiplication in human cells. *Proc Natl Acad Sci USA* 83: 5573–5577

52 Mossman K, Lee SF, Barry M, Boshkov L, McFadden G (1996) Disruption of M-T5, a novel myxoma virus gene member of poxvirus host range superfamily, results in dramatic attenuation of myxomatosis in infected European rabbits. *J Virol* 70: 4394–4410

53 Spehner D, Gillard S, Drillien R, and Kirn A (1988) A cowpox virus gene required for multiplication in Chinese hamster ovary cells. *J Virol* 62: 1297–1304

54 Camus-Bouclainville C, Fiette L, Bouchiha S, Pignolet B, Counor D, Filipe C, Gelfi J, Messud-Petit F (2004) A virulence factor of myxoma virus colocalizes with NF-κB in the nucleus and interferes with inflammation. *J Virol* 78: 2510–2516

55 Johnston JB, Wang G, Barrett JW, Nazarian SH, Colwill K, Moran M, McFadden G (2005) Myxoma virus M-T5 protects infected cells from the stress of cell cycle arrest through its interaction with host cell cullin-1. *J Virol* 79: 10750–10763

56 Antoine G, Scheiflinger F, Dorner F, Falkner FG (1998) The complete genomic sequence of the modified vaccinia Ankara strain: comparison with other orthopoxviruses. *Virology* 244: 365–396

57 Shchelkunov SN, Safronov PF, Totmenin AV, Petrov NA, Ryazankina OI, Gutorov VV, Kotwal GJ (1998) The genome sequence analysis of the left and right species-specific terminal region of a cowpox virus strain reveals unique sequences and a cluster of intact ORFs for immunomodulatory and host range proteins. *Virology* 243: 432–460

58 Kochneva G, Kolosova I, Maksyutova T, Ryabchikova E, Shchelkunov S (2005) Effects of deletions of kelch-like genes on cowpox virus biological properties. *Arch Virol* 150: 1857–1870

59 Tulman ER, Afonso CL, Lu Z, Zsak L, Sur J-H, Sandybaev NT, Kerembekova UZ, Zaitsev VL, Kutish GF, Rock DL (2002) The genomes of sheeppox and goatpox viruses. *J Virol* 76: 6054–6061

60 Pires de Miranda M, Reading PC, Tscharke DC, Mur Phy BJ, Smith GL (2003) The vaccinia virus kelch-like protein C2L affects calcium-independent adhesion to the extracellular matrix and inflammation in a murine intradermal model. *J Gen Virol* 84: 2459–2471

61 Kawagishi-Kobayashi M, Cao C, Lu J, Ozato K, Dever TE (2000) Pseudosubstrate inhibition of protein kinase PKR by swine pox virus C8L gene product. *Virology* 276: 424–434

62 Barcena J, Lorenzo MM, Sanchez-Puig JM, Blasco R (2000) Sequence and analysis of a swinepox virus homologue of the vaccinia virus major envelope protein P37 (F13L). *J Gen Virol* 81: 1073–1085

63 Feller JA, Massung RF, Turner PC, Gibbs EP, Bockamp EO, Beloso A, Talavera A, Vinuela E, Moyer RW (1991) Isolation and molecular characterization of the swinepox virus thymidine kinase gene. *Virology* 183: 578–585

64 Winslow BJ, Cochran MD, Holzenburg A, Sun J, Junker DE, Collisson EW

(2003) Replication and expression of a swinepox virus vector delivering feline leukemia virus gag and env to cell lines of swine and feline origin. *Virus Res* 98: 1–15

65 Barcena J, Blasco R (1998) Recombinant swinepox virus expressing beta-galactosidase: investigation of viral host range and gene expression levels in cell culture. *Virology* 243: 396–405

66 Hahn J, Park S-H., Song J-Y, An S-H, Ahn B-Y (2001) Construction of recombinant swinepox viruses and expression of the classical swine fever virus E2 protein. *J Virol Methods* 93: 49–56

67 Foley PL, Paul PS, Levings RL, Hanson SK, Middle LA (1991) Swinepox virus as a vector for the delivery of immunogens. *Ann NY Acad Sci* 646: 220–222

68 Tripathy DN (1999) Swinepox virus as a vaccine vector for swine pathogens. Adv Vet Med 41: 463–480

69 van der Leek ML, Feller JA, Sorensen G, Isaacson W, Adams CL, Borde DJ, Pfeiffer N, Tran T, Moyer RW, Gibbs EPJ (1994) Evaluation of swinepox virus as a vaccine vector in pigs using an Aujeszky's disease (pseudorabies) virus gene insert coding for glycoproteins gp50 and gp63. *Vet Rec* 134: 13–18

70 Winslow BJ, Kalabat DY, Brown SM, Cochran MD, Collisson EW (2005) Feline B7.1 and B7.2 proteins produced from swinepox virus vectors are natively processed and biologically active: Potential for use as non-chemical adjuvants. *Vet Microbiol* 111: 1–13

Poxviruses
ed. by Andrew A. Mercer, Axel Schmidt and Olaf Weber

Genus *Avipoxvirus*

David B. Boyle

CSIRO Livestock Industries, Australian Animal Health Laboratory, 5 Portarlington Road, Geelong, Victoria 3220, Australia

Abstract

Poxviruses identified in skin lesions of domestic, pet or wild birds are assigned largely by default to the *Avipoxvirus* genus within the subfamily *Chordopoxvirinae* of the family *Poxviridae*. Avipoxviruses have been identified as the causative agent of disease in at least 232 species in 23 orders of birds. Vaccines based upon attenuated avipoxvirus strains provide good disease control in production poultry, although with the large and intensive production systems there are suggestions and real risks of emergence of strains against which current vaccines might be ineffective. Sequence analysis of the whole genome has revealed overall genome structure and function resemblance to the *Chordopoxvirinae*; however, avipoxvirus genomes exhibit large-scale genomic rearrangements with more extensive gene families and novel host range gene in comparison with the other *Chordopoxvirinae*. Phylogenetic analysis places the avipoxviruses externally to the Chorodopoxvirinae to such an extent that in the future it might be appropriate to consider the *Avipoxvirus*es as a separate subfamily within the *Poxviridae*. A unique relationship exists between Fowlpox virus (FWPV) and reticuloendothelosis viruses. All FWPV strains carry a remnant long terminal repeat, while field strains carry a near full-length provirus integrated at the same location in the FWPV genome. With the development of techniques to construct poxviruses expressing foreign vaccine antigens, the avipoxviruses have gone from neglected obscurity to important vaccine vectors in the past 20 years. The seminal observation of their utility for delivery of vaccine antigens to non-avian species has driven much of the interest in this group of viruses. In the veterinary area, several recombinant avipoxviruses are commercially licensed vaccines. The most successful have been those expressing glycoprotein antigens of enveloped viruses, e.g. avian influenza, Newcastle diseases and West Nile viruses. Several recombinants have undergone extensive human clinical trials as experimental vaccines against HIV/AIDS and malaria or as treatment regimens in cancer patients. The safety profile of avipoxvirus recombinants for use as veterinary and human vaccines or therapeutics is now well established.

Introduction

Poxviruses identified in skin lesions of domestic, pet or wild birds are assigned largely by default to the *Avipoxvirus* genus within the subfamily *Chordopoxvirinae* of the family *Poxviridae* [1]. Disease is characterised by proliferative lesions of the skin ranging from small nodules to tumour or wart-like masses and rarely with proliferative or diphtheric membranes on mucous membranes of the respiratory tract, mouth and oesophagus. *Avipoxvirus*es have usually been assigned species names on the basis of the bird species from which the virus was isolated or at least described by light or electron microscopy of lesions. Our understanding of the relationships of these avipoxvirus species to each other and to the type species – Fowlpox virus (FWPV) – is rudimentary since detailed genomic information is currently available for two FWPV isolates [2, 3] and one Canarypox virus (CNPV) isolate [4]. The detailed study of FWPV and CNPV has been driven largely by their use as vaccine vectors for poultry and human vaccines [5].

Avipoxviruses have been identified as the causative agent of disease in a wide range of avian species – a review of available literature reveals natural infections described in at least 232 species in 23 orders of birds [6]. In some instances these infections have been of considerable concern as a threat to endangered species or species in captive breeding recovery programs. Disease caused by FWPV in domestic poultry, while not one of the major diseases of concern to commercial poultry production, can cause significant problems from time to time when conditions are favourable for transmission, predominantly mechanical transmission by mosquitoes. Attenuated strains of FWPV and other avipoxviruses are successfully and widely used to vaccinate susceptible species for disease control.

A detailed understanding of the molecular virology and relationships of avipoxviruses is largely restricted to FWPV and CNPV for which full-genome sequences are available [2–4]. These studies have revealed characteristic poxvirus morphology with a large double-stranded DNA genome (266–288 kbp for FWPV, 365 kbp for CNPV), cytoplasmic replication with gene expression regulatory elements in common with the *Chordopoxvirinae* and a genome that encodes in excess of 250 putative genes. The genomes of avipoxviruses exhibit large-scale genomic rearrangements, more extensive gene families and novel host range genes in comparison with other members of the *Chordopoxvirinae*. A unique relationship exists between FWPV and the avian retrovirus, reticuloendotheliosis virus (REV). All FWPV vaccine strains carry a remnant long terminal repeat (LTR), while field strains carry a near full-length provirus integrated at the same location [7]. The provirus gives rise to REV infection when the FWPV infects susceptible poultry. REV sequences have not been detected in other avipoxviruses.

Perhaps the greatest interest in avipoxviruses has been in their use as vaccine vectors, firstly to deliver vaccine antigens to poultry and secondly as vaccine vectors for non-avian species [5]. Many of the techniques developed for the construction of orthopoxvirus recombinants were readily adapted to the construction of avipoxvirus recombinants with appropriate changes to the cell substrate and selection protocols. Approaching a billion doses of recombinant FWPV (rFWPV)-avian influenza H5 vaccine have been used in the control of avian influenza in Mexico [8, 9]. The observation that FWPV and CNPV infect a wide range of mammalian cells without productive replication, while gene expression occurs at a level sufficient to induce antibody, cellular and protective immune responses to the recombinant antigen, is the driver for substantial interest in the use of avipoxviruses as vaccine vectors in non-avian species, including man [10]. The utility of the avipoxvirus vaccine vectors has been extended in prime-boost vaccination regimens [11] and for the delivery of cancer and immune-stimulatory/modulatory molecules for treatment regimens [12]. A number of avipoxvirus recombinants have undergone extensive preclinical and clinical trials, including vaccine candidates for the control of HIV/AIDS and malaria [13, 14]. The safety profile of such recombinants is now well established [15, 16].

Taxonomy and origins

The avipoxviruses are classified in the family *Poxviridae* subfamily *Chordopoxvirinae* genus *Avipoxvirus* [17]. The type species is the well known and characterised FWPV; many different isolates of FWPV have been described, including a wide range of commercial vaccines available globally. There are now ten official species accepted with several more tentative species in the genus (Tab. 1) [1]. Species demarcation is poorly defined but criteria include disease characteristics, origin host, growth characteristics in the chorioallantoic membrane of embryonated eggs or avian cell cultures, cross-protection in chickens against classical FWPV and restriction endonuclease analysis of genomic DNA and cross-hybridisation. Given the size and complexity of the avipoxviruses at the genome and virion level, our understanding of the extent and nature of relationships of the official and tentative species is at best rudimentary. Nucleotide sequence determination of selected conserved genes might provide a means of presumptive classification, and has been attempted using the 4b gene [18, 19]. However, relationships defined on this basis will fail to take into account variations in gene content arising from gene loss and gain during evolution [20, 21]. Avipoxviruses may well be the largest and most diverse genus in the *Chordopoxvirinae* [6]. Although the origin of birds is controversial they have probably been around in some form for at least 150 million years. The avipoxviruses have almost certainly co-evolved with their hosts and in the process acquired genes from the host that have assisted the virus to counter the host cellular and immune responses [20, 21]. Avipoxviruses that are accepted as species tend to be those which have been successfully cultivated in the laboratory.

Disease in production poultry

FWP in production chickens and turkeys tends to be slow-spreading with characteristic skin lesions ranging from small nodules to tumour or wart-

Table 1. Family *Poxviridae*, subfamily *Chordopoxvirinae*, genus *Avipoxvirus*

Genus *Avipoxvirus*	Type species	Other species	Assigned abbreviations	Full genome sequence: strain and accession no.
	Fowlpox virus		FWPV	FP9 – AJ581527[a] FPV – AF198100[b]
		Canarypox virus	CNPV	CNPV – AY318871[c]
		Juncopox virus	JNPV	
		Mynahpox virus	MYPV	
		Pigeonpox virus	PGPV	
		Psittacinepox virus	PSPV	
		Quailpox virus	QUPV	
		Sparrowpox virus	SRPV	
		Starlingpox virus	SLPV	
		Turkey pox	TKPV	
Tentative species		Crowpox virus	CRPV	
		Peacockpox virus	PKPV	
		Penguinpox virus	PEPV	

[a]Fowlpox virus FP9: plaque-purified, tissue culture-adapted, attenuated European virus [3].
[b]Fowlpox challenge virus; Animal Health Inspection Service Centre for Veterinary Biologicals, Ames Iowa [2].
[c]CNPV strain Wheatley; American Type Culture Collection (ATCC VR-111) [4].

like masses, which occur predominantly on unfeathered skin areas, e.g. the head and legs [22]. Mortality is low; however, a substantial transient drop in egg production can occur in laying birds. In young birds, growth rates can be significantly affected [23, 24]. The role that simultaneous REV infection arising from the provirus integrated into the FWPV genome might play in the expression of FWP is unknown. However, the potential effects of REV infection cannot be discounted since REV infection is known to lead to immunosuppression [25]. A severe diphtheritic form of FWP with proliferative lesions in the nasal, laryngeal and tracheal regions results in respiratory distress and higher mortality [23].

Disease control – vaccination and transmission control

Control of diseases caused by the avipoxviruses is best achieved by the prevention of transmission and by vaccination [23, 24]. There are no suitable or specific treatments available once infection is established. Transmission by biting insects, particularly mosquitoes, can be linked to seasonal and geographic incidence of disease, so appropriate screening and insect control programs for commercial poultry production can reduce the impacts of disease. Infection *via* cutaneous injuries or inhalation can be reduced by control of crowding and decontamination of premises following outbreaks. FWPV can survive in dried scabs for extended periods (weeks if not months), so attention to sanitation of housing, feed and water is essential for effective disease prevention. FWP is distributed worldwide in domestic poultry with the incidence variable in different geographic regions – related to management and hygiene practices, mosquito control and the use of prophylactic vaccination.

Prophylactic vaccination for the control of FWP in commercial poultry has been practiced for a considerable period of time [22]. The early history of vaccines for FWP, pigeonpox (PGP), turkeypox (TKP) and CNP was well documented by Beaudette in 1949 [22]; this reference provides fascinating insights into early attempts to vaccinate against avipox and to understand the relationships amongst the avipoxviruses. Since the late 1960s and early 1970s, modern commercial vaccines have been available in most regions of the world for the control of FWP. Other vaccines, e.g. against TKP, quailpox (QUP), CNP and PGP, are available in specific regions [23]. The virus strains used in the vaccines have been derived empirically by the passage of field isolates in embryonated eggs or chicken embryo-derived cell cultures. Selected on the basis of immunogenicity (protection against challenge) and attenuation (reduced pathogenicity) in comparison with the original field strain and on the basis of freedom from other avian pathogens, the vaccines have found widespread use for the control of avipox disease. The origins and history of many named vaccine strains are obscure because of commercial consideration or the loss of information with the passage of time [22].

Avipox vaccines are most effectively applied by wing web inoculation using single or two pronged needle inoculators. This makes the vaccines expensive to administer in commercial poultry as each bird needs to be handled. Vaccine take can be assessed by inspection of the inoculation site for the development of a characteristic pox lesion 5–10 days after vaccination. Administration by other routes, e.g. drinking water or spray is far less effective in the induction of protective immunity with much higher virus concentrations needed to achieve an acceptable level of protection [22, 26, 27]. *In ovo* vaccination at close to hatch date with highly attenuated or rFWPV strains may be a viable alternative to individual chick vaccination [28, 29]. Revaccination may be necessary to sustain protection in chickens used for egg production or subject to heavy challenge because of high mosquito populations. FWPV vaccine strains range from highly attenuated suitable for vaccination of 1-day-old chicks to others that have residual pathogenicity and are recommended for first use at 3–6 weeks of age or for revaccination immediately prior to commencement of lay.

FWPV vaccines provide little if any effective protection against TKPV, QUPV and CNPV, consequently it is essential to use the appropriate vaccine for disease control in these species [22, 23]. The poor cross-protection is probably related to the antigenic differences that exist between these viruses. Vaccination is sometimes practiced in the circumstance where a small proportion of birds are showing disease in an endeavour to limit further spread within a flock.

Humoral and cell-mediated immune responses play a role in immunity, although their relative contributions have not been thoroughly investigated [30, 31]. Humoral responses can be assessed by ELISA or virus neutralisation [32]. The utility of commercial poultry vaccines for the control of poxvirus diseases in other avian species is questionable, although on occasions their use has been attempted. Such uses are not without risks as the vaccines themselves should always be considered as having the potential to cause disease in the vaccinated species.

Many of the commercial vaccine strains of FWPV and CNPV have been used as the basis for the development of recombinant poxvirus vector-based vaccines for control of other avian diseases or for use in non-avian species [5]. FWPV vaccines were associated with the inadvertent spread of REV because of apparent vaccine contamination. Modern poultry vaccines rarely have the risks of spread of adventitious agents as the quality assurance processes for their production are well established [24]. Nonetheless, the association of FWPV with REV has turned out to be a unique relationship with the REV provirus integrated in the FWPV genome [7]. The availability of full-genome sequences for one FWPV strain and one CNPV opens the possibility of rational attenuation of viruses for the development of new avipox vaccines or to enhance specific immunogenicity characters where the avipoxviruses are used for the delivery of antigens and/or immunomodulators to avian and non-avian hosts [5]. We have recently removed the integrated REV provirus from FWPV vaccine and field strains to generate new vaccine strains (D. Boyle, unpublished).

Emergence of new strains

The scale and intensity of global production of commercial poultry has led to the emergence of new diseases principally caused by viruses and the emergence of variants of existing viruses. With this have come the pressures to develop new vaccines or to select new strains for inclusion in vaccines. Most of the challenges have come from the RNA genome viruses [e.g. infectious bronchitis virus, infectious bursal disease virus (IBDV) and avian influenza virus]; however, Marek's disease virus (MDV) has undergone substantial variation with many older vaccines providing poor or limited protection against the emerging MDV strains [33]. There are some reports of emerging FWPV strains causing unusual disease patterns or disease against which current vaccine may be ineffective [34–36]. The potential for emergence of new FWPV strains or the spread of other avipoxviruses into commercial poultry production systems is real; however, the timing and consequence of emergence of such viruses is not predictable.

Disease in wild birds and in threatened avian species

Avipoxviruses have been identified as the causative agent of disease in a wide range of avian species (for review see [6]). Mortalities approaching 80–100% on occasions have been reported in pigeons, quails and canaries with highly pathogenic strains [22–24]. Natural disease in wild and caged birds ranges from mild cutaneous lesion on feet and other unfeathered areas to severe disease and high mortality associated with cutaneous and diphtheritic disease. Poxvirus infections along with avian malaria are considered to be important factors in limiting and threatening endangered and unique populations of birds on the Hawaiian, Galapagos and Canary Islands [37, 38]. In other circumstances the introduction of poxvirus infections into captive breeding programs for endangered bird species has been of significant concern [39].

Poxvirus infection is generally diagnosed on clinical signs, histopathology, e.g. characteristic cytoplasmic inclusion bodies in infected cells, and electron microscopic detection of virus in lesions [24]. Where viruses have been isolated by inoculation of embryonated eggs or avian cell cultures, further studies have been possible [23, 24]. These studies usually involve cross-protection and pathogenesis studies in chickens in comparison with FWPV [37], restriction endonuclease analysis of genomic DNA [37, 39–42] or sequencing of PCR amplified genome regions [18, 19]. Complex patterns of relationships to FWPV are revealed with the avipoxviruses that are rarely pathogenic in chickens, providing poor cross protection against FWPV challenge and with significant differences in the restriction endonuclease profiles of the genomes [23]. The sources of poxvirus infections in such a wide range of avian species can only be speculated upon; virus infection could be enzootic and only manifests as disease under stress or other environmental factors; virus and disease might spill over from related species or from domestic poultry; and there is the possibility of extended persistence of virus in cutaneous warty lesions in some avian species [43]. Spread of poxvirus from one avian species to another because of habitat disruption or insect transmission has the potential to cause severe disease in the newly infected species. The full nature and complexity of the relationships of these avipoxviruses will only be revealed with detailed genome sequence analysis of a greater range of isolates.

Whole genome sequences

Genome sequences with analysis of putative gene functions and relationships are now available for a pathogenic FWPV US (FWP challenge virus;

Animal Health Inspection Centre for Veterinary Biologics, Ames, Iowa), a plaque-purified, tissue culture-adapted, attenuated European virus FWPV (FP9) and a CNPV virulent strain (Wheatley C93, American Type Culture Collection VR-111) [2–4]. Additionally, genome wide differences between the FWPV US and FP9 have been characterised in the HP1 strain, which is the progenitor virulent FWPV of FP9 [3]. FWPV genome sizes ranged from 266 kbp for FP9 to 288 kbp for the pathogenic FWP challenge strain. The CNPV genome (365 kbp) is 80–100 kbp larger than the FWPV genomes. Given the size and complexity of the genomes, it is not proposed to review individual genes and their relationships in detail. Readers are best referred to the original manuscripts for this level of analysis.

In the case of FWPV US, there is a resemblance to *Chordopoxvirinae* in overall genome structure and function with a centralised conserved core of genes whose functions are involved in the basic replicative mechanisms such as viral transcription and RNA modification, genome replication and the structure and assembly of mature virions; there are 65 conserved gene homologues involved in these functions [2]. The FWPV US genome contains inverted terminal repeats approaching 10 kbp in length. Gene expression regulatory elements, e.g. early, intermediate and late promoters, contain typical *Chordopoxvirinae* sequences. The early poxvirus transcription termination sequence (T5NT) is identifiable near the translational stop codon of many predicted early genes. However, there are marked differences in that genome co-linearity in comparison with the *Chordopoxvirinae* is disrupted in FWPV US by translocations and inversions, multiple and large gene families and novel cellular homologues. Much of the marked size difference between FWPV US and other *Chordopoxvirinae* is accounted for by the large numbers of cellular homologues and 10 multi-gene families. Most notably, in FWPV US, the ankyrin repeat family (31 genes), N1R/p28 family (10 genes) and the B22R family (6 genes) represent ~32% of the total genome [2]. There are a large number of putative cellular homologue genes involved in immune evasion, apoptosis, cell growth and tissue tropism. Other cellular homologues are involved in steroid biogenesis, antioxidant functions and vesicle trafficking. All of these suggest that there is a substantial modification of host cell function occurring upon virus infection. There is also a suggested photo-reactivation DNA repair pathway encoded by FWPV US. Gene acquisition by horizontal transfer appears to have played a significant role in the adaptation of FWPV US to its avian host [2].

A comparison of the attenuated, tissue culture-adapted European FP9 strain with FWPV US identified just 118 differences; 71 genes were affected by deletion (26 of 1–9334 bp), insertion (15 of 1–108 bp), substitution, termination or frame-shift [3]. FWPV FP9 is a derivative of a virulent European FWPV HP1 by passage in embryonated eggs and chicken embryo fibroblast cell culture (over 400 passages). Sequence determination of the HP1 at loci where differences exist between the FP9 and FWPV US showed that 68 of 118 loci differed from the FWPV US but were identical to FP9. More than half of the differences between the two geographic FWPV lineages represented differences between the parent virulent viruses – HP1 and FWPV US. Thus, more than half of the differences between FWPV US and FP9 represent differences between different viruses of the two geographic origins. A comparison of the attenuated European FP9 with its virulent parent FWPV HP1 showed that 50 of 118 loci were different – representing changes/mutations accumulated during the egg and tissue culture passage for attenuation. Twelve of the 46 open reading frames affected by the apparent passage-specific mutations encoded members of the ankyrin repeat family. The mechanisms by which such mutations lead to attenuation are as yet unclear [3].

Restriction endonuclease enzyme profiles of avipoxvirus genomes show significant variation in genome arrangements, suggesting the potential for marked differences in genome content [37, 40, 41]. Limited gene sequence data from CNPV Tokyo CG-2 strain indicated that, while CNPV and FWPV appeared to share regions of similar gene order, there are marked differences at the deduced amino acid level. Gene homologies between CNPV and FWPV ranged from 55% to 74%, a divergence that is comparable to that seen between the different *Chordopoxvirinae* genera [44]. The substantial differences between CNPV and FWPV were confirmed by full sequencing of the CNPV genome [4]. The CNPV is markedly larger than FWPV, with 365 kbp *versus* 266–288 kbp. Central regions of the CNPV genome contain homologues of the *Chordopoxvirinae* genes involved in the basic replicative mechanisms such as viral transcription, RNA modification, viral DNA replication, structure and assembly of virions. It has been shown that there are 106 conserved *Chordopoxvirinae* genes shared between CNPV and FWPV with an average of 70% amino acid identity. CNPV genome encodes 39 genes, the homologues for which are absent from the FWPV genome or fragmented, while CNPV lacks 15 genes present in the terminal genome regions of FWPV. Internal genome regions exhibit considerable variability between CNPV and FWPV in contrast with the relative overall conservation of central regions of genomes in other *Chordopoxvirinae*. Major genome variability is located near the junctions of genome rearrangements relative to the other *Chordopoxvirinae*. These regions contain genes that appear to be involved in virus-host interactions. The CNPV Wheatley C93 strain has a close relationship at the nucleotide (98%) and amino acid (91% to 100%) level to the CNPV Tokyo CG-2 strain in those regions for which there is comparable sequence available [4, 44]. This provides a level of confirmation of genome conservation for different isolates causing CNP and supports the designation of CNPV at the species level in the *Avipoxvirus* genus. Tulman et al. [4] concluded that "the genomic data and phylogenic analysis of individual open reading frames support a monophyletic origin of the two avipoxviruses relative to the other *Chordopoxvirinae*." The divergence between FWPV and CNPV appears to be as great as that between other *Chordopoxviridae* genera. The apparent divergence established by restriction endonuclease analysis of avipoxvirus genomes [37, 39–42] and nucleotide sequence of the 4b gene [18, 19] supports this conclusion, and suggests that there is potentially substantial and far ranging genomic diversity amongst the viruses that have been reported as causing disease in at least 232 species in 23 orders of birds. With substantial sequence data from a range of avipoxviruses, our understanding of the *Avipoxvirus* genus may be such that they constitute a separate subfamily within the *Poxviridae*.

Relationships to poxviruses in general

Complete genome sequences for 20 poxviruses have allowed genome wide analysis of phylogeny, genome structure and evolutionary pathways [20, 21]. Gene order and gene spacing are highly conserved within the *Chordopoxvirinae* with the exception of FWPV and CNPV [2, 4]. Phylogenetic analyses placed FWPV externally to the *Chordopoxvirinae* (and presumably CNPV, although a similar analysis has not yet been reported). Notwithstanding the conservation of overall genome composition and structure, including a central core of genes, inverted terminal repeats and a large numbers of functionally important orthologs, the FWPV and CNPV genomes exhibit large-scale genomic rearrangements with more extensive gene families and novel host range genes in comparison with the other *Chordopoxvirinae* [2, 3]. Gene loss and gain appears to be the dominant mechanism in the evolution of *Chordopoxvirinae* genomes. Many genes have been acquired by horizontal gene transfer from the host. FWPV has gained 94 genes since divergence from a common ancestor of the *Chordopoxvirinae* [20]. Of 34 gene families shared by *Chordopoxvirinae* with animal genomes, 8 are found only in FWPV [21]. Acquisition by horizontal gene transfer has been an important and perhaps dominant source of new genes for avipoxviruses in their evolution. Many of the acquired genes enable the virus to escape host cellular and immunological defences. It is perhaps an important challenge in poxvirus biology to understand the rate and mechanisms of gene transfer.

FWPV and REV

A unique relationship exists between the avian retrovirus, REV and FWPV [7]. A near full-length, infectious provirus of REV has been found in the genome of most if not all pathogenic isolates of FWPV. At least one vaccine strain, FPV-S, whose use was discontinued because it was the source of REV in poultry in Australia also carries the infectious provirus. Other FWPV vaccine strains known not to cause REV infection carry either a complete or partial LTR [7, 45–49]. The presence of full or partial LTRs in FWPV vaccine strains can be explained by the presence of tandem repeated LTRs of the provirus. Such structures are inherently unstable in poxvirus genomes with the intervening sequences rapidly lost by inter- or intramolecular recombination [50, 51]. Instability of tandem repeated sequences in poxviruses is exploited to construct recombinants using transient dominant selection methods [52, 53]. Since the 5' and 3' LTRs of the integrated provirus are different, the presence or absence of a full or partial LTR upon loss of the REV provirus would be dependent upon the cross-over site during the recombination event in the LTR leading to the provirus loss [45, 48].

A number of features of the REV integration into the FWPV genome suggest an ancient and unique event [46]. Provirus and LTR sequences have only been found at a single location in the FWPV genomes examined (between FPV201 and FPV203, FPV202 being mainly encompassed by the LTR sequences) [3]. Integration site sequence duplications that normally occur during provirus integration are absent. The 5′ LTR is complete, while the 3' LTR has deletions and rearrangements when the near full-length provirus is present. Provirus or LTRs have been identified in FWPV strains isolated well before the widespread use of FWPV vaccines in commercial poultry [46]. In Australia, FWPV field isolates made in late 1940s to early 1950s all carry the REV provirus (unpublished observations). FWPV strains carrying the REV sequences appear to be globally distributed.

Re-integration or recombination of REV into vaccine strains carrying LTR remnants appears an unlikely scenario. It has been speculated that this might lead to pathogenic FWPV arising from vaccine strains in the field and perhaps explain apparent vaccine failures. Given the complexity of the FWPV genome and the undoubted role of multiple gene products in determination of virulence and pathogenicity, the re-integration of REV alone is unlikely to be sufficient to restore full virulence to FWPV vaccine strains – many of which have undergone multiple passages in culture to generate attenuation with consequent gene loss, rearrangement and disruption [3]. There is no evidence for this occurring and it is important to remember the biology of FWPV and REV. Retrovirus integration takes place in the nucleus of infected cells by a well-defined pathway. FWPV DNA replication takes place in the cytoplasm of the infected cell and is unlikely to be a readily accessible target for REV integration. Given the physical and functional separation of REV and FWPV infection cycles in cells, integration is an unlikely rare event following co-infection of cells with FWPV and REV. Attempts to generate re-integration or recombination between the vaccine strain FPV-M3 and REV by co-infection and passage in CEF cells have been unsuccessful (Boyle, unpublished). It is difficult, however, to construct selection regimens that might allow rare events to be detected. In contrast, co-infection in cell culture with MDV and REV or avian leukosis virus (ALV) leads to rapid and numerous integration events in the MDV genome – a reflection that MDV replicates in the nucleus of the infected cell where it can be a ready target for REV or ALV integration [54].

The presence of REV provirus or LTR in other avipoxviruses has been explored to some extent. LTR sequences are absent from the completed genome sequence of CNPV in which the orthologous genes flanking REV sequences in FWPV are separated by 64 bp [4]. USA FWPV commercial vaccines (12 vaccines plus a parent strain and a recombinant FWPV) and 3 PGPV vaccines contain complete or incomplete REV LTRs [47], while 1 QUPV and 2 CNPV vaccines did not contain integrated REV sequences [47]. None of the FWPV vaccine strains contained a REV provirus. In contrast, 6 of 7 field isolates of FWPV made between 1949 and 1978 appeared to contain an integrated REV provirus – the remaining isolate appeared to have only a LTR remnant [46]. In this study, a CNPV and PGPV isolated in 1968 lacked integrated REV sequences. Our observations (unpublished) on 25 avipoxviruses isolated from native avifauna of Australia and New Zealand have shown that REV is absent from these isolates. The isolates were tested by both PCR and hybridisation for LTR and gag region sequences, which showed that REV sequences were absent throughout the genome, not just the homologous site identified in FWPV. Australian avipoxvirus isolates from poultry (chickens, turkeys, geese and pigeons) carried the provirus or a LTR.

Rapid loss of the REV provirus upon passage of field isolates in embryo cell culture might be expected due to the inherent instability of the provirus structure as discussed above. This has probably occurred in existing commercial vaccine strains during passage and selection. For the maintenance of the REV provirus in field strains of FWPV, a selective advantage must be conferred on the FWPV strains carrying the REV provirus. Equally intriguing is the mechanism of recovery of REV infection in chickens infected with FWPV strains carrying the REV provirus. We were unable to detect free REV in the vaccine strain FPV-S, yet this virus when inoculated into chickens gave rise to REV infection in all chickens [7]. Other FWPV isolates are undoubtedly contaminated with free infectious REV – perhaps a reflection of the co-isolation of FWPV and REV in the chicken embryo or cell culture used for isolation [55]. The integrated near full-length REV provirus is infectious since transfection of EcoRI-digested FWPV DNA into CEF cells results in the recovery of infectious REV [7]. Expression of the REV genome from the provirus 5' LTR promoter is unlikely since the promoter would not be recognised by the poxvirus transcription machinery. Expression of REV protein has been reported; however, the co-isolation of REV and FWPV in the culture systems could be an explanation for the apparent expression of REV genes from the FWPV carrying integrated REV provirus [45, 49].

The selective advantage conferred on FWPV strains carrying the REV provirus is probably related to the immunosuppression caused by the concurrent REV infection [25], leading to a longer and more severe FWP infection, thus extending the duration of possible transmission by contact or mosquitoes. Although it has been suggested that widespread FWPV vaccination might provide selection pressure for the retention of REV provirus in FWPV [48], this seems unlikely since REV provirus has been detected in isolates made before the widespread use of FWVP vaccines in poultry. Upon removal of the REV provirus from two field strains and FPV-S vaccine strain of FWPV, we have not been able to identify marked differences in disease produced in chickens infected at 3–4 week of age (Boyle, unpublished).

Removal of the REV LTR has been considered desirable by some for the use of FWPV strains for poultry vaccines or as vaccine vectors [5]. In the process of constructing complex FPV-M3/HIV vaccine vectors, we have removed the remnant LTR from FPV-M3 by using this locus for the insertion of HIV vaccine antigens. We did not observe any apparent impacts upon virus replication *in vitro* [53].

The relationship between FWPV and REV leads to a mechanism by which a retrovirus is transmitted through the infection cycle of a poxvirus, including mechanical transmission by biting insects. Earlier observations of REV transmission by biting insects might better be explained by transmission *via* FWPV. With FWPV, we are perhaps observing one example of a poxvirus gaining genetic information to its advantage from another virus. Equally, REV has gained significant advantage by being transmitted by mosquitoes.

Avipoxvirus vaccine vector technology

Upon the development of techniques for the construction of recombinant vaccinia viruses [56, 57] to deliver heterologous antigens as vaccines, a great deal of interest was generated in the potential to use species-specific poxviruses, e.g. FWPV and CNPV, in a similar manner. At the time there was a paucity of knowledge regarding the molecular biology of the avipoxviruses, consequently it was not obvious that the techniques developed for vaccinia virus recombinants would be directly applicable to the construction of avipox recombinants. The first attempts to construct rFWPV and rCNPV were directed to their use as vectors for the delivery of poultry vaccines [58, 59]. The novel finding that rFWPV and rCNPV could enter non-avian cell types, undergo an abortive (non-productive) replication cycle, express the foreign encoded vaccine antigen and thus induce immune responses in mammals led to an expanded interest in the avipoxviruses as vaccine vectors [10, 60–62]. It is generally accepted that avipoxviruses can cause productive infection and thus disease only in avian species. Early studies indicated that upon intranasal inoculation of mice there was an absence of replication and limited pathology [63] and that in cell cultures cytopathology occurs without replication [64]. For those avipoxviruses examined, there appears to be a general ability to enter most non-avian cells; however, the stage at which replication is blocked appears different depending upon cell type [65, 66].

Table 2. rFWPV and rCNPV delivered vaccines and therapeutics

Poultry vaccines	Veterinary vaccines (not poultry)	Human vaccines (non-cancer)	Cancer antigens and immuno-stimulatory/ modulatory molecules
Avian influenza virus H5, H7, H9, N1, NP	Bovine respiratory syncytial virus	Cytomegalovirus glycoprotein B	Bladder cancer
Avian leukosis virus	Bovine viral diahorrea virus	Hepatitis B virus	B7-1
Coccidiosis	Canine distemper virus	Hepatitis C virus	Melanoma
Duck hepatitis B virus	Equine herpes virus 1	HIV-1, HIV-2, SIV, SHIV	
Haemorrhagic enteritis of turkeys	Feline coronavirus	Japanese encephalitis virus	P53
Infectious bronchitis virus (avian coronavirus)	Feline leukaemia virus	Malaria *Plasmodium falciparum* *Plasmodium berghei*	Prostate antigen
Infectious bursal disease virus	Rabbit haemorrhagic disease virus	Measles irus	
Marek's disease virus	Rabies virus	*Mycobacterium* BCG	
Mycoplasma gallisepticum	West Nile virus	Rabies virus	
Newcastle disease virus			
Reticuloendotheliosis virus			
Turkey rhinotracheitis virus			

Detailed reference relating to studies using avipoxviruses expressing these antigens can be obtained by suitably structured search: http://www.ncbi.nlm.nih.gov/entrez

There has been a recent unconfirmed report of FWPV productive infection of baby hamster kidney (BHK-21) cell line [67]. A consequence of the abortive replication cycle is that avipoxvirus recombinants as vaccine vectors offer significant safety advantages when used to deliver vaccine antigens to mammalian species, in comparison with replication competent poxvirus vectors, e.g. vaccinia virus. A large number of rFWPV and rCNPV have now been described designed to express vaccine antigens for delivery to mammalian hosts. Many have progressed through veterinary and human clinical trials, including vaccine candidates against HIV/AIDS and malaria [13, 68] (Tab. 2). The safety profile of such recombinants is now well established, as a significant number of such recombinants have been subjected to regulatory required toxicology and safety trials in animals and man without reports of significant adverse events [69–71].

Construction technologies

A substantial understanding of the molecular biology of the orthopoxviruses was essential to the construction of the first vaccinia virus recombinants. It was subsequently shown that the avipoxviruses share many basic features with the orthopoxviruses, particularly in the control of gene expression, e.g. promoters and transcription termination sequences. The essential features required for the construction of avipoxvirus recombinants can be summarised as: (1) a poxvirus promoter for gene expression, (2) sites for insertion of foreign genes either within a non-essential gene or between genes, and (3) a suitable method for identification and selection of recombinants. Additionally, it is prudent to consider the removal of early poxvirus transcription terminator (T5NT) sequences from the gene(s) to be expressed, as their presence may abort or significantly attenuate early gene expression in cells. Impacts upon the induction of cell-mediated responses may also occur as it has been demonstrated in vaccinia virus that late gene expression may not induce cell-mediated immune responses [72]; this impact has not formally been shown for avipoxvirus recombinants to my knowledge. It might be argued that late gene expression in FWPV is less likely to affect cell-mediated immune responses since FWPV does not shut down host cell protein synthesis to the extent that vaccinia virus does [73]. Antigen processing into MHC class I antigen-presenting pathways has been shown to be the mechanism by which vaccinia virus inhibits cell-mediated immune response induction from late expressed gene products [74].

If avipoxvirus recombinants are intended for animal or human clinical trials, then it is essential to use a cell substrate acceptable for this purpose. Consequently, growth and plaquing must be undertaken in chicken embryo cell cultures derived from certified sources of specific pathogen-free embryonated eggs. Additionally, full documentation and traceability of all biological materials used during the construction and growth of the recombinants will be required for regulatory approval to test the recombinants in humans – the work essentially needs to be conducted under GLP (Good Laboratory Practice) protocols. Other cell substrates, e.g. transformed quail cell lines, are not acceptable for vaccines contemplated for clinical use, although they are suitable for the construction of recombinants for research purposes [75, 76]. The construction of recombinant avipoxviruses should not be embarked upon lightly since the time required to construct recombinants is many months in contrast with vaccinia virus recombinants which can be constructed in a few weeks. The time difference is a reflection of the much longer replication cycle of avipoxviruses in comparison with vaccinia virus [77].

Promoters

It has been generally demonstrated that promoter sequences from one poxvirus will operate across the genera in the *Chordopoxvirinae* retaining temporal regulation [78]. Promoters such as the vaccinia virus P 7.5 early/late promoter have been widely used for the construction of recombinant poxviruses including rFWPV and rCNPV. The choice of promoter appears to have been largely driven by convenience and access with endogenous FWPV and CNPV promoters frequently used along with vaccinia virus optimised synthetic early or early/late promoters. A rational choice of promoter for optimal gene expression in recombinant avipoxviruses is not entirely clear as only a few studies have attempted to compare promoters for levels of expression [78–82] and promoter optimisation by sequence modification has been undertaken only in vaccinia virus. There is a paucity of evidence to support the belief that higher gene expression levels necessarily lead to better immune responses. With certain antigens the nature of the antigen rather than the expression level achieved from recombinant avipoxviruses has a greater impact on the immunogenicity [83].

Insertion sites

The key features of insertion sites are that they do not disrupt gene functions that might affect *in vivo* or *in vitro* replication or gene expression, and that stable recombinants can be plaque purified. The large genome size [2–4, 84] of the avipoxviruses suggests that there are many potential insertion sites (far more than have been described to date [44, 85–87]) and that there is a large capacity to carry multiple gene insertions either at individual or multiple sites [53]. The thymidine kinase gene of FWPV has been used as a locus for the construction of recombinants; however, in some circumstance stable recombinants have proven difficult to obtain [88–90]. We have been able to obtain stable recombinants within the thymidine kinase gene; however, this may be a reflection of the FWPV strain (FPV M3) and cell type used (chicken embryo skin cells) [58]. Others have shown that inactivation of the thymidine kinase gene can affect efficient replication of rFWPV [88]. Use of the thymidine kinase site for insertions is perhaps best avoided as there are many other potential sites including immediately downstream of the thymidine kinase gene [53]. We have encountered difficulties in generating stable recombinants on very few occasions for the approximately 150 recombinants constructed. Instability appears related to the gene being inserted, although with so few unstable recombinants a common factor is difficult to identify.

Recombinant selection

Following the recombination event generated by infection of cell cultures with parent virus and transfection with suitably constructed plasmid, recombinants can be identified by gene hybridisation or expression; however, the proportion of recombinants is low (less 1/1000 of the virus yield), making plaque purification of recombinants challenging. Co-expression of the *Escherichia coli* xanthine guanine ribosyl transferase gene conferring resistance to mycophenolic acid is a convenient selection marker for amplification of recombinants [58]. Additionally, co-expression of the Lac Z gene allows convenient identification and plaque purification of recombinants on the basis of blue staining of plaques with suitable β-galactosidase enzyme substrate [53, 58]. With dominant selection, the selection and marker genes are retained in the final recombinant [53]. Their presence in recombinants intended for human clinical trials may be problematic at the stage of regulatory approval, although rFWPVs carrying such genes have been approved in some jurisdictions for human clinical trials. The use of transient dominant selection for insertion of vaccine or therapeutic genes into avipoxvirus recombinants should be considered, as the selection and marker genes are not retained in the final recombinant and the selection and marker genes can be reused to make additional insertions at different loci [53]. This allows the construction of complex recombinants carrying multiple antigen genes and immune modulators. Multiple rounds (at least three or four) of plaque purification are generally required to generate homogenous stable recombinants. Thereafter, in our hands, recombinants have been stable through multiple generations required for master and working seeds lots, and final trial vaccine batches in preparation for human clinical trials [91]. The availability of plasmid vectors and general selection and amplification techniques, for both dominant and transient dominant selection, facilitates the construction of complex rFWPVs for use in vaccine trials [53, 91].

Avipoxviruses for the recovery of other poxviruses from naked DNA

The description of bacterial artificial chromosome vectors for the construction of vaccinia virus recombinants is dependent upon the use of FWPV to recover infectious vaccinia virus from poxvirus DNA [92, 93]. Poxvirus DNA is non-infectious; however, non-genetic reactivation, whereby an infectious virus can be recovered from an inactivated poxvirus by co-infection with an unrelated poxvirus (infectious or inactivated in a different manner) provides the mechanism for recovery of infectious virus from naked poxvirus DNA [94, 95]. Since productive avipoxvirus infections are restricted to avian cells, FWPV non-genetic reactivation of poxviruses in avian or non-avian cells provides a facile mechanism for recovery of infectious poxvirus from naked DNA – the contaminating FWPV is simply removed by passage on non-avian cells [96]. Recovery of FWPV from DNA has not been demonstrated to date; however, it should be possible by the use of a poxvirus whose replication is non-permissive in avian cells or whose infectivity has been suitably inactivated. Conservation of poxvirus promoter and transcription elements across the poxvirus genera suggests a ready explanation for this mechanism. On occasions FWPV has been incorrectly described as providing packaging or helper virus function [97].

Reverse genetics of RNA viruses – T7 system

The use of T7 RNA polymerase for transient gene expression and for negative-strand RNA virus rescue was pioneered using vaccinia virus expressing T7 polymerase [98]. Replacement of vaccinia virus (wild type or modified vaccinia Ankara) with FWPV expressing T7 has the advantages of reduced cytopathic effects in non-avian cells, comparable levels of expression, handling safety and lack of productive infection. Recovery of the rescued virus is simplified since removal of the FWPV-T7 is achieved by passage on non-avian cell cultures [99–103].

Poultry vaccines

Avian influenza

Vaccination of poultry with rFWPV expressing H5 or H7 avian influenza haemagglutinin (HA) induces protection against experimental or natural infection with highly pathogenic avian influenza (HPAI) [59, 104–106]. Clinical disease and mortality are reduced or prevented even though haemagglutination inhibiting (HI) antibody titres following vaccination are low or undetectable [59, 104, 105]. rFWPV-expressed influenza nucleoprotein (NP) fails to provide protection [105]. Protection is antibody mediated [105] and HA-type specific [104, 105]. Interestingly, a recent report showed that rFWPV-H5-N1 provided protection against H5N1 and H7N1 HPAI challenge. Presumably the cross-protection was mediated *via* immunity to the common neuraminidase (N1) [107]. Shedding of avian influenza virus *via* respiratory and enteric routes is significantly reduced in vaccinated birds [9], thus reducing the potential for spread. Antibody responses to HA and NP rise rapidly following challenge, suggesting a substantial level of replication of challenge virus even though disease does not occur [104]. The restriction of antibody responses to the HA following vaccination and the induction of high titres of antibodies to both HA and NP following infection can be used to discriminate vaccinated birds or flocks from those in which avian influenza (HPAI or LPAI) may have circulated since the latter flocks will have antibodies to both HA and NP – so-called DIVA tests (differentiation of infected from vaccinated animals). Optimisation of the HA insert may not be necessary to provide effective field protection against H5 avian influenza, as a single rFWPV-H5 recombinant provided adequate protection against H5 influenza virus isolates from four continents over a 38-year period [108]. Prior vaccination or field exposure to FWPV may limit the usefulness of rFWPV-influenza vaccines as the protection afforded against avian influenza challenge is inconsistent in such circumstances [109, 110]. rFWPV-H5 alone or in combination with other avian influenza vaccines has been widely used in Mexico – approaching a billion doses of vaccine have been used [109]. HPAI H5N1 in Asia has had profound impacts on poultry production and is currently considered the greatest threat of emergence as pandemic human influenza [111]. rFWPV-influenza vaccines have the potential to find widespread application for poultry vaccination in Asia. Their use to date has only been documented in chickens and turkeys. Vaccine efficacy in ducks and water birds needs to be demonstrated.

Newcastle disease

rFWPV and rPGPV expressing haemagglutinin-neuraminidase (HN) and/or fusion (F) proteins from Newcastle disease virus (NDV) provide protection against challenge with virulent NDV [86, 112–118]. Efficacy may be enhanced by the expression of both HN and F and by the use of rFWPV in conjunction with conventional NDV vaccines in a prime-boost vaccination regimen [113]. NDV HI antibody responses were markedly elevated in chickens vaccinated with live or inactivated NDV vaccine prior to vaccination with rFWPV-HN (geometric mean NDV HI titres were 10–100-fold higher). In contrast, chickens previously vaccinated with non-recombinant FWPV vaccine failed to develop NDV (HI) antibodies following vaccination with rFWPV-HN and were not protected against challenge with virulent NDV.

Other poultry vaccine candidates

Candidate rFWPV vaccines against a number of poultry pathogens have been evaluated (Tab. 2). Vaccine successes have been achieved predominantly with glycoproteins from enveloped viruses, e.g. avian leukosis, avian influenza, MDV, NDV, REV, and turkey rhinotracheitis virus [119–126]. Exceptions have been infectious bursal disease virus (IBDV) and haemorrhagic enteritis of turkeys where rFWPVs expressing the VP2 protein or hexon, respectively, have been shown to induce protective immunity [127–131]. rFWPV vaccine candidates against coccidiosis [132] and infectious bronchitis virus ([133] and Boyle, unpublished observations) have had variable or limited success. Host genetics have been shown to play a role in the efficacy of rFWPV candidate vaccines in chickens against IBDV [128] and MDV [121]. Since these studies have been conducted using inbred chickens, it is not clear if genetic effects play a role in limiting efficacy in commercial production breeds. It is also not clear if the observed differences are related to an inherent feature of the antigens or to their delivery by rFWPV.

Enhancing poultry vaccines based on rFWPV

Heterologous prime-boost vaccination regimens and co-expression of immune-stimulators/modulators have found favour as mechanisms to improve immunogenicity of rFWPV-based vaccines [12, 134]. NDV HI antibody responses were markedly elevated in chickens vaccinated with live or inactivated NDV vaccine prior to vaccination with rFWPV-HN (geometric mean NDV HI titres were 10–100-fold higher) [113]. Sequential vaccination with recombinant MDV and rFWPV expressing the VP2 gene of IBDV markedly improved protection from gross lesions upon challenge with very virulent IBDV [135]. Chicken IL-18 co-expressed with VP2 gene of IBDV has been reported to significantly improve protection afforded against IBDV [5]. Co-expression in rFWPV of chicken type I interferon and NDV HN and F genes reduced post-vaccination body weight loss when the vaccine was used *in ovo* or shortly after hatching; however, the antibody responses to NDV were reduced by the co-expressed interferon [136]. *In ovo* vaccination of turkeys with rFWPV expressing HN and F of NDV and chicken type I or II interferons demonstrated earlier induction of antibodies to NDV without any adverse effects on hatchability. Treatment of chickens with rFWPV expressing chicken myelomonocytic growth factor (cMGF) prolonged survival times and reduced viraemia and tumour incidence when highly susceptible chickens were challenged with virulent MDV. In addition, rFWPV cMGF treatment improved vaccination protection provided by herpes virus of turkey vaccine. Both innate and acquired immune responses appeared enhanced following rFWPV cMGF treatment [137, 138].

Other veterinary vaccines delivered by recombinant avipoxviruses

The safety profile offered by rFWPV and rCNPV for delivering vaccines to non-avian species make them attractive vaccine vectors for a wide range of animal species (Tab. 2). In experimental studies, successful induction of protective immune responses has predominantly occurred with glycoprotein antigens of enveloped viruses. rFWPV and/or rCNPV expressing antigens from rabies, canine distemper, feline leukaemia and West Nile viruses provide effective protection against disease [139–147]. Expression of the rabies glycoprotein by rFWPV provided protection against disease in mice, cats and dogs [10, 139]. In a comparative study of vaccinia virus, rFWPV and rCNPV expressing the rabies glycoprotein, the rCNPV elicited better neutralising antibodies and was approximately 100 times more effective in inducing a protective immune response than rFWPV. Protection provided by immunisation with rCNPV was not significantly different from that induced by the replication competent vaccinia virus rabies glycoprotein recombinant [139]. Although the level of rabies glycoprotein expression was slightly higher from the rCNPV than rFWPV, the difference was not sufficient to account for the marked difference in protection induced. The greater efficacy of rCNPV was probably the motivation for the extensive development of CNPV (ALVAC) as a vaccine vector in preference to FWPV [148, 149]. It is not clear if these differences in immunogenicity would necessarily hold for other antigens expressed by rCNPV and rFWPV.

Canine distemper is an important disease and it provides a useful model for vaccine studies for the other morbilliviruses, e.g. rinderpest and measles. rCNPV (ALVAC) expressing HA and F of canine distemper virus provides high levels of protection against symptomatic disease in a ferret challenge model and in dogs [142, 143]. The rCNPV vaccine was safe and could be used in combination with other canine vaccines without detrimental effects on the performance of any of the vaccines [143]. Oral vaccine delivery was found to be an effective vaccination route inducing protective immunity in highly susceptible Siberian pole cats as a model for potential vaccine use in the endangered black-footed ferret [150]. Intranasal vaccination with rCNPV (ALVAC) and recombinant vaccinia virus expressing HA and F in young ferrets induced lower levels of neutralising antibodies and provided poorer protection than animals vaccinated parenterally [151]. rFWPV and vaccinia virus vaccines expressing rinderpest HN and F genes provided a modest level of protection against canine distemper in ferrets, demonstrating the ability to generate cross-reacting immunity to morbilliviruses [152].

The spread of West Nile virus into North America in 1999–2000 has led to substantial veterinary and public health issues. An effective vaccine for the control of West Nile disease in horses based upon rCNPV expressing prM/E proteins has been licensed for use in horses [145–147]. A single intramuscular dose of vaccine provided protection against the development of viraemia (eight out of nine horses) following challenge (day 26 post vaccination) using West Nile virus-infected mosquitoes even in the absence of measurable antibody responses in some of the horses [146]. Two doses of vaccine provided effective protection against the development of mosquito-transmitted viraemia for at least 1 year post vaccination [145]. A marked amnestic antibody response was observed in horses previously vaccinated with an inactivate West Nile virus vaccine and subsequently boosted with the rCNPV vaccine – a prime-boost vaccination regimen [147].

rCNPV expressing *env* and *gag* genes of feline leukaemia virus provides high level protection against oro-nasal challenge with feline leukaemia virus [144, 153]. Protection lasted for at least 1 year, was effective against severe contact challenge and was obtained in the absence of detectable antibodies to the env antigen. A high proportion of the cats failed to develop latent infections following challenge. When used in combination with other feline vaccines there were no impacts upon the performance of the rCNPV vaccine or the other vaccines.

Preclinical and clinical human vaccine trials

The search for an effective HIV/AIDS vaccine is perhaps the greatest biomedical research challenge existing today. It is in this area that rFWPV and rCNPV have been explored in great detail. It is not proposed to review this area extensively as it is well covered in specialised reviews [154]. Underlying this interest is the safety profile of avipoxviruses in non-avian hosts [70, 155, 156], the observations that heterologous prime-boost vaccination regimens can both enhance and direct the immune response to DNA vaccines and other poorly immunogenic vaccines [11, 13, 157, 158], and that co-expression of immunostimulatory/modulatory molecules can enhance or modify the nature of responses [159–161]. Much of the emphasis on rFWPV and rCNPV has been in their use in prime-boost vaccination regimens to generate enhanced cell-mediated immune responses [13, 157]. Studies in non-human primates have shown that this approach induces elevated levels of cellular immunity and provides effective levels of immunity against HIV/SHIV that can reduce peak and set viral loads, albeit without preventing infection. Regrettably, to date early phase human clinical trials with DNA/rFWPV prime-boost vaccination regimens have provided disappointing results [162, 163]. Co-expression of immunostimulatory/modulatory molecules in conjunction with HIV antigens, while attractive scientifically has, in our hands, faced substantial regulatory hurdles when proposed for use in non-HIV infected individuals. rFWPV expressing HIV antigens and human interferon-γ has been tested in Phase I/IIa therapeutic vaccination trials in HIV-positive individuals; however, the results have once again been disappointing [164]. In contrast to HIV/AIDS, the prime-boost vaccination regimen involving DNA vaccine and rFWPV has provided promising levels of T cell-mediated immunity to malaria including *Plasmodium falciparum* in pre-clinical and human clinical trials [14, 71, 165, 166]. rFWPV and rCNPV have been explored for the delivery of vaccines against cytomegalovirus, hepatitis B and C viruses, Japanese encephalitis virus, measles virus, rabies virus and mycobacterium (Tab. 2) [5].

In the cancer therapy area, rFWPV and rCNPV are being explored to see whether they can express cancer antigens and immunostimulatory/modulatory molecules to develop novel treatment regimens [167–171]. This is a large and growing area of research and is well covered in specialised literature. It is an area in which immunostimulatory/modulatory molecules can be explored since the safety concerns are overridden to the extent that, in the absence of any other treatment regimen, a higher level of risk can be accepted. This can include the direct intra-tumour injection of rFWPV or rCNPV expressing tumour antigens and immunostimulators in attempts to break self tolerance.

General conclusions

The avipoxviruses have gone from neglected obscurity to important vaccine vectors in the past 20 years. The seminal observation of their utility for delivery of vaccine antigens to non-avian species has driven much of the interest in this group of viruses to the extent that rFWPV and rCNPV have undergone extensive clinical trials in humans for vaccines against HIV/AIDS and in treatment regimens for cancer patients. Their application as vaccine vectors in avian and non-avian species has been most successful where glycoprotein antigens of enveloped viruses have been expressed. Interest in the human area has been driven by their safety profile, generation of enhanced and directed responses in prime-boost vaccination regimens and the ability to co-express immunostimulatory/modulatory molecules. Exploration of the basic molecular virology of the avipoxviruses has thrown light on the evolutionary pathways of the *Poxviridae* and in the future it may be necessary to consider the *Avipoxvirus* genus as a separate subfamily within the *Poxviridae* but outside the *Chordopoxvirinae*. The intriguing and unique relationship that exists between FWPV and REV is one of those fascinating stories that have emerged from our studies of this group of viruses.

To provide consistency and accuracy this manuscript has adopted the nomenclature and abbreviations used by the ICTV: 7th Report [1]. However, where referring to specific isolates or strains of virus, the nomenclature or abbreviation adopted by the publication where the isolate or strain was described have been used, e.g. FPV-M3, FP1.

References

1 van Regenmortel MHV, Fauquet CM, Bishop DHL, Carstens EB, Estes MK, Lemon SM, Maniloff J, Mayo MA, McGeoch DJ, Pringle CR, Wickner RB (2000) *Virus taxonomy: The Seventh Report of the International Committee on Taxonomy of Viruses*. Academic Press, New York

2 Afonso CL, Tulman ER, Lu Z, Zsak L, Kutish GF, Rock DL (2000) The genome of fowlpox virus. *J Virol* 74: 3815–3831

3 Laidlaw SM, Skinner MA (2004) Comparison of the genome sequence of FP9, an attenuated, tissue culture-adapted European strain of Fowlpox virus, with those of virulent American and European viruses. *J Gen Virol* 85: 305–322

4 Tulman ER, Afonso CL, Lu Z, Zsak L, Kutish GF, Rock DL (2004) The genome of canarypox virus. *J Virol* 78: 353–366

5 Skinner MA, Laidlaw SM, Eldaghayes I, Kaiser P, Cottingham MG (2005)

Fowlpox virus as a recombinant vaccine vector for use in mammals and poultry. *Expert Rev Vaccines* 4: 63–76
6 Bolte AL, Meurer J, Kaleta EF (1999) Avian host spectrum of avipoxviruses. *Avian Pathol* 28: 415–432
7 Hertig C, Coupar BE, Gould AR, Boyle DB (1997) Field and vaccine strains of fowlpox virus carry integrated sequences from the avian retrovirus, reticuloendotheliosis virus. *Virology* 235: 367–376
8 Webster RG, Taylor J, Pearson J, Rivera E, Paoletti E (1996) Immunity to Mexican H5N2 avian influenza viruses induced by a fowl pox-H5 recombinant. *Avian Dis* 40: 461–465
9 Swayne DE, Beck JR, Mickle TR (1997) Efficacy of recombinant fowl poxvirus vaccine in protecting chickens against a highly pathogenic Mexican-origin H5N2 avian influenza virus. *Avian Dis* 41: 910–922
10 Taylor J, Weinberg R, Languet B, Desmettre P, Paoletti E (1988) Recombinant fowlpox virus inducing protective immunity in non-avian species. *Vaccine* 6: 497–503
11 Ramsay AJ, Leong KH, Ramshaw IA (1997) DNA vaccination against virus infection and enhancement of antiviral immunity following consecutive immunization with DNA and viral vectors. *Immunol Cell Biol* 75: 382–388
12 Leong KH, Ramsay AJ, Boyle DB, Ramshaw IA (1994) Selective induction of immune responses by cytokines coexpressed in recombinant fowlpox virus. *J Virol* 68: 8125–8130
13 Kent SJ, Zhao A, Best SJ, Chandler JD, Boyle DB, Ramshaw IA (1998) Enhanced T-cell immunogenicity and protective efficacy of a human immunodeficiency virus type 1 vaccine regimen consisting of consecutive priming with DNA and boosting with recombinant fowlpox virus. *J Virol* 72: 10180–10188
14 Moorthy VS, Imoukhuede EB, Keating S, Pinder M, Webster D, Skinner MA, Gilbert SC, Walraven G, Hill AV (2004) Phase 1 evaluation of 3 highly immunogenic prime-boost regimens, including a 12-month reboosting vaccination, for malaria vaccination in Gambian men. *J Infect Dis* 189: 2213–2219
15 Tubiana R, Gomard E, Fleury H, Gougeon ML, Mouthon B, Picolet H, Katlama C (1997) Vaccine therapy in early HIV-1 infection using a recombinant canarypox virus expressing gp160MN (ALVAC-HIV): a double-blind controlled randomized study of safety and immunogenicity. *AIDS* 11: 819–820
16 Salmon-Ceron D, Excler JL, Finkielsztejn L, Autran B, Gluckman JC, Sicard D, Matthews TJ, Meignier B, Valentin C, El Habib R et al (1999) Safety and immunogenicity of a live recombinant canarypox virus expressing HIV type 1 gp120 MN MN tm/gag/protease LAI (ALVAC-HIV, vCP205) followed by a p24E-V3 MN synthetic peptide (CLTB-36) administered in healthy volunteers at low risk for HIV infection. AGIS Group and L'Agence Nationale de Recherches sur Le Sida. *AIDS Res Hum Retroviruses* 15: 633–645
17 Mayo MA, Maniloff J, Desselberger U, Ball LA, Fauquet CM (2004) *Virus Taxonomy: VIIIth Report of the International Committee on Taxonomy of Viruses*. Academic Press, New York
18 Luschow D, Hoffmann T, Hafez HM (2004) Differentiation of avian poxvirus strains on the basis of nucleotide sequences of 4b gene fragment. *Avian Dis* 48: 453–462

19 Weli SC, Traavik T, Tryland M, Coucheron DH, Nilssen O (2004) Analysis and comparison of the 4b core protein gene of avipoxviruses from wild birds: evidence for interspecies spatial phylogenetic variation. *Arch Virol* 149: 2035–2046

20 McLysaght A, Baldi PF, Gaut BS (2003) Extensive gene gain associated with adaptive evolution of poxviruses. *Proc Natl Acad Sci USA* 100: 15655–15660

21 Hughes AL, Friedman R (2005) Poxvirus genome evolution by gene gain and loss. *Mol Phylogenet Evol* 35: 186–195

22 Beaudette FR (1949) Twenty years of progress in immunization against virus diseases of birds. *J Am Vet Med Assoc* 115: 234–244

23 Tripathy DN (1993) Avipox viruses. In: JB McFerran, MS McNulty (eds): *Virus infections of birds*. Elsevier, London, 5–15

24 Tripathy DN (2004) *Fowl Pox. Manual of Diagnostic Tests and Vaccines for Terrestrial Animals*. OIE World Organisation for Animal Health, Paris

25 Walker MH, Rup BJ, Rubin AS, Bose HR Jr (1983) Specificity in the immunosuppression induced by avian reticuloendotheliosis virus. *Infect Immun* 40: 225–235

26 Nagy E, Maeda-Machang'u AD, Krell PJ, Derbyshire JB (1990) Vaccination of 1-day-old chicks with fowlpox virus by the aerosol, drinking water, or cutaneous routes. *Avian Dis* 34: 677–682

27 Deuter A, Southee DJ, Mockett AP (1991) Fowlpox virus: pathogenicity and vaccination of day-old chickens via the aerosol route. *Res Vet Sci* 50: 362–364

28 Sharma JM, Zhang Y, Jensen D, Rautenschlein S, Yeh HY (2002) Field trial in commercial broilers with a multivalent *in ovo* vaccine comprising a mixture of live viral vaccines against Marek's disease, infectious bursal disease, Newcastle disease, and fowl pox. *Avian Dis* 46: 613–622

29 Gagic M, St Hill CA, Sharma JM (1999) *In ovo* vaccination of specific-pathogen-free chickens with vaccines containing multiple agents. *Avian Dis* 43: 293–301

30 Tripathy DN, Hanson LE (1975) Immunity to fowlpox. *Am J Vet Res* 36: 541–544

31 Morita C (1973) Role of humoral and cell-mediated immunity on the recovery of chickens from fowlpox virus infection. *J Immunol* 111: 1495–1501

32 Isa G, Pfister K, Kaaden OR, Czerny CP (2002) Development of a monoclonal blocking ELISA for the detection of antibodies against fowlpox virus. *J Vet Med B Infect Dis Vet Public Health* 49: 21–23

33 Davison F, Nair V (2005) Use of Marek's disease vaccines: could they be driving the virus to increasing virulence? *Expert Rev Vaccines* 4: 77–88

34 Singh P, Kim TJ, Tripathy DN (2000) Re-emerging fowlpox : evaluation of isolates from vaccinated flocks. *Avian Pathol* 29: 449–455

35 Fatunmbi OO, Reed WM (1996) Evaluation of a commercial quail pox vaccine (Bio-Pox Q) for the control of "variant" fowl poxvirus infections. *Avian Dis* 40: 792–797

36 Fatunmbi OO, Reed WM (1996) Evaluation of a commercial modified live virus fowl pox vaccine for the control of "variant" fowl poxvirus infections. *Avian Dis* 40: 582–587

37 Tripathy DN, Schnitzlein WM, Morris PJ, Janssen DL, Zuba JK, Massey G,

Atkinson CT (2000) Characterization of poxviruses from forest birds in Hawaii. *J Wildl Dis* 36: 225–230
38 Smits JE, Tella JL, Carrete M, Serrano D, Lopez G (2005) An epizootic of avian pox in endemic short-toed larks (*Calandrella rufescens*) and Berthelot's pipits (*Anthus berthelotti*) in the Canary Islands, Spain. *Vet Pathol* 42: 59–65
39 Kim TJ, Schnitzlein WM, McAloose D, Pessier AP, Tripathy DN (2003) Characterization of an avianpox virus isolated from an Andean condor (*Vultur gryphus*). *Vet Microbiol* 96: 237–246
40 Ghildyal N, Schnitzlein WM, Tripathy DN (1989) Genetic and antigenic differences between fowlpox and quailpox viruses. *Arch Virol* 106: 85–92
41 Schnitzlein WM, Ghildyal N, Tripathy DN (1988) Genomic and antigenic characterization of avipoxviruses. *Virus Res* 10: 65–75
42 Shivaprasad HL, Kim TJ, Woolcock PR, Tripathy DN (2002) Genetic and antigenic characterization of a poxvirus isolate from ostriches. *Avian Dis* 46: 429–436
43 Kirmse P (1967) Host specificity and long persistence of pox infection in the flicker (*Colaptes auratus*). *Bull Wildlife Dis Assoc* 3: 14–20
44 Amano H, Morikawa S, Shimizu H, Shoji I, Kurosawa D, Matsuura Y, Miyamura T, Ueda Y (1999) Identification of the canarypox virus thymidine kinase gene and insertion of foreign genes. *Virology* 256: 280–290
45 Garcia M, Narang N, Reed WM, Fadly AM (2003) Molecular characterization of reticuloendotheliosis virus insertions in the genome of field and vaccine strains of fowl poxvirus. *Avian Dis* 47: 343–354
46 Kim TJ, Tripathy DN (2001) Reticuloendotheliosis virus integration in the fowl poxvirus genome: not a recent event. *Avian Dis* 45: 663–669
47 Moore KM, Davis JR, Sato T, Yasuda A (2000) Reticuloendotheliosis virus (REV) long terminal repeats incorporated in the genomes of commercial fowl poxvirus vaccines and pigeon poxviruses without indication of the presence of infectious REV. *Avian Dis* 44: 827–841
48 Singh P, Schnitzlein WM, Tripathy DN (2003) Reticuloendotheliosis virus sequences within the genomes of field strains of fowlpox virus display variability. *J Virol* 77: 5855–5862
49 Tadese T, Reed WM (2003) Detection of specific reticuloendotheliosis virus sequence and protein from REV-integrated fowlpox virus strains. *J Virol Methods* 110: 99–104
50 Ball LA (1987) High-frequency homologous recombination in vaccinia virus DNA. *J Virol* 61: 1788–1795
51 Kriajevska MV, Zakharova LG, Altstein AD (1994) Genetic instability of vaccinia virus containing artificially duplicated genome regions. *Virus Res* 31: 123–137
52 Falkner FG, Moss B (1990) Transient dominant selection of recombinant vaccinia viruses. *J Virol* 64: 3108–3111
53 Boyle DB, Anderson MA, Amos R, Voysey R, Coupar BE (2004) Construction of recombinant fowlpox viruses carrying multiple vaccine antigens and immunomodulatory molecules. *Biotechniques* 37: 104–111
54 Isfort RJ, Qian Z, Jones D, Silva RF, Witter R, Kung HJ (1994) Integration of

multiple chicken retroviruses into multiple chicken herpesviruses: herpesviral gD as a common target of integration. *Virology* 203: 125–133
55 Fadly AM, Witter RL (1997) Comparative evaluation of *in vitro* and *in vivo* assays for the detection of reticuloendotheliosis virus as a contaminant in a live virus vaccine of poultry. *Avian Dis* 41: 695–701
56 Panicali D, Davis SW, Weinberg RL, Paoletti E (1983) Construction of live vaccines by using genetically engineered poxviruses: biological activity of recombinant vaccinia virus expressing influenza virus hemagglutinin. *Proc Natl Acad Sci USA* 80: 5364–5368
57 Mackett M, Smith GL, Moss B (1982) Vaccinia virus: a selectable eukaryotic cloning and expression vector. *Proc Natl Acad Sci USA* 79: 7415–7419
58 Boyle DB, Coupar BE (1988) Construction of recombinant fowlpox viruses as vectors for poultry vaccines. *Virus Res* 10: 343–356
59 Taylor J, Weinberg R, Kawaoka Y, Webster RG, Paoletti E (1988) Protective immunity against avian influenza induced by a fowlpox virus recombinant. *Vaccine* 6: 504–508
60 Taylor J, Paoletti E (1988) Fowlpox virus as a vector in non-avian species. *Vaccine* 6: 466–468
61 Taylor J, Meignier B, Tartaglia J, Languet B, VanderHoeven J, Franchini G, Trimarchi C, Paoletti E (1995) Biological and immunogenic properties of a canarypox-rabies recombinant, ALVAC-RG (vCP65) in non-avian species. *Vaccine* 13: 539–549
62 Baxby D, Paoletti E (1992) Potential use of non-replicating vectors as recombinant vaccines. *Vaccine* 10: 8–9
63 Nelson JB (1941) The behaviour of poxviruses in the respiratory tract. IV. The nasal instillation of fowl pox virus in chickens and mice. *J Exp Med* 74: 203–211
64 Burnett JW, Frothingham TE (1968) The cytotoxic effect of fowlpox virus on primary human amniotic cell cultures. *Arch Gesamte Virusforsch* 24: 137–147
65 Somogyi P, Frazier J, Skinner MA (1993) Fowlpox virus host range restriction: gene expression, DNA replication, and morphogenesis in nonpermissive mammalian cells. *Virology* 197: 439–444
66 Stannard LM, Marais D, Kow D, Dumbell KR (1998) Evidence for incomplete replication of a penguin poxvirus in cells of mammalian origin. *J Gen Virol* 79: 1637–1646
67 Weli SC, Nilssen O, Traavik T (2004) Morphogenesis of fowlpox virus in a baby hamster kidney cell line. *Med Electron Microsc* 37: 225–235
68 Webster DP, Dunachie S, Vuola JM, Berthoud T, Keating S, Laidlaw SM, McConkey SJ, Poulton I, Andrews L, Andersen RF et al (2005) Enhanced T cell-mediated protection against malaria in human challenges by using the recombinant poxviruses FP9 and modified vaccinia virus Ankara. *Proc Natl Acad Sci USA* 102: 4836–4841
69 De Rose R, Chea S, Dale CJ, Reece J, Fernandez CS, Wilson KM, Thomson S, Ramshaw IA, Coupar BE, Boyle DB et al (2005) Subtype AE HIV-1 DNA and recombinant Fowlpoxvirus vaccines encoding five shared HIV-1 genes: safety and T cell immunogenicity in macaques. *Vaccine* 23: 1949–1956
70 Gilbert PB, Chiu YL, Allen M, Lawrence DN, Chapdu C, Israel H, Holman D,

Keefer MC, Wolff M, Frey SE (2003) Long-term safety analysis of preventive HIV-1 vaccines evaluated in AIDS vaccine evaluation group NIAID-sponsored Phase I and II clinical trials. *Vaccine* 21: 2933–2947
71 Moore AC, Hill AV (2004) Progress in DNA-based heterologous prime-boost immunization strategies for malaria. *Immunol Rev* 199: 126–143
72 Coupar BE, Andrew ME, Both GW, Boyle DB (1986) Temporal regulation of influenza hemagglutinin expression in vaccinia virus recombinants and effects on the immune response. *Eur J Immunol* 16: 1479–1487
73 Prideaux CT, Boyle DB (1987) Fowlpox virus polypeptides: sequential appearance and virion associated polypeptides. *Arch Virol* 96: 185–199
74 Townsend A, Bastin J, Gould K, Brownlee G, Andrew M, Coupar B, Boyle D, Chan S, Smith G (1988) Defective presentation to class I-restricted cytotoxic T lymphocytes in vaccinia-infected cells is overcome by enhanced degradation of antigen. *J Exp Med* 168: 1211–1224
75 Niikura M, Narita T, Mikami T (1991) Establishment and characterization of a thymidine kinase deficient avian fibroblast cell line derived from a Japanese quail cell line, QT35. *J Vet Med Sci* 53: 439–446
76 Cowen BS, Braune MO (1988) The propagation of avian viruses in a continuous cell line (QT35) of Japanese quail origin. *Avian Dis* 32: 282–297
77 Prideaux CT, Boyle DB (1987) Fowlpox virus polypeptides: sequential appearance and virion associated polypeptides. *Arch Virol* 96: 185–199
78 Prideaux CT, Kumar S, Boyle DB (1990) Comparative analysis of vaccinia virus promoter activity in fowlpox and vaccinia virus recombinants. *Virus Res* 16: 43–57
79 Boyle DB (1992) Quantitative assessment of poxvirus promoters in fowlpox and vaccinia virus recombinants. *Virus Genes* 6: 281–290
80 Srinivasan V, Schnitzlein WM, Tripathy DN (2003) A consideration of previously uncharacterized fowl poxvirus unidirectional and bidirectional late promoters for inclusion in homologous recombinant vaccines. *Avian Dis* 47: 286–295
81 Dhawale S, Beisel CE, Nazerian K (1990) Transient expression assay for qualitative assessment of gene expression by fowlpox virus. *Virus Genes* 3: 213–220
82 Kumar S, Boyle DB (1990) Activity of a fowlpox virus late gene promoter in vaccinia and fowlpox virus recombinants. *Arch Virol* 112: 139–148
83 Vazquez-Blomquist D, Gonzalez S, Duarte CA (2002) Effect of promoters on cellular immune response induced by recombinant fowlpox virus expressing multi-epitope polypeptides from HIV-1. *Biotechnol Appl Biochem* 36: 171–179
84 Coupar BE, Teo T, Boyle DB (1990) Restriction endonuclease mapping of the fowlpox virus genome. *Virology* 179: 159–167
85 Boulanger D, Baier R, Erfle V, Sutter G (2002) Generation of recombinant fowlpox virus using the non-essential F11L orthologue as insertion site and a rapid transient selection strategy. *J Virol Methods* 106: 141–151
86 Boursnell ME, Green PF, Campbell JI, Deuter A, Peters RW, Tomley FM, Samson AC, Emmerson PT, Binns MM (1990) A fowlpox virus vaccine vector with insertion sites in the terminal repeats: demonstration of its efficacy using the fusion gene of Newcastle disease virus. *Vet Microbiol* 23: 305–316
87 Spehner D, Drillien R, Lecocq JP (1990) Construction of fowlpox virus vectors

with intergenic insertions: expression of the beta-galactosidase gene and the measles virus fusion gene. *J Virol* 64: 527–533

88 Scheiflinger F, Falkner FG, Dorner F (1997) Role of the fowlpox virus thymidine kinase gene for the growth of FPV recombinants in cell culture. *Arch Virol* 142: 2421–2431

89 Nazerian K, Dhawale S (1991) Structural analysis of unstable intermediate and stable forms of recombinant fowlpox virus. *J Gen Virol* 72: 2791–2795

90 Letellier C (1993) Role of the TK^+ phenotype in the stability of pigeonpox virus recombinant. *Arch Virol* 131: 431–439

91 CouparBEH, Purcell DFJ, Thomson SA, Ramshaw IA, Kent SJ, Boyle DB (2006) Fowlpox virus vaccines for HIV and SHIV clinical and pre-clinical trials. *Vaccine* 24: 1378–1388

92 Domi A, Moss B (2002) Cloning the vaccinia virus genome as a bacterial artificial chromosome in *Escherichia coli* and recovery of infectious virus in mammalian cells. *Proc Natl Acad Sci USA* 99: 12415–12420

93 Domi A, Moss B (2005) Engineering of a vaccinia virus bacterial artificial chromosome in *Escherichia coli* by bacteriophage lambda-based recombination. *Nat Methods* 2: 95–97

94 Hanafusa H, Hanafusa H, Kamahora J (1959) Transformation phenomena in the pox group virus. II. Transformation between several members of pox group. *Biken J* 2: 85–91

95 Joklik WK, Woodroofe GM, Holmes IH, Fenner F (1960) The reactivation of poxviruses. I. Demonstration of the phenomenon and techniques of assay. *Virology* 11: 168–184

96 Harley VR, Hudson PJ, Coupar BE, Selleck PW, Westbury H, Boyle DB (1990) Vaccinia virus expression and sequence of an avian influenza nucleoprotein gene: potential use in diagnosis. *Arch Virol* 113: 133–141

97 Scheiflinger F, Dorner F, Falkner FG (1992) Construction of chimeric vaccinia viruses by molecular cloning and packaging. *Proc Natl Acad Sci USA* 89: 9977–9981

98 Fuerst TR, Niles EG, Studier FW, Moss B (1986) Eukaryotic transient-expression system based on recombinant vaccinia virus that synthesizes bacteriophage T7 RNA polymerase. *Proc Natl Acad Sci USA* 83: 8122–8126

99 Das SC, Baron MD, Barrett T (2000) Recovery and characterization of a chimeric rinderpest virus with the glycoproteins of peste-des-petits-ruminants virus: homologous F and H proteins are required for virus viability. *J Virol* 74: 9039–9047

100 Casais R, Thiel V, Siddell SG, Cavanagh D, Britton P (2001) Reverse genetics system for the avian coronavirus infectious bronchitis virus. *J Virol* 75: 12359–12369

101 Britton P, Green P, Kottier S, Mawditt KL, Penzes Z, Cavanagh D, Skinner MA (1996) Expression of bacteriophage T7 RNA polymerase in avian and mammalian cells by a recombinant fowlpox virus. *J Gen Virol* 77: 963–967

102 Das SC, Baron MD, Skinner MA, Barrett T (2000) Improved technique for transient expression and negative strand virus rescue using fowlpox T7 recombinant virus in mammalian cells. *J Virol Methods* 89: 119–127

103 Evans S, Cavanagh D, Britton P (2000) Utilizing fowlpox virus recombinants to

generate defective RNAs of the coronavirus infectious bronchitis virus. *J Gen Virol* 81: 2855–2865

104 Boyle DB, Selleck P, Heine HG (2000) Vaccinating chickens against avian influenza with fowlpox recombinants expressing the H7 haemagglutinin. *Aust Vet J* 78: 44–48

105 Webster RG, Kawaoka Y, Taylor J, Weinberg R, Paoletti E (1991) Efficacy of nucleoprotein and haemagglutinin antigens expressed in fowlpox virus as vaccine for influenza in chickens. *Vaccine* 9: 303–308

106 Swayne DE (2003) Vaccines for List A poultry diseases: emphasis on avian influenza. *Dev Biol* 114: 201–212

107 Qiao CL, Yu KZ, Jiang YP, Jia YQ, Tian GB, Liu M, Deng GH, Wang XR, Meng QW, Tang XY (2003) Protection of chickens against highly lethal H5N1 and H7N1 avian influenza viruses with a recombinant fowlpox virus co-expressing H5 haemagglutinin and N1 neuraminidase genes. *Avian Pathol* 32: 25–32

108 Swayne DE, Garcia M, Beck JR, Kinney N, Suarez DL (2000) Protection against diverse highly pathogenic H5 avian influenza viruses in chickens immunized with a recombinant fowlpox vaccine containing an H5 avian influenza hemagglutinin gene insert. *Vaccine* 18: 1088–1095

109 Swayne DE, Beck JR, Kinney N (2000) Failure of a recombinant fowl poxvirus vaccine containing an avian influenza hemagglutinin gene to provide consistent protection against influenza in chickens preimmunized with a fowl pox vaccine. *Avian Dis* 44: 132–137

110 Swayne DE, Perdue ML, Beck JR, Garcia M, Suarez DL (2000) Vaccines protect chickens against H5 highly pathogenic avian influenza in the face of genetic changes in field viruses over multiple years. *Vet Microbiol* 74: 165–172

111 Aldhous P, Tomlin S (2005) Avian flu special: Avian flu: Are we ready? *Nature* 435: 399

112 Boursnell ME, Green PF, Samson AC, Campbell JI, Deuter A, Peters RW, Millar NS, Emmerson PT, Binns MM (1990) A recombinant fowlpox virus expressing the hemagglutinin-neuraminidase gene of Newcastle disease virus (NDV) protects chickens against challenge by NDV. *Virology* 178: 297–300

113 Iritani Y, Aoyama S, Takigami S, Hayashi Y, Ogawa R, Yanagida N, Saeki S, Kamogawa K (1991) Antibody response to Newcastle disease virus (NDV) of recombinant fowlpox virus (FPV) expressing a hemagglutinin-neuraminidase of NDV into chickens in the presence of antibody to NDV or FPV. *Avian Dis* 35: 659–661

114 Letellier C, Burny A, Meulemans G (1991) Construction of a pigeonpox virus recombinant: expression of the Newcastle disease virus (NDV) fusion glycoprotein and protection of chickens against NDV challenge. *Arch Virol* 118: 43–56

115 Edbauer C, Weinberg R, Taylor J, Rey-Senelonge A, Bouquet JF, Desmettre P, Paoletti E (1990) Protection of chickens with a recombinant fowlpox virus expressing the Newcastle disease virus hemagglutinin-neuraminidase gene. *Virology* 179: 901–904

116 Ogawa R, Yanagida N, Saeki S, Saito S, Ohkawa S, Gotoh H, Kodama K, Kamogawa K, Sawaguchi K, Iritani Y (1990) Recombinant fowlpox viruses

inducing protective immunity against Newcastle disease and fowlpox viruses. *Vaccine* 8: 486–490
117 Taylor J, Christensen L, Gettig R, Goebel J, Bouquet JF, Mickle TR, Paoletti E (1996) Efficacy of a recombinant fowl pox-based Newcastle disease virus vaccine candidate against velogenic and respiratory challenge. *Avian Dis* 40: 173–180
118 Taylor J, Edbauer C, Rey-Senelonge A, Bouquet JF, Norton E, Goebel S, Desmettre P, Paoletti E (1990) Newcastle disease virus fusion protein expressed in a fowlpox virus recombinant confers protection in chickens. *J Virol* 64: 1441–1450
119 Nazerian K, Yanagida N (1995) A recombinant fowlpox virus expressing the envelope antigen of subgroup A avian leukosis/sarcoma virus. *Avian Dis* 39: 514–520
120 Heine HG, Foord AJ, Young PL, Hooper PT, Lehrbach PR, Boyle DB (1997) Recombinant fowlpox virus vaccines against Australian virulent Marek's disease virus: gene sequence analysis and comparison of vaccine efficacy in specific pathogen free and production chickens. *Virus Res* 50: 23–33
121 Lee LF, Bacon LD, Yoshida S, Yanagida N, Zhang HM, Witter RL (2004) The efficacy of recombinant fowlpox vaccine protection against Marek's disease: its dependence on chicken line and B haplotype. *Avian Dis* 48: 129–137
122 Nazerian K, Lee LF, Yanagida N, Ogawa R (1992) Protection against Marek's disease by a fowlpox virus recombinant expressing the glycoprotein B of Marek's disease virus. *J Virol* 66: 1409–1413
123 Omar AR, Schat KA, Lee LF, Hunt HD (1998) Cytotoxic T lymphocyte response in chickens immunized with a recombinant fowlpox virus expressing Marek's disease herpesvirus glycoprotein B. *Vet Immunol Immunopathol* 62: 73–82
124 Yanagida N, Ogawa R, Li Y, Lee LF, Nazerian K (1992) Recombinant fowlpox viruses expressing the glycoprotein B homolog and the pp38 gene of Marek's disease virus. *J Virol* 66: 1402–1408
125 Calvert JG, Nazerian K, Witter RL, Yanagida N (1993) Fowlpox virus recombinants expressing the envelope glycoprotein of an avian reticuloendotheliosis retrovirus induce neutralizing antibodies and reduce viremia in chickens. *J Virol* 67: 3069–3076
126 Qingzhong Y, Barrett T, Brown TD, Cook JK, Green P, Skinner MA, Cavanagh D (1994) Protection against turkey rhinotracheitis pneumovirus (TRTV) induced by a fowlpox virus recombinant expressing the TRTV fusion glycoprotein (F). *Vaccine* 12: 569–573
127 Butter C, Sturman TD, Baaten BJ, Davison TF (2003) Protection from infectious bursal disease virus (IBDV)-induced immunosuppression by immunization with a fowlpox recombinant containing IBDV-VP2. *Avian Pathol* 32: 597–604
128 Shaw I, Davison TF (2000) Protection from IBDV-induced bursal damage by a recombinant fowlpox vaccine, fpIBD1, is dependent on the titre of challenge virus and chicken genotype. *Vaccine* 18: 3230–3241
129 Boyle DB, Heine HG (1994) Influence of dose and route of inoculation on

responses of chickens to recombinant fowlpox virus vaccines. *Vet Microbiol* 41: 173–181

130 Heine HG, Boyle DB (1993) Infectious bursal disease virus structural protein VP2 expressed by a fowlpox virus recombinant confers protection against disease in chickens. *Arch Virol* 131: 277–292

131 Cardona CJ, Reed WM, Witter RL, Silva RF (1999) Protection of turkeys from hemorrhagic enteritis with a recombinant fowl poxvirus expressing the native hexon of hemorrhagic enteritis virus. *Avian Dis* 43: 234–244

132 Vermeulen AN (1998) Progress in recombinant vaccine development against coccidiosis. A review and prospects into the next millennium. *Int J Parasitol* 28: 1121–1130

133 Wang X, Schnitzlein WM, Tripathy DN, Girshick T, Khan MI (2002) Construction and immunogenicity studies of recombinant fowl poxvirus containing the S1 gene of Massachusetts 41 strain of infectious bronchitis virus. *Avian Dis* 46: 831–838

134 Boyle DB (1998) Diversified prime and boost protocols: the route to enhanced immune responses to recombinant DNA based vaccine? *Aust Biotechnol* 8: 96–98

135 Tsukamoto K, Sato T, Saito S, Tanimura N, Hamazaki N, Mase M, Yamaguchi S (2000) Dual-viral vector approach induced strong and long-lasting protective immunity against very virulent infectious bursal disease virus. *Virology* 269: 257–267

136 Karaca K, Sharma JM, Winslow BJ, Junker DE, Reddy S, Cochran M, McMillen J (1998) Recombinant fowlpox viruses coexpressing chicken type I IFN and Newcastle disease virus HN and F genes: influence of IFN on protective efficacy and humoral responses of chickens following *in ovo* or post-hatch administration of recombinant viruses. *Vaccine* 16: 1496–1503

137 Djeraba A, Musset E, Lowenthal JW, Boyle DB, Chausse AM, Peloille M, Quere P (2002) Protective effect of avian myelomonocytic growth factor in infection with Marek's disease virus. *J Virol* 76: 1062–1070

138 York JJ, Strom AD, Connick TE, McWaters PG, Boyle DB, Lowenthal JW (1996) *In vivo* effects of chicken myelomonocytic growth factor: delivery via a viral vector. *J Immunol* 156: 2991–2997

139 Taylor J, Trimarchi C, Weinberg R, Languet B, Guillemin F, Desmettre P, Paoletti E (1991) Efficacy studies on a canarypox-rabies recombinant virus. *Vaccine* 9: 190–193

140 Taylor J, Tartaglia J, Riviere M, Duret C, Languet B, Chappuis G, Paoletti E (1994) Applications of canarypox (ALVAC) vectors in human and veterinary vaccination. *Dev Biol Stand* 82: 131–135

141 Plotkin SA, Cadoz M, Meignier B, Meric C, Leroy O, Excler JL, Tartaglia J, Paoletti E, Gonczol E, Chappuis G (1995) The safety and use of canarypox vectored vaccines. *Dev Biol Stand* 84: 165–170

142 Stephensen CB, Welter J, Thaker SR, Taylor J, Tartaglia J, Paoletti E (1997) Canine distemper virus (CDV) infection of ferrets as a model for testing Morbillivirus vaccine strategies: NYVAC- and ALVAC-based CDV recombinants protect against symptomatic infection. *J Virol* 71: 1506–1513

143 Pardo MC, Bauman JE, Mackowiak M (1997) Protection of dogs against canine

distemper by vaccination with a canarypox virus recombinant expressing canine distemper virus fusion and hemagglutinin glycoproteins. *Am J Vet Res* 58: 833–836
144 Poulet H, Brunet S, Boularand C, Guiot AL, Leroy V, Tartaglia J, Minke J, Audonnet JC, Desmettre P (2003) Efficacy of a canarypox virus-vectored vaccine against feline leukaemia. *Vet Rec* 153: 141–145
145 Minke JM, Siger L, Karaca K, Austgen L, Gordy P, Bowen R, Renshaw RW, Loosmore S, Audonnet JC, Nordgren B (2004) Recombinant canarypoxvirus vaccine carrying the prM/E genes of West Nile virus protects horses against a West Nile virus-mosquito challenge. *Arch Virol* (Suppl) 18: 221–230
146 Siger L, Bowen RA, Karaca K, Murray MJ, Gordy PW, Loosmore SM, Audonnet JC, Nordgren RM, Minke JM (2004) Assessment of the efficacy of a single dose of a recombinant vaccine against West Nile virus in response to natural challenge with West Nile virus-infected mosquitoes in horses. *Am J Vet Res* 65: 1459–1462
147 Grosenbaugh DA, Backus CS, Karaca K, Minke JM, Nordgren RM (2004) The anamnestic serologic response to vaccination with a canarypox virus-vectored recombinant West Nile virus (WNV) vaccine in horses previously vaccinated with an inactivated WNV vaccine. *Vet Ther* 5: 251–257
148 Paoletti E, Tartaglia J, Taylor J (1994) Safe and effective poxvirus vectors – NYVAC and ALVAC. *Dev Biol Stand* 82: 65–69
149 Paoletti E, Taylor J, Meignier B, Meric C, Tartaglia J (1995) Highly attenuated poxvirus vectors: NYVAC, ALVAC and TROVAC. *Dev Biol Stand* 84: 159–163
150 Wimsatt J, Biggins D, Innes K, Taylor B, Garell D (2003) Evaluation of oral and subcutaneous delivery of an experimental canarypox recombinant canine distemper vaccine in the Siberian polecat (*Mustela eversmanni*). *J Zoo Wildl Med* 34: 25–35
151 Welter J, Taylor J, Tartaglia J, Paoletti E, Stephensen CB (2000) Vaccination against canine distemper virus infection in infant ferrets with and without maternal antibody protection, using recombinant attenuated poxvirus vaccines. *J Virol* 74: 6358–6367
152 Jones L, Tenorio E, Gorham J, Yilma T (1997) Protective vaccination of ferrets against canine distemper with recombinant pox virus vaccines expressing the H or F genes of rinderpest virus. *Am J Vet Res* 58: 590–593
153 Tartaglia J, Jarrett O, Neil JC, Desmettre P, Paoletti E (1993) Protection of cats against feline leukemia virus by vaccination with a canarypox virus recombinant, ALVAC-FL. *J Virol* 67: 2370–2375
154 Franchini G, Gurunathan S, Baglyos L, Plotkin S, Tartaglia J (2004) Poxvirus-based vaccine candidates for HIV: two decades of experience with special emphasis on canarypox vectors. *Expert Rev Vaccines* 3: S75–S88
155 Belshe RB, Stevens C, Gorse GJ, Buchbinder S, Weinhold K, Sheppard H, Stablein D, Self S, McNamara J, Frey S et al (2001) Safety and immunogenicity of a canarypox-vectored human immunodeficiency virus Type 1 vaccine with or without gp120: a phase 2 study in higher- and lower-risk volunteers. *J Infect Dis* 183: 1343–1352
156 de Bruyn G, Rossini AJ, Chiu YL, Holman D, Elizaga ML, Frey SE, Burke D,

Evans TG, Corey L, Keefer MC (2004) Safety profile of recombinant canarypox HIV vaccines. *Vaccine* 22: 704–713
157 Robinson HL, Montefiori DC, Johnson RP, Manson KH, Kalish ML, Lifson JD, Rizvi TA, Lu S, Hu SL, Mazzara GP et al (1999) Neutralizing antibody-independent containment of immunodeficiency virus challenges by DNA priming and recombinant pox virus booster immunizations. *Nat Med* 5: 526–534
158 Dale CJ, De Rose R, Stratov I, Chea S, Montefiori DC, Thomson S, Ramshaw IA, Coupar BE, Boyle DB, Law M, Kent SJ (2004) Efficacy of DNA and fowlpox virus priming/boosting vaccines for simian/human immunodeficiency virus. *J Virol* 78: 13819–13828
159 Leong KH, Ramsay AJ, Boyle DB, Ramshaw IA (1994) Selective induction of immune responses by cytokines coexpressed in recombinant fowlpox virus. *J Virol* 68: 8125–8130
160 Dale CJ, De Rose R, Wilson KM, Croom HA, Thomson S, Coupar BE, Ramsay A, Purcell DF, Ffrench R, Law M et al (2004) Evaluation in macaques of HIV-1 DNA vaccines containing primate CpG motifs and fowlpoxvirus vaccines co-expressing IFNgamma or IL-12. *Vaccine* 23: 188–197
161 Dale CJ, Zhao A, Jones SL, Boyle DB, Ramshaw IA, Kent SJ (2000) Induction of HIV-1-specific T-helper responses and type 1 cytokine secretion following therapeutic vaccination of macaques with a recombinant fowlpoxvirus co-expressing interferon-gamma. *J Med Primatol* 29: 240–247
162 Kelleher AD, Puls RL, Bebbington M, Boyle D, Ffrench R, Kent SJ, Kippax S, Purcell DFJ, Thomson S, Wand H et al (2006) A randomised, placebo-controlled Phase I trial of DNA prime, recombinant fowlpox virus boost prophylactic vaccine for HIV-1. *AIDS* 20: 294–297
163 Cohen J (2004) AIDS vaccines. HIV dodges one-two punch. *Science* 305: 1545–1547
164 Emery S, Workman S, Puls RL, Block M, Baker D, Bodsworth N, Anderson J, Crowe SM, French MAH, Aichelburg A et al on behalf of the NCHVR01 study team (2005) Randomised, placebo-controlled, phase I/IIa evaluation of the safety and immunogenicity of fowlpox virus expressing HIG gag-pol and intereferon-gamm in HIV-1 infected subjects. *Human Vaccines* 1: 232–238
165 Anderson RJ, Hannan CM, Gilbert SC, Laidlaw SM, Sheu EG, Korten S, Sinden R, Butcher GA, Skinner MA, Hill AV (2004) Enhanced $CD8^+$ T cell immune responses and protection elicited against *Plasmodium berghei* malaria by prime boost immunization regimens using a novel attenuated fowlpox virus. *J Immunol* 172: 3094–3100
166 Prieur E, Gilbert SC, Schneider J, Moore AC, Sheu EG, Goonetilleke N, Robson KJ, Hill AV (2004) A *Plasmodium falciparum* candidate vaccine based on a six-antigen polyprotein encoded by recombinant poxviruses. *Proc Natl Acad Sci USA* 101: 290–295
167 Hodge JW, Grosenbach DW, Schlom J (2002) Vector-based delivery of tumor-associated antigens and T-cell co-stimulatory molecules in the induction of immune responses and anti-tumor immunity. *Cancer Detect Prev* 26: 275–291
168 Hodge JW, Grosenbach DW, Aarts WM, Poole DJ, Schlom J (2003) Vaccine therapy of established tumors in the absence of autoimmunity. *Clin Cancer Res* 9: 1837–1849

169 Rosenberg SA, Yang JC, Schwartzentruber DJ, Hwu P, Topalian SL, Sherry RM, Restifo NP, Wunderlich JR, Seipp CA, Rogers-Freezer L et al (2003) Recombinant fowlpox viruses encoding the anchor-modified gp100 melanoma antigen can generate antitumor immune responses in patients with metastatic melanoma. *Clin Cancer Res* 9: 2973–2980

170 Triozzi PL, Aldrich W, Allen KO, Lima J, Shaw DR, Strong TV (2005) Antitumor activity of the intratumoral injection of fowlpox vectors expressing a triad of costimulatory molecules and granulocyte/macrophage colony stimulating factor in mesothelioma. *Int J Cancer* 113: 406–414

171 Triozzi PL, Strong TV, Bucy RP, Allen KO, Carlisle RR, Moore SE, Lobuglio AF, Conry RM (2005) Intratumoral administration of a recombinant canarypox virus expressing interleukin 12 in patients with metastatic melanoma. *Hum Gene Ther* 16: 91–100

Poxviruses
ed. by Andrew A. Mercer, Axel Schmidt and Olaf Weber

Subfamily *Entomopoxvirinae*

Marie N. Becker and Richard W. Moyer

Department of Molecular Genetics and Microbiology, College of Medicine, University of Florida, Gainesville, FL 32610, USA

Abstract

The subfamily *Entomopoxvirinae* is a related but distinct member of the family *Poxviridae*. These viruses share many biological features of the poxviruses of chordates, but instead infect the larvae of a number of insect families. The three genera that comprise the entomopoxviruses are the genus *Alphaentomopoxvirus*, infecting beetles; genus *Betaentomopoxvirus*, infecting butterflies, moths, grasshoppers, and locusts, and the genus *Gammaentomopoxvirus* infecting flies and mosquitoes. The entomopoxviruses, like their vertebrate counterparts, have a double-stranded linear DNA genome that is transcribed in a temporal fashion. Entomopoxviruses are occluded in a paracrystalline protein matrix, forming spheroids that protect the virus from environmental conditions. A number of genes are conserved between the entomopoxviruses and chordopoxviruses defining a minimal complement of poxvirus genes. The entomopoxviruses have some unique molecular features. This review covers pathogenesis, transcription, and molecular analysis of the entomopoxviruses.

Taxonomy and history

The family *Poxviridae* is comprised of two subfamilies, the *Chordopoxvirinae* and *Entomopoxvirinae*, which are viruses of vertebrates and insects, respectively. Classification of the entomopoxviruses (EVs) is based on the host insect, virion morphology, and genome size. Recently, the International Committee on Taxonomy of Viruses (ICTV) has renamed the genera within the *Entomopoxvirinae* and redefined the abbreviations used for viruses [1]. The former genera A, B, and C are now *Alphaentomopoxvirus*, whose members infect beetles (Coleoptera); *Betaentomopoxvirus*, viruses of moths and butterflies (Lepidoptera) as well as grasshoppers and locusts (Orthoptera), and the *Gammaentomopoxvirus*, viruses which infect flies (Diptera) and mosquitoes. There are viruses that remain unclassified. As a result of changing the genera names to single word descriptors, the abbreviations for viruses listed by the ICTV now eliminate the “P” from the abbreviations, thus

AmEPV is now AMEV. A number of EVs are documented in the literature but not listed in the ICTV list, thus the abbreviations for viruses may vary. For brevity, the terms Alpha, Beta, and Gamma may be used in this text to indicate each genus, respectively. EVs are named with the name of the host insect. Table 1 lists the viruses referenced in this chapter.

The size and shape of the virions vary for each genus. The alphaentomopoxvirus virions are about 450×250 nm with a unilateral concave core and a single lateral body. The virions tend to be ovoid. The genomic sizes of these viruses are 260–370 kb as determined by electron microscopy and sedimentation rates. No viruses from this genus have been sequenced or characterized in detail at a molecular level, partially due to the inability to manipulate these viruses in cell culture. The type species is *Melolontha melolontha entomopoxvirus* (MMEV).

The betaentomopoxviruses infect members of both the lepidopteran and orthopteran families. These virions are ovoid in shape and 250×350 nm in size. The core is cylindrical and there is a "sleeve-shaped" lateral body. One of the sequenced viruses in this genus is AMEV isolated from the larvae of a moth, *Amsacta moorei*. AMEV is the type species for the genus. The other sequenced EV was isolated from the grasshopper, *Melanoplus sanguinipes* (MSEV). While both viruses were originally classified as betaentomopoxviruses, as discussed further below, analysis of the genomic sequences has led the ICTV to remove MSEV from the genus *Betaentomopoxvirus* and reclassify it as an undesignated member of the subfamily *Entomopoxvirinae*. As more genomic sequence data accumulates it seems likely that the genus *Betaentomopoxvirus* may need to be further subdivided.

The virions of gammaentomopoxvirus are brick shaped rather than ovoid. Their size is 320×230×110 nm and they have a biconcave core with two lateral bodies. These viruses infect flies and mosquitoes and the type species is *Chironomus luridus entomopoxvirus*.

As a sub-family, EVs are the most distant relatives of the vertebrate poxviruses known. The first description of a pox-like virus in insects was by Vago [2], who examined the larvae of the common cockchafer, *Melolontha melolontha* (Coleoptera). Subsequently, additional insect poxviruses were discovered in different insects and, based on morphology in the electron microscope, were determined to be members of the family *Poxviridae*. More recently, the genomes of two EVs have been sequenced, allowing clear and positive assignment of these viruses as poxviruses as well as a molecular comparison of these viruses with their chordopoxvirus (CV) relatives [3–6]. This provided insights into several very important aspects of basic poxvirus biology; namely genome organization, the minimal complement of genes required for poxviruses, and a glimpse of the differences in evasion of host defenses, including the immune response by the different subfamilies of poxviruses.

EV genomes, like their vertebrate counterparts, are comprised of large double-stranded DNA molecules. However, the central co-linear core of common genes, a signature feature of the vertebrate poxviruses, is absent in

Table 1. Entomopoxvirus genera and selected members[a]

Genus	Virus name	Abbr.	Host species, common name
Alphaentomopoxvirus	*Anomala cuprea entomopoxvirus*	ACEV	Cupreous chafer
	Melolontha melolontha entomopoxvirus	MMEV	Common cockchafer
	Othnonius batesi entomopoxvirus	ObEPV	Scarab beetle
	Ips typographus entomopoxvirus	ItEPV	European spruce bark beetle
Betaentomopoxvirus	***Amsacta moorei entomopoxvirus 'L'***	AMEV	Red hairy caterpillar
	Choristoneura biennis entomopoxvirus 'L'	CBEV	Two year cycle spruce budworm
	Choristoneura fumiferana entomopoxvirus 'L'	CFEV	Spruce budworm
	Heliothis armigera entomopoxvirus 'L'	HAEV	Cotton bollworm
	Ocnogyna baetica 'L'		
	Elasmopalpus lignosellus 'L'	ElEPV	Lesser cornstalk borer
	Adoxophyes honmai 'L'	AhEPV	Smaller tea tortrix
	Psuedaletia unipuncta 'L'	PuEPV	Army worm
	Euxoa auxiliaris 'L'	EAEV	Army cutworm
Gammaentomopoxvirus	***Chironomus luridus entomopoxvirus***	CLEV	Midge
	Goeldichironomus haloprasimus entomopoxvirus	GHEV	Midge
Unassigned	*Melanoplus sanguinipes entomopoxvirus 'O'*	MSEV	Lesser migratory grasshopper

[a] Viruses listed in bold are the type species for each genus. Other listings can be found in the VIIIth edition of the ICTV report [1] and in the following review [75]

the EVs. Instead, these core genes are "scattered" throughout the genome as compared to their vertebrate counterparts [3, 4, 6]. Ignoring the different organizational strategies between vertebrate and insect poxviruses, the genomic sequence data from EVs has proved quite useful in determining the minimal complement of poxvirus genes [6] common to all members of the family. A second interesting point that has emerged from EV genomic sequence relates to the generally accepted concept that vertebrate poxviruses devote approximately 33% of their genome to genes which function to deflect the host response to infection. Many of these genes are nonessential for growth in cell culture and some control host range. This appears to be true for the EVs as well. However, the nature of the EV "nonessential" genes is quite distinct from the vertebrate poxviruses and many are completely unique. The distinctive character of the EV nonessential genes is undoubtedly reflective of the fact that insect response to infection is quite different and in a sense more primitive from that of the mammalian host and involves primarily innate immunity.

EVs replicate in the cytoplasm of infected cells and exhibit temporal regulation of gene expression typical of all poxviruses. The EVs differ in one significant fashion from most CVs in that they form paracrystalline occlusion bodies (OBs), also called spheroids, within the cytoplasm of the host cell. This is a parallel to the situation that exists in some orthopoxviruses, such as cowpox virus, which form A-type inclusion bodies; however, these are not paracrystalline [7]. A variable number of EV virions are occluded in the matrix of the spheroid, which is composed of a single protein. Ingestion of the spheroid by the insect is the normal means of transmission of the virus from host to host and it is believed that the spheroid serves to stabilize the virus in the environment. It is of interest that EV OBs are alkaline sensitive, consistent with their degradation in the insect gut following ingestion, whereas orthopoxvirus A-type inclusions, which probably serve a function similar to that of spheroids, are acid sensitive. Occluded virus is also found in the unrelated baculovirus family of insect viruses.

There have been a large number of EVs described in the literature. However, only a few EVs have been adapted to cell culture, a feature necessary to facilitate studies at the molecular level. HAEV, an EV of *Heliothis armigera*, has been reported to grow in cell culture [8], but only the EV from *Amsacta moorei* (AMEV) grows reproducibly well to high titer in cultured cells. AMEV is routinely grown in a *Lymantria dispar* cell line (Ld652), [9] but can also be propagated in EAA-BTI cells derived from *Estigmene acrea* [10]. It has been proposed that these viruses could be used for insect control purposes, which would require the ability to produce sufficient quantities of virus in a controlled environment.

Genome size and organization

Like their chordopox counterparts, the EVs have a large double-stranded DNA genome with inverted terminal repeats (ITRs). Langridge and Roberts [11] examined the DNA from AMEV, EAEV, ObEPV, and GHEV (Tab. 1) by electron microscopy and estimated the molecular masses to be 200×10^6 (GHEV); 251×10^6 (ObEPV) and 135×10^6 daltons (AMEV, EAEV). Sedimentation values gave a molecular mass estimate for CBEV of 142×10^6 [12]. Sedimentation coefficients and DNA melting techniques place the percent G+C in EVs at 16.3–26%, significantly lower than that of vaccinia virus (VV) [12, 13].

The lower G+C content of the EVs was an indication that, although related to the CVs, there might be relatively little homology at the DNA level. Indeed, Southern hybridization studies found little or no hybridization between VV and AMEV or MSEV [14, 15]. No hybridization was seen between AMEV and CBEV [16]. However, AMEV did show some homology to EAEV [14]. With dot blots, MSEV hybridized to two other orthopteran EVs, but not to EV from other hosts or VV. The restriction enzyme patterns for AMEV, CBEV, EAEV, MSEV, and ObEPV were also dissimilar [16].

More precise information became available with the sequencing of both the AMEV and MSEV genomes. AMEV has a genome size of 232 kb and a G+C content of 17.8% [3]. The MSEV genome was determined to be 236 kb and has a G+C content of 18.3% [4]. Among the orthopoxviruses, the central-most genome "core" consists of a highly conserved co-linear collection of conserved genes essential for growth of all poxviruses [6]. However, a comparison of the gene order of either AMEV or MSEV to VV reveals that these core genes, while conserved, are non-linear and dispersed throughout the genome [3, 4]. Furthermore, no common order of conserved genes is observed even between the two sequenced EVs. This implies that the EVs and vertebrate poxviruses diverged quite some time ago. Indeed, Gubser et al. [17] when examining the phylogeny of sequenced poxviruses, was unable to incorporate the EVs into the analysis due to the low average homology between the EVs and other poxviruses. The lack of correspondence between the two sequenced betaentomopoxviruses is one of the reasons that MSEV is no longer assigned to this genus and is considered for the time being as "unclassified".

Despite these dissimilarities, the value of sequence data from the EVs should not be underestimated. Upton et al. [6] determined that there are 90 gene families conserved within the CVs and 49 gene families that are conserved throughout the entire *Poxviridae* family. The inclusion of EVs in this sequence analysis thus refines the list of minimal genes required to define a poxvirus. Several genes that might be considered important are missing homologs in the EVs. The intermediate transcription factors, VITF1 and one subunit of VITF3, are not found in the EVs. Two late transcription factors (VLTF1 and VLTF4) are also not present within the EV genome. It may be that some aspects of EV transcription are controlled by host elements rather than virus-encoded ones. Perhaps most interestingly, several members of the RNA polymerase complex are absent from the two sequenced EVs. These include RPO30, RPO22, and RPO7 [6].

Pathology

EVs are typically pathogens of the larvae of insects rather than of adults. However, there have been reports of infected adults in laboratory settings

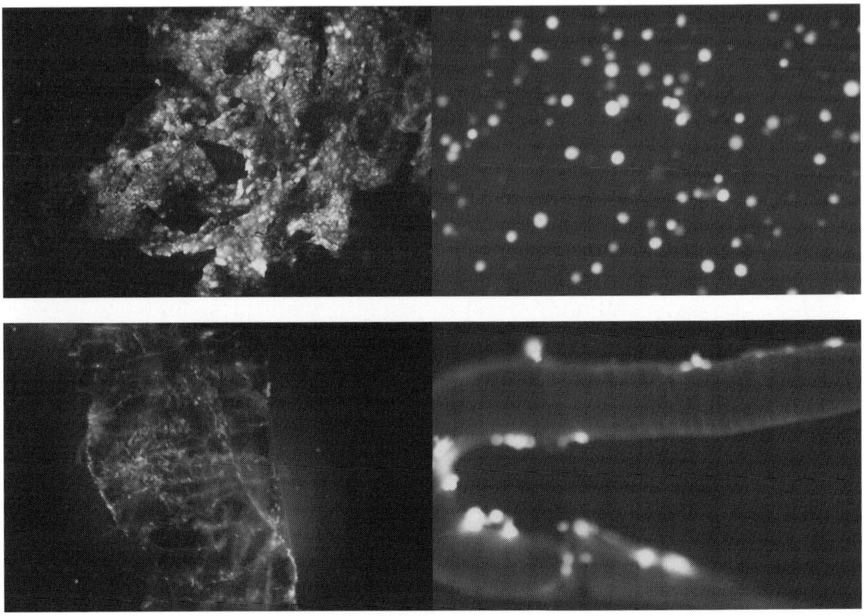
A B C D

Figure 1. AMEV-infected tissues from *Lymantria dispar* larvae. All photos show tissue infected with AMEV that contains the GFP gene under the control of the spheroidin promoter. The presence of virus is indicated by the white areas. (A) Fat body. (B) Hemocytes. (C) Silk gland. (D) Trachea with attached hemocytes. Photos courtesy of Basil Arif and Lillian Pavlik

[18] and one report of an EV infection in the adult bark beetle, *Ips typographus* [19]. In larvae, the pathogenesis of infection is similar for all EVs that have been examined. In nature, infection occurs through larval consumption of spheroids. The occluded virus is then dissolved from the spheroid by the alkaline environment of the insect gut. The virions that are released from the spheroid attach to the midgut epithelium and enter the cells through an undefined fusion mechanism. The primary site of virus replication is the fat body (Fig. 1A). In most infected insects, spheroids can be detected in the hemolymph. Some EVs appear to infect hemocytes, although others argue that this might be due to phagocytosis by the hemocytes (Fig. 1B) [20]. As the disease progresses the hemolymph fills with spheroids, turning it milky white, and the fat body begins to disintegrate, resulting in dissemination and generalized infection of many if not all tissues throughout the insect (Figs 1C, D and 2). For *Chironomus luridus* (genus Gamma) spheroids are also found in the epidermis, imaginal leg discs, genital discs, muscles, and the nervous system [21].

As the infection continues, the larvae routinely become lethargic, disoriented, and fail to eat. The time between instars is greatly increased. In some species the larvae turn white or white spotted [18, 21], due to the

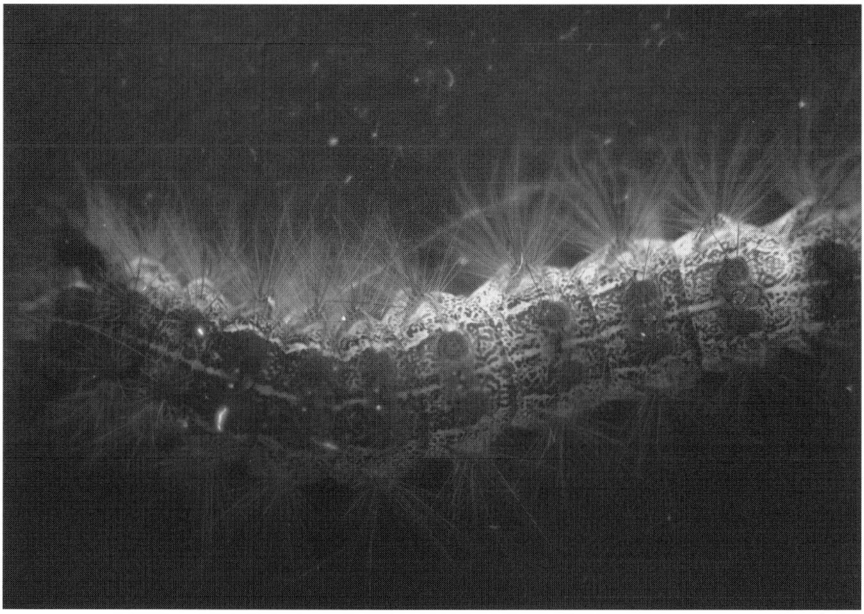

Figure 2. AMEV-infected *Lymantria dispar* larva. The larva was infected with AMEV expressing GFP. The GFP expression (white areas) is indicative of a disseminated infection. Photo courtesy of Basil Arif and Lillian Pavlik.

large number of spheroids present in the hemolymph [22]. *Estigmene acrea* larvae infected with AMEV have been reported to regurgitate or defecate material containing spheroids [23]. Many larvae become paralyzed before death. The time to death varies significantly with species of host and virus, and is affected greatly by the initial infectious dose of the virus. Lipa et al. [24] determined that the LD_{50} for *Ocnogyna baetica* EV (Lepidoptera) was approximately 6700 spheroids [24]; however, Mitchell et al. [22]determined an LD_{50} of 9–700 for *Elasmopalpus lignosellus entomopoxvirus* spheroids in the lesser cornstalk borer larvae (Lepidoptera), with the lower number for earlier and smaller instars. A very low LD_{50} of 2.4 spheroids was found for CFEV in fourth instar spruce budworms with an LT_{50} of 25.2 days [25].

The reason for the prolonged larval period and failure to pupate of infected larvae is not clear. It has been shown that both CFEV and *Adoxophyes honmai entomopoxvirus* increase the levels of juvenile hormone in infected larvae compared with uninfected larvae. Both viruses also decrease ecdysteroid levels [25, 26].

In addition to the spheroids formed by all known EVs, many EVs also produce a second type of structure called spindles comprised primarily of the protein fusolin [16]. The spindles are free of virions, although they may be incorporated into spheroids. Spindles are found predominantly in the Alpha and Beta genera but are absent in AMEV. More discussion about the nature and function of these spindles follows in a later section. Several EVs can infect related hosts, while others are relatively host restricted. MSEV has been shown to infect several other grasshopper species [27, 28].

Spheroids

Spheroids or OBs are composed predominately, if not exclusively, of a single protein, spheroidin (sph) [29] (Fig. 3). This large protein (100–115 kDa) is produced late during infection, and virion particles are incorporated into the assembling matrix. Hall and Moyer [30] demonstrated that the *sph* transcript has a 5' poly(A) head, which is characteristic of vaccinia transcripts. They characterized the promoter as a late promoter with several upstream early termination signals. There is a significant amount of homology (83–94%) at the protein level between spheroidin from EVs within the same host genus [31, 32]. The homology between the spheroidins from different host species genera is low, 22–40% [31–33]. The protein is believed to contain internal disulfide bonds and there are a number of conserved cysteines [33]. Although there is functional similarity to the polyhedron protein of baculoviruses, there is little homology between the polyhedron protein and spheroidin [30]. The role of spheroids is believed to be in protecting and stabilizing virus against the external environment. However, fully infectious virus is still formed when the spheroidin gene is deleted from AMEV [34, 35]. Some electron microscopic studies suggest that the final steps of infectious virus maturation occur within the spheroid; however, this clearly is not the case for AMEV, since fully infectious non-occluded virus can be found readily in the supernatant of infected cells in culture [36, 37] with both wild-type and sph-minus strains of virus. Virus particles are not required for spheroid formation as spheroidin protein produced in a recombinant baculovirus system forms empty spheroids [38]. This finding strongly implies that spheroidin is the major, if not only, protein constituent of the spheroid.

Infectious virions can be released from spheroids by treatments of sodium carbonate and thioglycolate at high pH [15, 39]. The number of virions found within a spheroid varies. There appears to be no defined orientation of the virions within the occlusions, but this has not been exhaustively studied.

An alkaline protease has been found to be associated with the spheroids of AMEV [40], CBEV, CFEV [29], and MSEV [41]. The pH optimum for these proteases ranges from 8.6 to 11. Bilimoria and Arif [29] hypothesized that this protease might be necessary for dissolution of the spheroid in an appropriate environment such as the alkaline midgut of the insect *in vivo*. Interestingly, Langridge and Roberts [40] reported that the alkaline protease was not associated with AMEV grown in culture. Whether this protease is viral or cellular in origin has not been determined.

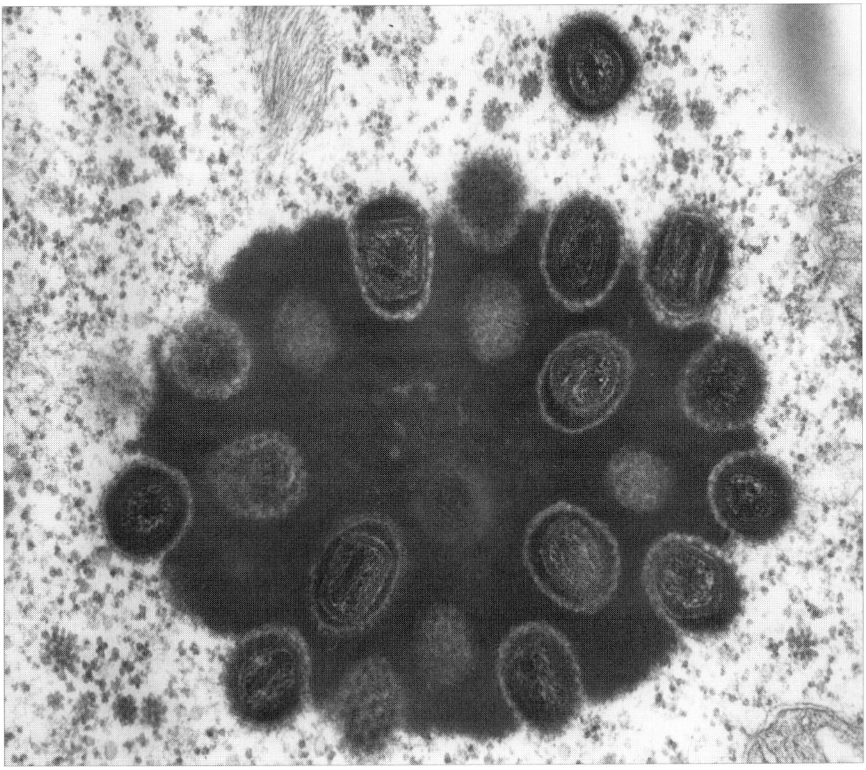

Figure 3. Electron micrograph of an AMEV occlusion body from an infected *Estigmene acrea* cell. Photo provided by Robert Granados.

Fusolin/spindles/enhancing factor

Many EVs produce a second macromolecular structure termed spindles. They are commonly found in the alphaentomopoxviruses, and many of the lepidopteran betaentomopoxviruses also produce spindles. However, spindles are rarely seen in the gammaentomopoxviruses or the orthopteran EVs [42]. Spindles do not contain virions, but may be incorporated in spheroids. The virus-encoded protein, fusolin (38 kDa), is the sole component of the crystalline spindles. Fusolin is synthesized late in infection and produced in large quantities. It is noteworthy that AMEV, although a betaentomopoxvirus, does not form spindles nor encodes a fusolin gene. Fusolin is believed to dimerize through N-terminal motifs and is thought to be glycosylated [43, 44]. Sequence comparison of fusolin genes shows that they are related to the gp37 protein of baculoviruses [16, 44] and different fusolin genes show about 40% homology to each other at the amino acid level [16].

Fusolin is thought to "enhance" EV infection. The absence of fusolin and spindles from AMEV, however, indicates successful infection of larvae does not depend on either fusolin or spindles. Most of the information on spindle function comes from the study of baculoviruses. Xu and Hukuhara first recognized that the spindles from the entomopoxvirus PsEPV can have an enhancing effect on the infection of *Psuedaletia unipuncta* baculovirus [45]. This observation has been repeatedly observed for different combinations of baculoviruses and EVs. Due to the difficulty in preparing purified spindles from spheroids, it was not clear whether the EV spheroids also had an enhancing mechanism for baculovirus infection. A number of groups have shown convincingly that the spindles alone or the purified fusolin protein [46, 47] is responsible for the enhancement of infection. Fusolin also increases the oral infectivity of non-occluded baculovirus, BmMNPV [48]. Several researchers have proposed that the mechanism for enhancement is through the fusolin-assisted dissolution of the non-cellular peritrophic membrane within the midgut of many insects. Mitsuhashi and Miyamoto demonstrated that if larvae were fed spindles and then immediately dissected, the peritrophic membrane was smaller or not present [49]. This effect was mitigated if the insects were allowed to recover for 24 hours after being fed a diet containing spindles. Others have proposed that fusolin increases the amount of baculovirus:cell fusion [46, 47]. The role of spindles during an EV infection remains relatively unexplored; however, the spindles from ACEV do increase the infectivity of ACEV as well as the infectivity of gammaentomopoxviruses that do not produce spindles [50, 51].

The molecular biology of entomopoxviruses

Much of what we know about the molecular biology of EVs is derived from AMEV, primarily because this virus can be grown in cell culture and there are methods for genetic manipulation of the virus [35, 52]. The length of the virus growth cycle is roughly 18–24 h at 26°C, not that dissimilar in time from that of VV. The protein expression profile for AMEV was examined *via* ^{35}S-labeling experiments [9]. The results of these experiments show that host protein synthesis is shut off by 9 h post infection (hpi). DNA synthesis is typically initiated by 6 hpi but the rate of synthesis increases until 12 hpi [9, 53]. Virus protein expression is temporal and changes during the course of infection with major changes in the expression pattern occurring in a viral DNA synthesis-dependent fashion. Winter et al. [9] examined the effect of several inhibitors of protein synthesis in AMEV. AraC inhibits late protein synthesis by blocking DNA synthesis in AMEV-infected cells. Both IBT and PAA also inhibit AMEV virus production. Some late proteins continue to be synthesized as late as 42 hpi. AMEV can not productively infect mammalian cells [54], but the virus binds to and enters mammalian cells and gene expression is limited to AMEV early genes. Similarly, VV can not productively infect insect cells, and, although gene expression (both early and late) appears relatively normal, no mature virus is formed [55]. These results indicate that there are environmental host-specific factors which govern the productive infection of both viruses within their own systems.

Transcription

The transcription patterns of EVs have not been extensively examined, although sequence analyses of the conserved genes as well as those cloned from both MSEV and AMEV allow one to predict many similarities to the vertebrate poxviruses. At least two classes of transcripts have been clearly defined. One class of transcripts (early) is initiated upon infection, and occurs prior to and independent of DNA synthesis. The second class of transcripts (late) is dependent on DNA synthesis for transcription. No intermediate genes have been described in AMEV, but most of the known VV intermediate genes have homologs in both AMEV and MSEV. The seven identified intermediate class genes in VV are: G8R, A1L, A2L, H7R, D12L, A6L, and A18R [56]. Not all of these genes have an established function; however, the ones that do are all involved in transcription regulation. Of this group, G8R (a late transcription factor), H7R and A6L (both of unknown function) are all missing in EVs. It is probable that the EVs do have intermediate genes and the formal definitions which distinguish intermediate and late genes derived for vertebrate poxviruses will apply as well to the EVs (for a review of poxvirus gene expression see [56]).

In VV, the early genes are transcribed upon entry into the cell. Early promoter requirements for initiation of transcription have been defined, as has a signal for early transcription termination (T_5NT). One early AMEV gene that has been extensively studied is the gene encoding the thymidine kinase (TK) protein. Northern blot analysis indicates that this gene is transcribed at 3–9 hpi [57]. Hence, the AMEV TK gene behaves as expected for a typical poxvirus early gene. The AMEV TK can functionally replace the TK gene of VV [58]. The early gene termination signal (T5NT) is present at the 3' end of the TK gene. The combination of an early gene promoter and the T5NT sequence are used together to predict early genes in both AMEV and MSEV [3, 4].

The late genes are transcribed after DNA replication. The late promoters in EVs are less well defined than in VV. The predicted late gene for MSEV DNA topoisomerase has a canonical promoter of TAAATG and an internal T_5NT early termination signal [59]. There is precedent for embedded T_5NT early transcription termination sequences, which are typically ignored late in infection, within VV late genes as well [56]. The promoter of the AMEV *sod* gene has a TAATG motif, and is expressed at late times during infection [57]. In VV, the majority of late transcripts are heterogeneous in length [60] due to 3'-variable extensions. In contrast, at least some of the randomly examined AMEV late genes are precise and discrete in length [57]. The presence of discrete 3' termini in AMEV late transcripts raises interesting questions about 3' end formation. Transcripts with precise 3′ termini, while rare, have been noted in VV [61, 62]. For at least two such genes, the VV F17L and the cowpox virus ATI transcript, discrete termini are formed by post-transcriptional cleavage of longer typically heterogeneous transcripts [61, 62]. In AMEV, where discrete late transcripts seem more common, the virus may use a similar post-transcriptional cleavage mechanism as for VV. However, a second alternative would be the presence of discrete late termination signals, recognized by virus-encoded transcription factors that have yet to be identified.

The *sph* gene, whose functional counterpart in cowpox virus is the ATI gene, deserves special mention. Inspection of the promoter sequence (TAAATG) of this AMEV gene would suggest that spheroidin is a late gene [30]. A hint that the spheroidin gene was regulated in a novel fashion came from studies which showed that when the gene and its putative promoter sequences were cloned into cowpox virus, expression was surprisingly poor. Examination of the transcripts produced indicated the use of several alternate start sites rather than precise 5' transcription initiation [35]. These results suggest that the spheroidin promoter from AMEV is not read correctly in orthopoxvirus-infected cells. It was later shown that efficient transcription requires sequences within the 5' coding region of the gene in addition to the classical promoter sequence for efficient transcription in AMEV-infected cells [35]. However, other late promoters, such as the MMEV fusolin promoter, function properly in VV-infected cells [16]. The transcript for the *sph* gene is expressed at later times post infection than other late genes, indicating that it might form a novel class of very late transcripts (M. N. Becker, R. W. Moyer, unpublished data). Spheroidin protein synthesis is not only initiated later than typical "late proteins" but continues to be synthesized well beyond that of typical late proteins [9]. Indeed, the levels of spheroidin continue to rise long after most protein synthesis in the cell has ceased. The unusually late kinetics of expression of the *sph* gene is reminiscent of the kinetics of polyhedron gene expression in baculoviruses. In that case, there is a novel baculovirus RNA polymerase synthesized late for this purpose [63]. By analogy, one possible explanation for the "very late" expression of spheroidin is that like the baculovirus polyhedron, spheroidin is synthesized by a novel or modified RNA polymerase. Interest in this question is heightened by the fact that EVs, like all other poxviruses, already synthesize and encapsidate a virus-specific RNA polymerase due to the cytoplasmic nature of poxviruses. Other possibilities include the synthesis of novel transcription initiation factors required for synthesis of a specific subset of late genes or remodeling of the "core" viral RNA polymerase itself.

Both MSEV and AMEV contain subunits of a conserved capping enzyme, and thus the 5' end of EV messages are predicted to have a cap 1 structure. In VV, both late and intermediate transcripts have a 5' poly(A) head. The spheroidin transcripts of AMEV, MMEV and CFEV have also all been shown to have a 5' poly(A) head [30, 33, 64].

The 3' end of EV transcripts is polyadenylated (M. N. Becker, R. W. Moyer, unpublished results). Polyadenylation is achieved in vertebrate poxviruses by a virus-encoded heterodimeric polyadenylating enzyme consisting of a large and small subunit. Both small and large subunits of the virus-encoded poly(A) polymerase are conserved in MSEV and AMEV. A small subunit of the poly(A) polymerase has been sequenced from HAEV as well. However, AMEV is unique and appears to encode two small subunits (AMV060 and AMV115) rather than only one. The AMV060 subunit exhibits somewhat greater similarity at the amino acid level to the VV J3 protein, which encodes the small subunit, but both AMV060 and AMV115 are clearly related. The VV J3 protein has three functions: as a processivity factor for polyadenylation in conjunction with the large poly(A) polymerase subunit; a 2'O-methyltransferase activity and as a transcription elongation factor [65–67]. It may be that these three functions are divided between the two putative subunits found in AMEV, or one subunit is a novel protein, or that there are different forms of the poly(A) polymerase used at different times after infection or in different tissues during infection.

Structural proteins and enzymes

Langridge and colleagues [15, 40, 53] used protein gels to determine that there were 36–37 structural proteins in the AMEV virion and 39–45 for MSEV. Virion morphogenesis in vertebrate poxviruses is heralded by proteolytic processing of structural protein precursors [68]. Interestingly, no proteolytic processing of the structural proteins was observed in AMEV-infected cells. Despite the failure to observe proteolytic processing in AMV-infected cells, the putative enzymes required for cleavage, the I7L and G1L homologs, are conserved in the AMEV genome. It may well be that the conditions used to detect protein processing during vertebrate poxvirus infection are not sufficiently sensitive to detect AMEV protein processing.

Among the unique genes found in both AMEV and MSEV is an NAD^+-dependent DNA ligase [69, 70]. Both of these enzymes lack the zinc finger motif typically found in such ligases as well as the C-terminal BRCT (BRCA1 C-terminal domain) structural domain. However, both enzymes have been demonstrated to be functional ligases and represent the first examples of NAD^+-dependent DNA ligases found outside of the eubacteria. In contrast, VV contains an ATP-dependent DNA ligase.

AMEV control of host responses to infection

The EVs clearly control the host immune response but probably in a fashion different from that of the CVs [71, 72]. VV, cowpox virus, myxoma virus, and other CVs contain a variety of genes to control both cellular and humoral immunity. There is no humoral immunity in insects. These differences are undoubtedly reflected in the complement of "nonessential" genes encoded by the vertebrate and insect poxviruses. For example, serine protease inhibitors (serpin), in many vertebrate poxviruses are thought to control the host response related to the immune response and apoptosis but are absent in EVs. EVs do, however, encode *inhibitor of apoptosis* (*iap*) genes. AMEV contains one *iap* gene and MSEV encodes two *iap* genes [4]. Vertebrate poxviruses do not encode *iap* genes. The AMEV IAP protein is functional as an apoptosis inhibitor, but is not essential for virus growth, indicating that there is probably another gene and/or alternative mechanism for controlling host cell apoptosis within the AMEV genome [73, 74]. The presence of *iap* genes is typical of complex DNA viruses of insects. The CVs also encode genes to target chemokine and interferon pathways; however, obvious homologs are missing in EVs.

VV and myxoma virus encode a nonessential, non-functional superoxide dismutase (SOD). AMEV encodes a SOD that is fully functional, and might act to overcome innate defenses in the insect gut. This gene is not required for growth in tissue culture, nor does it have an effect on virulence in *Lymantria dispar* larvae [57]. MSEV does not contain a *sod* gene, which reflects yet another difference between these two EVs, perhaps related to their hosts. These findings clearly indicate that, while control of the host response is important in all poxviruses, the details of how this is achieved in the two systems will continue to reveal insights into basic cell biology, which in the case of the insect poxviruses is most likely to target the innate immune response.

Summary

The EVs provide an important source of information regarding the evolution of poxviruses and the control of host responses. These viruses also provide interesting "twists" into the basic biology of this fascinating virus family as well as unique insights into the adaptations within the poxvirus family for evading host defenses. Further analysis of the regulation of transcription, protein synthesis and virus pathogenesis should prove both interesting and relevant to other aspects of poxvirus biology and how insect hosts counter effects of complex viruses in general.

Acknowledgements

The authors would like to thank Dr. Robert Granados, Cornell University; Dr. Basil Arif, and Ms. Lillian Pavlik, Canadian Forestry Service, Great Lakes Forestry Centre for the use of photographs.

References

1 Fauquet C, Mayo M, Maniloff J, Desselberger U, Ball L (2005) *Virus Taxonomy, VIIIth Report of the ICTV*. Elsevier/Academic Press, London, 117–133
2 Vago C (1963) A new type of insect virus. *J Insect Pathol* 5: 275–276
3 Bawden AL, Glassberg KJ, Diggans J, Shaw R, Farmerie W, Moyer RW (2000) Complete genomic sequence of the *Amsacta moorei* entomopoxvirus: analysis and comparison with other poxviruses. *Virology* 274: 120–139
4 Afonso CL, Tulman ER, Lu Z, Oma E, Kutish GF, Rock DL (1999) The genome of *Melanoplus sanguinipes* entomopoxvirus. *J Virol* 73: 533–552
5 Gubser C, Hue S, Kellam P, Smith GL (2004) Poxvirus genomes: a phylogenetic analysis. *J Gen Virol* 85: 105–117
6 Upton C, Slack S, Hunter AL, Ehlers A, Roper RL (2003) Poxvirus orthologous clusters: toward defining the minimum essential poxvirus genome. *J Virol* 77: 7590–7600
7 Patel DD, Pickup DJ, Joklik WK (1986) Isolation of cowpox virus A-type inclusions and characterization of their major protein component. *Virology* 149: 174–189
8 Fernon CA, Vera AP, Crnov R, Lai-Fook J, Osborne RJ, Dall DJ (1995) Replication of *Heliothis armigera* entomopoxvirus *in vitro*. *J Invertebr Pathol* 66: 216–233
9 Winter J, Hall RL, Moyer RW (1995) The effect of inhibitors on the growth of the entomopoxvirus from *Amsacta moorei* in *Lymantria dispar* (gypsy moth) cells. *Virology* 211: 462–473
10 Granados RR, Naughton M (1975) Development of *Amsacta moorei* entomopoxvirus in ovarian and hemocyte cultures from *Estigmene acrea* larvae. *Intervirology* 5: 62–68
11 Langridge WH, Roberts DW (1977) Molecular weight of DNA from four entomopoxviruses determined by electron microscopy. *J Virol* 21: 301–308
12 Arif BM (1976) Isolation of an entomopoxvirus and characterization of its DNA. *Virology* 69: 626–634
13 Langridge WH, Bozarth RF, Roberts DW (1977) The base composition of entomopoxvirus DNA. *Virology* 76: 616–620
14 Langridge WHR (1984) Detection of DNA base sequence homology between entomopoxviruses isolated from lepidoptera and orthoptera. *J Invertebr Pathol* 43: 41–46
15 Langridge WHR, Oma E, Henry JE (1983) Characterization of the DNA and structural proteins of entomopoxviruses from *Melanoplus sanguinipes*, *Arphia conspirsa*, and *Phoetaliotes nebrascensis* (Orthoptera). *J Invertebr Pathol* 42: 327–333
16 Gauthier L, Cousserans F, Veyrunes JC, Bergoin M (1995) The *Melolontha melolontha* entomopoxvirus (Mmepv) fusolin is related to the fusolins of Lepidopteran Epvs and to the 37K baculovirus glycoprotein. *Virology* 208: 427–436
17 Gubser C, Hue S, Kellam P, Smith GL (2004) Poxvirus genomes: a phylogenetic analysis. *J Gen Virol* 85: 105–117
18 Sutter GR (1972) Pox virus of army cutworm. *J Invertebr Pathol* 19: 375–382

19 Wegensteiner R, Weiser J (1995) A new entomopoxvirus in the bark beetle *Ips typographus* (Coleoptera: Scolytidae). *J Invertebr Pathol* 65: 203–205

20 Henry JE, Nelson BP, Jutila JW (1969) Pathology and development of grasshopper inclusion body virus in *Melanoplus sanguinipes*. *J Virol* 3: 605–610

21 Huger AM, Krieg A, Emschermann P, Gotz P (1970) Further studies on polypoxvirus Chironomi, an insect virus of pox group isolated from midge *Chironomus luridus*. *J Invertebr Pathol* 15: 253–261

22 Mitchell FL, Smith J (1985) Pathology and bioassays of the lesser cornstalk borer (*Elasmopalpus lignosellus*) entomopoxvirus. *J Invertebr Pathol* 45: 75–80

23 Roberts DW, Granados RR (1968) A poxlike virus from *Amsacta moorei* (Lepidoptera: Arctiidae). *J Invertebr Pathol* 12: 141–143

24 Lipa JJ, Aldebis HK, Vargas-Osuna E, Caballero P, Santiago-Alvarez C, Hernandez-Crespo P (1994) Occurrence, biological activity, and host range of entomopoxvirus B from *Ocnogyna baetica* (Lepidoptera: Arctiidae). *J Invertebr Pathol* 63: 130–134

25 Palli SR, Ladd TR, Tomkins WL, Shu S, Ramaswamy SB, Tanaka Y, Arif B, Retnakaran A (2000) Choristoneura fumiferana entomopoxvirus prevents metamorphosis and modulates juvenile hormone and ecdysteroid titers. *Insect Biochem Mol Biol* 30: 869–876

26 Nakai M, Shiotsuki T, Kunimi Y (2004) An entomopoxvirus and a granulovirus use different mechanisms to prevent pupation of *Adoxophyes honmai*. *Virus Res* 101: 185–191

27 Streett DA, Oma EA, Henry JE (1990) Cross infection of three grasshopper species with the *Melanoplus sanguinipes* entomopoxvirus. *J Invertebr Pathol* 56: 419–421

28 Levin DB, Adachi D, Williams LL, Myles TG (1993) Host specificity and molecular characterization of the entomopoxvirus of the lesser migratory grasshopper, *Melanoplus sanguinipes*. *J Invertebr Pathol* 62: 241–247

29 Bilimoria SL, Arif BM (1979) Subunit protein and alkaline protease of entomopoxvirus spheroids. *Virology* 96: 596–603

30 Hall RL, Moyer RW (1991) Identification, cloning, and sequencing of a fragment of *Amsacta moorei* entomopoxvirus DNA containing the spheroidin gene and three vaccinia virus-related open reading frames. *J Virol* 65: 6516–6527

31 Hernandez-Crespo P, Veyrunes JC, Cousserans F, Bergoin M (2000) The spheroidin of an entomopoxvirus isolated from the grasshopper *Anacridium aegyptium* (AaEPV) shares low homology with spheroidins from lepidopteran or coleopteran EPVs. *Virus Res* 67: 203–213

32 Mitsuhashi W, Saito H, Sato M, Nakashima N, Noda H (1998) Complete nucleotide sequence of spheroidin gene of *Anomala cuprea* entomopoxvirus. *Virus Res* 55: 61–69

33 Li X, Barrett JW, Yuen L, Arif BM (1997) Cloning, sequencing and transcriptional analysis of the *Choristoneura fumiferana* entomopoxvirus spheroidin gene. *Virus Res* 47: 143–154

34 Palmer CP, Miller DP, Marlow SA, Wilson LE, Lawrie AM, King LA (1995) Genetic modification of an entomopoxvirus: deletion of the spheroidin gene does not affect virus replication *in vitro*. *J Gen Virol* 76: 15–23

35 Hall RL, Li Y, Feller J, Moyer RW (1996) The *Amsacta moorei* entomopoxvirus spheroidin gene is improperly transcribed in vertebrate poxviruses. *Virology* 224: 427–436
36 Langridge WH (1983) Detection of *Amsacta moorei* entomopoxvirus and vaccinia virus proteins in cell cultures restrictive for poxvirus multiplication. *J Invertebr Pathol* 42: 77–82
37 Granados RR, Roberts DW (1970) Electron microscopy of a poxlike virus infecting an invertebrate host. *Virology* 40: 230–243
38 Marlow SA, Wilson LE, Lawrie AM, Wilkinson N, King LA (1998) Assembly of *Amsacta moorei* entomopoxvirus spheroidin into spheroids following synthesis in insect cells using a baculovirus vector. *J Gen Virol* 79: 623–628
39 McCarthy WJ, Granados RR, Sutter GR, Roberts DW (1975) Characterization of entomopox virions of the army cutworm, *Euxoa auxiliaris* (Lepidoptera: Noctuidae). *J Invertebr Pathol* 25: 215–220
40 Langridge WHR, Roberts DW (1982) Structural proteins of *Amsacta moorei*, *Euxoa auxiliaris*, and *Melanoplus sanguinipes* entomopoxviruses. *J Invertebr Pathol* 39: 346–353
41 Erlandson M (1991) Protease activity associated with occlusion body preparations of an entomopoxvirus from *Melanoplus sanguinipes*. *J Invertebr Pathol* 57: 255–263
42 Arif BM, Kurstak E (1991) The Entomopoxviruses. In: E Kurstak (ed): *Viruses of Invertebrates*. Marcel Dekker, New York, 179–195
43 Xu J, Hukuhara T (1994) Biochemical properties of an enhancing factor of an entomopoxvirus. *J Invertebr Pathol* 63: 14–18
44 Mitsuhashi W, Saito H, Sato M (1997) Complete nucleotide sequence of the fusolin gene of an entomopoxvirus in the cupreous chafer, *Anomala cuprea* Hope (Coleoptera: Scarabaeidae). *Insect Biochem Mol Biol* 27: 869–876
45 Xu J, Hukuhara T (1992) Enhanced infection of a nuclear polyhedrosis virus in larvae of the armyworm, *Pseudaletia separata*, by a factor in the spheroids of an entomopoxvirus. *J Invertebr Pathol* 60: 259–264
46 Hukuhara T, Wijonarko A (2001) Enhanced fusion of a nucleopolyhedrovirus with cultured cells by a virus enhancing factor from an entomopoxvirus. *J Invertebr Pathol* 77: 62–67
47 Hukuhara T, Hayakawa T, Wijonarko A (2001) A bacterially produced virus enhancing factor from an entomopoxvirus enhances nucleopolyhedrovirus infection in armyworm larvae. *J Invertebr Pathol* 78: 25–30
48 Furuta Y, Mitsuhashi W, Kobayashi J, Hayasaka S, Imanishi S, Chinzei Y, Sato M (2001) Peroral infectivity of non-occluded viruses of *Bombyx mori* nucleopolyhedrovirus and polyhedrin-negative recombinant baculoviruses to silkworm larvae is drastically enhanced when administered with *Anomala cuprea* entomopoxvirus spindles. *J Gen Virol* 82: 307–312
49 Mitsuhashi W, Miyamoto K (2003) Disintegration of the peritrophic membrane of silkworm larvae due to spindles of an entomopoxvirus. *J Invertebr Pathol* 82: 34–40
50 Mitsuhashi W (2002) Further evidence that spindles of an entomopoxvirus enhance its infectivity in a host insect. *J Invertebr Pathol* 79: 59–61
51 Mitsuhashi W, Sato M, Hirai Y (2000) Involvement of spindles of an entomo-

poxvirus (EPV) in infectivity of the EPVs to their host insect – Brief report. *Arch Virol* 145: 1465–1471
52 Li Y, Hall RL, Yuan SL, Moyer RW (1998) High-level expression of *Amsacta moorei* entomopoxvirus spheroidin depends on sequences within the gene. *J Gen Virol* 79: 613–622
53 Langridge WHR (1983) Virus DNA replication and protein synthesis in *Amsacta moorei* entomopoxvirus-infected *Estigmene acrea* cells. *J Invertebr Pathol* 41: 341–349
54 Li Y, HallRL, Moyer RW (1997) Transient, nonlethal expression of genes in vertebrate cells by recombinant entomopoxviruses. *J Virol* 71: 9557–9562
55 Li Y, Yuan S, Moyer RW (1998) The non-permissive infection of insect (gypsy moth) LD-652 cells by Vaccinia virus. *Virology* 248: 74–82
56 Moss B (2001) Poxviridae: The Viruses and Their Replication. In: DM Knipe, PM Howley (eds): *Fields Virology*. Lippincott Williams & Wilkins, Philadelphia, 2849–2883
57 Becker MN, Greenleaf WB, Ostrov DA, Moyer RW (2004) *Amsacta moorei* entomopoxvirus expresses an active superoxide dismutase. *J Virol* 78: 10265–10275
58 Gruidl ME, Hall RL, Moyer RW (1992) Mapping and molecular characterization of a functional thymidine kinase from *Amsacta moorei* entomopoxvirus. *Virology* 186: 507–516
59 Krogh BO, Cheng CH, Burgin A, Shuman S (1999) *Melanoplus sanguinipes* entomopoxvirus DNA topoisomerase: Site-specific DNA transesterification and effects of 5'-bridging phosphorothiolates. *Virology* 264: 441–451
60 Condit RC, Niles EG (2002) Regulation of viral transcription elongation and termination during vaccinia virus infection. *Biochim Biophys Acta* 1577: 325–336
61 D'Costa SM, Antczak JB, Pickup DJ, Condit RC (2004) Post-transcription cleavage generates the 3' end of F17R transcripts in vaccinia virus. *Virology* 319: 1–11
62 Patel DD, Pickup DJ (1987) Messenger RNAs of a strongly-expressed late gene of cowpox virus contain 5'-terminal poly(A) sequences. *EMBO J* 6: 3787–3794
63 Guarino LA, Xu B, Jin J, Dong W (1998) A virus-encoded RNA polymerase purified from baculovirus-infected cells. *J Virol* 72: 7985–7991
64 Sanz P, Veyrunes JC, Cousserans F, Bergoin M (1994) Cloning and Sequencing of the spherulin gene, the occlusion body major polypeptide of the *Melolontha melolontha* entomopoxvirus (Mmepv). *Virology* 202: 449–457
65 Schnierle BS, Gershon PD, Moss B (1992) Cap-specific mRNA (nucleoside-O2'-)-methyltransferase and poly(A) polymerase stimulatory activities of vaccinia virus are mediated by a single protein. *Proc Natl Acad Sci USA* 89: 2897–2901
66 Latner DR, Xiang Y, Lewis JI, Condit J, Condit RC (2000) The vaccinia virus bifunctional gene J3 (nucleoside-2'-O-)-methyltransferase and poly(A) polymerase stimulatory factor is implicated as a positive transcription elongation factor by two genetic approaches. *Virology* 269: 345–355
67 XiangY, Latner DR, Niles EG, Condit RC (2000) Transcription elongation

activity of the vaccinia virus J3 protein *in vivo* is independent of poly(A) polymerase stimulation. *Virology* 269: 356–369

68 Lee P, Hruby DE (1993) Trans processing of vaccinia virus core proteins. *J Virol* 67: 4252–4263

69 Sriskanda V, Moyer RW, Shuman S (2001) NAD^+-dependent DNA ligase encoded by a eukaryotic virus. *J Biol Chem* 276: 36100–36109

70 Lu J, Tong J, Feng H, Huang JM, Afonso CL, Rock DL, Barany F, Cao WG (2004) Unique ligation properties of eukaryotic NAD(+)-dependent DNA ligase from *Melanoplus sanguinipes* entomopoxvirus. *Biochim Biophys Acta* 1701: 37–48

71 Johnston JB, McFadden G (2003) Poxvirus immunomodulatory strategies: current perspectives. *J Virol* 77: 6093–6100

72 Seet BT, Johnston JB, Brunetti CR, Barrett JW, Everett H, Cameron C, Sypula J, Nazarian SH, Lucas A, McFadden G (2003) Poxviruses and immune evasion. *Annu Rev Immunol* 21: 377–423

73 Li Q, Liston P, Schokman N, Ho JM, Moyer RW (2005) *Amsacta moorei* Entomopoxvirus inhibitor of apoptosis suppresses cell death by binding Grim and Hid. *J Virol* 79: 3684–3691

74 Li Q, Liston P, Moyer RW (2005) Functional analysis of the inhibitor of apoptosis (iap) gene carried by the entomopoxvirus of *Amsacta moorei*. *J Virol* 79: 2335–2345

75 King LA, Wilkinson N, Miller DP, Marlow SA (1998) Entomopoxviruses. In: LK Miller, LA Ball (eds): *The Insect Viruses*. Plenum Publishing, New York, 1–29

Poxviruses
ed. by Andrew A. Mercer, Axel Schmidt and Olaf Weber

Immunomodulation by poxviruses

Steven H. Nazarian and Grant McFadden

Robarts Research Institute and, Department of Microbiology and Immunology, Schulich School of Medicine & Dentistry, The University of Western Ontario, London, ON N6G 2V4, Canada

Abstract

Large DNA viruses, such as poxviruses, encode an array of gene products, both secreted and intracellular, that systematically debilitate the various host responses to virus infection. The primary targets of the secreted gene products are members of the inflammatory innate immune system, such as the interferons, tumor necrosis factors, diverse interleukins, complement and the chemokine pathways. Poxvirus-infected cells also maintain a low profile to escape the cell-mediated arm of the adaptive immune response. Virulence factors that mediate this 'virostealth' are generally expressed intracellularly and interfere with host signaling processes or antigen presentation. Poxviruses also interfere with the cellular apoptotic response by regulating several key checkpoints within the cell. While many poxvirus virulence factors exhibit some sequence relationship with host proteins, suggesting that these genes may have been acquired from an ancestral host, others show no obvious similarity to any known host genes. Due to the intimate nature of the co-evolution with their hosts, poxviral immunomodulators have proved useful in examining diverse aspects of immunology, virology and cell biology.

Introduction

Poxviruses comprise a large family of double-stranded DNA viruses that are able to infect a wide spectrum of vertebrate (*Chordopoxvirinae*) and insect (*Entomopoxvirinae*) hosts. They are characterized by a characteristic large brick-shaped virion and the ability to replicate in the cytoplasm of infected cells, relatively autonomously from the host nuclear machinery. The poxvirus genomes range from 135 to 290 kbp, encode from 136 to 260 open reading frames that are arranged in a non-overlapping fashion (see www.poxvirus.org for comprehensive listings). Centrally located genes are the most conserved across poxviruses, and are generally required for replication or morphogenesis of the virus, while genes that map nearer to the genomic termini are more variable and encode a wide array of gene products dedicated for virus survival and replication within the host. Within these variable regions are inverted terminal repeats that typically contain few genes (less than ten) that are mirrored on either end of the poxvirus genome. Proteins encoded by genes from the variable region are generally required for virulence within a host and are very diverse in their functions. These proteins can be either cell-associated or secreted, usually as glycoproteins. Intracellular proteins have been shown to interfere with various cell-signaling pathways, including apoptosis, cytokine signaling and establishment of the antiviral state. Secreted immunomodulatory proteins include cytokine binding proteins, receptor homologs, complement binding proteins, and viral regulators of chemokines. These have been characterized as virokines (cytokine-like) or viroceptors (receptor-like). Some of these secreted proteins function as high affinity inhibitors of many important immune modulators, including proinflammatory cytokines [1].

Secreted immunomodulators: shaping the immuno-environment

Following poxvirus infection, there is a sequentially staged series of host responses designed to rid the body of the foreign pathogen. In the earliest stages, a nonspecific innate immune response is triggered [2]. The generation of an early proinflammatory microenvironment begins with the induction of chemokines, cytokines and interferons (IFNs) by the cells of the innate immune system: particularly neutrophils, macrophages, dendritic cells (DCs) and natural killer (NK) cells. These cell types are producers of key antiviral cytokines, including tumor necrosis factors (TNFs), IFNs, interleukin (IL)-1β, IL-18, and chemokines. This array of cytokines is not only important in recruiting migratory leukocytes to sites of virus infection but also in inducing a T helper type 1 (Th1) response, which is especially critical for poxvirus clearance [2]. This is a very complex response pathway and involves multiple cell types responding to the cues from many overlapping signals. However, poxviruses are able in many cases to micromanage key aspects of the host immune response by the cooperative actions of many virulence factors [1, 3]. The targets of many of these immunomodulators are summarized in the following sections.

Type I interferons

Type I IFNs are among the first antiviral proteins induced following a viral infection. Most types of cells are capable of producing IFN-α/β and the actions of these proteins on virus-infected cells and the surrounding tissues is ultimately to generate an antiviral state in responsive cells. This is accomplished through the recruitment and activation of the Janus kinases (JAKs) and phosphorylation of the signal transducers and activators of transcription (STATs), which are then translocated to the nucleus to drive the expression of IFN-stimulated genes (ISGs), such as the IFN-induced, dsRNA-activated protein kinase (PKR) and 2',5'-oligoadenylate synthetase (OAS), which are very effective at limiting viral replication [4]. Recently, the action of IFN has been attributed to the strict species barrier of *Myxoma virus* (MYXV), a leporipoxvirus that normally infects only rabbits. In this study, overcoming the Erk-dependent phosphorylation of IFN regulatory factor 3 (IRF3) and subsequent IFN-α/β expression and stimulation is key for productive replication of the virus in non-rabbit cells [5].

To counter the effects of type I IFNs, poxviruses encode a wide variety of intracellular (discussed later) and secreted proteins to counteract the IFN-stimulated antiviral responses. The secreted anti-IFN proteins exhibit sequence similarity to cellular IFN receptors or Ig-superfamily members and act by binding to and inhibiting the function of type I IFN in a competitive manner. *Vaccinia virus* (VACV) strain western reserve (WR) B18R encodes a secreted protein that contains an immunoglobulin domain that binds and inhibits IFN-α/β/δ/ω from various mammalian species [6, 7]. B18R is also able to bind to the cell surface of both non-infected and infected cells, an attribute that is likely important in maintaining a microenvironment conducive to viral replication [8]. Additionally, VACV deficient in B18R is attenuated in an intranasal and intracranial mouse model of infection [9], and is a potential candidate for vaccine development [10]. *Ectromelia virus* (ECTV) also encodes a type I IFN binding protein that inhibits both human and murine IFN-α and human IFN-β [11].

Type II interferons

IFN-γ is an integral component of both the innate and adaptive immune system that is produced only by certain cells of the immune system, including NK cells, $CD4^+$ T helper cells and $CD8^+$ cytotoxic T cells. The lack of IFN-γ expression in mice renders them especially susceptible to poxvirus infection, while injection of IFN-γ into VACV-infected mice increases their resistance to the infection [12]. Many poxviruses encode secreted proteins that bind to and inhibit the function of IFN-γ. While the binding of human and murine IFN-γ to their cognate receptor is highly species specific, orthopoxvirus IFN-γ binding proteins are able to bind to IFN from several species [13–15]. VACV, *Cowpox virus* (CPXV) and *Camelpox virus* IFN-γ binding proteins have been shown to exist as dimers in solution, possibly increasing the binding avidity and activity [16]. VACV deficient in B8R, which encodes the IFN-δ binding protein, has been shown to have a role in pathogenesis in a rabbit infection model, but surprisingly since it does not bind murine IFN-γ, it has also been shown to be a virulence factor in mouse models [10, 17, 18]. MYXV also encodes an IFN-γ binding protein, M-T7. Unlike the orthopoxvirus IFN-γ binding proteins, M-T7 exists as a trimer in solution and binds in a species-specific manner [19]. As expected, the M-T7 knockout virus is attenuated in infected rabbits [20]; however, the analysis is complicated by the fact that M-T7 has also been shown to interact with a variety of chemokines (discussed later).

IL-1β

The IL-1 family members comprise a group of potent pro-inflammatory cytokines that participate in the early signaling events leading to inflammation. IL-1β and IL-18 are members of this family and are both produced as inactive precursors (proIL-1β; proIL-18) lacking a signal peptide [21]. Like proIL-18, proIL-1β is cleaved by active caspase-1 (inhibition of this pathway is discussed later) to produce biologically active IL-1β that is then secreted. Several orthopoxvirus species encode secreted IL-1 receptor homologs. The gene products of VACV (strain WR) B15R, ECTV E191 and CPXV B14R are secreted proteins that bind to and inhibit the function of IL-1β [22–24]. These interactions are highly specific since these proteins bind neither to IL-1α nor the host IL-1 receptor antagonist. VACV lacking B15R is attenuated in mice after intracranial, but not intradermal, injection; however, after intranasal infection the symptoms are actually more severe [25, 26]. These studies show that IL-1β functions as the major pro-inflammatory molecule and B15R can suppress this response.

IL-18

IL-18 is a key proinflammatory cytokine that was previously known as IFN-γ-inducing factor, and which stimulates T cells, NK cells and macrophages [27]. It exerts its effect through a heterodimeric receptor complex composed of the binding chain, IL-18Rα, and the non-binding signaling chain, IL-18Rβ. Although IL-18 is thought to be primarily involved in inducing expression of IFN-γ, there is growing evidence that this is a very diverse effector molecule. It has been shown to up-regulate the expression of FasL on NK cells and consequently their Fas-FasL-mediated cytotoxicity.

ProIL-18 can be found in resting monocytes at both the RNA and protein level [28]. To regulate this potent inflammatory cytokine extracellularly, IL-18 binding protein (IL-18 BP), a high-affinity IL-18 antagonist distinct from cytokine receptors, is constitutively expressed [29]. At twofold molar excess, this inhibitor can completely abolish IFN-γ-inducing activity of IL-18 [30].

The poxviral IL-18 BPs are the most conserved virulence genes across members of the *Chordopoxvirinae* [1]. These viral proteins, like their mammalian counterparts, bind IL-18 and prevent IL-18R signaling. *Molluscum contagiosum virus* (MOCV) encodes three gene products (MC51L, 53L and

54L) that have sequence similarity to human (hu)IL-18 BP, but only one, 54L, is able to bind and inhibit IL-18 function [30, 31]. Amino acid residues critical for the high-affinity interaction of huIL-18 and huIL-18 BP have been elucidated. These residues correspond to residues found in MC54L and the ECTV IL-18 BP that are required for binding and are absent in MC51L and 53L [30, 32]. It has also been shown that the MC54L and the version from *Variola virus* (VARV), also bind glycosaminoglycans (GAGs) through their C-terminal tails [33, 34]. One study showed that MC054L protein can exist in two forms, one of which is a furin-cleaved form that contains only the IL-18 binding domain [33]. This class of virulence factor has also been shown to be important *in vivo*. The VACV IL-18 BP (C12L) has been shown to promote virulence in a murine intranasal model [35]. Additionally, the ECTV IL-18 BP has been shown to be important in down-regulating the NK cell response [36, 37].

Tumor necrosis factors

TNF is a potent proinflammatory molecule that is secreted by macrophages and activated T cells. There are three classes of TNF: TNF-α, lymphotoxin (LT) α and LTβ. This family of proteins forms trimers, and activates their cognate receptors TNFRI and TNFRII. Signaling through these receptors can have a variety of effects, such as induction of the antiviral state, cytolysis and inflammation, depending on the strength of signal and the type of ligand [38, 39].

Poxviruses encode a wide spread of TNF inhibitors, most of which mimic the cellular receptors [40]. However, there is another poxvirus protein, encoded by *Tanapox virus* (TANV), that shares no sequence homology to any known TNF receptor or binding protein [41]. There are two further subgroups within the receptor mimics: the T2 family of inhibitors expressed by leporipoxviruses and the cytokine response modifier (crm) family from orthopoxviruses. Both TNF receptor-mimic families share sequence similarity to TNFRI and TNFRII, including up to four cysteine-rich domains (CRDs). However, these viral proteins all lack any transmembrane domains as found in the cellular receptors and are expressed as oligomers that influence their activity [40].

MYXV T2 (M-T2) is expressed as an early glycosylated protein that specifically binds rabbit TNF with similar affinity to the rabbit TNFR [42, 43]. Additionally, this protein is able to function intracellularly as an inhibitor of apoptosis (discussed later). Virus disrupted in this M-T2 gene is significantly attenuated in rabbits susceptible to wild-type virus infection [44].

Orthopoxviruses encode several inhibitors of TNF; however, they are not all present in the same virus. CrmB, C, D and E are all TNF family inhibitors (crmA is an inhibitor of apoptosis and cytokine processing; discussed later). CrmB is an early protein that binds and inhibits both TNF and LTα.

CrmC inhibits TNF, while crmD inhibits both TNF and LTα [40]. CrmC is unique in this group since it is the only member that lacks the conserved C-terminal region shared among the other virus-encoded TNFRs (vTNFRs). It also has an additional function, in that it prevents TNF-mediated cytolysis [45]. Interestingly, crmD is absent in most CPXV strains, but it is encoded in orthopoxviruses if both crmB and crmC are missing [46]. CrmE is able to bind and inhibit rat, murine, and human TNF, but only protects against human TNF-mediated cytolysis. So far, only crmE from CPXV and VACV strain USSR have been shown to be functional [47]. CrmE from VACV strain USSR has also been shown to have both soluble and cell-associated vTNFR activity [48]. This activity is shared among crmC encoded by VACV strains Lister, USSR and Evans and mapping to A53R [49].

TANV encodes a TNF binding protein with no similarity to any host TNF receptor or binding protein [41]. Supernatants from TANV-infected cells were able to inhibit TNF-mediated induction of NF-kB and up-regulation of cell adhesion molecule expression [50, 51]. A subsequent study used human TNF to identify a high-affinity TNF binding protein corresponding to a 38-kDa glycoprotein. It was found that this protein maps to the 2L gene of TANV and has a high affinity (Kd=43 pM) to human TNF but no other family members or species. It is also able to inhibit human TNF-mediated cytolysis [41]. Finally, a homolog of CD30, a related TNFR superfamily member, has been identified in ECTV [52].

Chemokines

Chemotactic cytokines are rapidly induced at the site of virus infection and are critical for attracting immune cells from the blood vessel and into the infected tissue. As a testament to the importance of this group of proteins, poxviruses encode a variety of proteins to inhibit leukocyte chemotaxis mediated by chemokines. These include chemokine binding proteins (CBPs), chemokine receptor mimics, and homologs of chemokines themselves [53, 54].

Low-affinity CBPs

As previously mentioned, M-T7 of MYXV is a secreted IFN-γ binding protein that has the additional property that it can bind and inhibit a broad spectrum of C, CC and CXC chemokines [55]. M-T7 binds through the C-terminal heparin binding site present on many chemokines and likely functions by interfering with the ability of chemokines to bind to GAGs, thereby disrupting gradients, which are critical for effective taxis. Additionally, IFN-γ and chemokines likely bind to the same face of M-T7 since these interactions are mutually exclusive [55, 56].

The M-T7-knockout construct is attenuated in rabbits and characterized by an increase in the number of infiltrating leukocytes into sites of infection [56]. Since M-T7 is able to bind and inhibit both IFN-γ and chemokines, it is difficult to specifically attribute this property with either activity. However, it has been shown that M-T7 can reduce migration of inflammatory cells in rodent models of inflammation and angiogenesis [57, 58]. This can be attributed solely to chemokine binding function of M-T7, since it is not able to bind or inhibit murine IFN-γ.

High-affinity CBPs

This class of CBP, termed CBP-II, is more widespread across poxvirus genera. Both leporipoxviruses and orthopoxviruses encode CBP-II proteins that are able to bind and inhibit the function of a range of CC chemokines. Another feature that these proteins share is that they do not resemble any known host chemokine receptors or any other eukaryotic proteins. The basis by which these proteins are able to interact with so many different CC chemokines is due to a number of residues that are conserved in the cellular ligands. CBP-II proteins target these residues, which are in a region distinct from the heparin binding site, to promiscuously inhibit a broad variety of CC chemokines [1]. However, CBP-IIs are not able to bind and inhibit all CC chemokines. VACV CBP-II/35-kDa protein was shown to bind to most CC chemokines, out of those 80 that were tested [59]. In addition to its chemokine binding properties, MYXV CBP-II/M-T1 is capable of binding to GAGs, a property that allows this protein to bind cell surfaces and chemokines simultaneously [60]. MYXV and *Rabbitpox virus* require CBP-II for the inhibition of early leukocyte infiltration; however, these virulence genes alone are unable to reverse the ultimate outcome of disease progression [61]. The CBP-II family has also been used to treat a variety of animal models of inflammatory diseases that are dependent on chemokine activities [62].

Chemokine homologs

Surprisingly, a few poxviruses encode proteins that are mimics of host chemokines. To date the only chemokine homologs that have been identified are found in *Fowlpox virus* (FWPV) and MOCV; only the MOCV version has been characterized. MC148R is a homolog of IL-11 receptor α locus chemokine (ILC) [63]. This chemokine is specifically expressed in the skin, the same tissue distribution that MOCV itself adopts. While MC148R is structurally related to CC chemokines, there is a deletion in what would be the N-terminal portion of this family of protein. This region prior to the CC motif is required for transmission of signal through chemokine receptors.

Mechanistically, it has been shown that this protein is secreted and inhibits the binding and signaling of various CC and CXC chemokines through their cognate receptors, resulting in the inhibition of chemotaxis in various leukocytes [64]. It has also been shown that this protein acts by binding selectively to human CCR8, preventing signaling through occupied receptors [65]. However, MC148R is also effective in a murine model of allograft rejection, suggesting that it possesses additional functions [62, 66].

Multiple cytokine binding proteins

Orf virus (ORFV), a parapoxvirus that causes a contagious skin condition in sheep, goats and humans, encodes a secreted protein that is able to bind and inhibit both GM-CSF and IL-2 [67]. Termed GM-CSF/IL-2 inhibitory factor (GIF), this protein forms dimers and tetramers that bind at high affinity to ovine but not human or murine GM-CSF and IL-2 [68]. *In vivo*, GIF is able to affect the cell mediated immune (CMI) response measured by neutrophil and macrophage activation and maturation of and antigen presentation by DCs through IL-2 and GM-CSF, respectively. GIF has no sequence similarity to any known mammalian gene; however, it shares homology with A41L and members of the CBP-II class [68]. A41L is a related virulence factor encoded by VACV that is involved in the prevention of virus clearance and reduction of the infiltration of inflammatory cells into the infected area. While many chemokines and chemokine receptors were tested, no ligands have yet been identified for A41L [69]. TANV has also been demonstrated to express a multiple cytokine binding protein [50]. A secreted 38-kDa glycoprotein was isolated and shown to bind and inhibit TNF, IL-2, IL-5 and IFN-γ [50, 51]. TANV 2L is also a 38-kDa glycoprotein that binds and inhibits TNF-α; however, 2L does not bind IL-2, IL-5 or IFN-γ [41, 50]. The viral protein that binds these latter cytokines remains to be identified.

Cytokine homologs

Some cytokines transduce signals that inhibit proinflammatory signaling and CMI. IL-10 is a typical Th2-type cytokine associated with inhibition of the CMI response [70]. *Yaba-like disease virus* (YLDV), ORFV, and *Lumpy skin disease virus* (LSDV) exploit this and encode proteins that are homologous to IL-10 [1]. Of these, the ORFV IL-10 homolog was the first to be identified and characterized. It is most similar to IL-10 from sheep, cattle, humans and mice and has a similar function to ovine IL-10 in that it is able to stimulate murine thymocyte proliferation, mast cell growth, and suppress macrophage activation [71, 72]. More recently, the YLDV IL-10 homolog has also been characterized [73]. YLDV 134R encodes a secreted, monomeric glycoprotein that is actually more similar to IL-24 than IL-10. Purified protein was able to stimulate signal transduction from class II cytokine receptors. VACV expressing 134R exhibited reduced virulence in a murine intranasal model [73].

Anti-inflammatory serpins

Serine proteinase inhibitors (serpins) are characterized by a highly conserved secondary and tertiary structure. Generally, serpins are a highly versatile class of proteins and primarily, but not exclusively, act by irreversibly binding and inhibiting proteinases [74]. Inhibitory serpins are recognized as pseudosubstrates of their target proteinase. The mechanism by which serpins inhibit proteinases is based on their metastable conformation. The large amount of energy stored in the conformation of the protein allows it to function like a "mouse trap" for the target proteinase. Poxviruses are the only known viruses to encode functional serpins, and these show a remarkable array of different functions (the crmA/Spi-2 group of serpins will be discussed later). The secreted Serp-1 protein from MYXV is a 55–60-kDa glycoprotein that is expressed late in infection [75]. Serp-1 has been shown *in vitro* to form stable complexes and inhibit tissue-type plasminogen activator, plasmin, thrombin and urokinase [76]. MYXV deficient in Serp-1 results in increased inflammatory cell responses, attenuated virulence and a more rapid clearance [77].

In orthopoxviruses, a related class of proteins is termed Spi-3 and was originally linked to the inhibition of cell-cell fusion. However, Spi-3 has been shown to inhibit the same spectrum of proteinases as Serp-1 [78]. Nevertheless, Spi-3 cannot be functionally interchanged with Serp-1 [79]. Part of this functional difference may be attributed to the fact that Spl-3 is expressed early and the protein is tethered to cells *via* virally encoded hemagglutinin.

Complement

The complement system is a highly regulated cascade consisting of soluble and cell-surface-attached proteins. Activation of the complement system results in cleavage and activation of some of its early components, and the net effects of activation of this pathway are the formation of a membrane attack complex (MAC) and an inflammatory and chemoattractant microenvironment. MACs are able to pierce holes in lipid membranes which is an important mechanism of intracellular mature virus (IMV) and extracellular enveloped virus (EEV) neutralization [80]. Several poxviruses express secreted proteins that inhibit complement. VACV complement control protein (VCP), CPXV inflammation modulatory protein (IMP) and the smallpox inhibitor of complement enzymes (SPICE) are proteins that contain tandem short consensus repeat (SCR) motifs and act to inhibit the complement pathway through C3b and C4b [1]. During infection, VCP has been shown to have a significant role in the pathogenesis of the virus. In VCP-deficient virus, lesion sizes are smaller than in wild-type virus infection [81]. *In vitro,* VCP binds to C3b and C4b with higher affinity than the human C4b binding protein, and it can also act as a cofactor for the cleavage and inhibition of C3b and C4b by factor I, and increase the rate of decay for both classical and alternative C3 convertases [82–84]. The CPXV IMP protein has a similar role in pathogenesis, where it has been shown to play a role in inhibiting mononuclear cell infiltration, limiting tissue damage and the formation of lesions. Many of these symptoms are likely due to the inhibition of the release of chemoattractant and inflammatory cleavage fragments of the complement system, C4a, C3a, and C5a [85]. Additionally, the effectiveness of these interactions may be somewhat species specific since SPICE inhibits human C3b and C4b to a greater extent than VCP [86]. Other mechanisms of immune evasion of complement include the incorporation of host proteins, such as CD55 and CD59 that are regulators of complement in the lipid membrane surrounding the virus. The complement inhibitors have also been shown to have anti-inflammatory properties in a variety of animal models [62].

Inhibition of intracellular signaling

While the inhibition of extracellular signaling is critical for viral replication, a virus-infected cell needs to be also kept hidden from immune cells that have become activated. The most dire threats on a virus-infected cell are innate effector cells, such as NK cells, and educated effector cells, such as $CD8^+$ cytotoxic T lymphocytes (CTLs). To avoid detection by CTLs, poxviruses down-regulate MHC class I expression, which presents antigens to $CD8^+$ T cells. The extent to which poxviruses are able to exert this activity correlates well with the down-regulation of the CMI response [87, 88]. For example, orthopoxviruses are not associated with severe suppression of the CMI response, and cause only moderate down-regulation of MHC class I, while MYXV and *Rabbit fibroma virus* causes a rapid loss of MHC class I expression and systemic reduction in the CMI response [89]. The MYXV M153R gene product is responsible for down-regulation of MHC class I *in vitro*, and rabbits infected with virus deficient in M153R exhibit decreased symptoms and an increase in mononuclear infiltration at the site of infection [90]. M153R encodes a protein containing a distinctive motif known as a plant homeodomain or leukemia-associated protein motif [90, 91]. Potential orthologs of M153R exist in YLDV, LSDV, *Swinepox virus* (SWPV) and *Shope fibroma virus* (SFV). The mechanism of action is directly linked to the ability of this protein to localize to the endoplasmic reticulum (ER) *via* its transmembrane domains. It is postulated that M153R targets MHC class I molecules for retention and degradation *via* the late endosomal/lysosomal pathway, resulting in decreased levels of β2-microglobulin-associated MHC class I levels at the cell surface [90, 92]. One potential caveat with this down-regulation strategy is that the immune system already has contingency plans in place to deal with cells that lose MHC class I molecules. NK cells are able to nonspecifically kill cells that are unable to provide an MHC class I-dependent inhibitory signal. Homologs of MHC class I molecules have been identified from the genomes of several poxviruses, including MOCV and SWPV. MC80R has even been shown to form stable complexes with β2-microglobulin [93].

Another strategy that targets the CMI and humoral response is the down-regulation of CD4 expression on T lymphocytes. MYXV infection of T cells is able to deplete CD4 levels in a protein kinase C-independent fashion that involves internalization and degradation of the receptor, thereby down-regulating $CD4^+$ helper T cell function [92, 94].

Semaphorin

Semaphorins are members of a highly conserved family of regulatory molecules originally identified to induce axon steering and growth cone collapse [95, 96]. They are found in animals ranging from invertebrates to mammals, and may be secreted, glycosylphosphatidylinositol-anchored or be transmembrane molecules. They are defined by the presence of a SEMA domain, a large (500-amino acid) region within the extracellular region of the protein. It is now known that semaphorins participate in a wide variety of functions including: neuronal development, neuronal plasticity and repair, immunology, angiogenesis, and cancer [97, 98].

Several poxvirus-encoded proteins have been identified as having a SEMA domain, including VACV, ECTV, CPXV and FWPV. All but the fowlpox version of the protein also exhibit similarity with SemaA7A, a protein known to influence monocyte migration, T cell activation, B cell survival and the interactions between T cells, B cells and DCs [1]. The ECTV version of this protein has been shown to induce monocyte aggregation due to up-regulation of CD54 (ICAM-1) [99]. VACV A39R does not seem to be important in an intranasal model of infection; however, when A39R from strain Copenhagen was introduced into strain WR, lesions were larger and histology suggested an inflammatory role for this protein [100]. This protein has also been reported to bind plexin C1, a molecule expressed on neutrophils and DCs, and inhibited chemokine-induced migration of DCs *in vitro* [101]. In a separate study, A39R inhibited phagocytosis by DCs and neutrophils and inhibited the capacity of $CD8^+$ DC to take up apoptotic bodies [102].

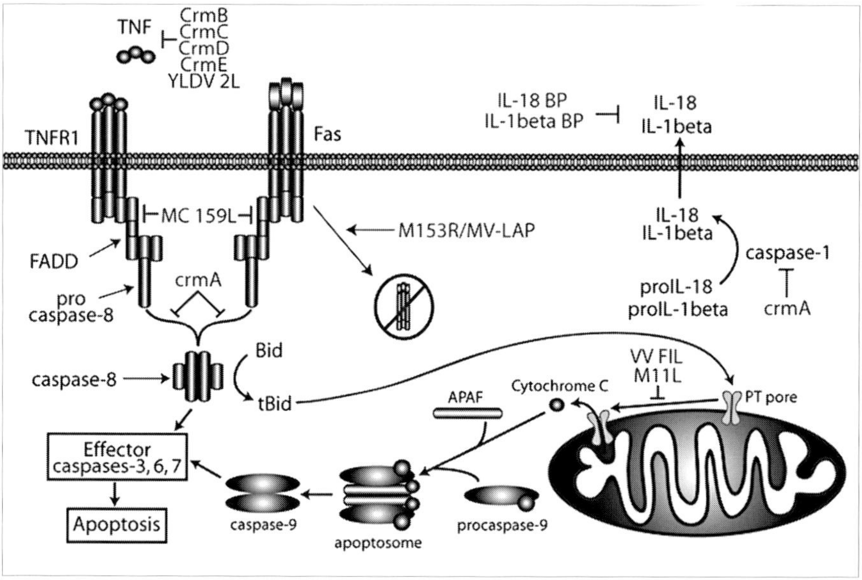

Figure 1. Inhibition of cellular proinflammatory processes and apoptosis by poxviral proteins. Cellular signals, such as TNF and Fas receptor signaling, can activate pro-apoptotic processes through recruitment of procaspase-8. Caspase-8 can cleave Bid to start the mitochondrial arm of the apoptotic pathway. Caspase-1 is most well known for its cytokine processing function. Once processed, IL-18 and IL-1β are secreted where they can act as a major proinflammatory cytokines. Illustrated are examples of inhibition of these processes by poxviral virulence factors (see [1] for a more detailed account.).

Inhibition of apoptosis

Apoptosis, a regulated form of cell death, is an important arm of the innate immune system. The induction of apoptotic death processes can be triggered by a variety of different stimuli; however, there are several key checkpoints in the cascade that poxviruses have learned to exploit. Cysteine-dependent aspartate-specific proteinases (caspases) and the mitochondria are both critical in the induction of apoptosis. One of the methods that poxviruses use to target this pathway is to directly inhibit caspase activation. Caspase-8 is frequently targeted and is an important mediator of TNF- or FasL-induced death signals (Fig. 1). Upon ligation, the TNF receptor and Fas/CD95/Apo-1 can recruit Fas-associated death domain (FADD) adaptor molecules. FADD contains two important domains, a death domain that interacts with the cytoplasmic portion of the death receptors, and a death effector domain (DED). This motif can recruit the inactive pro-caspase-8, which contains a DED motif in the pro domain. Transactivation of caspase-8 follows this recruitment. After activation of caspase-8, Bid can be cleaved to tBid and begin the induction of apoptosis through the mitochondrial arm of this pathway [1, 103].

Caspase inhibition

MOCV encodes two virulence factors that contain DEDs, designated MC159 and MC160. Both proteins are categorized as viral FLICE (caspase-8) inhibitory proteins (vFLIPs) that bind to FADD and procaspase-8 preventing its recruitment and subsequent activation. Most of the anti-apoptotic activity has been ascribed to MC159; however, MC160 is degraded by caspases when MC159 is not present. MC159 binds FADD and caspase-8 through the viral DED motifs [104, 105] Mutation within the DED region abolishes the anti-apoptotic properties. Surprisingly, mutations in adjacent hydrophobic regions that do not mitigate binding to FADD or caspase-8 also have deleterious effects on the ability of MC159 to inhibit apoptosis, suggesting that other protein interactions may be involved [104, 105].

The most common method of caspase inhibition is through direct interaction with the activated enzyme. Prior to the studies with the crmA gene from CPXV, all serpins were originally thought to inhibit only serine proteinases [106]. CrmA was originally discovered by examining mutations leading to white pock mutants of CPXV that arise spontaneously [107]. It has been extensively characterized and exhibits inhibition of caspase-8 and caspase-1 with high affinity, thus inhibiting both apoptosis and inflammation mediated by caspase-1 processing of proIL-1β and proIL-18 [108]. CrmA can also inhibit and form complexes with caspases-4, -5, -8, -9, and -10 and with granzyme B to some extent. This versatile serpin can block apoptosis induced by several pathways including serum deprivation, removal of nerve growth factor, detachment from the extracellular matrix, hypoxic conditions, TNF-α, and Fas ligation [1, 103].

CrmA is a very potent inhibitor of apoptosis in cultured cells but its role in the virus-infected host is less clear. This protein was predicted to be highly important to the fitness of the virus but, surprisingly, deletion of crmA leads to only modest attenuation of pathogenesis in a murine intranasal model and reduced inflammation [109]. Similarly, knocking out crmA/Spi-2 from VACV using a murine intranasal model had little or no effect on virulence or inflammation [110]. Double knockouts of crmA/Spi-2 and IL-1 soluble receptor (B15R) from VACV demonstrated that inhibition of IL-1β-mediated fever was controlled by the B15R protein, not crmA [111]. Intradermal inoculation of the VACV crmA/Spi-2 knockout, however, did result in a significant change in lesion size [26]. In contrast, Serp-2 from MYXV plays a critical role in the pathogenesis of the virus but is considerably less effective at inhibiting caspases [112]. The pathology showed a rapid inflammatory response and increased apoptosis of lymphocytes within lymph nodes [112]. This discrepancy suggests that inhibition of caspases is not alone sufficient to explain the role of these viral serpins in infection.

Inhibition of apoptosis at the mitochondrial checkpoint

Mitochondria are a regulated gateway in the apoptotic pathway. When mitochondria have received either intrinsic (e.g., unfolded protein response, oxidative stress or DNA damage) or certain extrinsic (e.g., a death ligand) signals, these are mediated by pro-apoptotic members of the Bcl-2 family, namely bid, bak and bax. Multimerization of bak and bax can cause the opening of the permeability transition pore (PTP) and cytochrome c release into the cytosol. Cytochrome c interacts with Apaf-1 and this complex can recruit and activate caspase-9, leading to apoptosis [113].

Both the leporipoxviruses and orthopoxviruses encode proteins (M11L and F1L, respectively) that localize to the mitochondria and inhibit apoptosis. M11L is an important virulence factor *in vivo*, and *in vitro* the knockout virus is unable to replicate in rabbit lymphocytes [114]. The mechanism of M11L function has been ascribed to both an interaction with the peripheral benzodiazepine receptor, a component of the PTP complex [115], and a constitutive interaction with bak [116]. VACV F1L may function in a related manner since its overall structure, motifs and localization is similar to M11L [117, 118].

Other anti-apoptotic poxvirus proteins

A number of poxvirus proteins target other arms of the apoptotic regulatory machine. M-T4, an ER resident protein expressed by MYXV, is thought to inhibit the unfolded protein response generated in the ER [119]. Additionally, the TNFR, M-T2 from MYXV (discussed previously), also exhibits anti-apoptotic properties within the cell. Through deletion mutagenesis, the anti-apoptotic regions have been mapped to the first two N-terminal CRDs, while TNF inhibition maps to the first three CRDs [120–122]. Recently, a MYXV protein, M-T5, with homology to the CPXV Chinese hamster ovary host range protein and which has anti-apoptotic properties, has been characterized to bind to human Cullin-1 [123]. This interaction has been shown to have the functional consequence of protecting virus-infected cells from apoptosis due to cell cycle arrest at the G0/G1 checkpoint [123]. The vast array of targets for inhibition of apoptosis points to its importance in the antiviral response.

Intracellular mechanisms of IFN inhibition

The inhibition of the IFN response is extremely critical for virus survival; as a result, secretion of potent inhibitors of IFN ligand is not enough to fully blunt IFN effects. Many poxviruses have evolved proteins that also target the downstream effector molecules of the IFN response [124]. Two major intracellular effectors that poxviruses have been characterized to target are PKR, a type I IFN-induced gene that is a dsRNA-activated serine/threonine protein kinase, and OAS/RNaseL, another dsRNA-activated pathway. Both of these effector arms have the net effect of inhibiting viral and host protein synthesis. PKR mediates its inhibitory effect by phosphorylating and inactivating eIF-2α, while OAS/RNaseL mediates mRNA degradation [1].

The most highly characterized poxvirus proteins that mediate inhibition of this IFN-regulated response are VACV E3L and K3L. Deletion of these genes in VACV renders virus-infected cells sensitive to IFN and severely attenuates the virus pathogenesis [125–129]. E3L is a dsRNA-binding protein that can sequester dsRNA to prevent activation of PKR and OAS/RNaseL [130, 131]. E3L can also bind to PKR, reducing its activity [132], to IRF3, blocking activation and subsequent up-regulation of IFN-β; and to IRF-7 and SUMO-1 [133, 134]. E3L has also been shown to reduce adenosine deaminase activity [135]. K3L and the related M156R from MYXV, are pseudosubstrate mimics of eIF-2α, which are able to competitively inhibit PKR-dependent eIF-2α phosphorylation [136–138]. Homologous genes have been identified in VARV, YLDV, SWPV, ORFV, MYXV and SFV. ECTV only encodes an E3L ortholog but not K3L [1].

Some poxviruses use additional strategies for inhibiting intracellular IFN signaling. VACV H1L encodes a phosphatase that acts on STAT-1, a transcription factor required for IFN action, thereby revising its activation [139]. MC159L, previously described as a vFLIP, may also inhibit some IFN-mediated events, including PKR-induced apoptosis and activation of NF-κB [140].

Conclusions

The number of strategies by which poxviruses manipulate the host immune responses continues to grow, and the affected pathways are increasingly complex. Figure 1 illustrates how just a few poxvirus proteins manipulate apoptosis and inflammation, but a comprehensive accounting of all the affected host pathways is beyond the scope of this chapter. Instead, we can regard poxviruses as master "anti-immunologists" and it is reasonable to predict that there are more modulatory pathways still to be uncovered.

References

1 Seet BT, Johnston JB, Brunetti CR, Barrett JW, Everett H, Cameron C, Sypula J, Nazarian SH, Lucas A, McFadden G (2003) Poxviruses and immune evasion. *Annu Rev Immunol* 21: 377–423

2 Smith SA, Kotwal GJ (2002) Immune response to poxvirus infections in various animals. *Crit Rev Microbiol* 28: 149–185

3 Alcami A, Koszinowski UH (2000) Viral mechanisms of immune evasion. *Immunol Today* 8: 447–455
4 Sen GC (2001) Viruses and interferon. *Annu Rev* Microbiol 55: 255–281
5 Wang F, Ma Y, Barrett JW, Gao X, Loh J, Barton E, Virgin HW, McFadden G (2004) Disruption of Erk-dependent type I interferon induction breaks the myxoma virus species barrier. *Nat Immunol* 5: 1266–1274
6 Symons JA, Alcami A, Smith GL (1995) Vaccinia virus encodes a soluble type I interferon receptor of novel structure and broad species specificity. *Cell* 81: 551–560
7 Vancova I, La Bonnardiere C, Kontsek P (1998) Vaccinia virus protein B18R inhibits the activity and cellular binding of the novel type interferon-delta. *J Gen Virol* 79: 1647–1649
8 Alcami A, Symons JA, Smith GL (2000) The vaccinia virus soluble alpha/beta interferon (IFN) receptor binds to the cell surface and protects cells from the antiviral effects of IFN. *J Virol* 74: 11230–11239
9 Colamonici OR, Domanski P, Sweitzer SM, Larner A, Buller RM (1995) Vaccinia virus B18R gene encodes a type I interferon-binding protein that blocks interferon alpha transmembrane signaling. *J Biol Chem* 270: 15974–15978
10 Jackson SS, Ilyinskii P, Philippon V, Gritz L, Yafal AG, Zinnack K, Beaudry KR, Manson KH, Lifton MA, Kuroda MJ et al (2005) Role of genes that modulate host immune responses in the immunogenicity and pathogenicity of vaccinia virus. *J Virol* 79: 6554–6559
11 Smith VP, Alcami A (2002) Inhibition of interferons by ectromelia virus. *J Virol* 76: 1124–1134
12 Katze MG, He Y, Gale M Jr (2002) Viruses and interferon: a fight for supremacy. *Nat Rev Immunol* 2: 675–687
13 Mossman K, Upton C, Buller RM, McFadden G (1995) Species specificity of ectromelia virus and vaccinia virus interferon-γ binding proteins. *Virology* 208: 762–769
14 Alcami A, Smith GL (1995) Vaccinia, cowpox, and camelpox viruses encode soluble gamma interferon receptors with novel broad species specificity. *J Virol* 69: 4633–4639
15 Bai HD, Buller RML, Chen NH, Green M, Nuara AA (2005) Biosynthesis of the IFN-gamma binding protein of ectromelia virus, the causative agent of mousepox. *Virology* 334: 41–50
16 Alcami A, Smith GL (2002) The vaccinia virus soluble interferon-g receptor is a homodimer. *J Gen Virol* 83: 545–549
17 Symons JA, Tscharke DC, Price N, Smith GL (2002) A study of the vaccinia virus interferon-gamma receptor and its contribution to virus virulence. *J Gen Virol* 83: 1953–1964
18 Sroller V, Ludvikova V, Maresova L, Hainz P, Nemeckova S (2001) Effect of IFN-gamma receptor gene deletion on vaccinia virus virulence. *Arch Virol* 146: 239–249
19 Mossman K, Upton C, McFadden G (1995) The myxoma virus-soluble interferon-γ receptor homolog, M-T7, inhibits interferon-γ in a species-specific manner. *J Biol Chem* 270: 3031–3038

20 Mossman K, Nation P, Macen J, Garbutt M, Lucas A, McFadden G (1996) Myxoma virus M-T7, a secreted homolog of the interferon-γ receptor, is a critical virulence factor for the development of myxomatosis in European rabbits. *Virology* 215: 17–30
21 Ghayur T, Banerjee S, Hugunin M, Butler D, Herzog L, Carter A, Quintal L, Sekut L, Talanian R, Paskind M et al (1997) Caspase-1 processes IFN-gamma-inducing factor and regulates LPS-induced IFN-gamma production. *Nature* 386: 619–623
22 Smith VP, Alcamí A (2000) Expression of secreted cytokine and chemokine inhibitors by ectromelia virus. *J Virol* 74: 8460–8471
23 Alcami A, Smith GL (1992) A soluble receptor for interleukin-1 beta encoded by vaccinia virus: a novel mechanism of virus modulation of the host response to infection. *Cell* 71: 153–167
24 Spriggs MK, Hruby DE, Maliszewski CR, Pickup DJ, Sims JE, Buller RM, VanSlyke J (1992) Vaccinia and cowpox viruses encode a novel secreted interleukin-1-binding protein. *Cell* 71: 145–152
25 Alcami A, Smith GL (1996) A mechanism for the inhibition of fever by a virus. *Proc Natl Acad Sci USA* 93: 11029–11034
26 Tscharke DC, Reading PC, Smith GL (2002) Dermal infection with vaccinia virus reveals roles for virus proteins not seen using other inoculation routes. *J Gen Virol* 83: 1977–1986
27 Dinarello CA (2000) Interleukin-18, a proinflammatory cytokine. *Eur Cytokine Netw* 11: 483–486
28 Puren AJ, Fantuzzi G, Dinarello CA (1999) Gene expression, synthesis, and secretion of interleukin 18 and interleukin 1beta are differentially regulated in human blood mononuclear cells and mouse spleen cells. *Proc Natl Acad Sci USA* 96: 2256–2261
29 Novick D, Kim SH, Fantuzzi G, Reznikov LL, Dinarello CA, Rubinstein M (1999) Interleukin-18 binding protein: a novel modulator of the Th1 cytokine response. *Immunity* 10: 127–136
30 Xiang Y, Moss B (1999) IL-18 binding and inhibition of interferon gamma induction by human poxvirus-encoded proteins. *Proc Natl Acad Sci USA* 96: 11537–11542
31 Xiang Y, Moss B (1999) IL-18 binding and inhibition of interferon γ induction by human poxvirus-encoded proteins. *Proc Natl Acad Sci USA* 96: 11537–11542
32 Esteban DJ, Buller RML (2004) Identification of residues in an orthopoxvirus interleukin-18 binding protein involved in ligand binding and species specificity. *Virology* 323: 197–207
33 Xiang Y, Moss B (2003) Molluscum contagiosum virus interleukin-18 (IL-18) binding protein is secreted as a full-length form that binds cell surface glycosaminoglycans through the C-terminal tail and a furin-cleaved form with only the IL-18 binding domain. *J Virol* 77: 2623–2630
34 Esteban DJ, Nuara AA, Buller RML (2004) Interleukin-18 and glycosaminoglycan binding by a protein encoded by variola virus. *J Gen Virol* 85: 1291–1299
35 Symons JA, Adams E, Tscharke DC, Reading PC, Waldmann H, Smith GL

(2002) The vaccinia virus C12L protein inhibits mouse IL-18 and promotes virus virulence in the murine intranasal model. *J Gen Virol* 83: 2833–2844

36 Born TL, Morrison LA, Esteban DJ, VandenBos T, Thebeau LG, Chen N, Spriggs MK, Sims JE, Buller RM (2000) A poxvirus protein that binds to and inactivates IL-18, and inhibits NK cell response. *J Immunol* 164: 3246–3254

37 Reading PG, Smith GL (2003) Vaccinia virus interleukin-18 binding protein promotes virulence by reducing gamma interferon production and natural killer and T-cell activity. *J Virol* 77: 9960–9968

38 Smith CA, Farrah T, Goodwin RG (1994) The TNF receptor superfamily of cellular and viral proteins: Activation, costimulation and death. *Cell* 76: 959–962

39 Locksley RM, Killeen N, Lenardo MJ (2001) The TNF and TNF receptor superfamilies: integrating mammalian biology. *Cell* 104: 487–501

40 Cunnion KM (1999) Tumor necrosis factor receptors encoded by poxviruses. *Mol Genet Metab* 67: 278–282

41 Brunetti CR, Paulose-Murphy M, Singh R, Qin J, Barrett JW, Tardivel A, Schneider P, Essani K, McFadden G (2003) A secreted high-affinity inhibitor of human TNF from Tanapox virus. *Proc Natl Acad Sci USA* 100: 4831–4836

42 Schreiber M, McFadden G (1994) The myxoma virus TNF-receptor homologue (T2) inhibits TNF α in a species-specific fashion. *Virology* 204: 692–705

43 Schreiber M, Rajarathnam K, McFadden G (1996) Mxyoma virus T2 protein, a tumor necrosis factor (TNF) receptor homolog, is secreted as a monomer and dimer that each bind rabbit TNFα, but the dimer is a more potent TNF inhibitor. *J Biol Chem* 271: 13333–13341

44 Upton C, Macen JL, Schreiber M, McFadden G (1991) Myxoma virus expresses a secreted protein with homology to the tumor necrosis factor receptor gene family that contributes to viral virulence. *Virology* 184: 370–382

45 Smith CA, Hu FQ, Smith TD, Richards CL, Smolak P, Goodwin RG, Pickup DJ (1996) Cowpox virus genome encodes a second soluble homologue of cellular TNF receptors, distinct from CrmB, that binds TNF but not LT alpha. *Virology* 223: 132–147

46 Loparev VN, Parsons JM, Knight JC, Panus JF, Ray CA, Buller RM, Pickup DJ, Esposito JJ (1998) A third distinct tumor necrosis factor receptor of orthopoxviruses. *Proc Natl Acad Sci USA* 95: 3786–3791

47 Saraiva M, Alcami A (2001) CrmE, a novel soluble tumor necrosis factor receptor encoded by poxviruses. *J Virol* 75: 226–233

48 Reading PC, Khanna A, Smith GL (2002) Vaccinia virus CrmE encodes a soluble and cell surface tumor necrosis factor receptor that contributes to virus virulence. *Virology* 292: 285–298

49 Alcami A, Khanna A, Paul NL, Smith GL (1999) Vaccinia virus strains Lister, USSR and Evans express soluble and cell-surface tumour necrosis factor receptors. *J Gen Virol* 80: 949–959

50 Essani K, Chalasani S, Eversole R, Beuving L, Birmingham L (1994) Multiple anti-cytokine activities secreted from tanapox virus-infected cells. *Microb Pathog* 17: 347–353

51 Paulose M, Bennett BL, Manning AM, Essani K (1998) Selective inhibition of TNF-alpha induced cell adhesion molecule gene expression by tanapox virus. *Microb Pathog* 25: 33–41

52 Saraiva M, Smith P, Fallon PG, Alcami A (2002) Inhibition of type 1 cytokine-mediated inflammation by a soluble CD30 homologue encoded by ectromelia (mousepox) virus. *J Exp Med* 196: 829–839
53 Murphy PM (2001) Viral exploitation and subversion of the immune system through chemokine mimicry. *Nat Immunol* 2: 116–122
54 Lalani AS, Barrett J, McFadden G (2000) Modulating chemokines: More lessons from viruses. *Immunol Today* 21: 100–106
55 Lalani AS, Graham K, Mossman K, Rajarathnam K, Clark-Lewis I, Kelvin D, McFadden G (1997) The purified myxoma virus IFN-γ receptor homolog, M-T7, interacts with the heparin binding domains of chemokines. *J Virol* 71: 4356–4363
56 Mossman K, Nation P, Macen J, Garbutt M, Lucas A, McFadden G (1996) Myxoma virus M-T7, a secreted homolog of the interferon-gamma receptor, is a critical virulence factor for the development of myxomatosis in European rabbits. *Virology* 215: 17–30
57 Liu LY, Lalani A, Dai E, Seet B, Macauley C, Singh R, Fan L, McFadden G, Lucas A (2000) The viral anti-inflammatory chemokine-binding protein M-T7 reduces intimal hyperplasia after vascular injury. *J Clin Invest* 105: 1613–1621
58 Boomker JM, Luttikhuizen DT, Veninga H, de Leij LFMH, The TH, de Haan A, van Luyn MJA, Harmsen MC (2005) The modulation of angiogenesis in the foreign body response by poxviral protein M-T7. *Biomaterials* 26: 4874–4881
59 Burns JM, Dairaghi DJ, Schall TJ (2001) Comprehensive mapping of poxvirus vCCI chemokine binding protein: expanded range of ligand interactions and unusual dissociation kinetics. *J Biol Chem* 277: 2785–2789
60 Seet BT, Barrett J, Robichaud J, Shilton B, Singh R, McFadden G (2001) Glycosaminoglycan-binding properties of the myxoma virus CC-chemokine inhibitor, M-T1. *J Biol Chem* 276: 30504–30513
61 Lalani AS, Masters J, Graham K, Liu L, Lucas A, McFadden G (1999) Role of the myxoma virus soluble CC-chemokine inhibitor glycoprotein, M-T1, during myxoma virus pathogenesis. *Virology* 256: 233–245
62 Lucas A, McFadden G (2004) Secreted immunomodulatory viral proteins as novel biotherapeutics. *J Immunol* 173: 4765–4774
63 Ishikawa-Mochizuki I, Kitaura M, Baba M, Nakayama T, Izawa D, Imai T, Yamada H, Hieshima K, Suzuki R, Nomiyama H, Yoshie O (1999) Molecular cloning of a novel CC chemokine, interleukin-11 receptor alpha-locus chemokine (ILC), which is located on chromosome 9p13 and a potential homologue of a CC chemokine encoded by molluscum contagiosum virus. *FEBS Lett* 460: 544–548
64 Damon I, Murphy PM, Moss B (1998) Broad spectrum chemokine antagonistic activity of a human poxvirus chemokine homolog. *Proc Natl Acad Sci USA* 95: 6403–6407
65 Luttichau HR, Stine J, Boesen TP, Johnsen AH, Chantry D, Gerstoft J, Schwartz TW (2000) A highly selective CC chemokine receptor (CCR)8 antagonist encoded by the poxvirus molluscum contagiosum. *J Exp Med* 191: 171–180
66 DeBruyne LA, Li K, Bishop DK, Bromberg JS (2000) Gene transfer of virally encoded chemokine antagonists vMIP-II and MC148 prolongs cardiac allograft survival and inhibits donor-specific immunity. *Gene Ther* 7: 575–582

67 Haig DM, McInnes C, Deane D, Reid H, Mercer A (1997) The immune and inflammatory response to orf virus. *Comp Immunol Microbiol Infect Dis* 20: 197–204
68 Deane D, McInnes CJ, Percival A, Wood A, Thomson J, Lear A, Gilray J, Fleming S, Mercer A, Haig D (2000) Orf virus encodes a novel secreted protein inhibitor of granulocyte-macrophage colony-stimulating factor and interleukin-2. *J Virol* 74: 1313–1320
69 Ng A, Tscharke DC, Reading PC, Smith GL (2001) The vaccinia virus A41L protein is a soluble 30 kDa glycoprotein that affects virus virulence. *J Gen Virol* 82: 2095–2105
70 Fickenscher H, Hor S, Kupers H, Knappe A, Wittmann S, Sticht H (2002) The interleukin-10 family of cytokines. *Trends Immunol* 23: 89–96
71 Fleming SB, McCaughan CA, Andrews AE, Nash AD, Mercer AA (1997) A homolog of interleukin-10 is encoded by the poxvirus orf virus. *J Virol* 71: 4857–4861
72 Fleming SB, Haig DM, Nettleton P, Reid HW, McCaughan CA, Wise LM, Mercer A (2000) Sequence and functional analysis of a homolog of interleukin-10 encoded by the parapoxvirus orf virus. *Virus Genes* 21: 85–95
73 Bartlett NW, Dumoutier L, Renauld JC, Kotenko SV, McVey CE, Lee HJ, Smith GL (2004) A new member of the interleukin 10-related cytokine family encoded by a poxvirus. *J Gen Virol* 85: 1401–1412
74 Silverman GA, Bird PH, Carrell RW, Church FC, Coughlin PB, Gettins PGW, Irving JA, Lomas DA, Luke CJ, Moyer RW, Pemberton PA, Remold-O'Donnell E, Salvesen GS, Travis J, Whisstock JC (2001) The serpins are an expanding superfamily of structurally similar but functionally diverse proteins. *J Biol Chem* 276: 33293–33296
75 Macen JL, Upton C, Nation N, McFadden G (1993) SERP-1, a serine proteinase inhibitor encoded by myxoma virus, is a secreted glycoprotein that interferes with inflammation. *Virology* 195: 348–363
76 Nash P, Whitty A, Handwerker J, Macen J, McFadden G (1998) Inhibitory specificity of the anti-inflammatory myxoma virus serpin, SERP-1. *J Biol Chem* 273: 20982–20991
77 Nash P, Lucas A, McFadden G (1997) SERP-1, a poxvirus-encoded serpin, is expressed as a secreted glycoprotein that inhibits the inflammatory response to myxoma virus infection. In: FC Church, DD Cunningham, D Ginsburg, M Hoffman, SR Stone, DM Tollefsen (eds): *Chemistry and Biology of Serpins*. Oxford University Press, New York, 195–205
78 Turner PC, Baquero MT, Yuan S, Thoennes SR, Moyer RW (2000) The cowpox virus serpin SPI-3 complexes with and inhibits urokinase-type and tissue-type plasminogen activators and plasmin. *Virology* 272: 267–280
79 Wang YX, Turner PC, Ness TL, Moon KB, Schoeb TR, Moyer RW (2000) The cowpox virus SPI-3 and myxoma virus SERP1 serpins are not functionally interchangeable despite their similar proteinase inhibition profiles *in vitro*. *Virology* 272: 281–292
80 Barrington R, Zhang M, Fischer M, Carroll MC (2001) The role of complement in inflammation and adaptive immunity. *Immunol Rev* 180: 5–15
81 Isaacs SN, Kotwal GJ, Moss B (1992) Vaccinia virus complement-control pro-

tein prevents antibody-dependent complement-enhanced neutralization of infectivity and contributes to virulence. *Proc Natl Acad Sci USA* 89: 628–632
82 Sahu A, Isaacs SN, Soulika AM, Lambris JD (1998) Interaction of vaccinia virus complement control protein with human complement proteins – factor I-mediated degradation of C3b to Ic3b(1) inactivates the alternative complement pathway. *J Immunol* 160: 5596–5604
83 Rosengard AM, Alonso LC, Korb LC, Baldwin WM, 3rd, Sanfilippo F, Turka LA, Ahearn JM (1999) Functional characterization of soluble and membrane-bound forms of vaccinia virus complement control protein (VCP). *Mol Immunol* 36: 685–697
84 Engelstad M, Howard ST, Smith GL (1992) A constitutively expressed vaccinia gene encodes a 42-kDa glycoprotein related to complement control factors that forms part of the extracellular virus envelope. *Virology* 188: 801–810
85 Miller CG, Shchelkunov SN, Kotwal GJ (1997) The cowpox virus-encoded homolog of the vaccinia virus complement control protein is an inflammation modulatory protein. *Virology* 229: 126–133
86 Rosengard AM, Liu Y, Nie Z, Jimenez R (2002) *Variola virus* immune evasion design: expression of a highly efficient inhibitor of human complement. *Proc Natl Acad Sci USA* 99: 8808–8813
87 Barry M, Bleackley RC (2002) Cytotoxic T lymphocytes: all roads lead to death. *Nat Rev Immunol* 2: 401–409
88 Buller RM, Palumbo GJ (1991) Poxvirus pathogenesis. *Microbiol Rev* 55: 80–122
89 Boshkov LK, Macen JL, McFadden G (1992) Virus-induced loss of class I major histocompatibility antigens from the surface of cells infected with myxoma virus and malignant rabbit fibroma virus. *J Immunol* 148: 881–887
90 Guerin JL, Gelfi J, Boullier S, Delverdier M, Bellanger FA, Bertagnoli S, Drexler I, Sutter G, Messud-Petit F (2002) Myxoma virus leukemia-associated protein is responsible for major histocompatibility complex class I and Fas-CD95 down-regulation and defines scrapins, a new group of surface cellular receptor abductor proteins. *J Virol* 76: 2912–2923
91 Fruh K, Bartee E, Gouveia K, Mansouri M (2002) Immune evasion by a novel family of viral PHD/LAP-finder proteins of gamma-2 herpesviruses and poxviruses. *Virus Res* 88: 55–69
92 Mansouri M, Bartee E, Gouveia K, Nerenberg BTH, Barrett J, Thomas L, Thomas G, McFadden G, Freu K (2003) The PHD/LAP-domain protein M153R of myxoma virus is a ubiquitin ligase that induces the rapid internalization and lysosomal destruction of CD4. *J Virol* 77: 1427–1440
93 Senkevich TG, Moss B (1998) Domain structure, intracellular trafficking, and beta2-microglobulin binding of a major histocompatibility complex class I homolog encoded by molluscum contagiosum virus. *Virology* 250: 397–407
94 Barry M, Lee SF, Boshkov L, McFadden G (1995) Myxoma virus induces extensive CD4 downregulation and dissociation of $p56^{lck}$ in infected rabbit $CD4^+$ T lymphocytes. *J Virol* 69: 5243–5251
95 Spriggs MK (1999) Shared resources between the neural and immune systems: semaphorins join the ranks. *Curr Opin Immunol* 11: 387–391

96 Tamagnone L, Comoglio PM (2000) Signalling by semaphorin receptors: cell guidance and beyond. *Cell Biol* 10: 377–383
97 Spriggs MK (1999) Shared resources between the neural and immune systems: semaphorins join the ranks. *Curr Opin Immunol* 11: 387–391
98 Tamagnone L, Comoglio PM (2000) Signalling by semaphorin receptors: cell guidance and beyond. *Trends Cell Biol* 10: 377–383
99 Comeau MR, Johnson R, DuBose RF, Petersen M, Gearing P, VandenBos T, Park L, Farrah T, Buller RM, Cohen JI et al (1998) A poxvirus-encoded semaphorin induces cytokine production from monocytes and binds to a novel cellular semaphorin receptor, VESPR. *Immunity* 8: 473–482
100 Gardner JD, Tscharke DC, Reading PC, Smith GL (2001) Vaccinia virus semaphorin A39R is a 50–55 kDa secreted glycoprotein that affects the outcome of infection in a murine intradermal model. *J Gen Virol* 82: 2083–2093
101 Walzer T, Galibert L, Comeau MR, De Smedt T (2005) Plexin C1 engagement on mouse dendritic cells by viral semaphorin A39R induces actin cytoskeleton rearrangement and inhibits integrin-mediated adhesion and chemokine-induced migration. *J Immunol* 174: 51–59
102 Walzer T, Galibert L, De Smedt T (2005) Poxvirus semaphorin A39R inhibits phagocytosis by dendritic cells and neutrophils. *Eur J Immunol* 35: 391–398
103 Barry M, Wasilenko ST, Stewart TL, Taylor JM (2004) Apoptosis regulator genes encoded by poxviruses. *Prog Mol Subcell Biol* 36: 19–37
104 Bertin J, Armstrong RC, Ottilie S, Martin DA, Wang Y, Banks S, Wang GH, Senkevich TG, Alnemri ES, Moss B et al (1997) Death effector domain-containing herpesvirus and poxvirus proteins inhibit both Fas- and TNFR1-induced apoptosis. *Proc Natl Acad Sci USA* 94: 1172–1176
105 Hu S, Vincenz C, Buller M, Dixit VM (1997) A novel family of viral death effector domain-containing molecules that inhibit both CD-95- and tumor necrosis factor receptor-1-induced apoptosis. *J Biol Chem* 272: 9621–9624
106 Komiyama T, Ray CA, Pickup DJ, Howard AD, Thornberry NA, Peterson EP, Salvesen G (1994) Inhibition of interleukin-1 beta converting enzyme by the cowpox virus serpin CrmA. An example of cross-class inhibition. *J Biol Chem* 269: 19331–19337
107 Martinez-Pomares L, Stern RJ, Moyer RW (1993) The ps/hr gene (B5R open reading frame homolog) of rabbitpox virus controls pock color, is a component of extracellular enveloped virus, and is secreted into the medium. *J Virol* 67: 5450–5462
108 Zhou Q, Snipas S, Orth K, Muzio M, Dixit VM, Salvesen GS (1997) Target protease specificity of the viral serpin CrmA. Analysis of five caspases. *J Biol Chem* 272: 7797–7800
109 Thompson JP, Turner PC, Ali AN, Crenshaw BC, Moyer RW (1993) The effects of serpin gene mutations on the distinctive pathobiology of cowpox and rabbitpox virus following intranasal inoculation of Balb/c mice. *Virology* 197: 328–338
110 Kettle S, Blake NW, Law KM, Smith GL (1995) Vaccinia virus serpins B13R (SPI-2) and B22R (SPI-1) encode M(r) 38.5 and 40K, intracellular polypeptides that do not affect virus virulence in a murine intranasal model. *Virology* 206: 136–147

111 Kettle S, Alcami A, Khanna A, Ehret R, Jassoy C, Smith GL (1997) Vaccinia virus serpin B13R (SPI-2) inhibits interleukin-1beta- converting enzyme and protects virus-infected cells from TNF- and Fas- mediated apoptosis, but does not prevent IL-1beta-induced fever. *J Gen Virol* 78: 677–685
112 Messud-Petit F, Gelfi J, Delverdier M, Amardeilh M-F, Py R, Sutter G, Bertagnoli S (1998) SERP-2, an inhibitor of the interleukin-1β-converting enzyme, is critical in the pathobiology of myxoma virus. *J Virol* 72: 7830–7839
113 Barry M, Wasilenko ST, Stewart TL, Taylor JM (2004) Apoptosis regulator genes encoded by poxviruses. *Prog Mol Subcell Biol* 36: 19–37
114 Everett H, Barry M, Lee SF, Sun X, Graham K, Stone J, Bleackley RC, McFadden G (2000) M11L: A novel mitochondria-localized protein of myxoma virus that blocks apoptosis in infected leukocytes. *J Exp Med* 191: 1487–1498
115 Everett H, Barry M, Sun X, Lee SF, Frantz C, Berthiaume LG, McFadden G, Bleackley RC (2002) The myxoma poxvirus protein, M11L, prevents apoptosis by direct interaction with the mitochondrial permeability transition pore. *J Exp Med* 196: 1127–1139
116 Wang G, Barrett JW, Nazarian SH, Everett H, Gao X, Bleackley C, Colwill K, Moran MF, McFadden G (2004) Myxoma virus M11L prevents apoptosis through constitutive interaction with Bak. *J Virol* 78: 7097–7111
117 Stewart TL, Wasilenko ST, Barry M (2005) Vaccinia virus F1L protein is a tail-anchored protein that functions at the mitochondria to inhibit apoptosis. *J Virol* 79: 1084–1098
118 Wasilenko ST, Stewart TL, Meyers AF, Barry M (2003) Vaccinia virus encodes a previously uncharacterized mitochondrial-associated inhibitor of apoptosis. *Proc Natl Acad Sci USA* 100: 14345–14350
119 Hnatiuk S, Barry M, Zeng W, Liu L, Lucas A, Percy D, McFadden G (1999) Role of the C-terminal RDEL motif of the myxoma virus M-T4 protein in terms of apoptosis regulation and viral pathogenesis. *Virology* 263: 290–306
120 Sedger L, McFadden G (1996) M-T2: A poxvirus TNF receptor homologue with dual activities. *Immunol Cell Biol* 74: 538–545
121 Schreiber M, McFadden G (1996) Mutational analysis of the ligand binding domain of M-T2 protein, the tumor necrosis factor receptor homologue of myxoma virus. *J Immunol* 157: 4486–4495
122 Schreiber M, Sedger L, McFadden G (1997) Distinct domains of M-T2, the myxoma virus TNF receptor homolog, mediate extracellular TNF binding and intracellular apoptosis inhibition. *J Virol* 71: 2171–2181
123 Johnston JB, Wang G, Barrett JW, Nazarian SH, Colvill K, Moran M, McFadden G (2005) Myxoma virus M-T5 protects infected cells from the stress of cell cycle arrest through its interaction with host cell cullin-1. *J Virol* 79: 10750–10763
124 Gil J, Esteban M (2004) Vaccinia virus recombinants as a model system to analyze interferon-induced pathways. *J Interferon Cytokine Res* 24: 637–646
125 Davies MV, Chang HW, Jacobs BL, Kaufman RJ (1993) The E3L and K3L vaccinia virus gene products stimulate translation through inhibition of the double-stranded RNA-dependent protein kinase by different mechanisms. *J Virol* 67: 1688–1692
126 Davies MV, Elroy-Stein O, Jagus R, Moss B, Kaufman RJ (1992) The vaccinia virus K3L gene product potentiates translation by inhibiting double-stranded-

RNA-activated protein kinase and phosphorylation of the alpha subunit of eukaryotic initiation factor 2. *J Virol* 66: 1943–1950

127 Kibler KV, Shors T, Perkins KB, Zeman CC, Banaszak MP, Biesterfeldt J, Langland JO, Jacobs BL (1997) Double-stranded RNA is a trigger for apoptosis in vaccinia virus- infected cells. *J Virol* 71: 1992–2003

128 Langland JO, Jacobs BL (2002) The role of the PKR-inhibitory genes, E3L and K3L, in determining vaccinia virus host range. *Virology* 299: 133–141

129 Brandt T, Heck MC, Vijaysri S, Jentarra GM, Cameron JM, Jacobs BL (2005) The N-terminal domain of the vaccinia virus E3L-protein is required for neurovirulence, but not induction of a protective immune response. *Virology* 333: 263–270

130 Chang HW, Watson JC, Jacobs BL (1992) The E3L gene of vaccinia virus encodes an inhibitor of the interferon- induced, double-stranded RNA-dependent protein kinase. *Proc Natl Acad Sci USA* 89: 4825–4829

131 Xiang Y, Condit RC, Vijaysri S, Jacobs B, Williams BRG, Silverman RH (2002) Blockade of interferon induction and action by the E3L double-stranded RNA binding proteins of vaccinia virus. *J Virol* 76: 5251–5259

132 Sharp TV, Moonan F, Romashko A, Joshi B, Barber GN, Jagus R (1998) The vaccinia virus E3L gene product interacts with both the regulatory and the substrate binding regions of PKR: implications for PKR autoregulation. *Virology* 250: 302–315

133 Smith EJ, Marie I, Prakash A, Garcia-Sastre A, Levy DE (2001) IRF3 and IRF7 phosphorylation in virus-infected cells does not require double-stranded RNA-dependent protein kinase R or Ikappa B kinase but is blocked by Vaccinia virus E3L protein. *J Biol Chem* 276: 8951–8957

134 Rogan S, Heaphy S (2000) The vaccinia virus E3L protein interacts with SUMO-1 and ribosomal protein L23a in a yeast two hybrid assay. *Virus Genes* 21: 193–195

135 Liu Y, Wolff KC, Jacobs BL, Samuel CE (2001) Vaccinia virus E3L interferon resistance protein inhibits the interferon-induced adenosine deaminase A-to-I editing activity. *Virology* 289: 378–387

136 Dar AC, Sicheri F (2002) X-ray crystal structure and functional analysis of vaccinia virus K3L reveals molecular determinants for PKR subversion and substrate recognition. Mol Cell 10: 295–305.

137 Ramelot TA, Cort JR, Yee AA, Liu F, Goshe MB, Edwards AM, Smith RD, Arrowsmith CH, Dever TE, Kennedy MA (2002) Myxoma virus immunolodulatory protein M156R is a structural mimic of eukaryotic translation initiation factor eIF2α. *J Mol Biol* 322: 943–954

138 Langland JO, Jacobs BL (2004) Inhibition of PKR by vaccinia virus: role of the N- and C-terminal domains of E3L. *Virology* 324: 419–429

139 Najarro P, Traktman P, Lewis JA (2001) Vaccinia virus blocks gamma interferon signal transduction: viral VH1 phosphatase reverses Stat1 activation. *J Virol* 75: 3185–3196

140 Gil J, Rullas J, Alcami J, Esteban M (2001) MC159L protein from the poxvirus molluscum contagiosum virus inhibits NF-kappaB activation and apoptosis induced by PKR. *J Gen Virol* 82: 3027–3034

Poxviruses
ed. by Andrew A. Mercer, Axel Schmidt and Olaf Weber

Immunomodulation by inactivated *Orf virus* (ORFV) – therapeutic potential

Olaf Weber[1], Percy Knolle[2] and Hans-Dieter Volk[3]

[1]Bayer Healthcare AG, Product-related Research, 42096 Wuppertal, Germany; [2]Institute for Molecular Medicine and Experimental Immunology, Universitätsklinikum Bonn, Rheinische Friedrich-Wilhelms-Universität, Sigmund-Freud-Str. 25 53105 Bonn; [3]Institute of Medical Immunology, Humboldt-Universität Berlin, Charité, Campus Mitte, 10098 Berlin, Germany

Abstract

Viruses manipulate the immune system either by bypassing or suppressing the immune reaction or by activation of the immune system.

Orf virus (ORFV) is an epitheliotropic DNA virus that belongs to the parapoxvirus genus of the poxvirus family. ORFV can repeatedly infect its host in spite of a vigorous inflammatory and complex host immune response. The viral genome encodes several immunomodulating genes, including orthologues of IL-10, and mammalian vascular endothelial growth factor (VEGF).

Novel immunomodulating agents that are based on active or inactivated poxviruses might have therapeutic potential in various diseases where the immune system is out of its balance; ORFV-based drugs are already used in veterinary medicine for prophylactic and therapeutic uses.

Inactivated ORFV showed strong effects on cytokine secretion by human immune cells which involved up-regulation of inflammatory and Th1-related cytokines as well as anti-inflammatory and Th2-related cytokines. This combination of suppressive and stimulating mechanisms could be exploited as a novel principle of therapeutic immunomodulation.

Current preclinical data, together with a favourable side effect profile, call for further investigation of ORFV for its potential use as a novel immunomodulatory agent.

Introduction

Immunomodulating agents and substances have been successfully used in medicine for centuries. Until recently, their use has been considered controversial and their mechanisms of action have not been fully understood. A poor understanding of immunology on one side and the complexity of the mode(s) of action(s) of immunomodulating agents on the other side contributed to this situation. However, the understanding of immunology has made significant progress during recent years and the knowledge about signaling pathways in the immune system and their molecular basis supports the rational use of immunomodulating agents today.

The number of immunomodulating agents has increased over the years. The spectrum of drugs is heterogeneous and ranges from traditional mistletoe [1–3] to recombinant cytokines [4, 5] and on to imidazochinolinamines like imiquimod or resiquimod. Well-established drugs are type I and II interferons (IFN). An innovative new strategy is the use of immunostimulatory CpG oligonucleotides.

The use of IFN-α as an immunomodulating agent has set standards in antiviral therapy [6]. However, despite its use as an antiviral and anti-cancer agent, the side effect profile of IFN-α is critical. In addition, viral resistance or escape mechanisms limit the use of IFN-α and responder rates are variable [7, 8].

Recently, CpG oligonucleotides have been introduced as a new experimental immunomodulating therapy [9]. CpG oligonucleotides are currently under investigation as adjuvants for vaccines or as anti-infective and anti-cancer agents. The CpG oligonucleotides are recognized by Toll-like receptor 9 and, possibly, by additional co-receptors. Upon binding, CpG oligonucleotides induce an immune cascade reaction that leads to improved presentation of antigens, and activates secretion of multiple chemokines and cytokines by B lymphocytes, natural killer (NK) cells, dendritic cells (DCs) and macrophages. The use of so-called "naked" DNA, however, is potentially associated with an increased risk of side effects like the induction of auto-DNA antibodies and autoimmune diseases [10]. In addition, repeated administration may lead to a systemic inflammatory syndrome [11]. Other investigators [12] have found liver necroses and ascites in mice that were treated chronically with high doses of CpG oligonucleotides. These findings indicate that the use of CpG oligonucleotides might be regarded as controversial.

Thus, there remains a need for new and safe immunotherapies.

Immunomodulation by parapoxvirus ovis

Viruses manipulate the immune system by bypassing and suppressing an immune reaction or by activation of the immune system [13]. Viral infections may modulate both positively and negatively the clinical course of concomitant infections by other pathogens. Immunodeficiency as a consequence of infection with human immunodeficiency virus (HIV) [14], Epstein-Barr-virus (EBV) [15] or cytomegalovirus (HCMV) [16, 17] is well described. In contrast, other viruses induce stimulatory effects on the immune system. Preclinical studies showed that a variety of viruses like adenoviruses, murine CMV and lymphocytic choriomeningitis virus activated the cellular immune responses in hepatitis B virus (HBV) transgenic mice and that this response had inhibitory effects on HBV replication [18, 19]. Importantly, these effects were accompanied by necro-inflammatory reactions in the liver.

Poxviruses use multiple strategies to manipulate the immune system [20]. *Orf virus* (ORFV) is an epitheliotropic DNA virus that belongs to the parapoxvirus genus of poxvirus family. ORFV causes orf, an acute skin disease of sheep and goats worldwide [21]. The virus is described in greater detail by Fleming and Mercer elsewhere in this volume.

Interestingly, ORFV can repeatedly infect its host in spite of a vigorous inflammatory host immune response [22–24]. Several viral and host factors contribute to the immune escape mechanisms of ORFV [25]. The viral IL-10 ortholog [26] may contribute to this phenomenon. ORFV may also directly interfere with antigen presentation. Induction of local CD95-mediated apoptosis has been described in antigen-presenting monocytes/macrophages [27]. Neutralizing antibodies have not been found for ORFV, although numerous attempts have been made [28–31].

ORFV induces phagocytosis, NK cell activity, release of IFN-α [32, 33], tumor necrosis factor-α (TNF-α), IL-2, and granulocyte-macrophage colony-stimulating factor (GM-CSF) [34, 35]. Several putative immunomodulating genes have been described for ORFV. These include the above-mentioned IL-10 ortholog [26] and viral orthologs of the mammalian vascular endothelial growth factor (VEGF) and of the vaccinia E3L gene that encodes an IFN resistance gene [36–38]. Recently, proteins that bind and inhibit GM-CSF and IL-2 have been described [39]. Most of these immunomodulating proteins are synthesized during viral replication and secreted by the infected cells.

Even before these findings were published, immunomodulation by ORFV had been the object of veterinary research. Mayr et al. studied the immunomodulatory activities of several poxviruses and suggested the use of ORFV as an immunomodulating agent [40, 41].

It is important to note that these authors used whole inactivated virus preparations to investigate immunomodulating activity of ORFV in numerous models *in vitro* and *in vivo*. A summary of functional tests as published by Mayr and Mayr [42] is depicted in Table 1. The data show that poxvirus-based immunomodulating agents might have therapeutic potential in various indications. In addition to the broad range of activity, these authors describe a favorable side effect profile. Table 2 shows a summary of poxvirus-induced cytokines. The picture that appeared in these investigations is heterogeneous, and is even more difficult to interpret because different species, times and conditions were used in these investigations. A summary of ORFV-mediated therapeutic effects in various disease models is provided in Table 3.

The evidence of immunomodulatory activity in various preclinical settings after administration of ORFV led to the development of a ORFV-based drug in veterinary medicine that was based on the ORFV-strain D1701. This drug was introduced as PIND-ORF and, later, sold under the brand name Baypamun®, or, again later, Baypamune® (Bayer Healthcare AG, Animal Health Division, Leverkusen, Germany). Today, Pfizer Ltd.

Table 1. Activity of poxvirus-based immunomodulators in functional assays *in vitro* (from [41])

Test	Method/read out	Result
Activity of granulocytes (flow cytometry)	Phagocytosis and respiratory burst	Increase [42, 43]
NK cell activity mouse, man	^{51}Chromium-release assay	Increase [31, 44]
Thymidine metabolism of hepatocytes	Activity of thymidine kinase, metabolites, regenerative capacity of liver after resection of 2/3 of liver	Increase of activity and regeneration [45, 46]
Tissue culture – virus challenge	Replication of VSV in pre-treated tissue cultures	Significant inhibition [47]

VSV: vesicular stomatitis virus

Table 2. Cytokines induced by poxvirus-based immunomodulators in various test systems (adapted from [41])

Test	Method/read out	Result
Interferon in cells of man, mouse, pig, sheep, horse, cattle	Stimulation of PBMC, ELISA, VSV-PRT with supernatant of stimulated cells	IFN-α and -β detected, active [31, 48, 49 50, 51]
IL-12	RT-PCR	Positive [52]
TNF-α	L929 cytotixicity assay with sera of stimulated rabbits and mice	Positive [33]
IL-2	Proliferation of CTLL2 clones (stimulated leukocytes from swine)	Increase [49]

sells the ORFV-based immunmodulator under the brand name Zylexis® for veterinary use. The drug has been used for prophylaxis, metaphylaxis and therapy of various diseases, including infectious diseases in pet and farm animals.

For example, Baypamune® was used to prevent stress-associated infections. Ziebell et al. [58] demonstrated activity in 4–10-month-old horses that were exposed to stress by weaning, transport and commingling with yearlings from different breeders (crowding). The clinical scores in the ORFV-treated group were significantly reduced by 40.3% ($p<0.05$) compared to the placebo group. The proportion of horses with purulent nasal discharge during the observation period (4 weeks) was also significantly reduced by 58.7% ($p<0.01$) in the Baypamune® group. Of the horses injected with Baypamune®, 50% showed no purulent nasal discharge and therefore no signs of complicated disease of the upper respiratory airways in contrast to

Table 3. Activity of poxvirus-based immunomodulators in disease models (from [41])

Test	Method/read out	Result
VSV, challenge of mice	survival	Positive [44]
Aujeszky virus, challenge of mice	survival	Positive [44]
Pseudomonas aeruginosa-wound infection in mice	survival	[39, 40]
Osteosarcoma model in mice	Take rate of tumors	[44, 53]
1. Cervix carcinoma 2. Osteosarcoma 3. Carcinoma of bladder	Tumor growth, glucose metabolism	Reduction in 1. and 2., no activity in 3. [54]
Irradiation mouse	1. Challenge of immunity 2. Regeneration of leukocytes	1. Restoration of immunosuppression [55] 2. Accelerated regeneration [56]
Stress (transport) in horses	Cortisone	No increase [57]

only 14.8% in the non-protected placebo group. Therapeutic efficacy has been described against bovine herpes virus I [59, 60]. Positive effects have also been observed in cats with chronic stomatitis [61], feline infectious peritonitis [62], in dogs with mammary tumors [63] and in other veterinary indications.

In addition, fundamental research [18, 19, 64, 65] supported the above concept and revived basic and applied research in the area of immunomodulators.

We have recently demonstrated that inactivated ORFV induces an autoregulatory cytokine response that involves the up-regulation of IL-12, IL-18, IFN-γ and other T helper (Th) 1 type cytokines and their subsequent down-regulation which is accompanied by induction of IL-4 [66]. We also found an increase in IL-10 expression in livers of ORFV-treated mice. ORFV protected mice from lethal herpes simplex virus (HSV-1) infection and guinea pigs from recurrent genital herpes disease. With dosages as low as 50000 viral particles, ORFV was more potent than the standard therapeutical 3TC (lamivudine, Glaxo Wellcome) in HBV-transgenic mice. We did not observe any signs of inflammation or any other side effects. In these studies, expression of the IFN-γ-inducing cytokine IL-12 was elevated in mice treated with ORFV to levels that were also observed after control administration of complete Freund's adjuvant (CFA), although CFA induced much less IFN-γ [66]. Moreover, CFA was not able to protect the mice against viral infections. IL-18, a cytokine shown to be a powerful inducer of IFN-γ [67], was induced only in ORFV-treated mice, an observation suggesting a role of IL-18 in the ORFV-mediated biological effects *in vivo*. Since administration of neutralizing antibodies against IFN-γ, but not against IL-12 or IL-18, abolished antiviral activity against HSV and reduced activity against HBV,

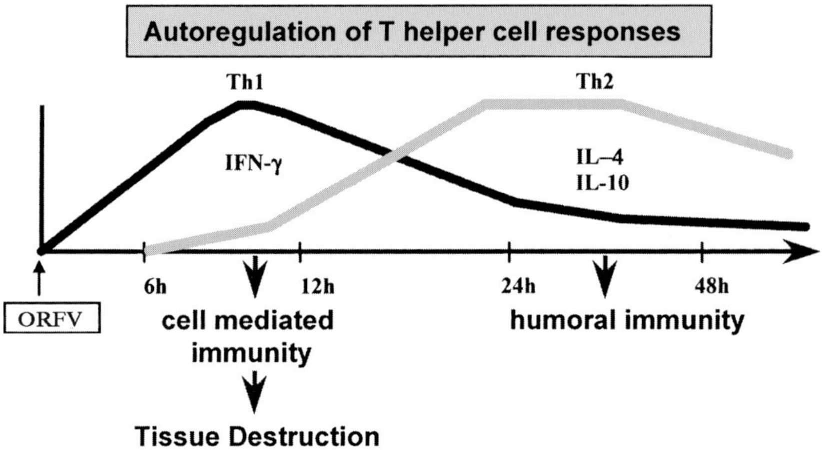

Figure 1. ORFV induces an autoregulatory cytokine response that involves the up-regulation of IFN-γ, IL-12, IL-18, and other Th1-type cytokines and their subsequent down-regulation which is accompanied by induction of IL-4 and IL-10. The Th2 response facilitates a silencing of the tissue-destructive cellular response and leads the organism back into a physiologically balanced situation.

a complementary scenario of IFN-γ induction is likely. Schijns and coworkers [68] demonstrated that following an infection with mouse hepatitis virus, mice with a targeted disruption of the IL-12p40 and/or p35 gene were still capable of producing a polarized Th1-type cytokine response, as evidenced by high IFN-γ and non-detectable IL-4 production. Therefore, IL-12 and IL-18 may complement each other in ORFV-mediated IFN-γ induction. The direct effects of IL-18 remain speculative, although a recent study supported direct antiviral activity of IL-18 in a HBV-transgenic mouse model [69]. In addition to its IFN-γ stimulating activity, IL-18 also has pro-Th2 effects. It has recently been reported that IL-18 enhances IL-4 production by ligand-activated NKT lymphocytes [70]. Therefore, IL-18 could also mediate the IL-4 increase. On the other hand, IL-4 has been demonstrated to down-regulate IL-18 receptor α chain, thereby negatively regulating IL-18 and IL-18-mediated effects [71]. We speculate that the ORFV-mediated IL-4 response might be part of cytokine networking and responsible for the down-modulation of the initial Th1 immune response (Fig. 1).

ORFV also induces IL-12 and IFN-γ in human peripheral blood leukocytes [72]. Inactivated ORFV has demonstrated strong effects on cytokine secretion by human immune cells that involve up-regulation of inflammatory and Th1-related cytokines (IFN-γ, TNF-α, IL-6, IL-8, IL-12, IL-18) as well as anti-inflammatory and Th2-related cytokines (IL-4, IL-10, IL-1ra).

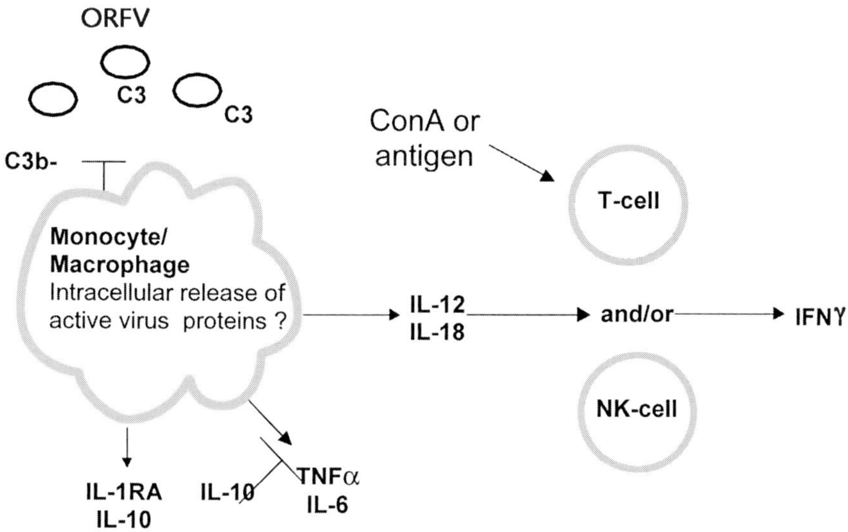

Figure 2. Monocytes/macrophages are the primary targets of inactivated ORFV. The scheme illustrates the mechanism(s) of ORFV-mediated immune modulation. ORFV particles that have been opsonized by complement 3b (C3b) induce secretion of several cytokines by monocytes/macrophages *via* a Toll-like receptor 2/4-independent pathway. Among the different cytokines, IL-12 and IL-18 secretion appears to play the key role in induction of IFN-γ by pre-activated T and NK cells. IFN-γ is essential for the antiviral effects *in vivo*. The induction of anti-inflammatory cytokines like IL-4, IL-10, and IL-1RA should prevent inflammatory side effects.

Experiments that focused on the mechanism of action revealed that the virus particles were the effective component of the preparation. According to our hypothesis, the virus particles might lead to an activation of monocytes *via* signaling over CD14 and a Toll-like receptor, and in addition *via* the intracellular presence of certain ORFV-specific viral components [72]. Activation of monocytes is followed by the release of early pro-inflammatory cytokines (TNF-α, IL-6, IL-8) as well as the Th1-inducing cytokines IL-12 and IL-18. The pro-inflammatory response is accompanied by the induction of anti-inflammatory and Th2 cytokines (IL-4, IL-10, IL-1ra) that exert a limiting effect on the inflammatory response induced by ORFV. A current working model for ORFV mode of action is shown in Figure 2.

Advantages of ORFV over existing cytokine monotherapies

Most of the immunomodulatory proteins of ORFV are synthesized during the replication cycle of the virus and are secreted from infected cells. However, the potential of ORFV to infect humans [21] would limit the use of non-inactivated ORFV as an immunomodulating agent. The therapeutic use of viruses that are not inactivated would bear certain risks and could lead to uncontrollable effects. The following conclusions can be drawn from the current preclinical data:

- Induction of a complex autoregulatory cytokine response.
- A favorable side effect profile after a single administration.
- A favorable side effect profile after repeated administration.
- No loss of activity after repeated administration.

These conclusions support the further investigation of ORFV for its potential use as a novel immunomodulatory agent. The induction of an autoregulatory cytokine response could explain the broad range of activities that has been described in the cited literature. Such a spectrum of activity is superior to that of several cytokines that have been investigated in preclinical models. In addition, the absence of notable side effects in preclinical models is surprising, but may be explained with the autoregulatory cytokine cascade that is induced by ORFV. Such a cascade might activate cells to exert their activity at the site of need but not in the entire organism (i.e., infected cell).

Our findings are encouraging, however, they will need to be confirmed in additional toxicological and clinical studies.

The antiviral activity that has been described for ORFV is consistent with the finding that inflammatory cytokines are capable of abolishing HBV replication and HBV gene expression [18, 19]. However, the application of therapeutic cytokines is limited. The half-life of recombinant IFN-γ is low and the protein would have to have been administered at high dosages which, in turn, would lead to serious side effects. In contrast to single systemic application of recombinant IFN-γ, ORFV appears to also up-regulate other effector cytokines (TNF, etc.) and, in parallel, it induces regulatory cytokines such as IL-4 detectable after 24–48 h in lymph nodes and IL-10 in the liver. This may explain the high efficiency in virus clearing without significant evidence for harmful tissue destruction particularly in transgenic mice. It has been shown that IL-12 administration is therapeutically useful in HBV-transgenic mice [19]. Most of the antiviral activity of IL-12 is mediated *via* IFN-γ induction with the longer *in vivo* half-life of IL-12 explaining its higher efficacy as compared to IFN-γ. Although we have observed a more pronounced Kupffer cell reaction in the livers of ORFV-treated HBV-transgenic mice, no signs of toxicity or inflammation have been observed histologically and liver enzymes were found in a normal range upon and after treatment with ORFV. IL-10, which was induced in the liver after ORFV administration, is known to down-regulate T cell activation by antigen-presenting liver sinusoidal cells [73]. The lack of any inflammation in the livers of ORFV-treated mice might be related to the prolonged induction of IL-10 expression.

We also did not find inflammation in pathological examinations of the HSV-infected guinea pigs. It has recently been described that IFN-γ is responsible for the clearance of viral infection from the central nervous system [74]. Using the guinea pig model of recurrent genital herpes, we could demonstrate three points: (i) the effects of ORFV are not mouse specific, (ii) infections could be targeted even at immune-privileged sites such as the CNS, and (iii) this method is possible without side effects and superior to existing therapies.

ORFV can be administered by different routes, and the antiviral effects are dose dependent. These are features that are needed for a drug candidate.

As pointed out earlier in this chapter, a favorable side effect profile after repeated administration and continuous activity after repeated administration are prerequisites for the therapeutic use of ORFV. We think that the constant efficacy after repeated dosing is due to the low immunogenicity of ORFV and, furthermore, could be supported by some of the unique immune escape mechanisms mediated by ORFV-encoded proteins [25–31].

Putative therapeutic options

Orf virus has a broad spectrum of gene products und functions that modulate the immune system. We conclude that this combination of suppressive and stimulatory mechanisms might not only be an effective viral survival strategy, but could also be used as a novel principle of immunomodulation. Such a therapeutic principle would offer some advantages over existing immunotherapies that primarily focus on either activation or suppression of the immune system.

In human cells, ORFV also induced the cytokine network comparable to that described in mice. It stimulates secretion of TNF-α and IL-12 and, in preactivated T cells, also IFN-γ. Therefore, ORFV might express similar protective effects in humans as in mice.

The existing data suggest that ORFV or related drugs might be effective in treatment of chronic viral infection without significant side effects. The autoregulatory cytokine cascade might also be active against viruses other than HBV or HSV. In addition, ORFV might be useful in other indications such as cancer or immune disorders.

References

1 Koch FE (1938) Experimentelle Untersuchungen über entzündungs- und nekroseerzeugende Wirkung von Viscum album. *Z Ges Exp Med* 103: 740–747

2 Luther P, Mehnert WH, Graffi A, Prokop O (1973) Reaktionen einiger antikörperähnlicher Strukturen aus Insekten (Prolektin) und Pflanzen (Lektine) mit Ascites-Tumorzellen. *Acta Biol Med Ger* 31: K11–K18

3 Kienle GS (1999) The story behind mistletoe: A european remedy from antroposophical medicine. *Altern Ther* 5: 34–37

4 Rosenberg SA, Yang JC, Topalian SL, Schwartzentruber DJ, Weber JS, Parkinson DR, Seipp CA, Einhorn JH, White DE (1994) Treatment of 283 consecutive patients with metastatic melanoma or renal cell cancer using high-dose bolus interleukin-2. *JAMA* 271: 907–913

5 Rosenberg SA (2000) Interleukin-2 and the development of immunotherapy for the treatment of patients with cancer. *Cancer J Sci Am* 6: 2–7

6 Hoofnagle JH, Lau D (1997) New therapies for chronic hepatitis B. *Viral Hepat* 4: 41–50

7 Michielsen P, Brenard R, Reynard H (2002) Treatment of hepatitis C: impact on the virus, quality of life and the natural history. *Acta Gastroenterol Belg* 65: 90–94

8 Indar A, Maxwell-Armstrong CA, Durrant LG, Carmichael J, Schelefield JH (2002) Current concepts in immunotherapy for the treatment of colorectal cancer. *JR Coll Surg Edinb* 47: 458–474

9 Krieg AM, Yi AK, Matson S, Waldschmidt TJ, Bishop GA, Teasdale R, Koretzky GA, Klinman DM et al (1995) CpG motifs in bacterial DNA trigger direct B-cell activation. *Nature* 374: 546–549

10 Pisetsky DS (1997) Immunostimulatory DNA: a clear and present danger? *Nat Med* 8: 829–831

11 Krieg AM (2003) CpG DNA: trigger of sepsis, mediator of protection, or both? *Scand J Infect Dis* 35: 653–659

12 Heikenwalder M, Polymenidou M, Junt T, Sigurdson C, Wagner H, Akira S, Zinkernagel R, Aguzzi A (2004) Lymphoid follicle destruction and immunsuppression after repeated CpG oligonukleotide administration. *Nat Med* 2: 187–192

13 Marrack P, Kappler J (1994) Subversion of immune system by pathogens. *Cell* 76: 323–332

14 Lane HC, Depper JM, Greene WC, Whalen G, Waldmann TA, Fauci AS (1985) Qualitative analysis of immune function in patients with the aquired immunodeficiency syndrome. Evidence for a selective defect in soluble antigen recognition. *N Engl J Med* 313: 79–84

15 Moore KW, Vieira P, Fiorentino DF, Trounstine ML, Khan TA, Mosmann TR (1990) Homology of cytokine synthesis inhibitory factor (IL-10) to the Epstein-Barr virus gene BCRF1. *Science* 248: 1230–1234

16 delVal M, Hengel H, Häcker H, Hartlaub U, Ruppert T, Lucin P, Koszinowski UH (1992) Cytomegalovirus prevents antigen presentation by blocking the transport of peptide-loaded major histocompatibility complex class I molecules into the medial-Golgi compartment. *J Exp Med* 176: 729–738

17 Yamashita Y, Shimokata K, Mizuno S, Yamaguchi H, Nishiyama Y (1993) Down-regulation of the surface expression of class I MHC antigens by human cytomegalovirus. *Virology* 193: 727–736

18 Guidotti LG, Borrow P, Hobbs MV, Matzke B, Gresser I, Oldstone MB, Chisari FV (1996) Viral cross talk: Intracellular inactivation of the hepatitis B virus during an unrelated viral infection of the liver. *Proc Natl Acad Sci USA* 93: 4589–4594

19 Cavanaugh VJ, Guidotti LG, Chisari FV (1998) Inhibition of Hepatitis B virus replication during adenovirus and cytomegalovirus infections in transgenic mice. *J Virol* 72 2630–2637
20 Pickup DJ (1994) Poxviral modifiers of cytokine responses to infection. *Infect Agents Dis* 3: 116–127
21 Haig DM, Mercer AA (1998) Ovine diseases. Orf. *Vet Res* 29: 311–326
22 McKeever DJ, Jenkinson DM, Hutchinson G, Reid HW (1988) Studies on the pathogenesis of orf virus infection in sheep. *Comp Pathol* 99: 317–328
23 Haig D, McInnes C, Deane D, Lear A, Myatt N, Reid H, Rothel J, Seow HF, Wood P, Lyttle D, Mercer A (1996) Cytokines and their inhibitors in orf virus infection. *Vet Immunol Immunopathol* 54: 261–267
24 Haig D, McInnes CJ, Deane D, Reid HW, Mercer AA (1997) The immune and inflammatory reponse to orf virus. *Comp Immunol Microbiol Infect Dis* 20: 197–204
25 Haig DM, McInnes CJ (2002) Immunity and counter-immunity during infection with the parapoxvirus orf virus. *Virus Res* 88: 3–16
26 Fleming SB, McCaughan CA, Andrews AE, Nash AD, Mercer AA (1997) A homolog of interleukin-10 is encoded by the poxvirus orf virus. *J Virol* 71: 4857–4861
27 Kruse N, Weber O (2001) Selective induction of apoptosis in antigen-presenting cells in mice by parapoxvirus ovis. *J Virol* 75: 4699–4704
28 McKeever DJ, Reid HW, Inglis NF, Herring AJ (1987) A qualitative and quantitative assessment of the humoral antibody response of the sheep to orf virus infection. *Vet Microbiol* 15: 229–241
29 Yirrell DL, Reid,HW, Howie S (1989)Immune response of lambs to experimental infection with orf virus. *Vet Immunol Immunopathol* 22: 321–332
30 Chand P, Kitching RP, Black DN (1994) Western blot analysis of virus-specific antibody responses for capripox and contagious pustular dermatitis viral infection in sheep. *Epidemiol Infect* 113: 77–85
31 Sullivan JT, Mercer AA, Fleming SB, Robinson AJ (1994) Identification and characterization of an orf virus homologue of the vaccinia virus gene encoding the major envelope antigen p37K. *Virology* 202: 968–973
32 Buettner M, Czerny CP, Lehner KH, Wertz K (1995) Interferon induction in peripheral blood mononuclear leukocytes of man and farm animals by poxvirus vector candidates and some poxvirus constructs. *Vet Immunol Immunopathol* 46: 237–250
33 Foerster R, Wolf G, Mayr A (1994) Highly attenuated poxviruses induce functional priming of neutrophils *in vitro*. *Arch Virol* 136: 219–226
34 Marsig E, Stickl H (1988) The effectiveness of immune modulatorsfrom microorganisms and of animal pox preparations against tumor cell lines *in vitro*. *Zentralbl Veterinaermed* 36: 81–99
35 Mayr A, Buettner M, Wolf G, Meyer H, Czerny C (1989) Experimental detection of the paraspecific effects of the purified and inactivated poxviruses. *Zentralbl Veterinaermed* 36: 81–99
36 Tzahar E, Moyer JD, Waterman H, Barbacci EG, Bao J, Levkowitz G, Shelly M, Strano S, Pinkas-Kramarski R, Pierce JH et al (1998) Pathogenic poxvi-

ruses reveal viral strategies to exploit the ErB signaling network. *EMBO J* 17: 5948–5963

37 Lyttle DJ, Frazer KM, Fleming SB, Mercer AA, Robinson AJ (1994) Homologs of vascular endothelial growth factor are encoded by the poxvirus orf virus. *J Virol* 68: 84–92

38 Haig DM, McInnes CJ, Thomson J, Wood A, Bunyan K, Mercer A (1998) The orf virus OV20.0L gene product is involved in interferon resistance and inhibits an interferon-inducible, double stranded RNA-dependent kinase. *Immunology* 93: 335–340

39 Dean D, McInnes CJ, Percival A, Wood A, Thomson J, Lear A, Gilray J, Fleming S, Mercer A, Haig D (2000) Orf virus encodes a novel secreted protein inhibitor of granulocyte-macrophage colony-stimulating factor and interleukin 2. *J Virol* 74: 1313–1320

40 Mayr A, Raettig H, Alexander M (1979) Paramunität, Paramunisierung, Paramunitätsinducer. Teil 1. Geschichtliche Entwicklung, Begriffsbestimmung und Wesen. *Fortschr Med* 97: 1159–1165

41 Mayr A, Raettig H, Alexander M (1979) Paramunität, Paramunisierung, Paramunitätsinducer. Teil 2.: Paramunitätsinducer, eigene Untersuchungen, Diskussion. *Fortschr Med* 97: 1205–1210

42 Mayr B, Mayr A (1995) Present state of preclinical research on the efficacy and safety of para immunity inducers from poxviruses. A study of the literature. *Tierarztl Prax* 23: 542–552

43 Förster RJ, Wolf G (1990) Phagozytosis of opsonized fluorescent microspheres by polymorphonuclear leukocytes. *J Vet Med B* 37: 481–490

44 Förster R, Wolf G, Mayr A (1994) Highly attenuated poxviruses induce functional priming of neutrophils *in vitro*. *Arch Virol* 136: 219–226

45 Mayr A, Buettner M, Pawlas S, Erfle V, Mayr B, Brunner R, Osterkorn K (1986) Vergleichende Untersuchungen über die immunstimulierende (paramunisierende) Wirksamkeit von BCG, Levamisol, *Corynebakterium parvum*, und Präparaten aus Pockenviren in verschiedenen *in vivo*- und *vitro*-Testen. *J Vet Med B* 33: 321–339

46 Altschuh CP (1985) *Untersuchungen über die Wirksamkeit des Paramunitätsinducers PIND-AVI als Leberschutzsubstanz*. Thesis, München

47 Haig DM, McInnes CJ (1983) *Influence of Immune modulators, liver inducing and protecting substances on thymidine metabolism of resting and regenerating hepatocytes*. Falk Symposium no. 38, Basel

48 Vilsmeier B (1995) *Entwicklung eines Zellkultur-Challenge-Tests zum Nachweis paramunisierender Aktivitäten verschiedener Präparationen aus Pockenviren*. Thesis, München

49 Leder P (1992) *Untersuchungen zur Anregung der Lymphozytenproliferation, Aktivität der natürlichen Killerzellen und Interferon-alpha Induktion in humanen peripheren Blutlymphozyten nach in vitro Stimulierung mit verschiedenen Parapocken-Kulturpassagen*. Thesis, München

50 Steinmassl G, Wolf G (1990) Bildung von Interleukin 2 und Interferon-γ durch mononukleäre Leukozyten des Schweines nach *in vitro*-Stimulation mit verschiedenen Viruspräparaten. *J Vet Med B* 37: 321–331

51 Thein P, Hechler H, Mayr A (1981) Vergleichende Untersuchungen zur

Wirksamkeit des Paramunitätsinducers PIND-AVI, des Mitogens PHA-P und von Rhinopneumonitisvirus auf die peripheren Lymphozyten des Pferdes. *Zentralbl Veterinarmed Med B* 28: 432–449
52 Belke G, Mayr A, Kaaden OR, Buettner M (1995) Induction and detection of mRNA, molecular clloning and sequencing of canine interleukin 12. The 4th International Veterinary Immunological Congress, Davis, CA, USA, July 15–21, 1995.
53 Mueller-Brunecker G, Erfle V, Mayr A (1984) Wirkungsvergleich von Paramunitätsinducern (PIND-AVI, PIND-ORF), Levamisol, BCG und *C. parvum* auf das Wachstum eines strahleninduzierten Osteosarkoms der Maus. *Tierärztl Umschau* 39: 366–368
54 Demel W (1992) Experimentelle Untersuchungen zur Biokinetik von Fluordeoxyglukose an Mäusen mit unterschiedlichen Tumoren. Thesis, München
55 Mayr A, Baljer G, Sailer J, Schels D (1980) Untersuchungen über eine Strahlenschutzwirkung des Paramunitätsinducers PIND-AVI am Modell Tetanusschutzimpfung Maus nach Röntgenbestrahlung. *Strahlentherapie* 156: 795–799
56 Breiter N, Ungemach FR, Beck G, Hegner D, Mayr A (1985) Untersuchungen über die Wirksamkeit der Paramunitätsinducer PIBD-AVI und PIND-ORF als Strahlenschutzsubstanzen. *Strahlentherapie* 161: 168–176
57 Mayr A, Siebert M (1990) Untersuchungen über die Wirksamkeit des Paramunitätsinducers PIND-ORF auf den durch Transportstress ausgelösten Kortisolanstieg beim Pferd. *Tierärztl Umschau* 45: 677–682
58 Ziebell KL, Steinmann H, Kretzdorn D, Schlapp T, Failing K, Schmeer N (1997) The use of Baypamun N in crowding associated infectious respiratory disease: efficacy of Baypamun N (freeze dried product) in 4–10 month old horses. *Zentralbl Veterinarmed B* 44: 529–536
59 Castrucci G, Ferrari M, Osburn BI, Frigeri F, Barreca F, Tagliati S, Cuteri V (1995) The use of a non-specific defence mechanism inducer in calves exposed to bovine herpesvirus-1 infection: preliminary trials. *Comp Immunol Microbiol Infect Dis* 18: 85–91
60 Castrucci G, Osburn BI, Ferrari M, Salvatori D, Lo Dico M, Barreca F (2000) The use of immunomudulators in the control of infectious bovine rhinotracheitis. *Comp Immunol Microbiol Infect Dis* 23: 163–173
61 Mayr B, Deininger S, Büttner M (1991) Treatment of chronic stomatitis of cats by local paramunization with PIND-ORF. *J Vet Med B* 38: 78–80
62 Bölcskeiv A, Bilkei G (1995) Langzeitstudie über die behandelte FIP – verdächtige Katzen. *Tierärztl Umschau* 50: 721–728
63 Berg G, Rüsse M (1994) Der Einsatz von Baypamun HK in der Mammatumorbehandlung der Hündin. *Tierärztl Umschau* 49: 476–480
64 Guidotti LG, Rochford R, Chung J, Shapiro M, Purcell R, Chisari FV (1999) Viral clearance without destruction of infected cells during acute HBV infection. *Science* 284: 825–829
65 Guidotti LG, Ishikawa T, Hobbs MV, Matzke B, Schreiber R, Chisari FV (1996) Intracellular inactivation of the hepatitis B virus by cytotoxic T lymphocytes. *Immunity* 4: 25–36

66 Weber O. Siegling A, Friebe A, Limmer A, Schlapp T, Knolle P, Mercer A, Schaller H, Volk HD (2003) Inactivated parapoxvirus ovis (orf virus) has antiviral activity against hepatitis B virus and herpes simplex virus. *J Gen Virol* 84: 1843–1852

67 Micallef MJ, Ohtsuki T, Kohno K, Tanabe F, Ushio S, Namba M, Tanimoto T, Torigoe K, Fuji M, Ikeda M, Fukuda S, Kurimoto (1996) Interferon-gamma-inducing factor enhances T-helper-1 cytokine production by interferon-gamma production. *Eur J Immunol* 26: 1647–1651

68 Schijns VECJ, Haagemans BL, Wierda ChMH, Kruithof B, Heijnen IA, Alber G, Horzinek MC (1998) Mice lacking IL-12 develop polarized Th1 cells during viral inection. *J Immunol* 160: 3958–3964

69 Kimura K, Kakimi K, Wieland S, Guidotti LG, Chisari FV (2002) Interleukin-18 inhibits hepatitis B virus replication in the livers of transgenic mice. *J Virol* 76: 10702–10707

70 Leite-de-Moraes MC, Hameg A, Pacilio M, Koezuka Y, Taniguchi M, Van Kaer L, Schneider E, Dy M, Herbelin A (2000) IL-18 enhances IL-4 production by ligand-activated NKT lymphocytes: a pro-Th2 effect of IL-18 exerted through NKT cells. *J Immunol* 166: 945–951

71 Smeltz RB, Chen J, Hu-Li J, Shevach EM (2001) Regulation of interleukin (IL)-18 receptor a chain expression on $CD4^+$ T cells during T helper (Th)1/Th2 differentiation: critical downregulatory role of IL-4. *J Exp Med* 194: 143–153

72 Friebe A, Siegling A, Friederichs S, Volk H-D, Weber O (2004) Immunomodulatory effects of inactivated parapoxvirus ovis (Orf-virus) on human peripheral immune cells – induction of cytokine secretion in monocytes and TH-1 like cells. *J Virol* 78: 9400–9411

73 Knolle PA, Uhrig A, Hegenbarth S, Loser E, Schmitt E, Gerken G, Lohse AW (1998) IL-10 down-regulates T cell activation by antigen-presenting liver sinusoidal endothelial cells through decreased antigen uptake via the mannose receptor and lowered surface expression of accessory molecules. *Clin Exp Immunol* 114: 427–433

74 Binder GK, Griffin DE (2001) Interferon-γ-mediated site-specific clearance of alphavirus from CNS neurons. *Science* 293: 303–306

Poxviruses
ed. by Andrew A. Mercer, Axel Schmidt and Olaf Weber

Recombinant poxvirus vaccines in biomedical research

Barbara S. Schnierle, Yasemin Suezer and Gerd Sutter

Paul-Ehrlich-Institut, Department of Virology, Paul-Ehrlich-Straße 51-59, 63225 Langen, Germany

Abstract

In biomedical research recombinant poxviruses are investigated as important candidate medicines to derive advanced options for prevention and/or treatment of infectious diseases or cancer. Genetically engineered viruses can readily synthesize biologically active heterologous proteins, serve to determine relevant targets of cell-mediated and humoral immunity, and identify types of immune responses needed for protection against a multitude of different specific diseases. Substantial progress in vaccine development is based on the availability of exceptionally safe but efficient carrier viruses, on increasingly versatile vector technologies and on the feasibility of large scale manufacturing. Moreover, advances in deciphering the molecular pathways regulating poxvirus-host interactions will provide additional means to potently activate innate immune stimulation upon vaccination and to derive vectors with specifically targeted replicative capacity for experimental tumor therapy.

Introduction

Poxviruses engineered to express foreign genes have been established as extremely valuable tools in modern biotechnology and for vaccine development in medical and veterinary research (for review see [1]). Compared to currently marketed vaccines, viral vectors appear still as futuristic option in vaccine development. Yet, many of today's health problems where vaccines are believed to become key medicines are likely not to be solved with existing technologies. Adequate biological and clinical safety, large packaging capacity for recombinant DNA, precise virus-specific control of target gene expression, high-level immunogenicity, lack of persistence or genomic integration in the host, and ease of vector and vaccine production are important features supporting the use of recombinant poxviruses as advanced tools for immunization. While making a multivalent poxvirus vector vaccine has been proposed as a particularly desirable medicinal product [2], recombinant poxviruses are primarily investigated as novel vaccines against major human and animal diseases that still lack effective intervention strategies. A major achievement has been the application of vector viruses providing extraordinary levels of safety with regard to protection of the non-target environment and use in possibly immunocompromised target populations [3, 4] (for review see [5, 6]). The substantial recent progress in conducting clinical research with candidate vaccines against AIDS, tuberculosis, malaria or tumor diseases may serve as an example. Poxviruses engineered as vector vaccines include viruses from multiple genera with the *Orthopoxvirus Vaccinia virus* (VACV) [7, 8] and *Avipoxvirus*es [9, 10] being the first and most frequently developed for applications in human and veterinary medicine. Other promising candidate vaccines against animal diseases are derived from *Parapox*- [11, 12], *Suipox*- [13], *Capripox*- [14], or *Leporipoxvirus*es [15, 16]. In this review, we attempt to provide an update on the state-of-the-art in poxvirus vector technologies and to sum up the recent progress in the development of prophylactic and therapeutic recombinant vaccines.

Generation of recombinant poxviruses

Poxviruses replicate within the cytoplasm of the infected cell and therefore their genome is not transcribed by cellular enzymes. The virus encodes its own transcription and replication machinery and its DNA is not infectious. The currently most frequently practiced strategy to generate recombinant poxviruses employs homologous DNA recombination in infected cells, a relatively frequent event during poxviral replication (0.1%). Recombination is typically directed by a plasmid-based transfer vector, containing the following features: an expression cassette, including a poxvirus-specific promoter, usually followed by a multiple cloning site to allow the insertion of the foreign gene of choice. In addition, selection or screening procedures are quite useful to ease the clonal isolation of recombinant viruses by plaque purification, which requires the additional insertion of selection marker gene expression cassettes. These heterologous DNA sequences are flanked by poxvirus DNA sequences that direct the recombination to a desired locus in a non-essential region of the poxviral genome (Fig. 1). A large variety of different natural and synthetic virus-specific promoters that are transcribed at early, intermediate or late times of VACV infection are available (for review see [17]). For vector construction tandem early and late promoters are commonly used to allow for moderate to strong target gene expression during the whole virus life cycle [18–20].

The standard insertion locus for generating recombinant VACV is the thymidine kinase (TK) locus, which allows the selection of recombinant virus by its TK-negative phenotype due to the insertional inactivation of TK in TK-deficient cells [18]. Recently, an improved dominant negative selection procedure has been developed. A recombinant VACV with an inserted *E. coli* TK/thymidylate kinase (tk/tmk) fusion gene, which converts 3'-azido-

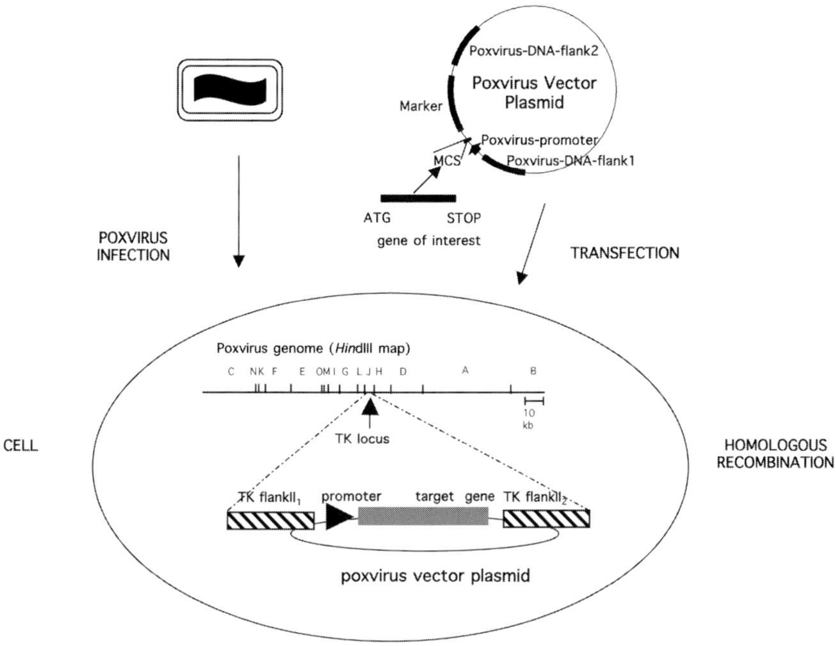

Figure 1. Generation of recombinant poxviruses by homologous recombination. Upper panel: A virus particle is shown on the left; on the right a schematic representation of a poxvirus vector plasmid is depicted. Viral DNA sequences adjacent to the genomic insertion site (flank1, flank2) are cloned in the plasmid and target genes are inserted between these sequences and placed under transcriptional control of poxvirus-specific promoters. Recombinant viruses are generated by infection and simultaneous transfection of cells with vector plasmid DNA, resulting in recombination between homologous DNA sequences of plasmid and virus. Lower panel: Poxvirus-infected, transfected cell. Schematic map of the viral genome and a plasmid designed for insertion of foreign DNA at the locus of the thymidine kinase (TK) gene. Sites of the restriction endonuclease *Hind*III within the virus genome are indicated at the top. The position of the TK gene is marked by an arrow. Virus DNA sequences adjacent to TK insertion locus (TK flank1, TK flank2) are contained in the plasmid.

2',3'-dideoxythymidine (AZT) into a toxic compound, has been used to construct recombinants. Inactivation of the tk/tmk gene by insertion of the transfer vector conveniently allows selection by AZT without the requirements of using TK-deficient cells [21].

Alternatively, the transfer vector contains an antibiotic selection marker or a reporter gene allowing the screening due to a change in phenotype such as co-expression of the *E. coli* β-galactosidase [22] and β-glucuronidase [23]. Among the co-expressed antibiotics, the *E. coli* gpt gene encoding the enzyme xanthine guanine phosphoribosyl transferase is frequently used for purification of recombinant viruses by dominant positive selection for resistance against mycophenolic acid [24].

Staining procedures require additional time of tissue culture, supplementation of agar overlays, and the use of chromogenic substrates and antibiotics. Complementation of a defect in virus production is a faster and more convenient method to obtain recombinant viruses. A first growth selection protocol was initiated using the VACV host range gene K1L to rescue mutant VACV replication in rabbit kidney RK-13 cells [25]. Blasco and colleagues [26, 27] introduced selection for plaque formation through co-insertion of the F13L gene. A VACV mutant and an appropriate complementing cell line enabled growth selection based on the essential D4R gene function [28]. Transient introduction of the K1L gene into the genome of severely growth-restricted modified VACV Ankara (MVA) is used for simple and efficient selection of recombinant MVA, because co-expression of K1L can also complement the defective MVA life cycle in RK-13 cells [29–31].

The large size and the covalently closed hairpin ends of the dsDNA poxvirus genome have been major hurdles for direct *in vitro* cloning of recombinant viruses. In addition, since poxviral DNA is not infectious, isolated poxvirus genomes require a helper poxvirus supplying essential enzymes that are needed to initiate transcription and replication of the recombinant virus. This helper virus should not recombine with the vector virus and not produce infectious progeny in the cells used for the generation of recombinant virus. Avian poxviruses or leporipoxviruses fulfill this requirement for reactivation of recombinant VACV [32, 33]. In one such approach, a unique restriction site was introduced into the VACV genome and the genome was cloned in two halves in lambda phages. Religation of the two halves together with the recombinant gene between them and direct transfection into helper virus-infected cells allowed the generation of recombinant poxviruses without cloning an intermediate DNA construct in *E. coli* [32, 34, 35]. Moreover, the efficient generation and reactivation of recombinant VACV from cells transfected with cloned DNA also enabled the construction of cDNA libraries [36].

Another elegant method to engineer poxvirus vectors has been pioneered recently [37]. The entire VACV genome was cloned into a bacterial artificial chromosome (BAC), which can be engineered in *E. coli* by homologous recombination with bacteriophage lambda-derived enzymes. The modified BAC clones can be used to produce pure recombinant poxvirus in mammalian cells with the initial assistance of a helper virus, but without further requirements for plaque purification.

Prophylactic recombinant poxvirus vaccines

Animal models for major viral diseases, such as influenza, hepatitis B, or rabies, have served to provide first strong proof-of-principle for protective

Table 1. Examples for infectious diseases in humans being targets of candidate poxvirus vector vaccines in recent clinical or preclinical research

Disease	Agent	Target antigens	Vector	Proposed use
AIDS	HIV-1, -2	Gag, Env, Nef, Tat, Rev	MVA, NYVAC, CPV, FPV	Prophylaxis / therapy
Hepatitis C	HCV	C, E1, E2, NS2, NS3, NS4, NS5	CPV, MVA	Prophylaxis / therapy
Cytomegalovirus infection	CMV	UL55, UL83, UL123	MVA	Prophylaxis / therapy
Tuberculosis	Mycobacteria	85A, Apa	MVA, FPV	Prophylaxis
Malaria	*P. falciparum*	TRAP, LSA-1, CS etc.	MVA, FPV, CPV, NYVAC	Prophylaxis
Leishmaniasis	*L. infantum*	LACK	VACV, MVA	Prophylaxis
Cervical carcinoma	HPV-16, 18	E2, E6, E7,L1	MVA	Prophylaxis / therapy

prophylactic vaccination with recombinant poxvirus vaccines [7, 8, 38, 39]. To prevent these diseases in humans, reasonably good and safe vaccines have been available, which has certainly contributed to a delay in the pharmaceutical development of poxvirus vectors for medical applications. In contrast, multiple poxvirus vector vaccines are already in use in veterinary medicine. Licensed products in Europe include vaccines based on recombinant VACV and recombinant *Canarypox virus* for prevention of rabies, equine influenza, and feline leukemia. Moreover, there is a steadily increasing interest to derive and test new vector vaccines, making veterinary medicine an important driving force in the development of advanced medicinal products [40–46]. In medical research and development, most ongoing efforts focus on the study of candidate vector vaccines against human diseases that are more "difficult" to prevent, e.g. those caused by newly emerging or chronic virus infections, or by bacterial infections, parasites or cancer (for overview see Tab. 1).

A safe and effective human immunodeficiency virus (HIV) vaccine is urgently needed to control the worldwide HIV epidemic. However, the development of a vaccine against AIDS represents a substantial scientific challenge related to HIV antigenic variability, the lacking understanding of immune correlates for protection, limitations of available animal models, and the enormous constraints associated with the probable need for multiple large-scale clinical trials in different parts of the world (for review see [47]). Moreover, the fragile immune system of HIV-infected individuals sets high standards for candidate vaccine safety. Recently, highly attenuated poxviruses have continued to play a major role in the international search for an AIDS vaccine, which also takes advantage of established technologies for vector vaccine production at an industrial scale. For example, safety-tested VACV strains MVA and NYVAC, and avirulent avipoxviruses are characterized by severe growth deficiencies in human cells; however, they can efficiently express recombinant genes and represent attractive candidate immunodeficiency virus-specific vaccines [48–50] (for review see [6, 51–55]). The data from clinical research with poxvirus recombinant vaccines so far demonstrate induction of humoral and cellular HIV antigen-specific immune responses in humans. In many preclinical experiments, varying degree of protection against homologous immunodeficiency virus infection has been found, predominantly depending on the challenge virus/animal model used for evaluation. However, HIV has an extraordinary genetic diversity and the "Holy Grail" AIDS vaccine would have to cross-protect against different HIV clades. A major scientific challenge is now to find appropriate antigens or epitopes that elicit a cross-protective immune response. For some time, induction of cellular immunity was the primary focus of HIV vaccine development but the generation of broadly neutralizing antibodies is also believed to be indispensable [56]. Concurrently, data from two studies in the macaque model showed that booster vaccinations with oligomeric or native Env proteins enhance Env-binding and virus-neutralizing antibody responses primed by recombinant MVA vaccines, and suggest that such antibodies are indeed likely to play a role in vaccine-induced protection [57, 58].

Hepatitis C is another global health problem caused by a chronic virus infection that still lacks a preventive vaccine, and substantial efforts are currently dedicated to preclinical research in animal model systems [59]. The immunogenicity of the first poxvirus vector vaccines based on recombinant *Canarypox virus* and recombinant MVA have been tested in HLA-transgenic mouse models [60, 61].

The threatening episode of suddenly emerging coronavirus infections in humans causing severe acute respiratory syndromes impressively demonstrated the suitability of recombinant poxvirus vaccines to quickly evaluate candidate vaccines against a previously unknown pathogen [62, 63]. Thus, in view of the current struggle to tune-up well established but rather too simple vaccine technologies for preparation against the global threat of an influenza pandemic, it is tempting to look into the possible usefulness of poxvirus vectors for development of more potent third generation influenza virus-specific vaccines.

In addition, recombinant poxviruses have proven to be excellent aspirants for vaccine development against other disastrous infectious diseases with global impact such as tuberculosis and malaria (for reviews see [64, 65]). The incidence of disease caused by *Mycobacterium tuberculosis* is steadily increasing often on the basis of poverty-impaired health services, widespread HIV infection, or the emergence of resistant *M. tuberculosis*. In recent efforts to elicit more potent anti-mycobacterial immunity, MVA vector viruses served to identify new promising target antigens and resulted in the development of the first subunit vaccines entering clinical testing

[66–68]. Similarly, an effective vaccine against malaria is urgently required and a variety of antigens from *Plasmodium falciparum* has been expressed and tested with recombinant VACV or avipoxviruses. First clinical trials have been initiated using recombinant MVA and fowlpox virus vectors and suggest the usefulness of prime-boost protocols for eliciting enhanced malaria-specific T cell immunity [69, 70].

Therapeutic application of recombinant poxviruses

In HIV-infected patients therapeutic immunization is considered as a possible means to achieve viral containment without maintenance of antiretroviral treatment. First data from clinical evaluation of recombinant canarypox virus and recombinant MVA vaccines are encouraging, with efficient expansion of vaccine-stimulated HIV antigen-specific $CD8^+$ and/or $CD4^+$ T cell responses and first evidence of improved virus control [71–74].

The identification of tumor-associated antigens (TAA), which are displayed by MHC molecules and recognized by specific T cells, showed that vaccination might serve as an effective therapy for a number of malignancies. The particular potential to activate robust cellular MHC class I- and II-restricted $CD8^+$ and $CD4^+$ T cell responses against recombinant antigens make poxvirus vectors attractive as vaccines for immunotherapeutic approaches against cancer. For experimental cancer therapy, virus antigen-associated malignancies seem to be predestined targets for vaccines because these TAA consist of non-self antigens and do not require breaking of immunotolerance. Taylor and co-workers [75] demonstrated the immunogenicity of an Epstein-Barr virus (EBV)-associated nasopharyngeal carcinoma vaccine by reactivating EBV-specific $CD8^+$ and $CD4^+$ memory T cells *in vitro*. There is evidence for the therapeutic efficacy of poxvirus vaccines delivering human papillomavirus (HPV) E2, E6 or E7 antigens against cervical cancer associated with HPV infection in Phase I/II clinical trials [76–80].

Several poxvirus vaccine candidates directed against auto-TAA are also in preclinical and clinical development, using carcinoembryonic antigen (CEA) [81, 82] and prostate-specific antigen (PSA) [83], and a number of melanoma-associated antigens [84, 85], like gp100, tyrosinase or Melan-A are the furthest developed vaccination strategies and are summarized by Kwak et al. in [86]. Often these strategies are combined with either cytokines like IL-2 [87, 88], costimulatory molecules such as B7-1 [89–91], CTLA-4 blockade [92] or cellular adjuvants like dendritic cells, to enhance immune responses against antigens that are likely tolerogenic self proteins [93, 94].

One approach in experimental cancer therapy is based on oncolytic viruses (OV) that were selected or engineered to replicate, propagate and spread exclusively in tumor cells, leading to their destruction, while not affecting normal cells. This targeting is possible because OV exploit the cellular defects that permit tumor cell growth. To date several types of OV have been developed and have entered clinical trials. These trials demonstrated an acceptable safety profile of OV, but limited therapeutic efficacy when used as monotherapy. However, improved performance was noted when OV were used in combination with traditional therapies (chemotherapy or radiation) (reviewed in [95]).

Replicating VACV is being developed as an oncolytic agent (for review see [96, 97]) because it is able to infect and spread in a large variety of cells and confers an anti-tumor effect by virus-mediated cell death. The first Phase I clinical trial with a VACV recombinant expressing granulocyte-macrophage colony-stimulating factor (GM-CSF) applied intratumorally showed that the vector is well tolerated and efficient to a limited extent in the treatment of cutaneous melanoma [98]. VACV variants have been engineered to improve safety by causing inefficient replication in normal cells but retaining high propagation efficiencies in tumor cells [99]. Deletions of the TK and vaccinia growth factor (VGF) genes were shown to decrease VACV virulence [100, 101]. TK/VGF-negative VACV double mutants are further attenuated and showed an enhanced growth capacity in tumor cells [102]. Preferential replication in tumor cells is attributed to the requirement of TTP for DNA synthesis from the nucleotide pool present in highly dividing cells and the activation of the epidermal growth factor receptor (EGFR) signaling pathway, a frequent abnormality in cancer cells. Another attenuation strategy makes use of the ability of cancer cells to evade the induction of apoptosis. The additional deletion of the viral anti-apoptotic genes SPI-1 and SPI-2 from the VACV genome resulted in a recombinant VACV that preferentially replicated in transformed or p53-negative cells and displayed a significant anti-tumor effect in mouse models [103]. A rabbit poxvirus, *Myxoma virus* (MV), which causes myxomatosis in European rabbits but is nonpathogenic in man, has also been developed as an oncolytic virus candidate. MV encodes proteins that counteract rabbit interferons but are unable to antagonize interferons of other species, including humans. In normal interferon-responsive human cells, MV replication is blocked [104]. However, MV productively infects a variety of human tumor cells, which are non-responsive to interferon [105]. Since the virus does not infect man there is no pre-existing immunity in the human population. This, together with the apparent inherent tropism for human tumor cells suggests the potential for exploiting MV as novel OV platform.

Outlook

Live poxviral vectors are particularly attractive because they mimic natural infections, while allowing for *de novo* synthesis of heterologous vaccine antigens. Hereby, poxviral vector vaccination is expected to elicit appropriate "danger" signals to the immune system resulting in a preferential recognition and presentation of target antigens. Concerns about the safety of poxviruses, including VACV as the former vaccine successfully used to eradicate human smallpox, have been addressed by the application of viruses that are replication defective and avirulent when tested *in vivo*. To date multiple types of poxvirus vectors have been developed and have entered clinical trials, particularly in the areas of HIV/AIDS or cancer vaccine development. Many results suggest satisfying safety and efficacy of poxvirus vector vaccines with regard to eliciting specific immune responses to selected target antigens in humans. Nevertheless, the complexity involved in inducing protective immunity against infections with immunodeficiency viruses or in eliciting potent immune responses against tumour-associated self-antigens suggests that the immunogenicity of candidate vaccines may still need a booster to achieve protective vaccination against AIDS, malaria or cancer. Hereby, exciting recent results from basic poxvirus research help to reveal an astonishing versatility of poxviral strategies to counteract the innate host immune response and will lead to the generation of optimized vectors and even better poxvirus vaccines [106–108].

Acknowledgements

This work was supported by the European Commission (grants LSHB-CT-2005-018700, LSHB-CT-2005-018680).

References

1 Moss B, Carroll MW, Wyatt LS, Bennink JR, Hirsch VM, Goldstein S, Elkins WR, Fuerst TR, Lifson JD, Piatak M et al (1996) Host range restricted, non-replicating vaccinia virus vectors as vaccine candidates. *Adv Exp Med Biol* 397: 7–13
2 Paoletti E (1996) Applications of pox virus vectors to vaccination: an update. *Proc Natl Acad Sci USA* 93: 11349–11353
3 Tartaglia J, Perkus ME, Taylor J, Norton EK, Audonnet JC, Cox WI, Davis SW, van der HJ, Meignier B, Riviere M (1992) NYVAC: a highly attenuated strain of vaccinia virus. *Virology* 188: 217–232
4 Sutter G, Moss B (1992) Nonreplicating vaccinia vector efficiently expresses recombinant genes. *Proc Natl Acad Sci USA* 89: 10847–10851
5 Drexler I, Staib C, Sutter G (2004) Modified vaccinia virus Ankara as antigen delivery system: how can we best use its potential? *Curr Opin Biotechnol* 15: 506–512
6 Franchini G, Gurunathan S, Baglyos L, Plotkin S, Tartaglia J (2004) Poxvirus-based vaccine candidates for HIV: two decades of experience with special emphasis on canarypox vectors. *Expert Rev Vaccines* 3: S75–S88
7 Smith GL, Mackett M, Moss B (1983) Infectious vaccinia virus recombinants that express hepatitis B virus surface antigen. *Nature* 302: 490–495

8 Panicali D, Davis SW, Weinberg RL, Paoletti E (1983) Construction of live vaccines by using genetically engineered poxviruses: biological activity of recombinant vaccinia virus expressing influenza virus hemagglutinin. *Proc Natl Acad Sci USA* 80: 5364–5368
9 Boyle DB, Coupar BE (1988) Construction of recombinant fowlpox viruses as vectors for poultry vaccines. *Virus Res* 10: 343–356
10 Taylor J, Paoletti E (1988) Fowlpox virus as a vector in non-avian species. *Vaccine* 6: 466–468
11 Fischer T, Planz O, Stitz L, Rziha HJ (2003) Novel recombinant parapoxvirus vectors induce protective humoral and cellular immunity against lethal herpesvirus challenge infection in mice. *J Virol* 77: 9312–9323
12 Marsland BJ, Tisdall DJ, Heath DD, Mercer AA (2003) Construction of a recombinant orf virus that expresses an *Echinococcus granulosus* vaccine antigen from a novel genomic insertion site. *Arch Virol* 148: 555–562
13 Tripathy DN (1999) Swinepox virus as a vaccine vector for swine pathogens. *Adv Vet Med* 41: 463–480
14 Romero CH, Barrett T, Chamberlain RW, Kitching RP, Fleming M, Black DN (1994) Recombinant capripoxvirus expressing the hemagglutinin protein gene of rinderpest virus: protection of cattle against rinderpest and lumpy skin disease viruses. *Virology* 204: 425–429
15 Kerr PJ, Jackson RJ (1995) Myxoma virus as a vaccine vector for rabbits: antibody levels to influenza virus haemagglutinin presented by a recombinant myxoma virus. *Vaccine* 13: 1722–1726
16 Bertagnoli S, Gelfi J, Le Gall G, Boilletot E, Vautherot JF, Rasschaert D, Laurent S, Petit F, Boucraut-Baralon C, Milon A (1996) Protection against myxomatosis and rabbit viral hemorrhagic disease with recombinant myxoma viruses expressing rabbit hemorrhagic disease virus capsid protein. *J Virol* 70: 5061–5066
17 Moss B (2001) Poxviridae: The viruses and their replication. In: Knipe DM, Howley PM, Griffin DE, Lamb RA, Martin MA, Roizman BE (eds): *Fields Virology*, vol. 2. Lippincott Williams & Wilkins, Philadelphia, 2849–2883
18 Mackett M, Smith GL, Moss B (1984) General method for production and selection of infectious vaccinia virus recombinants expressing foreign genes. *J Virol* 49: 857–864
19 Wyatt LS, Shors ST, Murphy BR, Moss B (1996) Development of a replication-deficient recombinant vaccinia virus vaccine effective against parainfluenza virus 3 infection in an animal model. *Vaccine* 14: 1451–1458
20 Chakrabarti S, Sisler JR, Moss B (1997) Compact, synthetic, vaccinia virus early/late promoter for protein expression. *Biotechniques* 23: 1094–1097
21 Holzer GW, Mayrhofer J, Gritschenberger W, Falkner FG (2005) Dominant negative selection of vaccinia virus using a thymidine kinase/thymidylate kinase fusion gene and the prodrug azidothymidine. *Virology* 337: 235–241
22 Chakrabarti S, Brechling K, Moss B (1985) Vaccinia virus expression vector: coexpression of beta-galactosidase provides visual screening of recombinant virus plaques. *Mol Cell Biol* 5: 3403–3409
23 Carroll MW, Moss B (1995) *E. coli* beta-glucuronidase (GUS) as a marker for recombinant vaccinia viruses. *Biotechniques* 19: 352–354, 356

24 Falkner FG, Moss B (1988) *Escherichia coli* gpt gene provides dominant selection for vaccinia virus open reading frame expression vectors. *J Virol* 62: 1849–1854

25 Perkus ME, Limbach K, Paoletti E (1989) Cloning and expression of foreign genes in vaccinia virus, using a host range selection system. *J Virol* 63: 3829–3836

26 Blasco R, Moss B (1995) Selection of recombinant vaccinia viruses on the basis of plaque formation. *Gene* 158: 157–162

27 Sanchez-Puig JM, Blasco R (2005) Isolation of vaccinia MVA recombinants using the viral F13L gene as the selective marker. *Biotechniques* 39: 665–666, 668, 670

28 Holzer GW, Gritschenberger W, Mayrhofer JA, Wieser V, Dorner F, Falkner FG (1998) Dominant host range selection of vaccinia recombinants by rescue of an essential gene. *Virology* 249: 160–166

29 Sutter G, Ramsey-Ewing A, Rosales R, Moss B (1994) Stable expression of the vaccinia virus K1L gene in rabbit cells complements the host range defect of a vaccinia virus mutant. *J Virol* 68: 4109–4116

30 Staib C, Drexler I, Ohlmann M, Wintersperger S, Erfle V, Sutter G (2000) Transient host range selection for genetic engineering of modified vaccinia virus Ankara. *Biotechniques* 28: 1137–1142

31 Staib C, Lowel M, Erfle V, Sutter G (2003) Improved host range selection for recombinant modified vaccinia virus Ankara. *Biotechniques* 34: 694–696

32 Scheiflinger F, Dorner F, Falkner FG (1992) Construction of chimeric vaccinia viruses by molecular cloning and packaging. *Proc Natl Acad Sci USA* 89: 9977–9981

33 Yao XD, Evans DH (2003) High-frequency genetic recombination and reactivation of orthopoxviruses from DNA fragments transfected into leporipoxvirus-infected cells. *J Virol* 77: 7281–7290

34 Merchlinsky M, Moss B (1992) Introduction of foreign DNA into the vaccinia virus genome by *in vitro* ligation: recombination-independent selectable cloning vectors. *Virology* 190: 522–526

35 Pfleiderer M, Falkner FG, Dorner F (1995) A novel vaccinia virus expression system allowing construction of recombinants without the need for selection markers, plasmids and bacterial hosts. *J Gen Virol* 76: 2957–2962

36 Smith ES, Shi S, Zauderer M (2004) Construction of cDNA libraries in vaccinia virus. *Methods Mol Biol* 269: 65–76

37 Domi A, Moss B (2005) Engineering of a vaccinia virus bacterial artificial chromosome in *Escherichia coli* by bacteriophage lambda-based recombination. *Nat Methods* 2: 95–97

38 Smith GL, Murphy BR, Moss B (1983) Construction and characterization of an infectious vaccinia virus recombinant that expresses the influenza hemagglutinin gene and induces resistance to influenza virus infection in hamsters. *Proc Natl Acad Sci USA* 80: 7155–7159

39 Kieny MP, Lathe R, Drillien R, Spehner D, Skory S, Schmitt D, Wiktor T, Koprowski H, Lecocq JP (1984) Expression of rabies virus glycoprotein from a recombinant vaccinia virus. *Nature* 312: 163–166

40 Perez-Jimenez E, Kochan G, Gherardi MM, Esteban M (2006) MVA-LACK as

a safe and efficient vector for vaccination against leishmaniasis. *Microbes Infect* 8: 810–822

41 Minke JM, Fischer L, Baudu P, Guigal PM, Sindle T, Mumford JA, Audonnet JC (2006) Use of DNA and recombinant canarypox viral (ALVAC) vectors for equine herpes virus vaccination. *Vet Immunol Immunopathol* 111: 47–57

42 Henkel M, Planz O, Fischer T, Stitz L, Rziha HJ (2005) Prevention of virus persistence and protection against immunopathology after Borna disease virus infection of the brain by a novel Orf virus recombinant. *J Virol* 79: 314–325

43 Karaca K, Swayne DE, Grosenbaugh D, Bublot M, Robles A, Spackman E, Nordgren R (2005) Immunogenicity of fowlpox virus expressing the avian influenza virus H5 gene (TROVAC AIV-H5) in cats. *Clin Diagn Lab Immunol* 12: 1340–1342

44 Mencher JS, Smith SR, Powell TD, Stinchcomb DT, Osorio JE, Rocke TE (2004) Protection of black-tailed prairie dogs (*Cynomys ludovicianus*) against plague after voluntary consumption of baits containing recombinant raccoon poxvirus vaccine. *Infect Immun* 72: 5502–5505

45 Breathnach CC, Clark HJ, Clark RC, Olsen CW, Townsend HG, Lunn DP (2006) Immunization with recombinant modified vaccinia Ankara (rMVA) constructs encoding the HA or NP gene protects ponies from equine influenza virus challenge. *Vaccine* 24: 1180–1190

46 Paillot R, Ellis SA, Daly JM, Audonnet JC, Minke JM, Davis-Poynter N, Hannant D, Kydd JH (2006) Characterisation of CTL and IFN-gamma synthesis in ponies following vaccination with a NYVAC-based construct coding for EHV-1 immediate early gene, followed by challenge infection. *Vaccine* 24: 1490–1500

47 Girard MP, Osmanov SK, Kieny MP (2006) A review of vaccine research and development: The human immunodeficiency virus (HIV). *Vaccine* 24: 4062–4081

48 Wyatt LS, Earl PL, Liu JY, Smith JM, Montefiori DC, Robinson HL, Moss B (2004) Multiprotein HIV type 1 clade B DNA and MVA vaccines: construction, expression, and immunogenicity in rodents of the MVA component. *AIDS Res Hum Retroviruses* 20: 645–653

49 De Rose R, Chea S, Dale CJ, Reece J, Fernandez CS, Wilson KM, Thomson S, Ramshaw IA, Coupar BE, Boyle DB et al (2005) Subtype AE HIV-1 DNA and recombinant Fowlpoxvirus vaccines encoding five shared HIV-1 genes: safety and T cell immunogenicity in macaques. *Vaccine* 23: 1949–1956

50 Goonetilleke N, Moore S, Dally L, Winstone N, Cebere I, Mahmoud A, Pinheiro S, Gillespie G, Brown D, Loach V et al (2006) Induction of multifunctional human immunodeficiency virus type 1 (HIV-1)-specific T cells capable of proliferation in healthy subjects by using a prime-boost regimen of DNA- and modified vaccinia virus Ankara-vectored vaccines expressing HIV-1 gag coupled to CD8+ T-cell epitopes. *J Virol* 80: 4717–4728

51 Sutter G, Staib C (2003) Vaccinia vectors as candidate vaccines: the development of modified vaccinia virus Ankara for antigen delivery. *Curr Drug Targets Infect Disord* 3: 263–271

52 Im EJ, Hanke T (2004) MVA as a vector for vaccines against HIV-1. *Expert Rev Vaccines* 3: S89–S97

53 Skinner MA, Laidlaw SM, Eldaghayes I, Kaiser P, Cottingham MG (2005) Fowlpox virus as a recombinant vaccine vector for use in mammals and poultry. *Expert Rev Vaccines* 4: 63–76

54 Gherardi MM, Esteban M (2005) Recombinant poxviruses as mucosal vaccine vectors. *J Gen Virol* 86: 2925–2936

55 Coupar BE, Purcell DF, Thomson SA, Ramshaw IA, Kent SJ, Boyle DB (2006) Fowlpox virus vaccines for HIV and SHIV clinical and pre-clinical trials. *Vaccine* 24: 1378–1388

56 Douek DC, Kwong PD, Nabel GJ (2006) The rational design of an AIDS vaccine. *Cell* 124: 677–681

57 Earl PL, Wyatt LS, Montefiori DC, Bilska M, Woodward R, Markham PD, Malley JD, Vogel TU, Allen TM, Watkins DI et al (2002) Comparison of vaccine strategies using recombinant env-gag-pol MVA with or without an oligomeric Env protein boost in the SHIV rhesus macaque model. *Virology* 294: 270–281

58 Quinnan GV Jr, Yu XF, Lewis MG, Zhang PF, Sutter G, Silvera P, Dong M, Choudhary A, Sarkis PT, Bouma P et al (2005) Protection of rhesus monkeys against infection with minimally pathogenic simian-human immunodeficiency virus: correlations with neutralizing antibodies and cytotoxic T cells. *J Virol* 79: 3358–3369

59 Shepard CW, Finelli L, Alter MJ (2005) Global epidemiology of hepatitis C virus infection. *Lancet Infect Dis* 5: 558–567

60 Abraham JD, Himoudi N, Kien F, Berland JL, Codran A, Bartosch B, Baumert T, Paranhos-Baccala G, Schuster C, Inchauspe G, Kieny MP (2004) Comparative immunogenicity analysis of modified vaccinia Ankara vectors expressing native or modified forms of hepatitis C virus E1 and E2 glycoproteins. *Vaccine* 22: 3917–3928

61 Pancholi P, Perkus M, Tricoche N, Liu Q, Prince AM (2003) DNA immunization with hepatitis C virus (HCV) polycistronic genes or immunization by HCV DNA priming-recombinant canarypox virus boosting induces immune responses and protection from recombinant HCV-vaccinia virus infection in HLA-A2.1-transgenic mice. *J Virol* 77: 382–390

62 Bisht H, Roberts A, Vogel L, Bukreyev A, Collins PL, Murphy BR, Subbarao K, Moss B (2004) Severe acute respiratory syndrome coronavirus spike protein expressed by attenuated vaccinia virus protectively immunizes mice. *Proc Natl Acad Sci USA* 101: 6641–6646

63 Chen Z, Zhang L, Qin C, Ba L, Yi CE, Zhang F, Wei Q, He T, Yu W, Yu J et al (2005) Recombinant modified vaccinia virus Ankara expressing the spike glycoprotein of severe acute respiratory syndrome coronavirus induces protective neutralizing antibodies primarily targeting the receptor binding region. *J Virol* 79: 2678–2688

64 Xing Z, Santosuosso M, McCormick S, Yang TC, Millar J, Hitt M, Wan Y, Bramson J, Vordermeier HM (2005) Recent advances in the development of adenovirus- and poxvirus-vectored tuberculosis vaccines. *Curr Gene Ther* 5: 485–492

65 Moore AC, Hill AV (2004) Progress in DNA-based heterologous prime-boost immunization strategies for malaria. *Immunol Rev* 199: 126–143

66 Kumar P, Amara RR, Challu VK, Chadda VK, Satchidanandam V (2003) The

Apa protein of *Mycobacterium tuberculosis* stimulates gamma interferon-secreting CD4+ and CD8+ T cells from purified protein derivative-positive individuals and affords protection in a guinea pig model. *Infect Immun* 71: 1929–1937

67 Goonetilleke NP, McShane H, Hannan CM, Anderson RJ, Brookes RH, Hill AV (2003) Enhanced immunogenicity and protective efficacy against *Mycobacterium tuberculosis* of bacille Calmette-Guerin vaccine using mucosal administration and boosting with a recombinant modified vaccinia virus Ankara. *J Immunol* 171: 1602–1609

68 McShane H, Pathan AA, Sander CR, Keating SM, Gilbert SC, Huygen K, Fletcher HA, Hill AV (2004) Recombinant modified vaccinia virus Ankara expressing antigen 85A boosts BCG-primed and naturally acquired antimycobacterial immunity in humans. *Nat Med* 10: 1240–1244

69 Webster DP, Dunachie S, Vuola JM, Berthoud T, Keating S, Laidlaw SM, McConkey SJ, Poulton I, Andrews L, Andersen RF et al (2005) Enhanced T cell-mediated protection against malaria in human challenges by using the recombinant poxviruses FP9 and modified vaccinia virus Ankara. *Proc Natl Acad Sci USA* 102: 4836–4841

70 McConkey SJ, Reece WH, Moorthy VS, Webster D, Dunachie S, Butcher G, Vuola JM, Blanchard TJ, Gothard P, Watkins K et al (2003) Enhanced T-cell immunogenicity of plasmid DNA vaccines boosted by recombinant modified vaccinia virus Ankara in humans. *Nat Med* 9: 729–735

71 Dorrell L, Yang H, Ondondo B, Dong T, di Gleria K, Suttill A, Conlon C, Brown D, Williams P, Bowness P et al (2006) Expansion and diversification of virus-specific T cells following immunization of human immunodeficiency virus type 1 (HIV-1)-infected individuals with a recombinant modified vaccinia virus Ankara/HIV-1 gag vaccine. *J Virol* 80: 4705–4716

72 Tubiana R, Carcelain G, Vray M, Gourlain K, Dalban C, Chermak A, Rabian C, Vittecoq D, Simon A, Bouvet E et al (2005) Therapeutic immunization with a human immunodeficiency virus (HIV) type 1-recombinant canarypox vaccine in chronically HIV-infected patients: The Vacciter Study (ANRS 094). *Vaccine* 23: 4292–4301

73 Harrer E, Bauerle M, Ferstl B, Chaplin P, Petzold B, Mateo L, Handley A, Tzatzaris M, Vollmar J, Bergmann S et al (2005) Therapeutic vaccination of HIV-1-infected patients on HAART with a recombinant HIV-1 nef-expressing MVA: safety, immunogenicity and influence on viral load during treatment interruption. *Antivir Ther* 10: 285–300

74 Cosma A, Nagaraj R, Buhler S, Hinkula J, Busch DH, Sutter G, Goebel FD, Erfle V (2003) Therapeutic vaccination with MVA-HIV-1 nef elicits Nef-specific T-helper cell responses in chronically HIV-1 infected individuals. *Vaccine* 22: 21–29

75 Taylor GS, Haigh TA, Gudgeon NH, Phelps RJ, Lee SP, Steven NM, Rickinson AB (2004) Dual stimulation of Epstein-Barr Virus (EBV)-specific CD4+- and CD8+-T-cell responses by a chimeric antigen construct: potential therapeutic vaccine for EBV-positive nasopharyngeal carcinoma. *J Virol* 78: 768–778

76 Garcia-Hernandez E, Gonzalez-Sanchez JL, Andrade-Manzano A, Contreras ML, Padilla S, Guzman CC, Jimenez R, Reyes L, Morosoli G, Verde ML,

Rosales R (2006) Regression of papilloma high-grade lesions (CIN 2 and CIN 3) is stimulated by therapeutic vaccination with MVA E2 recombinant vaccine. *Cancer Gene Ther* 13: 592–597

77 Valdez Graham V, Sutter G, Jose MV, Garcia-Carranca A, Erfle V, Moreno Mendoza N, Merchant H, Rosales R (2000) Human tumor growth is inhibited by a vaccinia virus carrying the E2 gene of bovine papillomavirus. *Cancer* 88: 1650–1662

78 Corona Gutierrez CM, Tinoco A, Navarro T, Contreras ML, Cortes RR, Calzado P, Reyes L, Posternak R, Morosoli G, Verde ML, Rosales R (2004) Therapeutic vaccination with MVA E2 can eliminate precancerous lesions (CIN 1, CIN 2, and CIN 3) associated with infection by oncogenic human papillomavirus. *Hum Gene Ther* 15: 421–431

79 Adams M, Borysiewicz L, Fiander A, Man S, Jasani B, Navabi H, Evans AS, Mason M (2001) Clinical studies of human papilloma vaccines in cervical cancer. *Adv Exp Med Biol* 495: 419–427

80 Kaufmann AM, Stern PL, Rankin EM, Sommer H, Nuessler V, Schneider A, Adams M, Onon TS, Bauknecht T, Wagner U et al (2002) Safety and immunogenicity of TA-HPV, a recombinant vaccinia virus expressing modified human papillomavirus (HPV)-16 and HPV-18 E6 and E7 genes, in women with progressive cervical cancer. *Clin Cancer Res* 8: 3676–3685

81 Hodge JW, Poole DJ, Aarts WM, Gomez YA, Gritz L, Schlom J (2003) Modified vaccinia virus ankara recombinants are as potent as vaccinia recombinants in diversified prime and boost vaccine regimens to elicit therapeutic antitumor responses. *Cancer Res* 63: 7942–7949

82 Marshall JL, Gulley JL, Arlen PM, Beetham PK, Tsang KY, Slack R, Hodge JW, Doren S, Grosenbach DW, Hwang J et al (2005) Phase I study of sequential vaccinations with fowlpox-CEA(6D)-TRICOM alone and sequentially with vaccinia-CEA(6D)-TRICOM, with and without granulocyte-macrophage colony-stimulating factor, in patients with carcinoembryonic antigen-expressing carcinomas. *J Clin Oncol* 23: 720–731

83 Eder JP, Kantoff PW, Roper K, Xu GX, Bubley GJ, Boyden J, Gritz L, Mazzara G, Oh WK, Arlen P et al (2000) A phase I trial of a recombinant vaccinia virus expressing prostate-specific antigen in advanced prostate cancer. *Clin Cancer Res* 6: 1632–1638

84 Smith CL, Dunbar PR, Mirza F, Palmowski MJ, Shepherd D, Gilbert SC, Coulie P, Schneider J, Hoffman E, Hawkins R et al (2005) Recombinant modified vaccinia Ankara primes functionally activated CTL specific for a melanoma tumor antigen epitope in melanoma patients with a high risk of disease recurrence. *Int J Cancer* 113: 259–266

85 van Baren N, Bonnet MC, Dreno B, Khammari A, Dorval T, Piperno-Neumann S, Lienard D, Speiser D, Marchand M, Brichard VG et al (2005) Tumoral and immunologic response after vaccination of melanoma patients with an ALVAC virus encoding MAGE antigens recognized by T cells. *J Clin Oncol* 23: 9008–9021

86 Kwak H, Horig H, Kaufman HL (2003) Poxviruses as vectors for cancer immunotherapy. *Curr Opin Drug Discov Devel* 6: 161–168

87 Liu M, Acres B, Balloul JM, Bizouarne N, Paul S, Slos P, Squiban P (2004)

Gene-based vaccines and immunotherapeutics. *Proc Natl Acad Sci USA* 101 Suppl 2: 14567–14571
88 Doehn C, Jocham D (2000) Technology evaluation: TG-1031, Transgene SA. *Curr Opin Mol Ther* 2: 106–111
89 Palena C, Foon KA, Panicali D, Yafal AG, Chinsangaram J, Hodge JW, Schlom J, Tsang KY (2005) Potential approach to immunotherapy of chronic lymphocytic leukemia (CLL): enhanced immunogenicity of CLL cells via infection with vectors encoding for multiple costimulatory molecules. *Blood* 106: 3515–3523
90 Oertli D, Marti WR, Zajac P, Noppen C, Kocher T, Padovan E, Adamina M, Schumacher R, Harder F, Heberer M, Spagnoli GC (2002) Rapid induction of specific cytotoxic T lymphocytes against melanoma-associated antigens by a recombinant vaccinia virus vector expressing multiple immunodominant epitopes and costimulatory molecules *in vivo*. *Hum Gene Ther* 13: 569–575
91 Hodge JW, Abrams S, Schlom J, Kantor JA (1994) Induction of antitumor immunity by recombinant vaccinia viruses expressing B7-1 or B7-2 costimulatory molecules. *Cancer Res* 54: 5552–5555
92 Espenschied J, Lamont J, Longmate J, Pendas S, Wang Z, Diamond DJ, Ellenhorn JD (2003) CTLA-4 blockade enhances the therapeutic effect of an attenuated poxvirus vaccine targeting p53 in an established murine tumor model. *J Immunol* 170: 3401–3407
93 Drexler I, Antunes E, Schmitz M, Wolfel T, Huber C, Erfle V, Rieber P, Theobald M, Sutter G (1999) Modified vaccinia virus Ankara for delivery of human tyrosinase as melanoma-associated antigen: induction of tyrosinase- and melanoma-specific human leukocyte antigen A*0201-restricted cytotoxic T cells *in vitro* and *in vivo*. *Cancer Res* 59: 4955–4963
94 Di Nicola M, Carlo-Stella C, Mortarini R, Baldassari P, Guidetti A, Gallino GF, Del Vecchio M, Ravagnani F, Magni M, Chaplin P et al (2004) Boosting T cell-mediated immunity to tyrosinase by vaccinia virus-transduced, CD34(+)-derived dendritic cell vaccination: a phase I trial in metastatic melanoma. *Clin Cancer Res* 10: 5381–5390
95 Parato KA, Senger D, Forsyth PA, Bell JC (2005) Recent progress in the battle between oncolytic viruses and tumours. *Nat Rev Cancer* 5: 965–976
96 Thorne SH, Hwang TH, Kirn DH (2005) Vaccinia virus and oncolytic virotherapy of cancer. *Curr Opin Mol Ther* 7: 359–365
97 McFadden G (2005) Poxvirus tropism. *Nat Rev Microbiol* 3: 201–213
98 Mastrangelo MJ, Maguire HC Jr, Eisenlohr LC, Laughlin CE, Monken CE, McCue PA, Kovatich AJ, Lattime EC (1999) Intratumoral recombinant GM-CSF-encoding virus as gene therapy in patients with cutaneous melanoma. *Cancer Gene Ther* 6: 409–422
99 Zeh HJ, Bartlett DL (2002) Development of a replication-selective, oncolytic poxvirus for the treatment of human cancers. *Cancer Gene Ther* 9: 1001–1012
100 Buller RM, Smith GL, Cremer K, Notkins AL, Moss B (1985) Decreased virulence of recombinant vaccinia virus expression vectors is associated with a thymidine kinase-negative phenotype. *Nature* 317: 813–815
101 Buller RM, Chakrabarti S, Cooper JA, Twardzik DR, Moss B (1988) Deletion

of the vaccinia virus growth factor gene reduces virus virulence. *J Virol* 62: 866–874

102 McCart JA, Ward JM, Lee J, Hu Y, Alexander HR, Libutti SK, Moss B, Bartlett DL (2001) Systemic cancer therapy with a tumor-selective vaccinia virus mutant lacking thymidine kinase and vaccinia growth factor genes. *Cancer Res* 61: 8751–8757

103 Guo ZS, Naik A, O'Malley ME, Popovic P, Demarco R, Hu Y, Yin X, Yang S, Zeh HJ, Moss B, Lotze MT, Bartlett DL (2005) The enhanced tumor selectivity of an oncolytic vaccinia lacking the host range and antiapoptosis genes SPI-1 and SPI-2. *Cancer Res* 65: 9991–9998

104 Wang F, Ma Y, Barrett JW, Gao X, Loh J, Barton E, Virgin HW, McFadden G (2004) Disruption of Erk-dependent type I interferon induction breaks the myxoma virus species barrier. *Nat Immunol* 5: 1266–1274

105 Lun X, Yang W, Alain T, Shi ZQ, Muzik H, Barrett JW, McFadden G, Bell J, Hamilton MG, Senger DL, Forsyth PA (2005) Myxoma virus is a novel oncolytic virus with significant antitumor activity against experimental human gliomas. *Cancer Res* 65: 9982–9990

106 Staib C, Kisling S, Erfle V, Sutter G (2005) Inactivation of the viral interleukin 1beta receptor improves $CD8^+$ T-cell memory responses elicited upon immunization with modified vaccinia virus Ankara. *J Gen Virol* 86: 1997–2006

107 Ishii KJ, Coban C, Kato H, Takahashi K, Torii Y, Takeshita F, Ludwig H, Sutter G, Suzuki K, Hemmi H et al (2006) A Toll-like receptor-independent antiviral response induced by double-stranded B-form DNA. *Nat Immunol* 7: 40–48

108 Clark RH, Kenyon JC, Bartlett NW, Tscharke DC, Smith GL (2006) Deletion of gene A41L enhances vaccinia virus immunogenicity and vaccine efficacy. *J Gen Virol* 87: 29–38

Poxviruses
ed. by Andrew A. Mercer, Axel Schmidt and Olaf Weber

Orthopoxvirus vaccines and vaccination

Lauren M. Handley, J. Paige Mackey, R. Mark Buller
and Clifford J. Bellone

Department of Molecular Microbiology and Immunology, Saint Louis University Health Sciences Center, St. Louis, MO 63104, USA

Abstract

Immunization procedures against *Variola virus*, from the historical perspective most often first credited to Edward Jenner in the late 18th century, helped finally to eradicate smallpox from the world. Since its eradication, the study of this disease and its pathology has been given little attention; however, with the emergence of *Monkeypox virus* into the human population and the potential use of smallpox as a bioterrorist weapon, the need for an option to vaccinate the world's population is once again a reality. The vaccines used during the eradication program were live, attenuated *Vaccinia virus* preparations of varying virulence that caused a significant number of adverse reactions in naïve subjects. Currently, immunosuppressed individuals, persons with certain skin diseases, and people with cardiovascular complications are contraindicated against receiving this type of vaccine. A new vaccine is needed. Until now, the only known correlate of immunity to the smallpox vaccine conveying protection has been the development of a scar at the site of vaccination. Characterizing the protective immune response established upon vaccination with Dryvax®, at both the innate and adaptive levels, would greatly enhance our understanding of the human immune response to the vaccine, and thus generate information for the production and evaluation of new and safer third- and fourth-generation vaccines.

History of smallpox vaccination

Early efforts at control

Variolation

Variolation describes the practice of inoculation of material from smallpox pustules into the mucosal or cornified epithelium. It was, for example, described in the Chinese literature in the 10th century [1]. Using a variety of recipes, the practitioner inactivated virus in scab material, ground the scab into a powder, and administered it by intranasal insufflation. During the 17th century, alternative variolation techniques were developed in India

[2]. This involved puncturing the cornified epithelium with a needle dipped in pus. From Asia and Africa, the practice spread to Europe and the New World. In the early 1700s, the Royal Society of London investigated both variolation techniques, and, by the late 1700s, the practice of variolation of the cornified epithelium was widespread in Great Britain. Variolation faced opposition as fatal cases occurred [1]. In addition, persons having undergone variolation were infectious and capable of transmitting "natural" smallpox to uninoculated, susceptible contacts. These two drawbacks gave the impetus for a further innovation, the substitution of *Variola virus* (VARV) with *Cowpox virus* (CPXV) and the discovery of vaccination.

Vaccination

The genesis of vaccination came in part from the observation that persons previously infected with cowpox virus as an occupational hazard, particularly milkmaids, were resistant to smallpox. Although others had reportedly claimed that individuals inoculated with CPXV were protected from smallpox, Edward Jenner is the first person documented to have inoculated an individual, James Phipps, with CPXV, challenge him with VARV, and publish the results [3]. Because cowpox produced a much less severe disease than did variolation, and because it did not result in transmission of natural smallpox to susceptible contacts, it gained rapid and widespread acceptance in Europe. Because the cow is an incidental host for CPXV, and the disease was sporadic in parts of Britain and Europe, Jenner and others used virus from lesions on horses suffering from a disease called "grease" as an alternative source of "vaccine" [4]. Grease was an inflammation of the fetlocks caused by a variety of agents, including horsepox. The use of horsepox virus instead of CPXV as vaccine was likely a widespread practice. None of the smallpox vaccines that have survived into the modern era, and were used by various countries during the smallpox eradication program, are composed of CPXV. Instead the smallpox "vaccine virus", known as *Vaccinia virus* (VACV), was shown to be biologically distinct from CPXV [5].

Vaccination as a principle to control disease (1900-1958)

Key components of what would become the smallpox eradication program were implemented during the first half of the 20th century [1]. Vaccine production was centralized within countries, quality control standards were implemented to assure uniform potency, and freeze-dried vaccine was developed. Vaccination techniques were refined for delivery of virus into the superficial layers of the skin *via* a single linear incision or scratch, or deeper through the use of a syringe and needle. Industrialized countries developed public health infrastructures that facilitated compulsory vaccination programs, and enabled the use of isolation and national and global quarantine practices to limit disease spread. International cooperation in the control of disease was initiated through the Health Organization of the League of Nations and continued through its successor, the World Health Organization (WHO). During this period, smallpox was eliminated from all the countries of Europe and North and Central America, lending credence to the idea that through a concerted effort global eradication of smallpox could be achieved.

Global smallpox eradication program (1959–1979)

In May of 1959, the 12th World Health Assembly adopted the goal of global eradication of smallpox; however, between 1959 and 1966 little progress was made due to lack of funds and personnel, and a preoccupation of many member States with malaria eradication. In 1966, the WHO committed to an intensification of the effort to globally eradicate smallpox. The strategic plan employed two critical components: (1) mass vaccination using freeze-dried vaccine of assured quality and potency, and (2) the development of an international surveillance system that both evaluated the vaccination programs and detected and contained outbreaks by vaccinating the contacts of smallpox cases in the form of a ring vaccination. The last natural case of smallpox occurred in Somalia in 1977, and the WHO certified the world free of smallpox on December 9, 1979.

Current concerns regarding re-exposure to poxviruses

With smallpox eradicated from the world, vaccination against the disease ended in the United States in 1980, with the exception of health professionals, research scientists and military recruits. A consequence of this process is that a significant number of the world's population has been rendered susceptible to any potential encounter with poxviruses. The recent bioterrorist attacks and the emergence of *Monkeypox virus* into the human population have re-introduced the potential need to vaccinate the world's population.

Vaccine-associated complications

While vaccination has been an effective tool for protection against smallpox disease, a certain frequency of adverse events have been associated with vaccination. Abnormally high mortality associated with primary immunization with VACV was documented in the U.K. in the early 1900s; however, it was not until later that immunization was recognized to be associated with adverse reactions [6]. Several determining factors were found to contribute to these complications.

Genetic basis for vaccine-associated complications

During the smallpox eradication program, vaccine-associated complications varied among countries due to differences in the diagnostic criteria, reporting requirements and strains of VACV used in the respective immunization programs. The importance of VACV strain to the frequency of complications was underscored when the frequency of deaths from post-vaccinial encephalitis was observed to decline with the replacement of the Copenhagen and the Bern strains in the Netherlands and Austria, respectively, with the Lister strain of VACV [7, 8]. Additional epidemiological investigations by Marennikova [9] showed higher levels of reported post-vaccinial complications with the Tashkent strain (18 per million immunizations) than the B-51 (10 per million immunizations) or EM-63 strains (7 per million immunizations). These findings were supported by clinical trials in which a number of VACV strains were compared, and the Lister and New York City Board of Health (NYCBH) strains were found to be less reactogenic than the Copenhagen and Bern strains [10, 11]. The genetic basis for virulence differences among vaccines may be explained by the significant number of polymorphisms detected in the coding regions of a number of the VACV vaccine strains including NYCBH, modified vaccinia virus Ankara (MVA), Copenhagen, Ankara and Tian Tan [12].

Type and frequency of complications

Fenner and colleagues [1] identified two major groups of VACV complications: abnormal skin eruptions [accidental infection, generalized vaccinia, eczema vaccinatum, erythema multiforme and progressive vaccinia (vaccinia necrosum)] and disorders affecting the central nervous system (encephalopathy and encephalitis). In the U.S., the frequency of VACV-associated complications (NYCBH strain) was thoroughly examined in 1968 through a national survey and a ten-state survey [13, 14]. The majority of vaccine-associated complications reported occurred after primary immunization and not re-vaccination, except in the case of progressive vaccinia. Using the ten-state survey, 1254 cases per million primary immunizations were observed for all ages. More specifically, for every million vaccinations, there were 936 serious, but not life-threatening reactions, 52 life-threatening reactions, and 1.5 deaths [14]. For a thorough description of these complications see the review by Fulginiti et al [15].

Contraindications to vaccination

Five conditions were traditionally accepted as contraindicators for immunization with VACV: immune disorders, young age (less than 2 years old), eczema, pregnancy, and disorders of the central nervous system [1]. Although cardiac complications associated with the vaccination were not considered significant during the 1960s, several cardiac complications reported in early 2003 prompted the Centers for Disease Control and Prevention (CDC) to revise their recommendations for contraindicators of vaccination to include heart disease [16]. Women who are breastfeeding, persons less than 18 years of age, and individuals with allergies to vaccine components have also been included as contraindicated to vaccination [17]. The current number of people afflicted with the contraindicated conditions has significantly increased since the eradication program. Thus, in the event of a bioterrorist attack or the emergence of *Monkeypox virus* into the human population, it is inevitable that the number of adverse events associated with a mass vaccination would be considerably more than during the eradication process. For this reason, a major thrust in the poxvirus field is directed toward the design and evaluation of safer vaccines. Evaluation of the newer vaccines will require that we know much more about lasting and protective immunity to orthopoxviruses.

Smallpox and immunity to natural infection and vaccination

Correlates of immunity

Little is known about the cellular and molecular basis of the immune response to smallpox, as the disease was eradicated prior to the emergence of modern cellular and molecular immunology. Also, little is known regarding the important aspects of the immune response that are essential for, and therefore predictive of, successful immunity after vaccination. The vaccination scar, the only correlate with protection from severe smallpox, correlated with a tenfold reduction in mortality and less severe disease in previously infected survivors after the primary infection [18, 19]. With the absence of well-characterized animal models that mimic smallpox, and the lack of knowledge of immune correlates of protection with the vaccines used in the smallpox eradication program, the efficacy of new vaccines can only be evaluated by showing bio-equivalency with the Dryvax® vaccine and information gained from survivors of VARV infection.

Primary immune response to orthopoxvirus infections

Primary encounter with poxviruses, whether by natural infection or vaccination, is thought to stimulate both early and late phase host defense mechanisms consisting of the innate and adaptive immune systems, respectively. Once believed to be independent systems, it is now known that both systems work in a coordinated fashion to establish long-lasting protection against viruses. Identifying and characterizing the essential components of the primary immune response to orthopoxviruses, both at the innate and adaptive levels, is essential information for the design of future vaccines.

Innate immune response

Over the past 15 years there has been an explosion of knowledge about the innate immune system and its importance in overall immunity. The studies have led to an appreciation of the involvement of the innate immune system in the overall formation of a protective adaptive immune response [20, 21]. The innate system not only controls the nature and extent of the initial infection, but also the subsequent adaptive immune response. Thus, any discussion of vaccine development for a specific infectious agent must take into account the interaction of the innate system with the particular organism in question.

The initial interactions of an orthopoxvirus with the innate system involve dendritic cells, macrophages, granulocytes, natural killer (NK) cells, and γδ-T cells. All of these early responding cells act to produce an anti-viral state, mainly through the production of chemokines and type I (Th1) cytokines, which serve to limit the infection in a nonspecific manner. Much of this insight into the role of the innate system in the control of orthopoxvirus infection has come from the discovery of viral molecules designed to subvert these innate anti-viral mechanisms. The viral modulators target cytokines or their receptors (i.e., tumour necrosis factor-α (TNF-α) [22, 23], interferon (IFN)-γ [24, 25], IFN-α/β [26–28], interleukin (IL)-1β [29–31], and IL-18 [32, 33]), CC chemokines [34, 35], complement [36], Toll-like receptors [30, 37], and intracellular cytokine receptor signaling [37, 38] (see the review by Seet et al [39] for a thorough review of the poxvirus immune modulators).

Further insight into the role of innate immunity against poxvirus infection has come from ectopic expression of cytokines and chemokines at the time of infection. This is accomplished by the insertion of host innate genes into the poxvirus genome, or the co-administration of cytokines and/or chemokines along with virus at the site of infection. Expression of the type I cytokines IL-12 [40], IL-18 [40, 41], TNF-α [42, 43], and IFN-γ [42] in this manner appear to effectively enhance host protection. On the other hand, the type II cytokine IL-4 cripples both innate and adaptive immunity, allowing poxvirus infection to cause severe pathology and death in otherwise resistant hosts [44]. In addition, the deletion of either the IL-12 [45] or IFN-γ [46] genes in mice renders them highly susceptible to VACV or *Ectromelia virus* (ECTV) infection, corroborating the importance of these cytokines in host protection against these viruses.

The cell types of the innate system shown to play a role in the control of host viral infections in general, most often in concert with cytokines and/or chemokines, include dendritic cells, NK cells, NKT cells, γδ-T cells, monocytes/macrophages, and granulocytes. However, there is relatively little known regarding their role(s) in the control of orthopoxvirus infection and the development of anti-poxvirus adaptive immunity. Dendritic cells undoubtedly play a key role in the initiation of the adaptive response to the orthopoxviruses. Although poxviruses, as do many viruses in general, shut down many of the dendritic cell functions, early gene expression results in antigen presentation *via* the classical endogenous class I pathway. On the other hand, late gene products stimulate $CD8^+$ cytotoxic T lymphocytes (CTL) through cross presentation pathways [47, 48] *via* the uptake of apoptotic poxvirus-infected dendritic cells by healthy dendritic cells that have escaped viral infection and eventual death by apoptosis. The importance of NK cells *in vivo* is shown in NK cell depletion experiments where the removal of NK cells significantly shortens the mean time of death [49]. Virtually nothing is known regarding the role of NK cells in the development of a memory adaptive response. Reports examining the role of γδ-T cells show that γδ-T cell expansion, predominantly $V\gamma9^+$, is induced in human volunteers immunized with *Canarypox virus* [50], and the loss of γδ-T cells in mice results in higher VACV titers and increased mortality [51]. Virtually nothing has been published on the role of NKT cells or granulocytes on host protection after poxvirus infection.

Humoral immune response

The critical role for the humoral response in clearing acute poxvirus infections is indicated by adverse reactions seen in both humans and animal models with deficient B cell function. In human subjects presenting with hypogammaglobulinemia, primary vaccination was generally tolerated [52, 53], and rare adverse reactions typically resolved [52, 54–56]. However, fatal infections often developed in children under the age of 1 year presenting with hypogammaglobulinemia or agammaglobulinemia [57–60], again often in combination with other immunodeficiencies [52, 61]. In the mouse model, $IgH^{-/-}$ and MHC class $II^{-/-}$ animals, both of which are Ig compromised, show increased signs of disease and a decreased ability to clear virus upon infection with vaccinia virus as compared to control mice [62]. In addition, Fang et al. [63] showed that $CD40^{-/-}$ mice infected with ECTV present with delayed mousepox disease due to persistent ECTV infection, and eventually succumb to death despite a sustained early $CD8^+$ T cell response. Because these symptoms are seen less frequently in patients with an intact humoral immune system, it is likely that the antibody response to initial infection aids in the clearance of poxvirus infection, both for natural infection and vaccination.

Characterizing the immune response to natural infection with VARV was mostly measured by serological assays, due to the limited technology available during the time of endemic smallpox. Assays measuring hemagglutinin inhibition (HI) antibody titers detected antibody as early as 2 days after the onset of illness (~12 days post infection) in some patients, and all were positive by 7 days [64–66]. Complement fixation (CF) and neutralizing antibody titers, as well as precipitin formation, were also detected in unvaccinated smallpox patients, but they were present in low titers [65–67]. Neutralizing antibody was present after 6 days, while CF titers began to appear 8–10 days after the onset of illness with a maximum titer around day 14 [65, 66]. Precipitating antibodies were present after 8 days of illness in a few patients [66]. Variability was seen between case studies regarding reported titers and frequency among patients, likely due to inconsistencies in the assays used.

Primary vaccine recipients mount a robust antibody response to the vaccine [68–73] with neutralizing and HI antibodies detected as early as 10 days after vaccination [68, 74, 75], which is slightly earlier than seen in natural infection. Fewer recipients presented CF titers, or these titers were very low [68, 76, 77]. The peak neutralizing antibody titer in primary vaccine recipients is 28 days after vaccination [70]. Neutralizing antibody titers persist longer than HI or CF antibodies [68, 74] and remain remarkably stable, being detected up to 75 years after vaccination [78]. With the exception of a tenfold drop within the first 10 years of immunization, VACV-specific memory B cells also remain very stable, and can be detected more than 50 years after vaccination [79].

The protective nature of immune sera is apparent when VACV immune gamma-globulin (VIG), pooled sera from vaccinated military recruits, is used as a prophylaxis for vaccine-associated complications and contacts of smallpox cases [80–86]. VIG has been able to confer protection from morbidity and mortality in many adult cases for such complications as accidental autoinoculation [87], eczema vaccinatum [85, 87], generalized vaccinia, and severe local vaccinial reactions [85]. VIG has been shown to confer protection even with adverse reactions to vaccination typically associated with T cell deficiencies, such as progressive vaccinia [14, 88]. In addition, one case study showed that contacts exposed to smallpox cases were significantly protected if treated with VIG (with 1.5%, 5 of 326 smallpox contacts, developing disease) compared to those untreated (with 5.5%, 21 of 379 smallpox contacts, developing disease) [82]. Several animal model studies also showed that passive transfer of immune sera to naïve recipients resulted in complete protection against poxvirus challenge [89–93].

Cell-mediated immune response

Very little information is available on cell-mediated immunity (CMI) and its role in protecting humans upon infection with VARV. The only study describing CMI in VARV infection was conducted by Jackson et al. [94] in

1977, who quantified the number of T and B cells in the peripheral blood of 17 smallpox patients in Bangladesh (vaccination history not reported). This study showed lower T cell counts in smallpox patients compared to controls, and fatal cases had low B cell counts but high "null cell" counts (cells not identified as either T or B cells). Additional information regarding CMI can be extrapolated from the responses of PBMCs *in vitro* from recently vaccinated individuals.

Mass vaccination during the eradication program resulted in severe complications in children with T cell deficiencies, adults with leukemia, and adults with undiagnosed HIV [52, 95, 96]. These types of complications after vaccination led to the recognition of an important role for CMI in the immune response to vaccination.

In healthy individuals, primary vaccination induces a VACV-specific cell-mediated immune response with a strong Th1 bias [97]. While both $CD4^+$ and $CD8^+$ T cells demonstrate CTL activity and IFN-γ production in response to VACV [73, 78, 97–102], $CD8^+$ T cells mediate the majority of the VACV-specific cytolytic activity and IFN-γ production [97, 99]. In a $CD8^+$ T cell depletion study, 64–100% of the VACV-specific cytolytic activity was abrogated, while depleting $CD4^+$ T cells only accounted for a 0–17% loss [99]. Similarly, IFN-γ production peaks 2 weeks after vaccination with $CD8^+$ T cells (geometric mean frequency, 1.37%) representing two- to fourfold more $CD3^+$ IFN-γ^+ T cells than $CD4^+$ T cells (geometric mean frequency, 0.33%) [97]. Helper activity of $CD4^+$ T cells after vaccination has not been fully investigated in humans; however, they are known to be necessary in other viral systems in mouse models for protective antiviral antibody responses and optimal cytolytic activity at the memory level [103–107]

Notably, there is a preferential persistence of $CD4^+$ T cells over $CD8^+$ T cells several years after vaccination [78, 97]. Hammarlund et al. [78] showed that 100% (16/16) of people receiving a primary vaccination maintained $CD4^+$ T cell activity 20 years after vaccination, whereas only 50% (8/16) of this population maintained $CD8^+$ T cell activity. Furthermore, another study shows different contraction kinetics between $CD4^+$ (twofold) and $CD8^+$ T cells (sevenfold) within 12 weeks after primary vaccination [97].

Animal studies have confirmed the dependence on CMI for survival from poxvirus infection [42, 49, 62, 90]. Mice deficient in $CD4^+$ T cells have incomplete viral clearance, but do survive challenge, whereas mice depleted of $CD8^+$ T cells do not survive VACV or ECTV virus challenge [49, 62, 63]. Additionally, resistance to ECTV in C57BL/6 mice is wholly dependent on an early type I cytokine response (IFN-γ, IL-2, and TNF-α) in conjunction with strong CTL activity [42]. In contrast, mousepox-susceptible mouse strains lack the development of a Th1 response to ECTV, namely very little CTL activity, resulting in diminished viral clearance and death despite generating a Th2 immune response [42].

Targets of the humoral immune response

In addition to characterizing the immune response to poxvirus infection, identifying the targets of the immune response to VACV is essential for the design of future vaccines, especially subunit or DNA vaccines that will ideally include only those epitopes that elicit immune memory.

Neutralizing antibody inhibits different stages of cellular uptake of poxviruses by targeting membrane proteins of both the intracellular mature virions (IMV) and the extracellular enveloped virus (EEV). It has long been known that antibodies are generated against the proteins located within both the IMV and EEV, but antibodies raised against EEV appear most critical for protection [89, 108]. Antibodies against the EEV proteins A33R and B5R prevent long-range dissemination of the virus [109]. While B5R has been shown to be the main target of neutralizing antibody found in VIG [110], A33R is a target of non-neutralizing antibodies [93]. The ability of antibody against A33R to prevent cell-to-cell spread, has been suggested to be a result of antibodies against A33R reacting with complement to lyse the EEV, exposing the IMV to neutralizing antibody [111]. Neutralizing antibodies generated against the IMV proteins D8L [112, 113], L1R [114, 115], H3L [116], and A27L [112, 117] inhibit attachment and/or penetration into host cells [113–117]. Antibodies against D8L have also been shown to be immunodominant in vaccinated patients [112].

Targets of the CMI response

Targets of $CD8^+$ T CMI have recently received a great deal of attention, largely due to the use of epitope prediction algorithms for MHC class I molecules [118–121]. These programs allow the search for potentially reactive peptides to become quickly focused, and activity is left to functional screening assays. Early studies restricted their search to proteins that were predicted to bind only one HLA type, HLA-A*0201, which is present in about half the American population. Using this strategy, $CD8^+$ T cell responses to epitopes in the viral proteins H3L (peptide VP35#1) [122], C16L [amino acids (aa) 79–87] [123] and C7L (aa 74–82) [123] (also reported as host range protein 2 [HRP2 (74–82)] [124]) were identified. These peptides were found to stimulate splenocytes from HLA-A*0201 transgenic mice and/or peripheral blood mononuclear cells (PBMC) of immunized HLA-A*0201-positive human volunteers within 1–2 weeks after immunization. Specifically, IFN-γ-producing PBMC specific to C7L and C16L represented 6-35% of the total VACV-specific IFN-γ-producing cells in three volunteers 2 weeks after immunization [123]. Snyder et al. [124] also showed that epitopes A26L(6–14) and VACV early transcription factor (VETF) small subunit [VETFsm(498–506)] were able to stimulate IFN-γ production from HLA-A*0201 transgenic mouse splenocytes 4 weeks after immunization. Of these peptides that stimulated $CD8^+$ T cell activity in the context of human HLA, two peptides were tested for *in vivo* protection. Immunizing HLA-A*0201 transgenic mice with HRP2(74–82) [124], but not H3L(VP35#1) [122], provided protection against lethal VACV strain Western Reserve (WR) challenge by the intranasal route.

Identifying targets of $CD8^+$ T cells has more recently been expanded to screen for epitope targets across multiple HLA supertypes, including HLA-A1, A2, A3, A24, B7, and B44 [125, 126]. Using CTL from VACV-infected HLA transgenic mice, Pasquetto et al. [126] screened for cytolytic activity against 2889 peptides predicted to bind various HLA supertypes. They identified 14 HLA-A*0201-, 4 HLA-A*1101-, and 3 HLA-B*0702-restricted $CD8^+$ T cell determinants over 20 distinct proteins, including the epitopes H3L (VP35#1) [122] and HRP2(74–82) [124] previously identified by other groups. Some of these peptides were able to bind several A2, A3 and B7 supertype HLA molecules. In another study, Oseroff et al. [125] screened 6000 peptides from 258 putative VACV open reading frames (ORF), and found 48 epitopes from 35 VACV antigens (including B8R, D1R, D5R, C10L, C19L, C7L, F12L, and O1L) capable of simulating IFN-γ production from PBMC of immunized volunteers. Several of these targets contained multiple epitopes recognized by several volunteers in the context of different HLA types.

In contrast to the array of epitopes targeted by the human CMI response, the mouse response to VACV is more restricted to relatively few viral determinants. Using the bioinformatics approach, Matthew et al. [127] identified two targets of the MVA strain, A47L and J6R, which stimulated IFN-γ production and CTL activity, respectively, from splenocytes of VACV-immunized (NYCBH strain) C57BL/6 mice. In another approach, Tscharke et al. [128] identified five additional $CD8^+$ T cell epitopes using a VACV expression library to screen each of the 258 predicted ORF. These five epitopes were found in the viral proteins B8R (aa 20–27), A19L (aa 47–55), A47L (138–146), A42R (aa 88–96), and K3L (aa 6–15) – in order of immunodominance – and represent almost half of the total VACV-specific $CD8^+$ T cell response in B6 mice [128]. In that study, immunization with the B8R epitope provided protection from lethal ECTV challenge. Tscharke et al. also notes an important variation in immunodominance hierarchy depending on the poxvirus strain used and route of infection, suggesting that the immunodominance of a peptide in vaccinia does not guarantee its immunodominance in variola. To date, no publications have appeared which identify epitopes targeted by $CD4^+$ T cells.

Memory immunity following immunization or infection

Jenner was the first to demonstrate the principle of memory immunity as a result of cross-protection when he infected James Phipps with VARV 2 months after inoculating him with CPXV [129]. Jenner also observed that memory immunity worked in both directions, as persons recovered from smallpox were resistant to infection with CPXV [129]. Similarly, immunization of human populations with VACV protected against severe smallpox and human monkeypox [1, 130]. Characterizing this protective memory immune response will also yield critical information for the design of future vaccines.

Humoral memory immunity

The memory immune response to variola infection in vaccinated patients is distinguished by the detection of antibody titers earlier in infection and in higher titers [65, 66]. In these patients, neutralizing antibody titers [65–67] and HI titers [65, 66] were present within 6–7 days after the onset of illness. CF [65–67] and precipitin formation [66, 67] did not appear until a couple of days later. While none of these assays demonstrated titers that absolutely correlated with protection, multiple case studies found the development of high neutralizing antibody titers to be the strongest serological correlation with survival [65, 66, 131, 132]. Many of the patients with high neutralizing antibody titers also developed CF titers, with a peak titer around day 14 of illness [65, 66]. Of note, the majority of fatal cases had low titers by both tests [66]. Precipitin formation correlated with high neutralizing and CF antibody titers, while HI titers did not correlate with either [66]. Although HI titers were usually detectable earlier than the other antibody types after infection [65], HI titers were weak correlates of protection [66, 131].

Similarly, contacts of smallpox patients were protected from developing disease if they had a pre-existing neutralizing antibody titer of >1:20 [132] or >1:32 [131]. Again, HI titers were not a reliable indicator of protection [131]. In these two studies, 0 of 41 and 1 of 130 vaccinated contacts developed disease compared to 6 of 16 and 2 of 12 unvaccinated contacts, respectively [131, 132].

Re-vaccination as secondary exposure to virus also stimulates early antibody production. Prior to re-vaccination, a majority of patients have detectable neutralizing antibody titers [68, 70, 133] as well as residual antibody-dependent cell-mediated cytotoxicity (ADCC) [134]. Neutralizing antibody titers increase as early as 7 days after re-vaccination [68], and peak within 12–15 days [70, 133]. McCarthy et al. [68] show very few patients producing significant CF or HI antibody titers after re-vaccination, regardless of the neutralizing antibody response. In general, multiple vaccinations do not affect either the titer or persistence of neutralizing antibody [78, 133, 135].

The protection afforded by previous vaccination, however, was found to decrease with time. In one case study, the severity of disease and mortality associated with VARV infection in individuals vaccinated at birth increased with age [18]. Greatest protection from severe disease was between 3 and

5 years after immunization, and death was found only in individuals vaccinated greater than 20 years previous to infection [18]. Additionally, one study immunizing volunteers with the Lister strain of VACV found that the length of time between vaccinations, along with preexisting antibody titers, directly affected the development of a successful clinical take and seroconversion [136]. Together, these observations correlate with the selective decline found for neutralizing antibodies against EEV greater than 20 years after vaccination [135] and the selective loss of $CD8^+$ T cells discussed earlier [78].

Cell-mediated memory immunity

Re-vaccination stimulates a recall proliferative [73, 98, 134] and cytolytic response [73, 137] in addition to IFN-γ production [73, 97, 98]. Proliferation and IFN-γ production, measured by ELISPOT, are detected earlier (day 7) than primary vaccine recipients, as expected for a memory response upon re-vaccination [73]. Both $CD4^+$ and $CD8^+$ T cells contribute to the proliferation and IFN-γ production [78, 97, 98]. Two weeks after re-vaccination, both $CD4^+$ and $CD8^+$ T cells expand in response to antigen stimulation with similar geometric mean frequencies, 0.22% and 0.34%, respectively [97]. However, by 12 weeks after receiving the booster vaccination, $CD8^+$ T cells have contracted 5.5-fold, whereas $CD4^+$ T cells have contracted only 2-fold, similar to the contraction kinetics after primary vaccination [97]. There is no significant correlation found between the magnitude of the immune response before re-vaccination to the magnitude of the peak effector response [97, 134]. In addition, neither the magnitude of the CMI response nor the persistence of these cells was significantly affected by multiple vaccinations [78, 97].

Vaccines

First generation vaccines – Live, animal passaged and virulent

First generation vaccines evolved from a locally produced product that gained regional and/or national prominence through efficacy. These vaccines were neither clonal nor highly purified and could be contaminated with microorganisms, as they were serially propagated on domesticated animals, most often calves or sheep (at least in the early years). Four major vaccines were used during the smallpox eradication program: Dryvax® (prepared from the NYCBH strain of VACV, USA), Lister (United Kingdom, Europe, Africa, Asia, Oceania), Temple of Heaven (China), and EM-63 (USSR). During the intensified smallpox eradication program, these vaccines were prepared locally to a uniform potency of 1×10^8 PFU/ml that gave a presented dose of ~2.5×10^5 PFU per vaccination site when used with a bifurcated needle. Although vaccines regardless of source gave similar levels of protection from severe smallpox, they varied in the severity of post-vaccination complications (see section *Vaccine-associated complications*).

Second generation vaccines – Live, tissue culture produced and virulent

With the increased threat of bioterrorism in the 21st century, the U.S. government contracted the procurement of ~209 million doses of a cloned, cell-culture vaccine to supplement the existing stockpile of 15 million doses of Dryvax® that recent clinical trial data indicated could be diluted 1:5 and still generate a "take" [71, 72, 138]. Together, sufficient vaccine is available to provide one dose for each citizen. The new vaccine, designated ACAM2000, was developed and produced by Acambis in a partnership with Baxter BioScience. ACAM2000 had a similar vaccination rate and antibody response to Dryvax® [139]. Since ACAM2000 was cloned from Dryvax®, the two vaccines will likely share a similar safety profile [139]. A second cell-cultured smallpox vaccine derived from Connaught Laboratories is being manufactured by DynPort Vaccine Company for the armed forces [140].

Third generation vaccines – Live, tissue culture produced and attenuated

MVA

To overcome the hazards of replicating virus, a highly attenuated strain of VACV, MVA, was developed by growing the Ankara strain of VACV for greater than 500 passages on chicken embryo fibroblasts. This resulted in a loss of about 15% of the genome, which correlated with a loss of replication capacity in most mammalian cells [141], thus reducing the risk of dissemination and transmission following vaccination [142]. In addition, MVA no longer encodes many of the soluble inhibitors of cytokine and chemokine function as well as other immune evasion factors that may result in a more vigorous immune response against the virus [143–145]. Epitopes known to elicit neutralizing antibodies [93, 115] are present, and three human $CD8^+$ CTL epitopes have been identified and conserved in MVA [122, 123]. Previous work with MVA demonstrated its safety and its ability to protect against poxvirus infections in several animal models [146–148]. For example, MVA vaccination provided protection against lethal pulmonary vaccinia virus challenge of mice, and, after an initial priming immunization with MVA, enhanced immunogenicity was observed following a booster immunization with MVA or Dryvax® [149]. Other attenuated strains have been produced, such as LC16m8, but MVA has the most extensive history of safety in humans.

LC16m8

The unacceptable level of vaccine-associated complications observed with the Ikeda vaccine in Japan during the first half of the 20th century underscored the need for a safer vaccine. LC16m8 was isolated through serial passage of the Lister strain in primary baby rabbit kidney cells, and the selection of a temperature-sensitive clone that produced smaller pocks on chorioallantoic membranes [150]. The small-pock phenotype of LC16m8 was attributed to a mutation in the *B5R* gene, which encodes an EEV surface protein [151] and is essential for optimal formation of EEV. LC16m8 was shown to be highly attenuated in animal models, and was tested in over 10 000 children [150, 152]. The efficacy of LC16m8 was comparable to Dryvax® as determined by humoral immune responses and protection against lethal disease in rabbitpox and mousepox models [153].

Fourth generation vaccines – Non-infectious and safe

A series of studies have suggested that vaccines containing immunogens from the surfaces of both the IMV and EEV may provide the best protection from a challenge with a virulent orthopoxvirus [89, 93, 116, 154–156]. These findings stimulated others to evaluate the efficacy of active immunization with IMV and EEV proteins and genes in mouse and nonhuman primate challenge models. Hooper and co-workers [157] showed a DNA vaccine composed of two IMV-specific genes (L1R and A27L) and two EEV-specific genes (A33R and B5R) offered complete protection for mice against a lethal intranasal dose of VACV, and was immunogenic in nonhuman primates. This DNA vaccine also protected rhesus macaques from severe disease after a lethal challenge dose of monkeypox virus [158]. Fogg and colleagues found that three immunizations with a three-protein combination of proteins from the surface of IMV and EEV (A33 + B5 + L1) provided complete protection from an intranasal challenge of mice with VACV strain WR [159].

Acknowledgements

This work was funded through NIAID Contract No. N01-AI-15436 (R. M. L. B.).

References

1 Fenner F, Henderson DA, Arita I, Jezek Z, Ladnyj ID (1988) *Smallpox and its eradication.* World Health Organization, Geneva

2 Coult R (1731) *Operation of inoculation of the smallpox as performed in Bengall* [from R. Coult to Dr Oliver Coult in An account of the diseases of Bengall (dated Calcutta, Feb 10. 1731]. Reprinted in: Dharampal (1971) *Indian science and technology in the eighteenth century*. Impex, Delhi, 141–143

3 Jenner E (1801) *The origin of the vaccine inoculation*. Shury, London

4 Crookshank EM (1889) *History and pathology of vaccination*, vols. 1 and 2. Lewis, London

5 Downie AW (1939) The immunological relationship of the virus of spontaneous cowpox to vaccinia virus. *Br J Exp Pathol* 20: 158–176

6 Ministry of Health for England and Wales (1924) *Smallpox and vaccination. Reports on public health and medical subjects, No. 8*. H.M. Stationery Office, London

7 Berger KAHW (1973) Decrease in postvaccinial deaths in Austria after introducing a less pathogenic virus strain. In: *International Symposium on Smallpox Vaccine, Bilthoven, the Netherlands, 11–13 October 1972: Symposia Series in Immunobiological Standardization, vol. 19*. Karger, Basel, 199–203

8 Polak MF (1973) Complications of smallpox vaccination in the Netherlands, 1959–1970. In: *International Symposium on Smallpox Vaccine, Bilthoven, the Netherlands, 11–13 October 1972: Symposia Series in Immunobiological Standardization*, vol. 19. Karger, Basel, 235–242

9 Marennikova SS (1973) Evaluation of vaccine strains by their behavior in vaccinated animals and possible implication of the revealed features for smallpox vaccination practice. In: *International Symposium on Smallpox Vaccine, Bilthoven, the Netherlands, 11–13 October 1972: Symposia Series in Immunobiological Standardization*, vol. 19. Karger, Basel, 253–260

10 Galasso GJ, Mattheis MJ, Cherry JD, Connor JD, McIntosh K, Benenson AS, Alling DW (1977) Clinical and serologic study of four smallpox vaccines comparing variations of dose and route of administration. *J Infect Dis* 135: 183–186

11 Polak MF, Beunders BJ, Van Der Werff AR, Sanders EW, Van Klaveren J, Brans LM (1963) A comparative study of clinical reaction observed after application of several smallpox vaccines in primary vaccination of young adults. *Bull World Health Organ* 29: 311–322

12 Poxvirus Bioinformatics Resource Center (2004) http://www. biovirus. org

13 Lane JM, Ruben FL, Neff JM, Millar JD (1969) Complications of smallpox vaccination, 1968. *N Engl J Med* 281: 1201–1208

14 Lane JM, Ruben FL, Neff JM, Millar JD (1970) Complications of smallpox vaccination, 1968: results of ten statewide surveys. *J Infect Dis* 122: 303–309

15 Fulginiti VA, Papier A, Lane JM, Neff JM, Henderson DA (2003) Smallpox vaccination: a review, part II. Adverse events. *Clin Infect Dis* 37: 251–271

16 CDC (2006) Frequently asked questions about smallpox vaccine. http://www.bt.cdc.gov/agent/smallpox/vaccination/faq.asp

17 Cono J, Casey CG, Bell DM (2003) Smallpox vaccination and adverse reactions. Guidance for clinicians. *MMWR Recomm Rep* 52: 1–28

18 Hanna W, Baxby D (2002) Studies in smallpox and vaccination. 1913. *Rev Med Virol* 12: 201–209

19 Mack TM (1972) Smallpox in Europe, 1950–1971. *J Infect Dis* 125: 161–169

20 Fearon DT, Locksley RM (1996) The instructive role of innate immunity in the acquired immune response. *Science* 272: 50–53
21 Pasare C, Medzhitov R (2004) Toll-like receptors: linking innate and adaptive immunity. *Microbes Infect* 6: 1382–1387
22 Alcami A, Khanna A, Paul NL, Smith GL (1999) Vaccinia virus strains Lister, USSR and Evans express soluble and cell-surface tumour necrosis factor receptors. *J Gen Virol* 80: 949–959
23 Cunnion KM (1999) Tumor necrosis factor receptors encoded by poxviruses. *Mol Genet Metab* 67: 278–282
24 Karupiah G, Fredrickson TN, Holmes KL, Khairallah LH, Buller RM (1993) Importance of interferons in recovery from mousepox. *J Virol* 67: 4214–4226
25 Smith GL, Symons JA, Alcami A (1998) Poxviruses: interfering with interferon. *Semin Virol* 8: 409–418
26 Smith VP, Alcami A (2002) Inhibition of interferons by ectromelia virus. *J Virol* 76: 1124–1134
27 Symons JA, Alcami A, Smith GL (1995) Vaccinia virus encodes a soluble type I interferon receptor of novel structure and broad species specificity. *Cell* 81: 551–560
28 Colamonici OR, Domanski P, Sweitzer SM, Larner A, Buller RM (1995) Vaccinia virus B18R gene encodes a type I interferon-binding protein that blocks interferon alpha transmembrane signaling. *J Biol Chem* 270: 15974–15978
29 Alcami A, Smith GL (1992) A soluble receptor for interleukin-1 beta encoded by vaccinia virus: a novel mechanism of virus modulation of the host response to infection. *Cell* 71: 153–167
30 Bowie A, Kiss-Toth E, Symons JA, Smith GL, Dower SK, O'Neill LA (2000) A46R and A52R from vaccinia virus are antagonists of host IL-1 and toll-like receptor signaling. *Proc Natl Acad Sci USA* 97: 10162–10167
31 Spriggs MK, Hruby DE, Maliszewski CR, Pickup DJ, Sims JE, Buller RM, VanSlyke J (1992) Vaccinia and cowpox viruses encode a novel secreted interleukin-1-binding protein. *Cell* 71: 145–152
32 Reading PC, Smith GL (2003) Vaccinia virus interleukin-18-binding protein promotes virulence by reducing gamma interferon production and natural killer and T-cell activity. *J Virol* 77: 9960–9968
33 Born TL, Morrison LA, Esteban DJ, VandenBos T, Thebeau LG, Chen N, Spriggs MK, Sims JE, Buller RM (2000) A poxvirus protein that binds to and inactivates IL-18, and inhibits NK cell response. *J Immunol* 164: 3246–3254
34 Graham KA, Lalani AS, Macen JL, Ness TL, Barry M, Liu LY, Lucas A, Clark-Lewis I, Moyer RW, McFadden G (1997) The T1/35kDa family of poxvirus-secreted proteins bind chemokines and modulate leukocyte influx into virus-infected tissues. *Virology* 229: 12–24
35 Smith CA, Smith TD, Smolak PJ, Friend D, Hagen H, Gerhart M, Park L, Pickup DJ, Torrance D, Mohler K, Schooley K, Goodwin RG (1997) Poxvirus genomes encode a secreted, soluble protein that preferentially inhibits beta chemokine activity yet lacks sequence homology to known chemokine receptors. *Virology* 236: 316–327
36 Howard J, Justus DE, Totmenin AV, Shchelkunov S, Kotwal GJ (1998)

Molecular mimicry of the inflammation modulatory proteins (IMPs) of poxviruses: evasion of the inflammatory response to preserve viral habitat. *J Leukoc Biol* 64: 68–71

37 Stack J, Haga IR, Schroder M, Bartlett NW, Maloney G, Reading PC, Fitzgerald KA, Smith GL, Bowie AG (2005) Vaccinia virus protein A46R targets multiple Toll-like-interleukin-1 receptor adaptors and contributes to virulence. *J Exp Med* 201: 1007–1018

38 Harte MT, Haga IR, Maloney G, Gray P, Reading PC, Bartlett NW, Smith GL, Bowie A, O'Neill LA (2003) The poxvirus protein A52R targets Toll-like receptor signaling complexes to suppress host defense. *J Exp Med* 197: 343–351

39 Seet BT, Johnston JB, Brunetti CR, Barrett JW, Everett H, Cameron C, Sypula J, Nazarian SH, Lucas A, McFadden G (2003) Poxviruses and immune evasion. *Annu Rev Immunol* 21: 377–423

40 Gherardi MM, Ramirez JC, Esteban M (2003) IL-12 and IL-18 act in synergy to clear vaccinia virus infection: involvement of innate and adaptive components of the immune system. *J Gen Virol* 84: 1961–1972

41 Tanaka-Kataoka M, Kunikata T, Takayama S, Iwaki K, Ohashi K, Ikeda M, Kurimoto M (1999) *In vivo* antiviral effect of interleukin 18 in a mouse model of vaccinia virus infection. *Cytokine* 11: 593–599

42 Chaudhri G, Panchanathan V, Buller RM, van den Eertwegh AJ, Claassen E, Zhou J, de Chazal R, Laman JD, Karupiah G (2004) Polarized type 1 cytokine response and cell-mediated immunity determine genetic resistance to mousepox. *Proc Natl Acad Sci USA* 101: 9057–9062

43 Ruby J, Bluethmann H, Peschon JJ (1997) Antiviral activity of tumor necrosis factor (TNF) is mediated via p55 and p75 TNF receptors. *J Exp Med* 186: 1591–1596

44 Jackson RJ, Ramsay AJ, Christensen CD, Beaton S, Hall DF, Ramshaw IA (2001) Expression of mouse interleukin-4 by a recombinant ectromelia virus suppresses cytolytic lymphocyte responses and overcomes genetic resistance to mousepox. *J Virol* 75: 1205–1210

45 van Den Broek M, Bachmann MF, Kohler G, Barner M, Escher R, Zinkernagel R, Kopf M (2000) IL-4 and IL-10 antagonize IL-12-mediated protection against acute vaccinia virus infection with a limited role of IFN-gamma and nitric oxide synthetase 2. *J Immunol* 164: 371–378

46 Ramshaw IA, Ramsay AJ, Karupiah G, Rolph MS, Mahalingam S, Ruby JC (1997) Cytokines and immunity to viral infections. *Immunol Rev* 159: 119–135

47 Norbury CC, Basta S, Donohue KB, Tscharke DC, Princiotta MF, Berglund P, Gibbs J, Bennink JR, Yewdell JW (2004) $CD8^+$ T cell cross-priming via transfer of proteasome substrates. *Science* 304: 1318–1321

48 Serna A, Ramirez MC, Soukhanova A, Sigal LJ (2003) Cutting edge: efficient MHC class I cross-presentation during early vaccinia infection requires the transfer of proteasomal intermediates between antigen donor and presenting cells. *J Immunol* 171: 5668–5672

49 Karupiah G, Buller RM, Van Rooijen N, Duarte CJ, Chen J (1996) Different roles for $CD4^+$ and $CD8^+$ T lymphocytes and macrophage subsets in the control of a generalized virus infection. *J Virol* 70: 8301–8309

50 Worku S, Gorse GJ, Belshe RB, Hoft DF (2001) Canarypox vaccines induce

antigen-specific human gammadelta T cells capable of interferon-gamma production. *J Infect Dis* 184: 525–532

51 Selin LK, Santolucito PA, Pinto AK, Szomolanyi-Tsuda E, Welsh RM (2001) Innate immunity to viruses: control of vaccinia virus infection by gamma delta T cells. *J Immunol* 166: 6784–6794

52 Fulginiti V, Kempe CH, Hathaway WE, Pearlman DS, Sieber OF, Eller JJ, Joyner JJ Sr, Robinson A (1968) Progressive vaccinia in immunologically-deficient individuals. *Birth Defects Orig Artic Ser* 4: 129–145

53 Good RA, Varco RL (1955) A clinical and experimental study of agammaglobulinemia. *J Lancet* 75: 245–271

54 CDC (1982) Vaccinia necrosum after smallpox vaccination-Michigan. *MMWR Morb Mortal Wkly Rep* 31: 501–502

55 Freed ER, Duma RJ, Escobar MR (1972) Vaccinia necrosum and its relationship to impaired immunologic responsiveness. *Am J Med* 52: 411–420

56 Mihailescu R, Topciu V, Dogaru D, Petrovici A, Plavosin L, Stanciu N, Moldovan E, Roth L (1979) Laboratory diagnosis in a case of fatal progressive vaccinia due to manifest immunologic deficiencies. *Zentralbl Bakteriol B* 169: 510–518

57 White CM (1963) Vaccinia gangrenosa due to hypogammaglobulinemia. *Lancet* 1: 969–971

58 Somers K (1957) Vaccinia gangrenosa and agammaglobulinaemia. *Arch Dis Child* 32: 220–225

59 Kozinn PJ, Sigel MM, Gorrie R (1955) Progressive vaccinia associated with agammaglobulinemia and defects in immune mechanism. *Pediatrics* 16: 600–608

60 Carson MJ, Donnell GN (1956) Vaccinia gangrenosa; a case in a child with hypogammaglobulinemia. *Calif Med* 85: 335–339

61 Olding-Stenkvist E, Nordbring F, Larsson E, Lindblom B, Wigzell H (1980) Fatal progressive vaccinia in two immunodeficient infants. *Scand J Infect Dis* Suppl 24: 63–67

62 Xu R, Johnson AJ, Liggitt D, Bevan MJ (2004) Cellular and humoral immunity against vaccinia virus infection of mice. *J Immunol* 172: 6265–6271

63 Fang Mand Sigal LJ (2005) Antibodies and $CD8^+$ T cells are complementary and essential for natural resistance to a highly lethal cytopathic virus. *J Immunol* 175: 6829–6836

64 Collier WA, Smit AM, von Heerde AF (1950) Demonstration of antihemagglutinins as an aid in the diagnosis of smallpox. *Z Hyg Infektionskr* 131: 555–567

65 Downie AW, McCarthy K (1958) The antibody response in man following infection with viruses of the pox group. III. Antibody response in smallpox. *J Hyg (Lond)* 56: 479–487

66 Downie AW, Saint VL, Goldstein L, Rao AR, Kempe CH (1969) Antibody response in non-haemorrhagic smallpox patients. *J Hyg (Lond)* 67: 609–618

67 Herrlich A, Mayr A, Mahnel H (1959) Antibody picture of variola vaccine infection. II. Serological studies on variola patients. *Zentralbl Bakteriol [Orig]* 175: 163–182

68 McCarthy K, Downie AW, Bradley WH (1958) The antibody response in man following infection with viruses of the pox group. II. Antibody response following vaccination. *J Hyg (Lond)* 56: 466–478

69 Belshe RB, Newman FK, Frey SE, Couch RB, Treanor JJ, Tacket CO, Yan L (2004) Dose-dependent neutralizing-antibody responses to vaccinia. *J Infect Dis* 189: 493–497

70 Frey SE, Newman FK, Yan L, Lottenbach KR, Belshe RB (2003) Response to smallpox vaccine in persons immunized in the distant past. *JAMA* 289: 3295–3299

71 Frey SE, Couch RB, Tacket CO, Treanor JJ, Wolff M, Newman FK, Atmar RL, Edelman R, Nolan CM, Belshe RB (2002) Clinical responses to undiluted and diluted smallpox vaccine. *N Engl J Med* 346: 1265–1274

72 Frey SE, Newman FK, Cruz J, Shelton WB, Tennant JM, Polach T, Rothman AL, Kennedy JS, Wolff M, Belshe RB, Ennis FA (2002) Dose-related effects of smallpox vaccine. *N Engl J Med* 346: 1275–1280

73 Kennedy JS, Frey SE, Yan L, Rothman AL, Cruz J, Newman FK, Orphin L, Belshe RB, Ennis FA (2004) Induction of human T cell-mediated immune responses after primary and secondary smallpox vaccination. *J Infect Dis* 190: 1286–1294

74 Downie AW, Hobday TL, St Vincent L, Kempe CH (1961) Studies of smallpox antibody levels of sera from samples of the vaccinated adult population of Madras. *Bull World Health Organ* 25: 55–61

75 Downie AW, Saint VL, Rao AR, Kempe CH (1969) Antibody response following smallpox vaccination and revaccination. *J Hyg (Lond)* 67: 603–608

76 Herrlich A, Mayr A, Munz E (1956) Antibody picture of variola vaccine infection. I. Varying antibody formation in the vaccine infection of rabbits, monkeys and humans. *Zentralbl Bakteriol [Orig]* 166: 73–83

77 Kempe CH, Benenson AS (1953) Vaccinia; passive immunity in newborn infants. I. Placental transmission of antibodies. II. Response to vaccinations. *J Pediatr* 42: 525–531

78 Hammarlund E, Lewis MW, Hansen SG, Strelow LI, Nelson JA, Sexton GJ, Hanifin JM, Slifka MK (2003) Duration of antiviral immunity after smallpox vaccination. *Nat Med* 9: 1131–1137

79 Crotty S, Felgner P, Davies H, Glidewell J, Villarreal L, Ahmed R (2003) Cutting edge: long-term B cell memory in humans after smallpox vaccination. *J Immunol* 171: 4969–4973

80 Barbero GJ, Gray A, Scott TF, Kempe CH (1955) Vaccinia gangrenosa treated with hyperimmune vaccinal gamma globulin. *Pediatrics* 16: 609–618

81 Kempe CH, Berge TO, England B (1956) Hyperimmune vaccinal gamma globulin; source, evaluation, and use in prophylaxis and therapy. *Pediatrics* 18: 177–188

82 Kempe CH, Bowles C, Meiklejohn G, Berge TO, St Vincent L, Babu BV, Govindarajan S, Ratnakannan NR, Downie AW, Murthy VR (1961) The use of vaccinia hyperimmune gamma-globulin in the prophylaxis of smallpox. *Bull World Health Organ* 25: 41–48

83 Marennikova SS (1962) The use of hyperimmune antivaccinia gamma-globulin for the prevention and treatment of smallpox. *Bull World Health Organ* 27: 325–330

84 Peirce ER, Melville FS, Downie AW, Duckworth MJ (1958) Anti-vaccinial gamma-globulin in smallpox prophylaxis. *Lancet* 2: 635–638

85 Sharp JC, Fletcher WB (1973) Experience of anti-vaccinia immunoglobulin in the United Kingdom. *Lancet* 1: 656–659
86 Hopkins RJ, Lane JM (2004) Clinical efficacy of intramuscular vaccinia immune globulin: a literature review. *Clin Infect Dis* 39: 819–826
87 Kempe CH (1960) Studies on smallpox and complications of smallpox vaccination. *Pediatrics* 26: 176–189
88 Neff JM, Lane JM, Pert JH, Moore R, Millar JD, Henderson DA (1967) Complications of smallpox vaccination. I. National survey in the United States, 1963. *N Engl J Med* 276: 125–132
89 Appleyard G, Hapel AJ, Boulter EA (1971) An antigenic difference between intracellular and extracellular rabbitpox virus. *J Gen Virol* 13: 9–17
90 Belyakov IM, Earl P, Dzutsev A, Kuznetsov VA, Lemon M, Wyatt LS, Snyder JT, Ahlers JD, Franchini G, Moss B, Berzofsky JA (2003) Shared modes of protection against poxvirus infection by attenuated and conventional smallpox vaccine viruses. *Proc Natl Acad Sci USA* 100: 9458–9463
91 Czerny CP, Mahnel H (1990) Structural and functional analysis of orthopoxvirus epitopes with neutralizing monoclonal antibodies. *J Gen Virol* 71: 2341–2352
92 Edghill-Smith Y, Golding H, Manischewitz J, King LR, Scott D, Bray M, Nalca A, Hooper JW, Whitehouse CA, Schmitz JE, Reimann KA, Franchini G (2005) Smallpox vaccine-induced antibodies are necessary and sufficient for protection against monkeypox virus. *Nat Med* 11: 740–747
93 Galmiche MC, Goenaga J, Wittek R, Rindisbacher L (1999) Neutralizing and protective antibodies directed against vaccinia virus envelope antigens. *Virology* 254: 71–80
94 Jackson TM, Zaman SN, Huq F (1977) T and B rosetting lymphocytes in the blood of smallpox patients. *Am J Trop Med Hyg* 26: 517–519
95 O'Connel CJ, Karzon DT, Barron AL, Plaut ME, Ali VM (1964) Progressive vaccinia with normal antibodies. A case possibly due to deficient cellular immunity. *Ann Intern Med* 60: 282–289
96 Redfield RR, Wright DC, James WD, Jones TS, Brown C, Burke DS (1987) Disseminated vaccinia in a military recruit with human immunodeficiency virus (HIV) disease. *N Engl J Med* 316: 673–676
97 Amara RR, Nigam P, Sharma S, Liu J, Bostik V (2004) Long-lived poxvirus immunity, robust CD4 help, and better persistence of CD4 than CD8 T cells. *J Virol* 78: 3811–3816
98 Combadiere B, Boissonnas A, Carcelain G, Lefranc E, Samri A, Bricaire F, Debre P, Autran B (2004) Distinct time effects of vaccination on long-term proliferative and IFN-gamma-producing T cell memory to smallpox in humans. *J Exp Med* 199: 1585–1593
99 Ennis FA, Cruz J, Demkowicz WE Jr, Rothman AL, McClain DJ (2002) Primary induction of human $CD8^+$ cytotoxic T lymphocytes and interferon-gamma-producing T cells after smallpox vaccination. *J Infect Dis* 185: 1657–1659
100 Hsieh SM, Pan SC, Chen SY, Huang PF, Chang SC (2004) Age distribution for T cell reactivity to vaccinia virus in a healthy population. *Clin Infect Dis* 38: 86–89

101 Littaua RA, Takeda A, Cruz J, Ennis FA (1992) Vaccinia virus-specific human $CD4^+$ cytotoxic T-lymphocyte clones. *J Virol* 66: 2274–2280

102 Abate G, Eslick J, Newman FK, Frey SE, Belshe RB, Monath TP, Hoft DF (2005) Flow-cytometric detection of vaccinia-induced memory effector CD4(+), CD8(+), and gamma delta TCR(+) T cells capable of antigen-specific expansion and effector functions. *J Infect Dis* 192: 1362–1371

103 von Herrath MG, Yokoyama M, Dockter J, Oldstone MB Whitton JL (1996) CD4-deficient mice have reduced levels of memory cytotoxic T lymphocytes after immunization and show diminished resistance to subsequent virus challenge. *J Virol* 70: 1072–1079

104 Janssen EM, Lemmens EE, Wolfe T, Christen U, von Herrath MG, Schoenberger SP (2003) $CD4^+$ T cells are required for secondary expansion and memory in $CD8^+$ T lymphocytes. *Nature* 421: 852–856

105 Shedlock DJ, Shen H (2003) Requirement for CD4 T cell help in generating functional CD8 T cell memory. *Science* 300: 337–339

106 Sun JC, Bevan MJ (2003) Defective CD8 T cell memory following acute infection without CD4 T cell help. *Science* 300: 339–342

107 Sun JC, Williams MA, Bevan MJ (2004) $CD4^+$ T cells are required for the maintenance, not programming, of memory $CD8^+$ T cells after acute infection. *Nat Immunol* 5: 927–933

108 Appleyard G, Andrews C (1974) Neutralizing activities of antisera to poxvirus soluble antigens. *J Gen Virol* 23: 197–200

109 Law M, Smith GL (2001) Antibody neutralization of the extracellular enveloped form of vaccinia virus. *Virology* 280: 132–142

110 Bell E, Shamim M, Whitbeck JC, Sfyroera G, Lambris JD, Isaacs SN (2004) Antibodies against the extracellular enveloped virus B5R protein are mainly responsible for the EEV neutralizing capacity of vaccinia immune globulin. *Virology* 325: 425–431

111 Lustig S, Fogg C, Whitbeck JC, Moss B (2004) Synergistic neutralizing activities of antibodies to outer membrane proteins of the two infectious forms of vaccinia virus in the presence of complement. *Virology* 328: 30–35

112 Demkowicz WE, Maa JS, Esteban M (1992) Identification and characterization of vaccinia virus genes encoding proteins that are highly antigenic in animals and are immunodominant in vaccinated humans. *J Virol* 66: 386–398

113 Hsiao JC, Chung CS, Chang W (1999) Vaccinia virus envelope D8L protein binds to cell surface chondroitin sulfate and mediates the adsorption of intracellular mature virions to cells. *J Virol* 73: 8750–8761

114 Ichihashi Y, Oie M (1996) Neutralizing epitope on penetration protein of vaccinia virus. *Virology* 220: 491–494

115 Wolffe EJ, Vijaya S, Moss B (1995) A myristylated membrane protein encoded by the vaccinia virus L1R open reading frame is the target of potent neutralizing monoclonal antibodies. *Virology* 211: 53–63

116 Lin CL, Chung CS, Heine HG, Chang W (2000) Vaccinia virus envelope H3L protein binds to cell surface heparan sulfate and is important for intracellular mature virion morphogenesis and virus infection *in vitro* and *in vivo*. *J Virol* 74: 3353–3365

117 Rodriguez JF, Janeczko R, Esteban M (1985) Isolation and characterization of neutralizing monoclonal antibodies to vaccinia virus. *J Virol* 56: 482–488
118 Doolan DL, Southwood S, Freilich DA, Sidney J, Graber NL, Shatney L, Bebris L, Florens L, Dobano C, Witney AA et al (2003) Identification of *Plasmodium falciparum* antigens by antigenic analysis of genomic and proteomic data. *Proc Natl Acad Sci USA* 100: 9952–9957
119 Parker KC, Bednarek MA, Hull LK, Utz U, Cunningham B, Zweerink HJ, Biddison WE, Coligan JE (1992) Sequence motifs important for peptide binding to the human MHC class I molecule, HLA-A2. *J Immunol* 149: 3580–3587
120 Parker KC, Bednarek MA, Coligan JE (1994) Scheme for ranking potential HLA-A2 binding peptides based on independent binding of individual peptide side-chains. *J Immunol* 152: 163–175
121 Rammensee H, Bachmann J, Emmerich NP, Bachor OA, Stevanovic S (1999) SYFPEITHI: database for MHC ligands and peptide motifs. *Immunogenetics* 50: 213–219
122 Drexler I, Staib C, Kastenmuller W, Stevanovic S, Schmidt B, Lemonnier FA, Rammensee HG, Busch DH, Bernhard H, Erfle V, Sutter G (2003) Identification of vaccinia virus epitope-specific HLA-A*0201-restricted T cells and comparative analysis of smallpox vaccines. *Proc Natl Acad Sci USA* 100: 217–222
123 Terajima M, Cruz J, Raines G, Kilpatrick ED, Kennedy JS, Rothman AL, Ennis FA (2003) Quantitation of $CD8^+$ T cell responses to newly identified HLA-A*0201-restricted T cell epitopes conserved among vaccinia and variola (smallpox) viruses. *J Exp Med* 197: 927–932
124 Snyder JT, Belyakov IM, Dzutsev A, Lemonnier F, Berzofsky JA (2004) Protection against lethal vaccinia virus challenge in HLA-A2 transgenic mice by immunization with a single $CD8^+$ T-cell peptide epitope of vaccinia and variola viruses. *J Virol* 78: 7052–7060
125 Oseroff C, Kos F, Bui HH, Peters B, Pasquetto V, Glenn J, Palmore T, Sidney J, Tscharke DC, Bennink JR et al (2005) HLA class I-restricted responses to vaccinia recognize a broad array of proteins mainly involved in virulence and viral gene regulation. *Proc Natl Acad Sci USA* 102: 13980–13985
126 Pasquetto V, Bui HH, Giannino R, Mirza F, Sidney J, Oseroff C, Tscharke DC, Irvine K, Bennink JR, Peters B et al (2005) HLA-A*0201, HLA-A*1101, and HLA-B*0702 transgenic mice recognize numerous poxvirus determinants from a wide variety of viral gene products. *J Immunol* 175: 5504–5515
127 Mathew A, Terajima M, West K, Green S, Rothman AL, Ennis FA, Kennedy JS (2005) Identification of murine poxvirus-specific $CD8^+$ CTL epitopes with distinct functional profiles. *J Immunol* 174: 2212–2219
128 Tscharke DC, Karupiah G, Zhou J, Palmore T, Irvine KR, Haeryfar SM, Williams S, Sidney J, Sette A, Bennink JR, Yewdell JW (2005) Identification of poxvirus CD8+ T cell determinants to enable rational design and characterization of smallpox vaccines. *J Exp Med* 201: 95–104
129 Jenner E (1798) *An inquiry into the causes and effects of the variolae vaccinae, a disease discovered in some of the western counties of England, particularly Gloucestershire, and known by the name of the cow pox, London Classics of medicine and surgery*. Dover, New York, 213–240

130 Jezek Z, Fenner F (1988) *Human Monkeypox. Monographs in Virology,* No. 17. Karger, Basel

131 Mack TM, Noble J Jr, Thomas DB (1972) A prospective study of serum antibody and protection against smallpox. *Am J Trop Med Hyg* 21: 214–218

132 Sarkar JK, Mitra AC, Mukherjee MK (1975) The minimum protective level of antibodies in smallpox. *Bull World Health Organ* 52: 307–311

133 Stienlauf S, Shoresh M, Solomon A, Lublin-Tennenbaum T, Atsmon Y, Meirovich Y, Katz E (1999) Kinetics of formation of neutralizing antibodies against vaccinia virus following re-vaccination. *Vaccine* 17: 201–204

134 Moller-Larsen A, Haahr S (1978) Humoral and cell-mediated immune responses in humans before and after revaccination with vaccinia virus. *Infect Immun* 19: 34–39

135 Viner KM, Isaacs SN (2005) Activity of vaccinia virus-neutralizing antibody in the sera of smallpox vaccinees. *Microbes Infect* 7: 579–583

136 Orr N, Forman M, Marcus H, Lustig S, Paran N, Grotto I, Klement E, Yehezkelli Y, Robin G, Reuveny S et al (2004) Clinical and immune responses after revaccination of Israeli adults with the Lister strain of vaccinia virus. *J Infect Dis* 190: 1295–1302

137 Moller-Larsen A, Haahr S, Heron I (1978) Lymphocyte-mediated cytotoxicity in humans during revaccination with vaccinia virus. *Infect Immun* 21: 687–695

138 Monath TP, Caldwell JR, Mundt W, Fusco J, Johnson CS, Buller M, Liu J, Gardner B, Downing G, Blum PS et al (2004) ACAM2000 clonal Vero cell culture vaccinia virus (New York City Board of Health strain) – a second-generation smallpox vaccine for biological defense. *Int J Infect Dis* 8 (Suppl 2): S31–S44

139 Artenstein AW, Johnson C, Marbury TC, Morrison D, Blum PS, Kemp T, Nichols R, Balser JP, Currie M, Monath TP (2005) A novel, cell culture-derived smallpox vaccine in vaccinia-naive adults. *Vaccine* 23: 3301–3309

140 Greenberg RN, Kennedy JS, Clanton DJ, Plummer EA, Hague L, Cruz J, Ennis FA, Blackwelder WC, Hopkins RJ (2005) Safety and immunogenicity of new cell-cultured smallpox vaccine compared with calf-lymph derived vaccine: a blind, single-centre, randomised controlled trial. *Lancet* 365: 398–409

141 Drexler I, Staib C, Sutter G (2004) Modified vaccinia virus Ankara as antigen delivery system: how can we best use its potential? *Curr Opin Biotechnol* 15: 506–512

142 Carroll MW, Moss B (1997) Host range and cytopathogenicity of the highly attenuated MVA strain of vaccinia virus: propagation and generation of recombinant viruses in a nonhuman mammalian cell line. *Virology* 238: 198–211

143 Staib C, Kisling S, Erfle V, Sutter G (2005) Inactivation of the viral interleukin 1beta receptor improves $CD8^+$ T-cell memory responses elicited upon immunization with modified vaccinia virus Ankara. *J Gen Virol* 86: 1997–2006

144 Blanchard TJ, Alcami A, Andrea P, Smith GL (1998) Modified vaccinia virus Ankara undergoes limited replication in human cells and lacks several immunomodulatory proteins: implications for use as a human vaccine. *J Gen Virol* 79: 1159–1167

145 Antoine G, Scheiflinger F, Dorner F, Falkner FG (1998) The complete genomic sequence of the modified vaccinia Ankara strain: comparison with other orthopoxviruses. *Virology* 244: 365–396

146 Werner GT, Jentzsch U, Metzger E, Simon J (1980) Studies on poxvirus infections in irradiated animals. *Arch Virol* 64: 247–256
147 Mayr A, Stickl H, Muller HK, Danner K, Singer H (1978) The smallpox vaccination strain MVA: marker, genetic structure, experience gained with the parenteral vaccination and behavior in organisms with a debilitated defence mechanism (author's transl). *Zentralbl Bakteriol B* 167: 375–390
148 Hochstein-Mintzel V, Hanichen T, Huber HC, Stickl H (1975) An attenuated strain of vaccinia virus (MVA). Successful intramuscular immunization against vaccinia and variola (author's transl). *Zentralbl Bakteriol [Orig A]* 230: 283–297
149 Meseda CA, Garcia AD, Kumar A, Mayer AE, Manischewitz J, King LR, Golding H, Merchlinsky M, Weir JP (2005) Enhanced immunogenicity and protective effect conferred by vaccination with combinations of modified vaccinia virus Ankara and licensed smallpox vaccine Dryvax in a mouse model. *Virology* 339: 164–175
150 Hashizume S, Yoshizawa H, Morita M, Suzuki K (1985) Properties of Attenuated Mutant of Vaccinia Virus, LC16m8, Derived from the Lister Strain. In: G Quinnan (ed): *Vaccinia viruses as vectors for vaccine antigens*. Elsevier, New York, 87–99
151 Takahashi-Nishimaki F, Funahashi S, Miki K, Hashizume S, Sugimoto M (1991) Regulation of plaque size and host range by a vaccinia virus gene related to complement system proteins. *Virology* 181: 158–164
152 Yamaguchi M, Kimura M, Hirayama M (1975) Report of the National Smallpox Vaccination Research Committee: study of side effects, complications and their treatments. *Clin Virol* 3: 269–278 (in Japanese)
153 Empig C, Kenner JR, Perret-Gentil M, Youree BE, Bell E, Chen A, Gurwith M, Higgins K, Lock M, Rice AD et al (2005) Highly attenuated smallpox vaccine protects rabbits and mice against pathogenic orthopoxvirus challenge. *Vaccine* 24: 3686–3694
154 Boulter EA, Zwartouw HT, Titmuss DH, Maber HB (1971) The nature of the immune state produced by inactivated vaccinia virus in rabbits. *Am J Epidemiol* 94: 612–620
155 Lai CF, Gong SC, Esteban M (1991) The purified 14-kilodalton envelope protein of vaccinia virus produced in *Escherichia coli* induces virus immunity in animals. *J Virol* 65: 5631–5635
156 Law M, Putz MM, Smith GL (2005) An investigation of the therapeutic value of vaccinia-immune IgG in a mouse pneumonia model. *J Gen Virol* 86: 991–1000
157 Hooper JW, Custer DM, Thompson E (2003) Four-gene-combination DNA vaccine protects mice against a lethal vaccinia virus challenge and elicits appropriate antibody responses in nonhuman primates. *Virology* 306: 181–195
158 Hooper JW, Thompson E, Wilhelmsen C, Zimmerman M, Ichou MA, Steffen SE, Schmaljohn CS, Schmaljohn AL, Jahrling PB (2004) Smallpox DNA vaccine protects nonhuman primates against lethal monkeypox. *J Virol* 78: 4433–4443
159 Fogg C, Lustig S, Whitbeck JC, Eisenberg RJ, Cohen GH, Moss B (2004) Protective immunity to vaccinia virus induced by vaccination with multiple recombinant outer membrane proteins of intracellular and extracellular virions. *J Virol* 78: 10230–10237

Poxviruses
ed. by Andrew A. Mercer, Axel Schmidt and Olaf Weber

Poxvirus diagnostics

Martin Pfeffer and Hermann Meyer

Bundeswehr Institute of Microbiology, Neuherbergstr. 11, 80937 München, Germany

Abstract

Members of the family *Poxviridae* form a large group of viruses that can infect humans as well as animals including the major domestic animal species (cattle, sheep, goat, swine, dog, cat and chicken). Poxviruses can be highly pathogenic for humans (i.e., *Variola virus*), of zoonotic importance (e.g., *Monkeypox virus*) or highly contagious among animal populations (e.g., *Sheeppox virus*). Therefore, laboratory confirmation of the specific poxvirus involved is, indeed, essential. This is especially true for the most notorious member, *Variola virus*, the smallpox virus, which might reemerge as a weapon, and also for those "exotic" poxviruses which are absent in many countries but still enzootic in other parts of the world. Today, poxvirus diagnostics covers the entire spectrum of either traditional (such as inoculation of embryonated eggs) or more advanced laboratory tests (such as genome sequencing or microarray assays). This chapter presents methods of sample collection and handling, and reviews techniques used in the diagnosis of poxvirus infections by briefly describing the principle and procedure of the method, and critically weighting the pros and cons as well as providing some examples of application for each method.

Introduction

Specific diagnosis of poxviruses can be achieved by one of three procedures: (i) isolation and characterization of the causative agent, (ii) direct demonstration of virions, viral antigens, or viral nucleic acids in tissues, secretions or excretions, and (iii) detection and measurement of antibodies. Each group of methods has its place depending on the specific needs.

Historically, biological properties of the causative agent have been used to identify and differentiate poxviruses: although growth characteristics in tissue cultures or embryonated chicken eggs may allow specific identification of a particular poxvirus, these techniques are labor- and time-consuming, and require a high level of skills and expertise.

For decades now, electron microscopy has become a first-line technique allowing a fast identification of poxvirus particles. However, an identification of the respective genus or even the species involved is usually not possible because of their similar morphology. Poxvirus genera can be identified and differentiated by virus neutralization tests (NTs) with hyperimmune sera: within a given genus, poxviruses are antigenically closely related so that serological tests are insufficiently discriminatory to distinguish between the species.

Nowadays, polymerase chain reaction (PCR) is regarded as the method of choice for a fast, sensitive and specific identification. Various target regions on the viral genome have been investigated and different approaches have been made to verify authenticity of the amplicons. Among these, nucleotide sequencing or rather the use of specific fluorogenic DNA probes in real-time PCR assays are the methods of choice today. In particular, sequencing allows comparison with existing data and thus enables molecular epidemiological and evolutionary studies. On the other hand, viral DNA can be quantified in real-time PCR assays and – given the proper design of an assay – a further differentiation of species in a generic test is feasible. Various methods have been employed for poxvirus serology over the years, but only virus neutralization in tissue cultures and enzyme-linked immunosorbent assays (ELISAs) are suitable in terms of sensitivity and specificity to be used in retrospective analyses of poxvirus infections.

As with any other viral disease, poxvirus diagnostic methods should fulfill five criteria: speed, simplicity, sensitivity, specificity and low cost. In contrast to other viruses there is a lack of commercially available standardized diagnostic tests and reagents for poxvirus diagnostics.

Sample collection and handling

Before taking samples, careful consideration should be given to the purpose for which they are required. This will determine the type and number of samples needed. Mostly, a combination of blood samples for serology and tissues/scabs/vesicle fluids for virus isolation, antigen detection and pathological examination will be required. Whenever handling such biological material from either live or dead animals, the risk of zoonotic disease should be kept in mind. Arrangements should be made for appropriate safe disposal of animal carcasses and tissues (for example see www.cdc.gov/ncidod/monkeypox/diagspecimens.htm and ditto/necropsy.htm). In case of vesicular lesions, affected epithelial tissue should be sampled aseptically and placed in buffer. Additionally, vesicular fluids should be aspirated with a syringe and placed in a separate sterile tube without any buffer. Blood samples may sometimes be taken for culture, in which case anticoagulants, such as ethylenediamine tetraacetic acid (EDTA) or heparin are necessary. In most cases blood samples will be taken for serology, which requires serum. To establish the significance of antibody titers, paired serum samples will often need to be collected 7–14 days apart. An alternative method for collecting and transporting blood is to place a drop of blood onto filter paper, the blood is dried at room temperature and the sample can then be shipped unrefrigerated.

In any case it is crucial that individual samples are clearly identified using appropriate methods. The necessary information and the case history should be placed in a plastic envelope on the outside of the shipping container and also inside the shipping container (www.hms.Harvard.edu/orsp/coms/BiosafetyResources/Shipping-Regulations-Explaned.pdf).

A complete case history, also listing the suspected disease and the requested tests would be beneficial. It is advisable to contact the receiving laboratory to determine if it has a submission form that it would like to have submitted along with the samples or if other information, any special packaging or shipping requirements are needed. A special import permit will usually be required for shipment of any biological material to other countries. It must be obtained in advance and placed in an envelope on the outside of the parcel. Shipments must be made in accordance with the dangerous goods rules for the particular mode of transport. Air transport has to be arranged according to the International Air Transport Association (IATA) Dangerous Goods Regulations. The shipper is responsible for checking and following these guidelines. The specimens should be forwarded to the laboratory by the fastest method available. If they may not reach the laboratory within 48 h, samples should be sent refrigerated. If dry ice is used, the additional packaging requirements must be met. In some countries, there are similar requirements for ground shipments and postal services, these requirements should be reviewed before shipping, especially since they are a frequent subject of sometimes important changes (see also: www.cdc.gov/od/ohs/biosfty/bmbl4/b4ac.htm).

Morphological methods

Electron microscopy

Electron microscopy is regarded as the first-line method for laboratory diagnosis of poxvirus infections, because of the typical morphology of the virion and a usually high amount of particles present in poxvirus-induced lesions. After transmission electron microscopy became a standard method in diagnostic virology in the 1950s, it was widely used during the smallpox eradication era. Because the clinical diagnosis of a poxvirus infection, particularly in humans, is now infrequent, electron microscopy observations may provide one of the first clues to the cause of an unknown rash illness today [1, 2].

All poxvirus genera other than parapoxviruses (e.g., ortho-, capri-, avi-, lepori-, swine-, yata- and molluscipoxviruess) share a brick-shaped virion morphology, which is irregularly covered with short tubular elements resembling small stretches of tape. The size may vary from 250 nm × 290 nm up to 280 nm × 350 nm. In sheep and goats, two poxviruses might cause disease: capripoxviruses, causing sheep- and goatpox, and a parapoxvirus, *Orf virus*, causing contagious pustular dermatitis. Both clinical entities can be easily differentiated by electron microscopy: the virions of capripoxviruses are indistinguishable from the other poxvirus genera, whereas the virions of parapoxviruses are smaller (140 nm × 170 nm up to 220 nm × 300 nm), oval in shape, and each is covered in a single continuous tubular element, which appears as striations over the virion.

Although poxviruses cannot be morphologically distinguished to the genus level, they are easily separated from herpesviruses, which are important differential diagnoses in affected humans (e.g., chickenpox caused by varicella zoster virus), in mammals (e.g., pseudo-lumpy skin disease caused by *Bovine herpesvirus 2*) or in birds (e.g., infectious laryngotracheitis caused by *Gallid herpesvirus 1*).

Because poxviruses are tightly associated within the cellular matrix, samples have to be properly prepared to allow their examination by electron microscopy [3]. Scabbed or minced material from lesions or neoplasia (fowlpox) can be ground in a mortar with sterile sand or pulverized after being frozen in liquid nitrogen. Commercially available systems (lysing matrices in combination with bead beater or mixing mills) are of advantage as they allow standardization of the procedure. Alternatively, the steel shot method using BB-sized shots can be applied on a common laboratory vortex. It has to be taken into account that these treatments produce kinetic energy that may lead to heat-inactivation of the virus, which is not relevant for electron microscopy, but may interfere with attempts to isolate virus in cell cultures. After this initial step, two cycles of freeze-thawing and/or a sonicating step (30 s at 80 Hz) facilitate disruption of cells and will further enhance release of virions. After centrifugation of the slurry (1000 g for 2 min), a drop of the supernatant is placed on the grid. This grid can be either activated with pileoform-carbon substrate by glow discharge in pentylamine vapor, or by covering with poly-L-lysine. Alternatively, a drop of the supernatant can be placed on parafilm for the activated grid to float on. After 2–5 min at room temperature the grid is dipped briefly into a drop of Tris-EDTA buffer (10 mM/1 mM; pH 7.8) and then covered with a drop of 1% or 2% phosphotungstic acid (in sterile water, pH 7.2). After 10–100 s, the fluid is removed using filter paper, air-dried and placed in the electron microscope. With this so-called negative staining, the electron beams penetrate the virion, but surface structures will be visible by the contrast of the embracing electron-dense tungsten that appears black.

A minimum of 10^5 virus particles is required for the diagnosis, and, as mentioned earlier, a particular virus species cannot be differentiated.

Preparation and examination of samples requires patience and experience. Even when brick-shaped poxvirus particles are found rather quickly, it is worthwhile examining the sample further, because additional viruses might be present. Simultaneous infections of camels with both, orthopox- and parapoxviruses, have been described [4]. Depending on the number of particles, it may need up to 30 min for examination, so that electron microscopy can yield results within 2 h after receipt of the samples.

Histology and inclusion bodies

Infections with poxviruses are often associated with cutaneous or diphtheritic lesions that temporarily consist of epithelial hyperplasia, but some of the poxviruses of interest, i.e., various avipoxviruses, *Orf virus* and *Molluscum contagiosum virus*, can induce neoplasias with a tumor-like tissue texture. In particular, cells infected by *Molluscum contagiosum virus* are hypertrophied and contain acidophilic masses called molluscum bodies. These consist of a sponge-like matrix with masses of viral particles.

Conventional hematoxylin and eosin (HE) staining (alternatively acridine orange or Giemsa stains) of thin sections of the skin eruptions is useful to judge the histomorphology of the affected tissues. In affected cells, poxviruses induce round or oval inclusion bodies, called Guarnieri's bodies. Guarnieri's bodies are slightly basophilic and are composed of viral particles and proteins; each body is the locus of viral replication and assembly. In addition, some poxviruses induce a second type of cytoplasmic inclusion bodies, which are acidophilic, so-called acidophilic-type inclusion (ATI) bodies. These inclusions exclusively appear in the cytoplasm and thus allow differentiation to other virus infections with intranuclear inclusion bodies, as can be found, for example, in herpesvirus-infected cells. All orthopoxviruses contain the gene coding for the ATI body protein. However, due to deletions in the respective open reading frames, visible ATIs are only found in cowpox virus- and mousepox virus-infected cells [5, 6]. This feature, the formation of ATI, is still used as a pathognomic marker to differentiate cowpox virus infections from other human orthopoxvirus infections, such as caused by *Variola*, *Vaccinia* or *Monkeypox virus*. *Sheeppox virus* and *Goatpox virus* also produce large intracytoplasmic inclusion bodies. In fowlpox virus-infected epithelial cells, the large intracytoplasmic inclusion bodies are called Bollinger bodies and contain smaller elementary bodies (Borrel bodies). The inclusions appear red, are approximately 0.2–0.3 μm in size and can be demonstrated in sections of cutaneous and/or smears of diphtheritic lesions using HE, acridine orange, Sudan red or Giemsa stains [7]. Borrel bodies appear red, while the remaining tissue stays in the counterstained malachite green.

Biological methods

Virus isolation in chick embryos and animals

The use of chick embryos for poxvirus diagnostics was first described in 1937 [8] and since then has become a valuable tool in poxvirus diagnostics. The only human poxviruses that produce pocks on the chorioallantoic membrane (CAM) of chicken eggs are four species of the genus *Orthopoxvirus* (*Variola virus*, *Monkeypox virus*, *Cowpox virus* and *Vaccinia virus*), whereas parapoxviruses, yatapoxviruses and molluscipoxviruses, which are also able to infect humans, do not form pocks. Differences in the pock morphology seen in 12-day-old embryos incubated at 34.5–35°C were useful in differentiating the orthopoxvirus species mentioned above and, consequently, the CAM assay was widely and successfully used during the smallpox eradication campaign: lesion material of suspected smallpox patients was inoculated onto the CAM and following inspection of the pock morphology the causative agent could be identified as either *Variola virus*, *Cowpox virus* or *Vaccinia virus* and the respective measures could be applied [2]. As a result of international collaboration under the WHO eradication program, smallpox was declared eradicated in 1980. Nevertheless, *Variola virus* is considered to be a potential biowarfare agent or terrorist weapon due to a high morbidity and mortality and because much of the human population is now susceptible after cessation of routine smallpox vaccination. Taking into account the serious consequences of the diagnosis "smallpox" or even the consequences of a misdiagnosis, there is a need to unambiguously, rapidly and reliably identify smallpox and to differentiate it from other similar clinical entities. In this context rapid molecular techniques have been developed recently that have replaced the rather time-consuming and experience-requiring CAM assay.

Other poxviruses that are capable of forming pocks are the avipox-, leporipox- and capripoxviruses. Especially for isolation of avipoxviruses the inoculation of the CAM is still the method of choice [9]. Approximately 0.1 ml of tissue suspension of skin or diphtheritic lesions, with the appropriate concentration of antibiotics, is inoculated onto the CAM of chicken embryos. These are further incubated at 37°C for 5–7 days, and then examined for focal white pock lesions or generalized thickening of the CAMs. Histopathological examination of the CAM lesions will reveal eosinophilic intracytoplasmic inclusion bodies following staining with HE in case of infection with avipoxvirues.

Inoculation of animals should be avoided since alternative methods are available for identification of the respective agent. Where all other methods have failed, it is an option to use the putative natural host animal to "isolate" virus. In the past, the intradermal inoculation of rabbits has been used to distinguish *Rabbit fibroma virus* (with its simple fibromatous local lesion) from *Myxoma virus* (capable of causing generalized infection in adult rabbits). In suspected cases of sheeppox and goatpox clarified biopsy preparation supernatants have also been used for intradermal inoculation into susceptible lambs to monitor for evidence of typical skin reactions.

Virus isolation in cultured cells

Despite new techniques allowing demonstration of virus, viral antigen, or viral nucleic acid in specimens taken directly from the patient or animal, it is still true that few of them achieve the sensitivity of virus isolation in cultured cells. Virus isolation remains the "gold standard" against which other/newer methods must be compared. Moreover, it can detect the unexpected, i.e., identify a totally unforeseen virus. This is especially of importance when biological samples (such as known vector or reservoir animals) are routinely screened for the presence of any virus they are capable to transmit. Finally, virus culture is the only method of producing a supply of live virus for further examination.

Although poxviruses grow satisfactorily in chick embryos, this is not commonly used because cell culture is generally the simpler option. Orthopoxviruses can be grown in a variety of established cell lines, including Vero, BSC-1, HeLa, chicken embryo fibroblasts, and MRC-5 human diploid fibroblast cells and a detectable cytopathic effect is seen within a day or two. To propagate *Fowlpox virus*, primary chicken embryo fibroblasts, chicken embryo kidney cells, chicken embryo dermal cells, or the permanent quail cell line QT-35 can be used [10]. For *Swinepox virus*, porcine kidney (PK15) cells, and for *Myxoma virus*, rabbit kidney (RK13) cells are the cell lines of choice.

The adaptation of virus strains to cell cultures is an important requirement to perform plaque reduction assay for the quantification of neutralizing antibodies. As not all strains will form plaques initially some rounds of "blind" passaging are needed before cytopathic effects become evident. Unfortunately, some poxviruses could not be adapted to a cell culture system thus far, e.g., *Molluscum contagiosum virus* or parapoxvirus of camels. Extended passaging often results in an attenuated phenotype for a given poxvirus and, by this approach, promising vaccine candidates have been obtained.

Serological methods for antigen detection

Enzyme-linked immunosorbent assay

Antigen-capture ELISAs for poxviruses are designed as sandwich assays with specific polyclonal (hyperimmune antiserum) or monoclonal antibody preparations immobilized on the bottom of microtiter plates for capturing the antigen. Detection is accomplished by use of hyperimmune sera raised against the respective poxvirus and an anti-IgG horseradish-peroxidase (POD) or alkaline phosphatase (AP) conjugate or – if available – with monoclonal antibodies and an anti-mouse-IgG-POD/AP conjugate. Washing steps are performed between incubations to avoid unspecific binding of antibodies and/or the POD conjugate. The reaction is rendered visible using a substrate. Results of an antigen-capture ELISA can be obtained usually within 3 h. Low costs, easy handling and a rather rapid performance makes the ELISA the method of choice in the field if fully equipped laboratory capabilities are out of reach. An antigen-capture ELISA has been described for orthopoxviruses [11] with a detection limit in the range of 10^4–10^5 $TCID_{50}$/ml. Thus, this assay is about ten times more sensitive than electron microscopy. An antigen-capture ELISA has also been described for capripoxviruses [12]. Both assays use genus-reactive reagents, thus allowing the detection of all poxviruses belonging to the respective genus, a differentiation of species is not possible. For leporipoxviruses, a radioimmunoassay can differentiate between strains of *Myxoma virus* [13].

Following the cloning of the highly antigenic capripoxvirus structural protein p32, the expressed recombinant antigen was used for the production of diagnostic reagents, including raising of p32 monospecific polyclonal antiserum and monoclonal antibodies. These reagents have facilitated the development of a highly specific ELISA for the detection of capripoxvirus antigen from biopsy suspensions or tissue culture supernatants [12].

Immunodiffusion

In agar gel diffusion, also called immunodiffusion assays, a sample suspected to contain viral antigen is placed in a well cut in agar opposite a similar well containing the respective antibody. The fluids diffuse towards each other and form a visible line of precipitation if the correct antigen is present. This assay was used for capripoxviruses (i.e., *Sheeppox virus*, *Goatpox virus*, and *Lumpy skin disease virus*). However, discrimination of the latter was only possible based on its different geographic distribution. Because of this lack of specificity as well as the cross-reaction with parapoxviruses, this test format was abandoned in favor of the p32 antigen-capture ELISA.

Immunohistochemistry and immunofluorescence assay

Viral antigen itself can be detected in affected tissues by immunohistochemistry. Usually the samples have been fixed in formalin and embedded in paraffin according to standard procedures. Otherwise, cryosections of approximately 3-μm thickness are cut and placed on glass slides. Deparaffinized and dehydrated sections are treated with H_2O_2 (3% in distilled water) for 5 min before washing with phosphate-buffered saline (PBS). Slides are incubated for 60 min at 37°C with a proper dilution of POD-conjugated specific polyclonal antibody. However, in most applications, specific staining is obtained when either polyclonal or monoclonal antibodies are used in an indirect test using a labeled second anti-species antibody conjugate. Various combinations of conjugate and substrate are commercially available, but the primary anti-poxvirus polyclonal or monoclonal antibodies may be not as easily purchased. In these cases the reference centers listed by the O.I.E. will help to provide the required reagents (www.oie.int). The most common procedures of immunohistological staining are adapted from the ABC technique described by Hsu et al. [14]. Results are normally obtained 2 days after receiving the samples. In addition to the diagnosis, immunohistochemistry is of particular interest for pathohistologists, because it visualizes the morphological changes induced by the virus and the distribution of poxviral antigen in the respective tissue layers. Another advantage of this method is that embedded tissue blocks can be investigated years after they have been made, thus making it suitable in retrospective studies. Further, sections can be examined with the light microscope and can be stored for an extended period without loss of color. The conjugate can also be labeled with fluorescein-isothiocyanate and the test performed as direct or, more likely, indirect immunofluorescence assay (IFA) to visualize the specific intracytoplasmic fluorescence. IFA can also be used for the identification of particular poxviruses after their isolation in cell culture. IFA is highly dependent on the quality of the specimen and should not be applied to scabs or other tissue samples showing the first stages of autolysis. In comparison with POD-labeled conjugate, the IFA is more sensitive and a few cells containing fluorescence of the right color and expected antigen distribution allow a firm diagnosis. However, IFA requires highly skilled personnel to examine the specimens, in particular when unspecific binding of the anti-poxvirus antibodies increases due to fading conditions of the sample.

DNA-based methods

The rapid development in nucleic acid research in recent years has facilitated many options of DNA-based detection methods in poxvirus diagnostics. Because sequencing techniques became automated and affordable, PCR, real-time PCR, microarrays and – to a lesser extent – genome sequencing are not restricted to a few dedicated laboratories any longer. However, we have to keep in mind that there may well be a difference between developing an assay *in silico* and a robust performance of the assay in practice. The best way to prove the specificity of an assay is to test it with as many strains as possible. DNA-based diagnostic procedures offer a high level of discrimination, which is often required for differentiating poxvirus species and strains. An appropriate starting point may be the analysis of restriction fragment length polymorphisms (RFLP).

Restriction fragment length polymorphism

The RFLP approach is based on the fact that the genomes of even closely related pathogens are defined by variation in sequence. Thus, the recognition sequence of a specific restriction enzyme in one genome may be absent in the genome of a closely related strain or isolate. In practice, the RFLP procedure consists of isolating the target virus, extracting DNA and then digesting the nucleic acid with one or a panel of restriction enzymes. The individual fragments within the digested DNA are then separated within an agarose gel by electrophoresis and visualized by staining with, for example, ethidium bromide. Ideally, each strain will reveal a unique pattern, or fingerprint. Many different restriction enzymes may be considered for a new setup, so that analyses of many molecular fingerprints from digestions with several individual restriction enzymes may be undertaken and combination of the best set of results will allow a comprehensive differentiation between strains or isolates.

RFLPs generated with *Hind*III have been used to investigate orthopoxvirus species [15, 16]. Naidoo et al. [17] were the first to confirm that the genomes of cowpox viruses isolated from cats in England are closely related to those originating from cows and their handlers. Minor differences found in the isolates did not correlate with the geographic origin of the strains. German cowpox viruses from cats, humans, elephants, and a cow were more variable, and seem to reflect a geographically independent evolution of these viruses in defined rodent reservoirs [18]. *Goatpox virus* and *Sheeppox virus* strains have been characterized by comparing the genome fragments generated by *Hind*III digestion. Differences have been identified between isolates from the different animal species, but these are not consistent and there is evidence for the movement of strains between species and recombination between strains in the field. Likewise, a differentiation of field isolates and vaccine strains of *Fowlpox virus* is possible.

However, RFLP of genomic DNA requires lengthy virus culture to generate suitable quantities of high quality DNA. To overcome these burdens, a modification to the basic RFLP technique has been applied whereby PCR is incorporated as a preliminary step to amplify a specific region of the genome (known to be variable in sequence between pathogens), which then serves as the template DNA for the RFLP technique.

PCR-RFLP offers a greater sensitivity for the identification of pathogens. PCR-RFLP was applied in an analysis of a panel of 45 variola viruses that were selected based on varied geographic distribution and year of isolation. Twenty consensus primer pairs were used to produce 20 overlapping amplicons, which cover 99.9% of the variola virus genome. Upon digestion with *Bst*UI or *Hpa*II the resulting patterns were compared. A composite dendrogram of all amplicon RFLP profiles differentiates variola major from variola minor, and the sub-clades within variola major were generally clustered according to their geographic location and/or epidemiological history. Likewise, less virulent *Monkeypox virus* strains from Western Africa could be separated from Central African strains using PCR-RFLP [19]. However, despite the impressive advances made with this technique, the pace of progress in DNA sequencing may circumvent its usefulness in the near future.

Polymerase chain reaction

PCR exploits natural DNA replication mechanisms and results in the production *in vitro* of large quantities of a desired sequence of DNA from a complex mixture of heterogeneous sequences. PCR can amplify a selected region of 50 to several thousand base pairs into billions of copies. Amplification of DNA is accomplished *via* a cyclic succession of incubation steps at different temperatures. These steps are repeated 30–40 times, resulting in the amplification of target DNA sequences. The key to the logarithmic amplification of target DNA sequences is the selection of paired primers that, when extended, will create additional reciprocal primer-annealing sites for primer extension in subsequent cycles. Any PCR product generated has, by definition, a characteristic size. Its identity is generally confirmed using DNA hybridization probes or restriction digests or more commonly *via* direct sequencing. The sensitivity of a PCR may be enhanced by the use of a second set of primers to amplify a sub-fragment from the PCR product of the first reaction. This technique is referred to as nested PCR; however, the use of nested PCR can increase the rate of false-positive results and thus should be avoided for routine diagnostics.

PCR is a highly sensitive procedure for detecting nucleic acid of an agent in host tissues and vectors, even when only a small number of host cells are infected. However, it does not differentiate between viable and nonviable organisms or incomplete pieces of genomic DNA, and this may complicate interpretation of results and affect the applicability of PCR in this role. When PCR is used for diagnosis, a great deal of care is required to avoid contamination of the samples because this can easily lead to false-positive results. Systems have been developed to deal with this problem, for example the dUTP-UNG system (desoxyuridine triphosphate and uracil-*N*-glycosylase). It is also important to control for potential 'negative' results caused by the presence of interfering substances in the PCR reaction mixture or patient's sample by the inclusion of a template known to produce a PCR product. Use of these precautions allows the PCR to become a realistic option for the diagnostician. PCRs have now been developed for the detection of almost any poxvirus. Its advantages in terms of speed, sensitivity and specificity have by far outreached the costs of the equipment needed, and procedures are in place to prevent the danger of contamination leading to false-positive results. Today, PCR is clearly the method of choice in poxvirus diagnostics. PCR protocols to identify and differentiate orthopoxviruses are available based on sequences of the hemagglutinin (HA), the cytokine response modifier B (crmB) or the A-type inclusion (ATI) protein gene [6, 20, 21]. In these assays, PCR is done using primers amplifying a sequence that is present in any orthopoxvirus. The amplicon is digested with an appropriate restriction enzyme and gel electrophoresis is used to discriminate species by comparison of the resulting patterns. On the other hand, when a large set of especially cowpox viruses was analyzed, heterogeneity of the restriction fragment patterns became evident, making interpretation of results rather ambiguous. A PCR assay has been described to detect the capripoxvirus sequences in biopsy or tissue culture samples relying on primers for the viral attachment protein gene and the viral fusion protein gene that are specific for capripoxvirus. The identity of resulting PCR products is confirmed using restriction enzyme recognition sites and a differentiation of *Sheeppox virus* and Lumpy skin virus is possible [22]. Differentiation of five avipoxvirus species was possible by use of PCR followed by nucleotide sequence analysis, which showed a nucleotide similarity of 72–100% among the different species [23]. PCR assays for analysis of clinical specimens have also been described for parapoxviruses, leporipoxviruses and molluscipoxviruses [24–26].

Real-time PCR

Conventional PCR methods are now being complemented and in some cases replaced with real-time PCR assays. Real-time PCR monitors the accumulation of the PCR product during the amplification reaction, thus enabling identification of the cycles during which near-logarithmic PCR product generation occurs. In other words, the assay can be used to reliably quantify the DNA content in a given sample. In contrast to conventional PCR, real-time PCR combines amplification and detection of target DNA in one vessel, thereby eliminating any time-consuming post-PCR procedures and, by this, decreasing the risk of cross-contamination. Real-time PCR is highly sensitive and specific, and provides quantitative information. The recent development of portable real-time PCR machines and assays raises the exciting prospect of these techniques being used for rapid (less than 2 h) diagnosis of disease outbreaks in the field.

The many advantages of the real-time PCR technique led to its introduction into the field of poxvirus diagnostics to rapidly and unambiguously identify smallpox and to differentiate it from other rash-causing illnesses [27–33]. A screening assay for real-time PCR identification of variola virus DNA was compiled in a kit system under ‘good manufacturing practice’ (GMP) conditions with standardized reagents [33]. A single nucleotide mismatch resulting in a unique amino acid substitution in smallpox virus was used to design a hybridization probe pair with a specific sensor probe that allows reliable differentiation of *Variola virus* from other orthopoxviruses *via* melting curve analysis. The applicability was demonstrated by successful amplification of 120 strains belonging to the *Orthopoxvirus* species *Variola virus*, *Vaccinia virus*, *Camelpox virus*, *Ectromelia virus*, *Cowpox virus* and *Monkeypox virus*. Nevertheless, it needs to be stressed that a positive *Variola virus* PCR result must be confirmed by amplifying other parts of the genome. Another recent application of real-time PCR was the development of an assay for the detection of *Tanapox virus* and *Yaba-like disease virus* [34].

Oligonucleotide microarray analysis

Recently, methods have been described to discern PCR-amplified, fluorescence-labeled DNA fragments by hybridization to orthopoxvirus species-specific DNA immobilized on a microchip [35, 36]. The assay described by Laassri et al. [36] detects and simultaneously discriminates between four orthopoxviruses species pathogenic for humans (*Variola virus*, *Vaccinia virus*, *Cowpox virus* and *Monkeypox virus*) and distinguishes them from chickenpox virus (varicella zoster virus (*Human herpes virus 3*)). To ensure redundancy and robustness the microchip contains several unique oligonucleotide probes specific for each virus species.

Sequencing

Sequencing of various PCR amplicons in a diagnostic setting enables allocation of a sample to known relatives after comparison with the respective data base. Sequences of the hemagglutinin gene of more than 120 orthopoxviruses are available and have been proven useful for phylogenetic studies. These studies confirm the current concept of established species within the genus orthopoxvirus, which historically was based on the different phenotype of the respective species.

Direct viral genome sequencing has become more important and has contributed to our understanding of poxvirus genome organization [37]. A total of 52 poxvirus genome sequences are accessible at www.poxvirus.org, representing all eight genera of the subfamily *Chordopoxvirinae*, including two major and one alastrim minor variola virus isolate. Genome sequencing was applied when a mild form of human monkeypox was first recognized outside Africa in 2003 during an outbreak in the USA. This outbreak was of major concern and the causative virus could be traced to imported monkeypox virus-infected West African rodents. In this context, genomic sequencing confirmed the existence of two clades of monkeypox virus and permitted prediction of viral proteins that could cause the observed differences in human pathogenicity [38]. Progress in sequencing technologies will certainly make this method a valuable forensic tool should smallpox reemerge, since this is the only way to clearly verify a deliberate release.

Serological methods for antibody detection

Although cell-mediated immune responses play an important role in poxvirus infections, and are believed to be crucial for long-term immunity, routine testing for T cell response is not convenient. Traditionally, serological testing in poxvirus diagnostics has focused on measuring the specific humoral immune responses only. However, antibodies are cross-reacting among members of each poxvirus genus, rendering serology nonspecific for a given virus species. Antibody detection has been performed mostly for orthopox- and capripoxviruses.

Neutralization test

In the NT, a fourfold rise in antibody titer between serum samples taken during acute and convalescent phases is usually considered positive for a poxvirus infection. A variety of serum neutralizing assays has been used to assess the antibody responses of humans and animals to *Vaccinia virus*. These assays include the use of pock formation on scarified rabbit skin, inoculation of the CAMs of embryonated chicken eggs, or determination of the cytopathic effect of serum-virus mixtures on primary rhesus monkey kidney tissue culture cells. Each of the aforementioned techniques is a variation of the plaque reduction neutralization test (PRNT). The PRNT has evolved from early methods using the scarification of rabbit skin further to CAM inoculation and then to the use of a variety of tissue culture systems. During its evolution, the PRNT has been dissected and reassembled numerous times using a variety of diluents, cell substrates, media, and incubation times and temperatures, but the principle of viewing the neutralizing effect of serum antibodies on a particular destructive viral effect remained. Most commonly, tissue cultures are used nowadays. A test serum can either be titrated against a constant titer of poxvirus or a standard virus strain can be titrated against a constant dilution of test serum to calculate a neutralization index. Usually, a serum is titrated against a fixed amount of viable virus which allows an easy readout in the cell culture system used. Thus, in 96-well plates or in a 24-well format the constant viral seed for each well is usually about 100 $TCID_{50}$ (50% tissue culture infective dose) or 50 PFU (plaque-forming units) depending on the counting system used. However, PFU will provide more accurate results, because all viable viruses are measured. Because of the variable sensitivity of tissue cultures to poxviruses, and the consequent difficulty of ensuring the use of the infectious dose, the neutralization index is the preferred method. This index is the log titer difference between the titer of the virus in the negative serum and in the test serum. An index greater than or equal to 1.5 is positive. To make sure that this index is statistically significant, the test has to be performed at least in quadruplicate and the results have to be calculated using a formula, e.g., the one developed by Kaerber [39]. After poxviruses have replicated within the cytoplasm of the cell, the progeny viruses infect the neighboring cells *via* cell-to-cell spread. Although the initially infected cell dies through programmed cell death, only a small fraction of the produced virus is released into the tissue culture medium. One effect of this centrifugal progression of lysing cells is the formation of visible plaques. In contrast to many other viruses, there is no need for the use of agarose or nitrocellulose overlays in plaque assays and consequently in the PRNT in poxvirus serology. As mentioned earlier, there is an extensive cross-reactivity within a given poxvirus genus. Although this hampers the specificity for the serological diagnosis, it has the advantage of choosing the least pathogenic member of a genus as antigen in the PRNT. This could be a vaccine strain or a member known to be incapable of human infections. Another feature of the PRNT should be kept in mind: in contrast to a simple antigen-antibody binding, as in an ELISA (see below) the PRNT provides biological information about the capability of a given serum to indeed neutralize virus. This makes the PRNT the method of choice when the success of vaccinations needs to be monitored.

Hemagglutination inhibition and agar gel immunodiffusion

Two techniques have been intensively used in the past because of their low cost and simple performance: hemagglutination inhibition (HI) and agar gel immunodiffusion. With both assays a secondary anti-species antibody is not required, making them suitable for antibody detection in any host species. Therefore, HI was the method of choice for screening mammalian blood samples in the search for natural reservoirs for *Monkeypox virus* and *Cowpox virus*. The principle is based on the existence of a hemagglutinin gene whose protein is capable of agglutinating erythrocytes of a particular animal species. Avipoxviruses, for example, agglutinate sheep and horse red blood cells, orthopoxviruses agglutinate chicken erythrocytes, whereas parapoxviruses do not agglutinate red blood cells. To demonstrate specific antibodies in a serum of interest, the serum (or dilutions thereof) is incubated with red blood cells and a certain amount of the respective poxviral antigen (usually four hemagglutinating units). If specific antibodies are present, they prevent agglutination of the virus and thus allow sedimentation of the red blood cells. The highest dilution of serum that inhibits the agglutination by the standardized amount of virus represents the hemagglutination titer of the serum.

HI is usually more sensitive but of the same poor specificity as agar gel immunodiffusion. The readout of the latter is the formation of a precipitation line or zone in solidified 1% agar where virus antigen and specific serum antibodies meet. The test material is positive if a precipitation line develops with the serum sample that is confluent with that produced by the positive control antigen. This assay has also been intensively used as a screening method for the diagnosis for avipoxviruses, orthopoxviruses and leporipoxviruses, but was abandoned because of its low sensitivity and the time required (2–3 days) before results are obtained.

Enzyme-linked immunosorbent assay

ELISAs are the serological assays of choice for the qualitative and quantitative determination of antibodies. Many in-house assays exist that rely on coating the wells of 96-well microtiter plates with the purified poxvirus of interest. Positive and negative sera are included and cutoff limits are calculated by the reactivity of the controls. ELISAs are preferably used in epidemiological studies or in surveillance programs for endemic and exotic diseases. A capripoxvirus antibody ELISA has been developed using the expressed structural protein p32 to circumvent the use of live capripoxvirus, which is not desirable in countries such as Australia where the virus is exotic. This ELISA was specific for capripoxvirus as only sera from sheep infected with capripoxvirus reacted with the capripoxvirus p32 antigen, thus overcoming the cross-reactions with sera from orf- or vaccinia virus-infected sheep [22].

A double-sandwich blocking-ELISA using a genus-specific neutralizing monoclonal antibody against the vaccinia virus 32-kDa adsorption protein can also be used in various animal species and human samples to detect orthopoxvirus-specific antibodies. The assay format is of advantage since no animal species-specific conjugates are needed. This assay was applied to 2173 feline serum samples and 2% reacted positive [40]. Recently, an orthopoxvirus-specific IgM assay was described and applied to determine acute-phase humoral immunity to *Monkeypox virus* in the 2003 US outbreak. IgM antibody detection allows a broader window for sample collection beyond the rash stage of illness, which is of advantage for demonstrating disease retrospectively and/or from remote locations [41].

Western blot assay

The Western blot assay is slow, expensive and technically demanding. However, this assay is regarded as a "gold standard" because of its capacity to identify antibodies to specific poxvirus proteins. This is of utmost importance especially in surveillance programs if suspected exotic poxvirus (i.e., capripoxvirus) infections have to be confirmed. The Western blot assay uses various antigens, including purified virus and sometimes the concentrate of culture fluid from infected cells. A Western blot has been described [22] using capripoxvirus-infected cell lysates. Positive test samples produce a pattern based on the reaction with the major structural proteins of capripoxvirus, whereas negative serum samples do not show such a pattern. Hyperimmune serum prepared against parapoxvirus reacts with some of the capripoxvirus proteins, but not with the 32-kDa protein that is specific for capripoxvirus.

References

1 Damon IK, Esposito JJ (2003) Poxviruses that infect humans. In: PR Murray, EJ Baron, JH Jorgensen, MA Pfaller, MH Yolker (eds): *Manual of clinical microbiology*, 8th edn. ASM Press, Washington DC, 1583-1591
2 Henderson DA, Inglesby TV, Bartlett JG, Ascher MS, Eitzen E, Jahrling PB, Hauer J, Layton M, McDade J, Osterholm TM et al (1999) Smallpox as a biological weapon: medical and public health management. Working Group on Civilian Biodefense. *JAMA* 281: 2127–2137
3 Hazelton PR, Gelderblom HR (2003) Electron microscopy for rapid diagnosis of infectious agents in emergent situations. *Emerg Infect Dis* 9: 294–303
4 Renner-Müller IC, Meyer H, Munz E (1995) Characterization of camelpoxvirus isolates from Africa and Asia. *Vet Microbiol* 45: 371–381
5 Downie AW (1939) A study of the lesions produced experimentally by cowpox virus. *J Pathol* 48: 361–378
6 Meyer H, Ropp SL, Esposito JJ (1997) Gene for A-type inclusion body protein is useful for a polymerase chain reaction assay to differentiate orthopoxviruses. *J Virol Methods* 64: 217–221
7 Tripathy DN, Hanson LE (1976) A smear technique for staining elementary bodies of fowlpox. *Avian Dis* 20: 609–610
8 Lazarus AS, Eddie A, Meyer KF (1937) Propagation of variola virus in the developing egg. *Proc Soc Exp Biol Med* 36: 7–8
9 Samour JH, Kaaden OR, Wernery U, Bailey TA (1996) An epornitic of avian pox in houbara bustards (*Chlamydotis undulata macqueenii*). *Zentralbl Veterinaermed* B 43: 287–292
10 Niikura M, Narita T, Mikami T (1991) Establishment and characterization of a thymidine kinase deficient avian fibroblast cell line derived from a Japanese quail cell line, QT35. *J Vet Med Sci* 53: 439–446
11 Czerny C-P, Meyer H, Mahnel H (1989) Establishment of an ELISA for the detection of orthopox viruses based on neutralizing monoclonal and polyclonal antibodies. *Zentralbl Veterinarmed* B 36: 537–546
12 Carn VM (1995) An antigen trapping ELISA for the detection of capripoxvirus in tissue culture supernatant and biopsy samples. *J Virol Methods* 51: 95–102
13 Bults HG, Brandon MR (1982) An immunological method to determine antigenic variation in three strains of myxoma virus. *J Virol Methods* 5: 21–26

14 Hsu SM, Raine L (1981) Protein A, avidin, and biotin in immunohistochemistry. *J Histochem Cytochem* 29: 1349–1353

15 Mackett M, Archard LC (1979) Conservation and variation in orthopoxvirus genome structure. *J Gen Virol* 45: 683–701

16 Esposito JJ, Knight JC (1985) Orthopoxvirus DNA: a comparison of restriction profiles and maps. *Virology* 143: 230–251

17 Naidoo J, Baxby D, Bennett M, Gaskell RM, Gaskell CJ (1992) Characterization of orthopoxviruses isolated from feline infections in Britain. *Arch Virol* 125: 261–272

18 Meyer H, Schay C, Mahnel H, Pfeffer M (1999) Characterization of orthopoxviruses isolated from man and animals in Germany. *Arch Virol* 144: 491–501

19 Neubauer H, Reischl U, Ropp S, Esposito JJ, Wolf H, Meyer H (1998) Specific detection of monkeypox virus by polymerase chain reaction. *J Virol Methods* 74: 201–207

20 Ropp SL, Jin Q, Knight JC, Massung RF, Esposito JJ (1995) PCR strategy for identification and differentiation of small pox and other orthopoxviruses. *J Clin Microbiol* 33: 2069–2076

21 Loparev VN, Massung RF, Esposito JJ, Meyer H (2001) Detection and differentiation of old world orthopoxviruses: restriction fragment length polymorphism of the crmB gene region. *J Clin Microbiol* 39: 94–100

22 Heine HG, Stevens MP, Foord AJ, Boyle DB (1999) A capripoxvirus detection PCR and antibody ELISA based on the major antigen P32, the homolog of the vaccinia virus H3L gene. *J Immunol Methods* 30: 187–196

23 Luschow D, Hoffmann T, Hafez HM (2004) Differentiation of avian poxvirus strains on the basis of nucleotide sequences of 4b gene fragment. *Avian Dis* 48: 453–462

24 Nunez A., Funes JM, Agromayor M, Moratilla M, Varas AJ, Lopez-Estebaranz JL, Esteban M, Martin-Gallardo A (1996) Detection and typing of molluscum contagiosum virus in skin lesions by using a simple lysis method and polymerase chain reaction. *J Med Virol* 50: 342–349

25 Thompson CH (1997) Identification and typing of molluscum contagiosum virus in clinical specimens by polymerase chain reaction. *J Med Virol* 53: 205–211

26 Torfason EG, Gunadottir S (2002) Polymerase chain reaction for laboratory diagnosis of orf virus infections. *J Clin Virol* 24: 79–84

27 Espy MJ, Cockerill IF, Meyer RF, Bowen MD, Poland GA, Hadfield TL, Smith TF (2002) Detection of smallpox virus DNA by LightCycler PCR. *J Clin Microbiol* 40: 1985–1988

28 Ibrahim MS, Esposito JJ, Jahrling PB, Lofts RS (1997) The potential of 5' nuclease PCR for detecting a single-base polymorphism in orthopoxvirus. *Mol Cell Probes* 11: 143–147

29 Ibrahim MS, Kulesh DA, Saleh SS, Damon IK, Esposito JJ, Schmaljohn AL, Jahrling PB (2003) Real-time PCR assay to detect smallpox virus. *J Clin Microbiol* 41: 3835–3839

30 Panning M, Asper M, Kramme S, Schmitz H, Drosten C (2004) Rapid detection and differentiation of human pathogenic orthopox viruses by a fluorescence resonance energy transfer real-time PCR assay. *Clin Chem* 50: 702–708

31 Nitsche A, Ellerbrok H, Pauli G (2004) Detection of orthopoxvirus DNA by real-time PCR and identification of variola virus DNA by melting analysis. *J Clin Microbiol* 42: 1207–1213
32 Kulesh DA, Baker RO, Loveless BM, Norwood D, Zwiers SH, Mucker E, Hartmann C, Herrera R, Miller D, Christensen D et al (2004) Smallpox and pan-orthopox virus detection by real-time 3'-minor groove binder TaqMan assays on the Roche LightCycler and the Cepheid smart Cycler platforms. *J Clin Microbiol* 42: 601–609
33 Olson VA, Laue T, Laker MT, Babkin IV, Drosten C, Shchelkunov SN, Niedrig M, Damon IK, Meyer H (2004) Real-time PCR system for detection of orthopoxviruses and simultaneous identification of smallpox virus. *J Clin Microbiol* 42: 1940–1946
34 Zimmermann P, Thordsen I, Frangoulidis D, Meyer H (2005) Real-time PCR assay for the detection of tanapox virus and yaba-like disease virus. *J Virol Methods* 130: 149–153
35 Lapa S, Mikheev M, Shchelkunov S, Mikhailovich V, Sobolev A, Blinov V, Babkin L, Guskov A, Sokunova E, Zasedatelev A et al (2002) Species-level identification of orthopoxviruses with an oligonucleotide microchip. *J Clin Microbiol* 40: 753–757
36 Laassri M, Chizhikov V, Mikheev M, Shchelkunov S, Chumakov K (2003) Detection and discrimination of orthopoxviruses using microarrays of immobilized oligonucleotides. *J Virol Methods* 112: 67–78
37 Gubser C, Hue S, Kellam P, Smith GL (2004) Poxvirus genomes: a phylogenetic analysis. *J Gen Virol* 85: 105–117
38 Likos AM, Sammons SA, Olson VA, Frace AM, Li Y, Olsen-Rasmussen M, Davidson W, Galloway R, Khristova ML, Reynolds MG et al (2005) A tale of two clades: monkeypox viruses. *J Gen Virol* 86: 2661–2672
39 Kaerber G (1931) Beitrag zur kollektiven Behandlung pharmakologischer Reihenversuche. *Arch Exp Pathol Pharmakol* 162: 480
40 Czerny C-P, Wagner K, Gessler K, Mayr A, Kaaden O-R (1996) A monoclonal blocking ELISA for detection of orthopox virus antibodies in feline sera. *Vet Microbiol* 52: 185–200
41 Karem KL, Reynolds M, Braden Z, Lou G, Bernard N, Patton J, Damon IK (2005) Characterization of acute-phase humoral immunity to monkeypox: use of immunoglobulin M enzyme-linked immunosorbent assay for detection of monkeypox infection during the 2003 North American outbreak. *Clin Diag Lab Immunol* 12: 867–872

Poxviruses
ed. by Andrew A. Mercer, Axel Schmidt and Olaf Weber

Therapy of poxvirus infections

Robert Snoeck, Graciela Andrei and Erik De Clercq

Rega Institute for Medical Research, Katholieke Universiteit Leuven, B-3000, Belgium

Abstract

Poxviruses have been recognized for centuries as a threat for human health. The most dreadful representative of the family, *Variola virus*, responsible for smallpox, was eradicated last century, after a wide and intensive campaign of vaccination. Meanwhile, the importance of other poxviruses has been recognized in human pathology, as well as the possible use of microbial agents, including smallpox, by bioterrorists. Together with the development of safer vaccination approaches, the research on antivirals has already led to the discovery of several families of active therapeutic compounds. The increased understanding of the viral replication and pathogenicity, as well as improvements in pharmacokinetics has led to the development of new and promising classes of compounds. These new molecules are either prodrugs giving better bioavailability, or compounds interfering with new molecular targets, both viral and cellular. Over the last few years, these latter developments have opened new opportunities for the treatment of poxvirus infections, and are discussed in this chapter.

Introduction

Research into the development of new therapies as well as novel approaches for prophylaxis for poxvirus infections has been stimulated over the last few years by the growing concern over the possible release of such viruses as weapons of mass destruction by bioterrorists [1]. The most important human pathogen in this family is *Variola virus* (VARV), which has been the first human virus to be definitely eradicated, after a mass vaccination programme under the control of the World Health Organisation. The last not-accidental case of smallpox was described in October 1977, and widespread vaccination was stopped in 1978 [2, 3]. Meanwhile, all the remaining strains of VARV in all the laboratories around the world have been centralized in two reference centers in the United States and Russia (former USSR). It was decided by the World Health Assembly that these stocks had to be destroyed, signing the final eradication of the virus. Unfortunately, based on a possible release of infectious agents from repositories, VARV, among many other viruses and bacteria, has been considered as one of the possible threats in a world population with a majority of people non-immunized and the others with an immunity that has not been boosted for several decades. It was, therefore, decided to intensify the development of better diagnostic tools, to generate new classes of vaccines responding to the actual rules of safety and finally to search for new and potent antiviral drugs. In order to reach these objectives, the destruction of the different stocks of VARV has been postponed to allow the characterization of the different strains and to establish and validate different surrogate models using other (ortho)poxviruses for diagnostic, vaccines and antiviral drugs.

In the meantime, other poxviruses for which no particular treatment is currently available have been recognized as important for human health, such as *Monkeypox virus* or *Orf virus* [4]. Similarly, some animal species-specific poxviruses, such as *Camelpox virus* or *Orf virus* could be of economical importance for some regions of the world.

Drugs active against poxviruses, mostly nucleoside analogues [5], have already been described but none of them has been used systemically on a large scale. Therefore, there is a clear need to enlarge the armamentarium of antiviral molecules, by further studying the different family members of already known drugs for improved activity and pharmacokinetics, and by searching for new classes of compounds with a different and original mechanism of action.

The search for antiviral agents started more than 50 years ago, using poxviruses (VACV) as a target. The first molecule shown to be active against VACV was a tuberculostatic, thiosemicarbazone, which also proved to be active *in vivo*. An analogue of thiosemicarbazone, methisazone, was found to reduce the smallpox attack rate by 75–95% in several trials in India [6, 7]. Despite these results, and also because the vaccination had proved efficient, this type of compounds was never further developed for the treatment of poxvirus infections, and their antiviral mechanism of action was never studied in any detail.

Now, under the pressure of the circumstances, several classes of compounds with anti-poxvirus activity have been revisited or newly developed and their activity and mechanism of action investigated.

Poxviruses are among the largest viruses, with genomes encoding a large number of viral proteins, each of them being a potential target for antiviral therapy. Such targets may include viral proteins that are essential for the viral replicative cycle. Several such encoded viral enzymes and factors are packaged in the infectious virion and are directly involved in mRNA synthesis and modification by capping and methylation. Also, many viral proteins are involved in processes required for virus replication, such as viral entry, uncoating, viral gene expression, DNA replication, virion assembly, maturation and release. Most of the selective anti-poxvirus agents that have been described are targeted at the viral DNA polymerase. Reviews on these compounds have been published [5, 8, 9]. Recently, novel promising targets have been uncovered that are complementary to those already known.

Compounds targeted at cellular enzymes

Nucleoside analogues

Many compounds that have been discovered to inhibit the replication of poxviruses do not inhibit a specific viral process or protein, but instead, are targeted at cellular enzymes. The most ancient inhibitors of poxviruses so far described are classified among these molecules, and target the following enzymes: inosine 5'-monophosphate (IMP) dehydrogenase, S-adenosylhomocysteine (SAH) hydrolase, orotidine 5'-monophosphate (OMP) decarboxylase, CTP synthetase and thymidylate synthetase. These nucleoside analogues and their mechanisms of action have been extensively reviewed [5].

The nucleoside analogues that have been described as inhibitors of VACV replication *in vitro* are ribavirin, EICAR, (*S*)-DHPA, (*RS*)-AHPA, c^3Ado, C-c^3Ado, neplanocin A, 3-deazaneplanocin A, DHCeA, c^3DHCeA, DHCaA, c^3DHCaA, F-C-Ado, 5'-noraristeromycin, 3 deaza-5'-noraristeromycin, (*R*)-6'-C-methylneplanocin A, pyrazofurin, cyclopentenylcytosine (Ce-Cyd), 5-substituted 2'-deoxyuridines, and the recently described 4',4'-difluoro-5'-noraristeromycin [10]. The chemical structures of some of the most representative compounds are depicted in Figures 1 and 2. Several compounds have emerged as potent inhibitors of VACV replication *in vitro*, with effective concentrations within the range of 0.01–0.1 μg/ml, i.e., neplanocin A, 3-deazaneplanocin A, DHCaA, c^3DHCaA, (–)-5'-noraristeromycin, (*R*)-6'C-methyl neplanocin A and cyclopentenylcytosine (Ce-Cyd) [5]. For some of these compounds their activity has been tested *in vivo* (for a summary see [5, 11]).

Inhibitors of cellular kinases

The genomes of all orthopoxviruses encode a growth factor (GF). The smallpox growth factor (SPGF) is expressed by VARV and the vaccinia growth factor (VGF) is induced by VACV. VGF binds to and activates the ErbB-1 kinase, a member of the epidermal GF receptor family of tyrosine kinases [12, 13]. Since the poxvirus-encoded GFs facilitate viral replication [14, 15], a well-tolerated interference with the cellular GF receptor might be a useful approach to inhibit poxvirus infection. Drugs that target the ErbB-signaling pathways represent a promising new class of antiviral agents against poxviruses [16].

Yang and colleagues [17] have recently reported that low molecular weight organic inhibitors of ErbB-1 kinases (i.e., CI-1033 and related 4-ani-

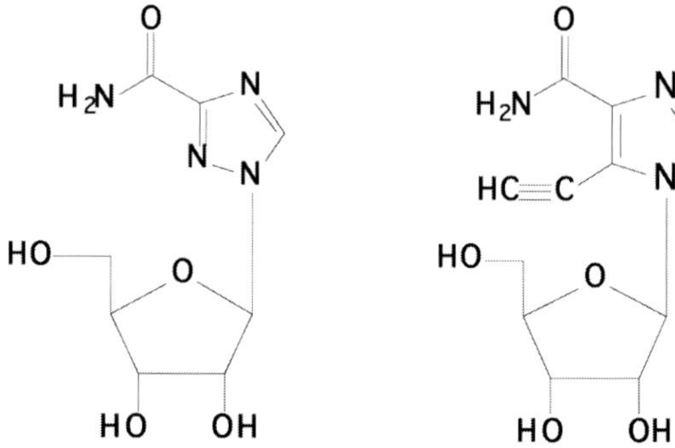

Ribavirin **EICAR**

Figure 1. IMP dehydrogenase inhibitors ribavirin and EICAR.

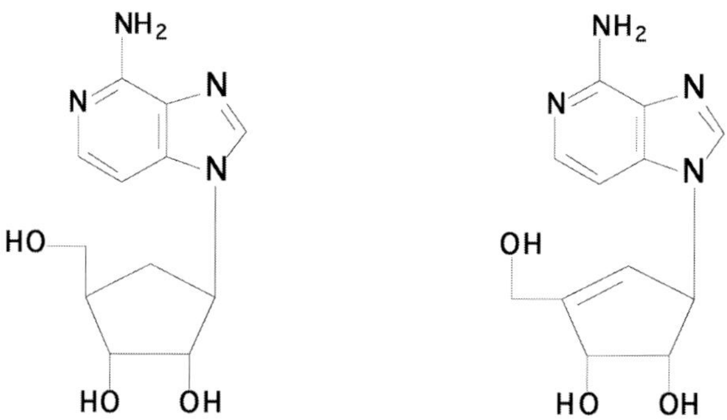

C-c³Ado (X = CH_2) **3-Deazaneplanocin A (X = CH)**

Figure 2. SAH hydrolase inhibitors carbocyclic deazaadenosine (C-c³Ado) and 3-deazaneplanocin A

linoquinazolines) (Fig. 3) might function as antiviral agents against smallpox. Furthermore, they provided new insight into the role of the poxvirus-encoded GFs in viral pathogenesis, suggesting that poxvirus GFs may play a direct role in virus replication. Previous studies demonstrated that VGF acts on cells to stimulate metabolism, increasing the number of cells capable of supporting efficient viral replication [14]. When Yang et al. [17] examined the effect of the ErbB inhibitor CI-1033 on the growth of VARV and VACV *in vitro*, they found that the drug had no effect on the overall yield of newly made virus in cell cultures when all the cells were infected simultaneously,

Erb B tyrosine kinase inhibitors

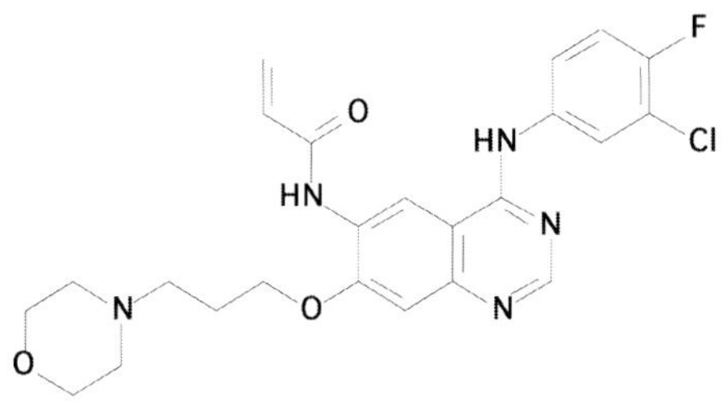

CI-1033

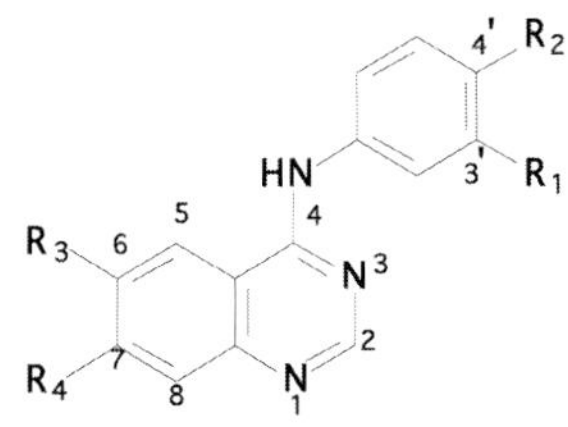

4-anilinoquinazoline

Other tyrosine kinase inhibitors

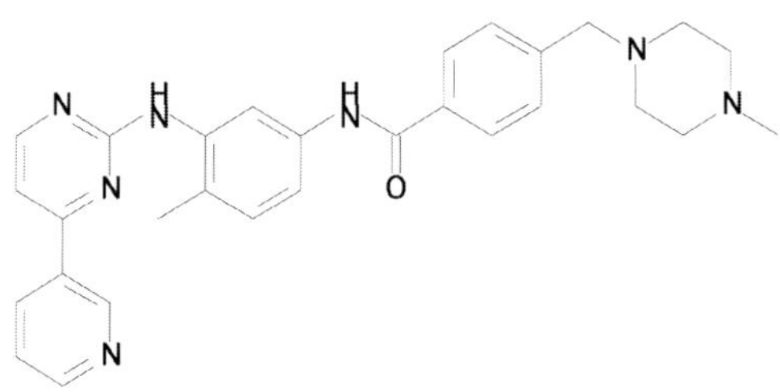

STI-571. (Imatinib)

Figure 3. Compounds targeted at cellular kinases.

but it did have an effect on the appearance of plaques arising from the initial infection of a single cell, which requires local spread of the virus from the infected cell to surrounding uninfected cells.

The morphogenesis of poxviruses in the cytoplasm of infected cells is a complex process and involves the generation of two distinct forms of virus, intracellular mature virus (IMV) and extracellular enveloped virus (EEV), which are surrounded by different numbers of lipid membranes and have different surface proteins [18]. Whereas some enveloped viruses complete virus assembly by budding through the plasma membrane, infectious poxvirus particles are produced within the cytoplasm. IMV particles are either further enveloped by intracellular membranes to form intracellular enveloped virus (IEV) that are transported to the cell surface on microtubules and released by exocytosis, or are released after cell lysis. If the enveloped virion remains attached to the cell surface it is called cell-associated enveloped virus (CEV) and is propelled into surrounding cells by growing actin tails beneath the plasma membrane. Alternatively, some CEV particles are released from the cells as EEV particles, which rapidly disseminate the infection. The four distinct forms of VACV particles are infectious (IMV, IEV, CEV and EEV), but the main mechanism responsible for dissemination of the virus is the release of EEV from infected cells.

Yang et al. [17] have shown that the ErbB inhibitor CI-1033 greatly reduces the release of EEV from VACV- or VARV-infected cells. CI-1033 can block the phosphorylation of ErbB-1 and subsequent activation of c-Src and the actin polymerization complex, which play a role in viral extrusion. Interestingly, a deletion of the GF gene from VACV has an effect on the release of EEV similar to that of CI-1033 on wild-type cells, suggesting that the reduction in EEV release is likely due, at least in part, to inhibition of the viral GF activation of the ErbB-signaling pathways. However, the drug appears to have additional antiviral effects since a reduction in the size of the plaques was also observed in cells infected with a VGF-mutant virus. CI-1033 may also interfere with events that render cells permissive for viral replication [16].

Yang et al. [17] also demonstrated that interference with the signal transduction pathway mediated by ErbB-1 can lead to the control of VACV *in vivo*. In a lethal VACV-infection model in mice, CI-1033 alone promoted survival of animals, augmented systemic T cell immunity and, in conjunction with a single dose of anti-L1R IMV particle-specific mAb, afforded nearly complete viral clearance of the lungs of infected animal at 8 days post infection.

The tyrosine kinase inhibitor Gleevec^{TM} (also called STI-571, imatinib mesylate or Glivec^{TM}) (Fig. 3), currently used to treat chronic myeloid leukemia, can also function as an antiviral drug to treat poxvirus infections. Reeves et al. [19] have recently shown that Gleevec^{TM} has the ability to block the egress of poxviruses from infected cells.

The cytoplasmic trafficking of the intracellular forms of poxviruses is mediated by microtubules, whereas extrusion of the cell-associated form at the cell surface occurs through the polymerization of actin tails, which facilitates cell-cell spread of the virus and promotes virus dissemination in the infected host [20]. The VACV protein A36R is located in the membrane surrounding the IEV, and is required for actin polymerization [21] and virulence [22]. A study in 1999 reported that A36R is tyrosine phosphorylated by host Src-family kinases, and is necessary for virus motility and virus egress [23]. The findings of Reeves et al. [19] indicate that CEV particles use Abl and Src family tyrosine kinases for actin motility, and these kinases act in a redundant fashion. Thus, multiple cellular kinases, including Src, Fyn, Yes, Abl and Arg all localize to the growing actin tails underneath CEV, but no single member is exclusively responsible for actin polymerization. Pyrido(2,3-d)-pyrimidine (PD) drugs, which occlude the ATP-binding domain of Abl and Src family kinases, reduced actin-based VACV motility, plaque formation and virus spread to neighboring cells. Additionally, release of CEV from the cells was shown to require the Abl, but not Src, family tyrosine kinases, and was blocked by Gleevec^{TM}, an inhibitor of a variety of Abl family tyrosine kinases, but not of Src, family kinases. This result indicated that the disengagement of EEV from infected cells is under control of the Abl family kinases, unlike the actin tail polymerization, which is triggered by both Abl and Src family kinases. Gleevec^{TM} was also able to reduce viral dissemination and promoted survival in infected mice, suggesting possible use of this drug in the treatment of smallpox or complications associated with vaccination.

The use of kinase inhibitors may prove generally efficacious in treating viral infections that rely on host kinases, and, because the drugs target host and not viral proteins, this strategy is much less likely to elicit drug resistance.

Compounds targeted at viral enzymes

Nucleoside analogues

There are several nucleoside analogues (Fig. 4) that may be postulated to target viral DNA synthesis. One example is adenine arabinoside (ara-A), which *in vitro* is about 10-fold more potent against VACV than against HSV-1 or-2. Its triphosphate form is believed to enter into competition with dATP, the natural substrate [24, 25]. Ara-A has been evaluated in different animal models [11], but does not actually represent a valuable alternative for human therapy.

Cytosine arabinoside (ara-C) inhibits VACV replication and host DNA synthesis at roughly the same concentrations; therefore, it cannot be considered a selective antiviral agent. Compounds such as 3'-C-methyladenosine and 3'-C-methylcytidine have demonstrated activity against VACV *in vitro* and *in vivo* [5, 26]. Of a series of 2-,6- and 8-alkylated adenosine analogues, the 8-methyladenosine emerged as a potent and selective inhibitor of VACV. Further studies, for example *in vivo*, will be needed to confirm the potential of this molecule [27].

Another compound of particular interest is an acyclic derivative of purine, 2 amino-7-(1,3-dihydroxy-2-propoxymethyl)purine, also known as S2242. This compound is a potent and selective inhibitor of virtually all herpesviruses and is an efficient inhibitor of VACV replication. The exact mode of action of S2242 has not been established, but it was demonstrated that the compound is phosphorylated intracellularly to its triphosphate, suggesting that as such, it could interfere selectively with the viral DNA polymerase [28, 29]. H-961, the diacetate ester of S2242, is an oral prodrug, displaying activity similar to the mother compound in animal models [11, 30, 31].

Finally, 5'-iodo-2'deoxyuridine, a drug used only topically, because of systemic toxicity, for the treatment of herpesviruses infections was shown to be active against VACV replication *in vitro* and *in vivo* [5, 32].

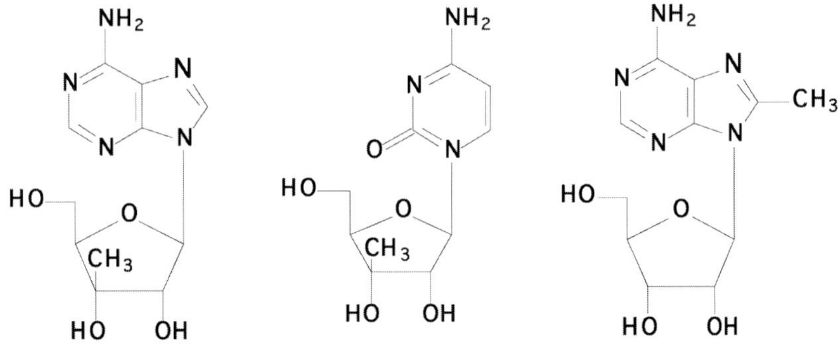

3'-*C*-methyl Ado **3'-*C*-methyl Cyt** **8-Methyl Ado**

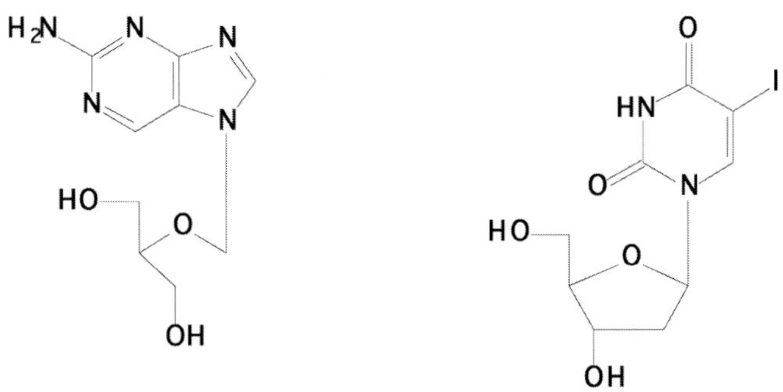

S2242 **IDU**

Figure 4. Nucleoside analogue inhibitors of viral DNA polymerase, 3'-C-methyladenosine, 3'-C-methylcytidine, 8-methyladenosine, S2242 and IDU.

Nucleotide analogues

(*S*)-9-(3-hydroxy-2-phosponylmethoxypropyl)adenine [(*S*)-HPMPA], the prototype of the acyclic nucleoside phosphonates, can be regarded as a hybrid molecule between (*S*)-DHPA and phosphonoacetic acid (PAA). (S)-DHPA and PAA inhibit the replication of VACV in cell culture at an IC_{50} of 20 and 30 μg/ml, respectively. In contrast, (*S*)-HPMPA inhibits the virus in similar conditions at a 100-fold lower concentration [33, 34].

(*S*)-HPMPA was found active against a broad range of DNA viruses, including herpesviruses, adenoviruses and hepadnaviruses, besides poxviruses. (*S*)-HPMPA does not need a virus-specific thymidine kinase to be

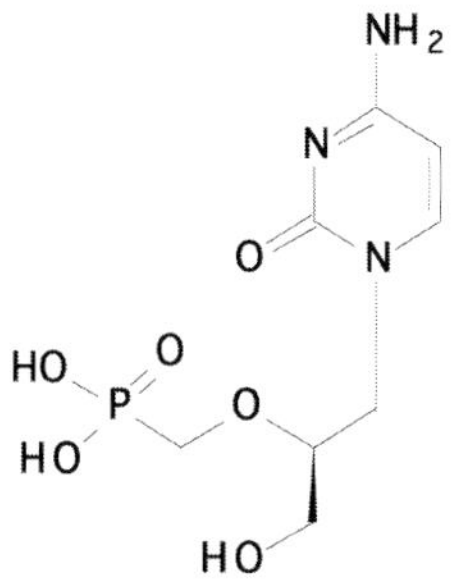

HPMPC (cidofovir)

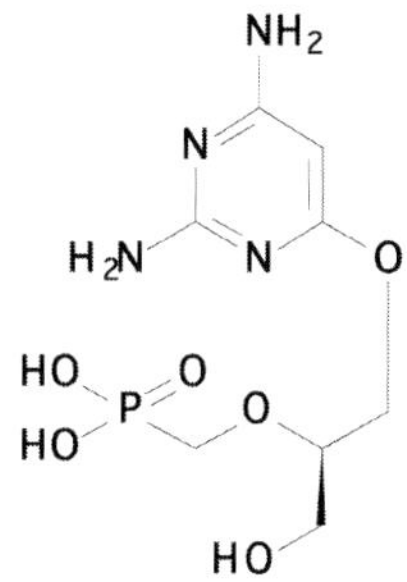

(*S*)-HPMPO-DAPy

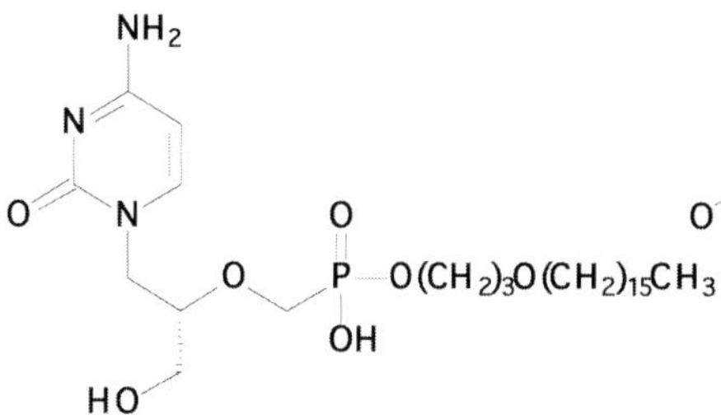

Hexadecyloxypropyl-cidofovir

(HDP-cidofovir)

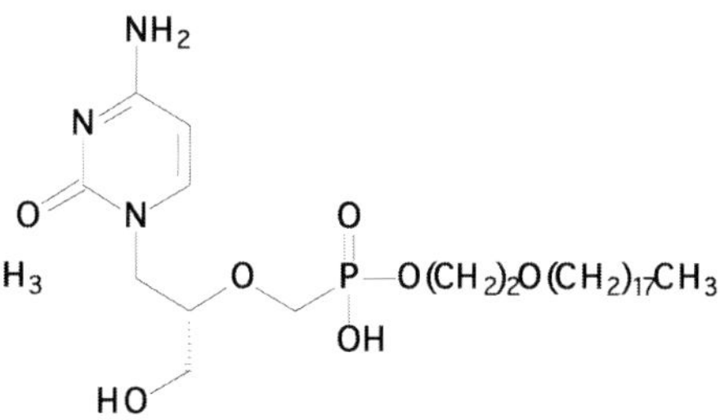

Octadecyloxyethyl-cidofovir

(ODE-cidofovir)

Figure 5. Nucleotide analogue inhibitors of viral DNA polymerase.

activated as is the case for other molecules such as acyclovir. The compound is phosphorylated by cellular enzymes to its diphosphate form, which then acts as an inhibitor of viral DNA synthesis.

(*S*)-1-(3-hydroxy-2-phosphonylmethoxypropyl)cytosine [(*S*)-HPMPC, cidofovir, Vistide^{TM}] (Fig. 5), the cytosine counterpart of (*S*)-HPMPA, has an activity spectrum similar to that of (*S*)-HPMPA. Its activity spectrum encompasses all DNA viruses, in particular papillomaviruses, polyomaviruses, adenoviruses, herpesviruses and poxviruses [34–37].

(*S*)-HPMPC confers a pronounced and prolonged inhibition of viral replication, lasting at least 7 days, after an exposure time as short as 6 h post infection. This long-lasting antiviral action is a unique property of cidofovir that allows prophylactic use and infrequent dosing of the drug. The long-lasting antiviral action may be attributed to the long half-life of its metabolites [i.e., (*S*)-HPMPCp, (*S*)-HPMPCpp, (*S*)-HPMPCp-choline]; in particular, (*S*)-HPMPCp-choline may serve as an intracellular depot of (*S*)-HPMPC since its intracellular half-life is extremely long (48 h). This mechanism of action has been extensively reviewed elsewhere [8, 35, 37].

Further studies have been performed on the poxvirus DNA polymerase. The results revealed that (*S*)-HPMPCpp can be used by the VACV DNA polymerase as a dCTP analogue. The compound inhibits both chain extension and the associated 3'-to-5'exonuclease activity (which has a critical role in minimizing replication errors), and probably also catalyzes virus genetic recombination [38].

Cidofovir has been licensed for the treatment of CMV retinitis in AIDS patients, but it also has therapeutic potential, on either systemic or topical administration, in the treatment of various other herpesvirus, polyomavirus, papillomavirus, adenovirus and poxvirus infections [8].

Cidofovir and (*S*)-HPMPA were first shown to be active *in vitro* against vaccinia virus and later found to be active against various other orthopoxviruses, including *Cowpox virus*, *Camelpox virus*, *Monkeypox virus*, and against parapoxviruses (*Orf virus*). At first, most of these experiments were performed in monolayer cell culture assay [8, 30, 37]. More recently, VACV, *Cowpox virus* and *Orf virus* were shown to replicate efficiently in three-dimensional epithelial raft cultures, using either human or lamb keratinocytes, giving histological pictures comparable to that described for the skin biopsy specimens of the corresponding diseases. In these conditions, cidofovir and several acyclic nucleoside phosphonate analogues exhibited the expected selective antiviral activity [39, 40].

Among the most recently synthesized phosphonates, the 6-[2-(phosphonomethoxy)alkoxy-2,4-diaminopyrimidines were the most promising. The alkylpurine counterparts of (*S*)-HPMPDAP, PMEA and (*R*)-PMPA, named respectively HPMPO-DAPy, PMEO-DAPy and (*R*)-PMPO-DAPy, exhibit an antiviral activity spectrum and potency that is similar to that of their parent compounds. HPMPO-DAPy (Fig. 5) was found to inhibit different poxviruses (i.e., VACV, *Cowpox virus*, and *Orf virus*) at a similar potency as cidofovir [9, 40–42].

Cidofovir is poorly bioavailable and therefore administered by the intravenous route, which require hospitalization to pre-and post-hydrate the patients and to administer probenecid to reduce the risk of nephrotoxicity associated with cidofovir [43,44].

Poxviruses resistant to cidofovir have been described after selection *in vitro* [45, 46]. Such selection is difficult and requires much time. The resistant viruses need still to be molecularly characterized.

Since an oral drug would be needed in the case of a smallpox outbreak, cidofovir prodrugs were made, consisting of a series of lipid conjugates, in which cidofovir was covalently coupled to an alkoxyalkanol such as hexadecylpropanediol (HDP-cidofovir) or octadecylethanediol (ODE-cidofovir) (Fig. 5) to form an ether-lipid-cidofovir conjugate. The conjugates were made to mimic the natural lipids that are absorbed by the gastrointestinal tract and distributed *via* plasma and/or lymph. The concentrations reached in the different organs that are potential target sites of a poxviral infection, particularly liver, spleen and lungs, are considerably higher after the administration of the lipid prodrugs compared to cidofovir. Interestingly, exposure in the kidney, the site of cidofovir toxicity is considerably reduced, suggesting that the cidofovir conjugates could have a better toxicological profile [47, 48].

The lipophilic prodrugs are also associated with a better cellular uptake, reflected by higher intracellular concentrations of the different metabolites of cidofovir (HPMPC-p and HPMPC-pp) [49]. This increased level of the different metabolites is associated with an enhanced activity compared to cidofovir against poxvirus replication *in vitro* [50, 51]. Similar observations have been reported for adenovirus [52] and both human and murine cytomegaloviruses [53].

The *in vivo* activity of cidofovir against VACV infection was first reported in 1993 in a model of prevention and treatment of lethal infections in severe combined immunodeficiency (SCID) mice [54]. Cidofovir could be given as a single dose from as early as 7 days before infection and significantly delayed mortality. Similar results were obtained for treatments started up to 6 days post infection. These results have been confirmed subsequently in other studies [55, 56]. When mice were challenged with aerosol containing *Cowpox virus*, cidofovir given systemically [57, 58] or aerosolized [59] was effective in treating the infection.

In a mouse model, in which the mice were infected with *Ectromelia virus* (mousepox) encoding interleukin-4 (IL-4), a highly immunosuppressive cytokine, cidofovir failed to protect the animals; only the higher doses used could delay the mortality of the animals [60].

Cidofovir also demonstrated activity in monkeys infected experimentally with *Monkeypox virus*, in an attempt to establish a surrogate model that was related as closely as possible to VARV infection in humans [11, 57]. The use of these primate models has been restricted to few well-equipped centers in the world, where some trials were performed using smallpox [11]. Extensive reviews of the different animal models in which cidofovir and other antivirals have been tested have been published [5, 8, 11, 35, 37].

Among the other phosphonates, HPMPO-DAPy was also investigated for its *in vivo* activity. The results obtained in different models of VACV infections in mice demonstrated activity similar to that of cidofovir, making HPMPO-DAPy a good candidate for the treatment of poxviral infections in humans [61].

The lipophilic prodrugs of phosphonates were recently extensively evaluated in different animal models, including the safety evaluation of intraocular injections of hexadecyloxypropyl-cyclic cidofovir in a guinea

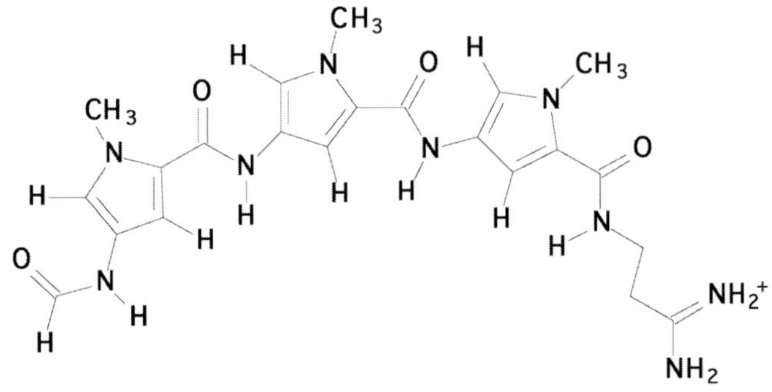

Figure 6. Inhibitors of post-DNA replicative mRNA synthesis.

pig model. The different results confirmed the potential of these prodrugs for the systemic treatment of DNA viruses and particularly poxviruses [62–65].

Cidofovir was also used in the clinic to treat patients with different presentations of poxvirus infections. The molecule has proved active in AIDS patients with recalcitrant molluscum contagiosum [66, 67], as well as for the treatment of echtyma contagiosum (orf) in a renal transplant patient [68]. Recently, monkeypox has been considered as an emerging zoonosis after the virus was introduced into the U.S., and infected prairie dogs had contaminated clusters of patients in the Midwest. While there is no clear clinical data on the usefulness of cidofovir in such cases, cidofovir was the only drug available if one of those cases had to be treated [4, 69, 70].

Inhibitors of post-replicative mRNA synthesis

Distamycin A (Fig. 6) has been described as an inhibitor of the cellular pathogenesis of VACV in culture. The compound targets the minor groove of DNA, preferentially binding DNA sequences that have five consecutive A-T pairs, with affinity that varies with the particular sequence [71]. Transcriptional promoter regions contain close to 90% A-T in VACV, making them ideal targets for the antibiotic. Early gene transcription and DNA synthesis appeared to proceed normally in the presence of the antibiotics, while VACV intermediate and late gene transcription was inhibited [72]. Although distamycin may be too toxic for therapeutic purposes, other minor-groove ligands with specificity for VACV and other poxviral promoters may be developed.

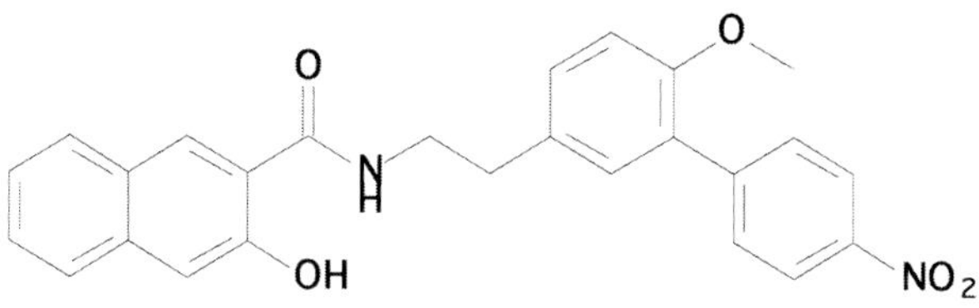

TTP-6171

Figure 7. Inhibitors of viral morphogenesis.

Inhibitors of viral morphogenesis

In an attempt to discover inhibitors of viral morphogenesis Byrd et al. [73] developed a structural model of the VACV I7L proteinase using a homology-based bioinformatics approach. This protein has been shown to be the cysteine proteinase responsible for the cleavage of the core protein precursors that occur during the stage of viral morphogenesis [74, 75]. Morphogenesis proteolysis occurs in the stage between the formation of the infectious IMV from the noninfectious intracellular virus. Byrd et al. [73] identified a new class of small molecule inhibitors, the prototype being compound TTP-6171 (Fig. 7), that were modeled to fit in the predicted active site pocket of I7L. Investigation of the mechanism of action of TTP-6171 indicated that early stages of VACV replication were unaffected, while cleavage of the major core protein precursors and subsequent maturation of the immature viral intermediates into infectious IMVs were blocked. To confirm the hypothesis that the I7L catalytic activity is the target of TTP-6171, drug-resistant mutants were selected and mutations within the I7L gene were shown to be responsible for the resistant phenotypes.

Inhibitors of viral release

Most drugs developed for the treatment of poxvirus infections are nucleoside analogues, and act by interfering with DNA viral polymerase activity; however, compounds that act by a different mechanism of action are needed. Yang et al. [76] have recently described a potent and specific inhibitor of orthopoxvirus replication, ST-246 {4-trifluoromethyl-N-(3,3a,4,4a,5,5a,6,6a-octahydro-1,3-dioxo-4,6-ethenocycloprop[f]isoindol-2-[1H]-yl)-benzamide} (Fig. 8), which is active against several species of orthopoxviruses, including VARV. Resistance mapping studies indicated that ST-246 targets the cowpox virus V061 gene, which encodes a major envelope protein homologous to the VACV F13L gene product. VACV F13L encodes a 37-kDa palmitylated peripheral membrane protein that participates in the enveloping of

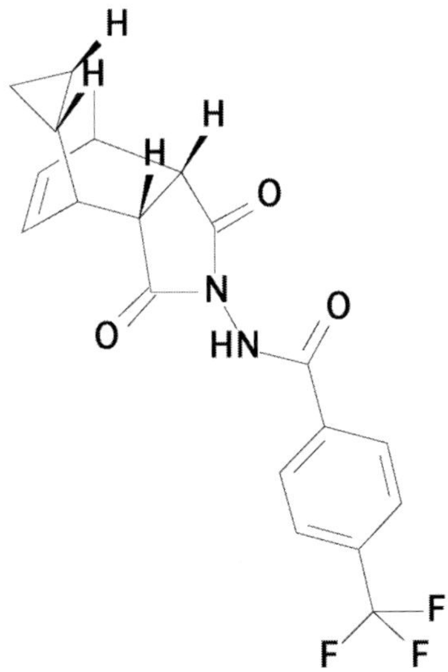

ST-246

Figure 8. Inhibitors of viral release.

IMV particles and is required for extracellular virus formation [77, 78]. In cell culture, ST-246 inhibited plaque formation and virus-induced cytopathic effect, and reduced extracellular virus formation, while having little effect on the production of intracellular virus. Oral delivery of ST-246 protected mice from lethal orthopoxvirus challenge and prevented VACV-induced disease. Maximal protective effect required 14 days of dosing. The requirement for extended dosing is consistent with a compound that targets a virulence factor. Unlike cidofovir, which accumulates inside the cells and targets viral DNA polymerase, ST-246 inhibits virus spread by targeting an enzyme involved in extracellular virus formation [76]. Therefore, a maximal therapeutic benefit can be achieved only if the drug is present continuously to inhibit virus spread and allows the host immune response to clear the infection.

Interferon

Interferon (IFN) constitutes one of the most potent first-line host defenses against virus infection, and can induce direct antiviral effects as well as promote T helper cell type 1 (Th1) responses [79]. Poxviruses are sensitive to IFN-α/β and IFN-γ *in vivo*, as mice lacking IFN-α/β or IFN-γ are highly susceptible to poxvirus infections [80, 81].

IFN and the IFN inducers polyacrylic acid and poly(inosinic acid). poly(cytidylic acid) (poly IC) have been recognized for a long time as inhibitors of VACV both *in vitro* and *in vivo* [5]. Prophylactic administration of IFN and IFN inducers afforded a pronounced protection in the mouse VACV tail lesion model [5]. Monkeys treated with daily intramuscular or intravenous injections of leukocyte IFN from day –1 before to day +1 after VACV infection were completely protected and the severity of the skin lesions was decreased. An inverse correlation between score lesions and dose of IFN was observed [82].

Recently, Liu et al. [83] reported the prevention of lethal respiratory VACV infections in mice with IFN-α and IFN-γ. Intranasal administration of IFN-α and IFN-γ (days –1 to +3) were effective in protecting mice from viral replication in lungs, and the associated mortality.

The actions of IFNs are effective at controlling the spread of poxviruses at a variety of extracellular and intracellular levels [79]. These mechanisms target intracellular responses activated by dsRNA produced within infected cells during virus transcription, such as the IFN-dependent enzymatic cascades mediated by dsRNA-dependent protein kinase R (PKR) and the 2',5'-oligoadenylate synthetase (OAS). In addition to directly inhibiting the PKR and OAS pathways, some poxviruses may also act indirectly by diminishing the antiviral state induced by IFN, such as by targeting the transcription factors that transduce the biological effects of IFN-inducible genes.

Besides the intracellular mechanisms of IFN inhibition, many poxviruses also target the IFN system at the extracellular level [79]. These viruses encode soluble versions of cytokine receptors that intercept the normal activities of the target cytokines, e.g., proteins that bind to and prevent IFN-α/β and IFN-γ from binding to their respective receptors on the cell membrane [84, 85]. An important virulence factor of poxviruses is the B8R protein, which is a homolog of the extracellular domain of the IFN-γ receptor and can therefore bind to intact IFN-γ and prevents its interaction with the receptor [86]. Ahmed et al. [87] have recently developed peptide agonists/mimetics of IFN-γ. These mimetics do not act through recognition of the extracellular domain of IFN-γ receptor but rather bind to the cytoplasmic domain of the receptor chain 1, IFNGR-1, and thereby initiate cellular signaling. These mimetics bypass the poxvirus virulence factor B8R protein, and, in contrast to human IFN-γ, the mimetics do not bind poxvirus B8R protein, a homolog of the IFN-γ receptor extracellular domain. In addition, the mimetics, but not IFN-γ, inhibited VACV replication *in vitro*, suggesting that small mimetics of IFN-γ could be potential candidates for antivirals against smallpox.

IFN inducers (and/or IFN) can be considered as interesting therapeutic and/or prophylactic agents for the treatment and prevention of poxvirus infections. In addition, compounds that target viral proteins responsible for inhibition of IFN-induced functions likely represent selective targets for therapeutic intervention.

Acknowledgements

We thank C. Callebaut for her dedicated editorial help.

References

1 Berche P (2001) The threat of smallpox and bioterrorism. *Trends Microbiol* 9: 15–18
2 Breman JG, Arita I (1980) The confirmation and maintenance of smallpox eradication. *N Engl J Med* 303: 1263–1273
3 Behbehani AM (1983) The smallpox story: life and death of an old disease. *Microbiol Rev* 47: 455–509
4 Di Giulio DB, Eckburg PB (2004) Human monkeypox: an emerging zoonosis. *Lancet Infect Dis* 4: 15–25
5 De Clercq E (2001) Vaccinia virus inhibitors as a paradigm for the chemotherapy of poxvirus infections. *Clin Microbiol Rev* 14: 382–397
6 Bauer DJ, St. Vincent L, Kempe CH, Downie AW (1963) Prophylactic treatment of smallpox contacts with *N*-methylisatin β-thiosemicarbazone. *Lancet* ii: 494–496
7 Hamre D, Brownlee KA, Donovick R (1951) Studies on the chemotheray of vaccinia virus. II. The activity of some thiosemicarbazones. *J Immunol* 67: 305–312
8 De Clercq E (2003) Clinical potential of the acyclic nucleoside phosphonates cidofovir, adefovir, and tenofovir in treatment of DNA virus and retrovirus infections. *Clin Microbiol Rev* 16: 569–596
9 De Clercq E (2005) Recent highlights in the development of new antiviral drugs. *Curr Opin Microbiol* 8: 552–560
10 Roy A, Schneller SW, Keith KA, Hartline CB, Kern ER (2005) The 4',4'-difluoro analog of 5'-noraristeromycin: a new structural prototype for possible antiviral drug development toward orthopoxvirus and cytomegalovirus. *Bioorg Med Chem* 13: 4443–4449
11 Smee DF, Sidwell RW (2003) A review of compounds exhibiting anti-orthopoxvirus activity in animal models. *Antiviral Res* 57: 41–52
12 Kim M, Yang H, Kim SK, Reche PA, Tirabassi RS, Hussey RE, Chishti Y, Rheinwald JG, Morehead TJ, Zech T et al (2004) Biochemical and functional analysis of smallpox growth factor (SPGF) and anti-SPGF monoclonal antibodies. *J Biol Chem* 279: 25838–25848
13 Tzahar E, Moyer JD, Waterman H, Barbacci EG, Bao J, Levkowitz G, Shelly M, Strano S, Pinkas-Kramarski R, Pierce JH et al (1998) Pathogenic poxviruses reveal viral strategies to exploit the ErbB signaling network. *EMBO J* 17: 5948–5963

14 Buller RM, Chakrabarti S, Cooper JA, Twardzik DR, Moss B (1988) Deletion of the vaccinia virus growth factor gene reduces virus virulence. *J Virol* 62: 866–874
15 Opgenorth A, Nation N, Graham K, McFadden G (1993) Transforming growth factor alpha, Shope fibroma growth factor, and vaccinia growth factor can replace myxoma growth factor in the induction of myxomatosis in rabbits. *Virology* 192: 701–709
16 Fauci AS, Challberg MD (2005) Host-based antipoxvirus therapeutic strategies: turning the tables. *J Clin Invest* 115: 231–233
17 Yang H, Kim S-K, Kim M, Reche PA, Morehead TJ, Damon IK, Welsh RM, Reinherz EL (2005) Antiviral chemotherapy facilitates control of poxvirus infections through inhibition of cellular signal transduction. *J Clin Invest* 115: 379–387
18 Smith GL, Law M (2004) The exit of vaccinia virus from infected cells. *Virus Res* 106: 189–197
19 Reeves PM, Bommarius B, Lebeis S, McNulty S, Christensen J, Swimm A, Chahroudi A, Chavan R, Feinberg MB, Veach D et al (2005) Disabling poxvirus pathogenesis by inhibition of Abl-family tyrosine kinases. *Nat Med* 11: 731–739
20 McFadden G (2005) Gleevec casts a pox on poxviruses. *Nat Med* 11: 711–712
21 Wolffe EJ, Weisberg AS, Moss B (1998) Role for the vaccinia virus A36R outer envelope protein in the formation of virus-tipped actin-containing microvilli and cell-to-cell virus spread. *Virology* 244: 20–26
22 Parkinson JE, Smith GL (1994) Vaccinia virus gene A36R encodes a M(r) 43–50 K protein on the surface of extracellular enveloped virus. *Virology* 204: 376–390
23 Frischknecht F, Moreau V, Rottger S, Gonfloni S, Reckmann I, Superti-Furga G, Way M (1999) Actin-based motility of vaccinia virus mimics receptor tyrosine kinase signalling. *Nature* 401: 926–929
24 Hasobe M, McKee JG, Borcherding DR, Borchardt RT (1987) 9-(*Trans*-2', *trans*-3'-dihydroxycyclopent-4'-enyl)-adenine and -3-deazaadenine: analogs of neplanocin A which retain potent antiviral activity but exhibit reduced cytotoxicity. *Antimicrob Agents Chemother* 31: 1849–1851
25 Neyts J, De Clercq E (2003) Therapy and short-term prophylaxis of poxvirus infections: historical background and perspectives. *Antiviral Res* 57: 25–33
26 Walton E, Jenkins SR, Nutt RF, Holly FW, Nemes M (1969) Branched-chain sugar nucleosides. V. Synthesis and antiviral properties of several branched-chain sugar nucleosides. *J Med Chem* 12: 306–309
27 Van Aerschot A, Mamos AP, Weyns NJ, Ikeda S, De Clercq E, Herdewijn P (1993) Antiviral activity of C-alkylated purine nucleosides obtained by cross-coupling with tetraalkyltin reagents. *J Med Chem* 36: 2938–2942
28 Neyts J, Andrei G, Snoeck R, Jähne G, Winkler I, Helsberg M, Balzarini J, De Clercq E (1994) The N-7-substituted acyclic nucleoside analog 2-amino-7-[(1,3-dihydroxy-2-propoxy)methyl]purine is a potent and selective inhibitor of herpesvirus replication. *Antimicrob Agents Chemother* 38: 2710–2716
29 Neyts J, Balzarini J, Andrei G, Chaoyong Z, Snoeck R, Zimmerman A, Mertens T, Karlsson A, De Clercq E (1998) Intracellular metabolism of the N7-substituted

acyclic nucleoside analog 2-amino-7-(1,3-dihydroxy-2-propoxymethyl)purine, a potent inhibitor of herpesvirus replication. *Mol Pharmacol* 53: 157–165

30 Neyts J, Jähne G, Andrei G, Snoeck R, Winkler I , De Clercq E (1995) *In vivo* antiherpesvirus activity of N-7-substituted acyclic nucleoside analog 2-amino-7[(1,3-dihydroxy-2-propoxy)methyl]purine. *Antimicrob Agents Chemother* 39: 56–60

31 Neyts J, De Clercq E (2001) Efficacy of 2-amino-7-[(1,3-dihydroxy-2-propoxy)methyl]purine for the treatment of vaccinia (orthopox-) virus infections in mice. *Antimicrob Agents Chemother* 45: 84–87

32 Neyts J, De Clercq E (2002) Effect of 5-iodo-2'-deoxyuridine on vaccinia virus (orthopoxvirus) infections in mice. *Antimicrob Agents Chemother* 46: 2842–2847

33 De Clercq E, Holý A, Rosenberg I, Sakuma T, Balzarini J, Maudgal PC (1986) A novel selective broad-spectrum anti-DNA virus agents. *Nature* 323: 464–467

34 De Clercq E, Sakuma T, Baba M, Pauwels R, Balzarini J, Rosenberg I, Holý A (1987) Antiviral activity of phosphonylmethoxyalkyl derivatives of purine and pyrimidines. *Antiviral Res* 8: 261–272

35 De Clercq E, Neyts J (2004) Therapeutic potential of nucleoside/nucleotide analogues against poxvirus infections. *Rev Med Virol* 14: 289–300

36 Naesens L, Snoeck R, Andrei G, Balzarini J, Neyts J, De Clercq E (1997) HPMPC (cidofovir), PMEA (adefovir) and related acyclic nucleoside phosphonate analogues: a review of their pharmacology and clinical potential in the treatment of viral infections. *Antiviral Chem Chemother* 8: 1–23

37 De Clercq E (2002) Cidofovir in the treatment of poxvirus infections. *Antiviral Res* 55: 1–13

38 Magee WC, Hostetler KY, Evans DH (2005) Mechanism of inhibition of vaccinia virus DNA polymerase by cidofovir diphosphate. *Antimicrob Agents Chemother* 49: 3153–3162

39 Snoeck R, Holý A, Dewolf-Peeters C, Van Den Oord J, De Clercq E, Andrei G (2002) Antivaccinia activities of acyclic nucleoside phosphonate derivatives in epithelial cells and organotypic cultures. *Antimicrob Agents Chemother* 46: 3356–3361

40 Dal Pozzo F, Andrei G, Holý A, Van Den Oord J, Scagliarini A, De Clercq E, Snoeck R (2005) Activities of acyclic nucleoside phosphonates against orf virus in human and ovine cell monolayers and organotypic ovine raft cultures. *Antimicrob Agents Chemother* 49: 4843–4852

41 Hocková D, Holý A, Masojidková M, Andrei G, Snoeck R, De Clercq E, Balzarini J (2004) Synthesis and antiviral activity of 2,4-diamino-5-cyano-6-[2-(phosphonomethoxy)ethoxy]pyrimidine and related compounds. *Bioorg Med Chem* 12: 3197–3202

42 Balzarini J, Pannecouque C, Naesens L, Snoeck R, De Clercq E, Hocková D, Holý A (2004) 6-[(Phosphonomethoxy)alkoxy]-2,4-diaminopyrimidines, a new class of acyclic pyrimidine nucleoside phosphonates with antiviral activity. *Nucleosides Nucleotides Nucleic Acids* 23: 243–249

43 Lalezari JP, Stagg RJ, Kuppermann BD, Holland GN, Kramer F, Ives DV, Youle M, Robinson MR, Drew WL, Jaffe HS (1997) Intravenous cidofovir for periph-

eral cytomegalovirus retinitis in patients with AIDS. A randomized, controlled trial. *Ann Intern Med* 126: 257–263
44 Lacy SA, Hitchcock MJM, Lee WA, Tellier P, Cundy KC (1998) Effect of oral probenecid coadministration on the chronic toxicity and pharmacokinetics of intravenous cidofovir in cynomolgus monkeys. *Toxicol Sci* 44: 97–106
45 Smee DF, Sidwell RW, Kefauver D, Bray M, Huggins JW (2002) Characterization of wild-type and cidofovir-resistant strains of camelpox, cowpox , monkeypox, and vaccinia viruses. *Antimicrob Agents Chemother* 46: 1329–1335
46 Smee DF, Wandersee MK, Bailey KW, Hostetler KY, Holý A, Sidwell RW (2005) Characterization and treatment of cidofovir-resistant vaccinia (WR strain) virus infections in cell culture and mice. *Antiviral Chem Chemother* 16: 203–211
47 Painter GR, Hostetler KY (2004) Design and development of oral drugs for the prophylaxis and treatment of smallpox infection. *Trends Biotechnol* 22: 423–427
48 Ciesla SL, Trahan J, Wan WB, Beadle JR, Aldern KA, Painter GR, Hostetler KY (2003) Esterification of cidofovir with alkoxyalkanols increases oral bioavailability and diminishes drug accumulation in kidney. *Antiviral Res* 59: 163–171
49 Aldern KA, Ciesla SL, Winegarden KL, Hostetler KY (2003) Increased antiviral activity of 1-0-hexadecyloxopropyl-[2-14C] cidofovir in MRC-5 human lung fibroblasts is explained by unique cellular uptake and metabolism. *Mol Pharmacol* 63: 678–681
50 Keith KA, Wan WB, Ciesla SL, Beadle JR, Hostetler KY, Kern ER (2004) Inhibitory activity of alkoxyalkyl and alkyl esters of cidofovir and cyclic cidofovir against orthopoxvirus replication *in vitro*. *Antimicrob Agents Chemother* 48: 1869–1871
51 Kern ER, Hartline C, Harden E, Keith K, Rodriguez N, Beadle JR, Hostetler KY (2002) Enhanced inhibition of orthopoxvirus replication *in vitro* by alkoxyalkyl esters of cidofovir and cyclic cidofovir. *Antimicrob Agents Chemother* 46: 991–995
52 Hartline CB, Gustin KM, Wan WB, Ciesla SL, Beadle JR, Hostetler KY, Kern ER (2005) Ether lipid-ester prodrugs of acyclic nucleoside phosphonates: activity against adenovirus replication *in vitro*. *J Infect Dis* 191: 396–399
53 Wan WB, Beadle JR, Hartline C, Kern ER, Ciesla SL, Valiaeva N, Hostetler KY (2005) Comparison of the antiviral activities of alkoxyalkyl and alkyl esters of cidofovir against human and murine cytomegalovirus replication *in vitro*. *Antimicrob Agents Chemother* 49: 656–662
54 Neyts J, De Clercq E (1993) Efficacy of (*S*)-1-(3-hydroxy-2-phosphonylmethox ypropyl)cytosine for the treatment of lethal vaccinia virus infections in severe combined immune deficiency (SCID) mice. *J Med Virol* 41: 242–246
55 Smee DF, Bailey KW, Sidwell RW (2001) Treatment of lethal vaccinia virus respiratory infections in mice with cidofovir. *Antiviral Chem Chemother* 12: 71–76
56 Smee DF, Bailey KW, Wong MH, Sidwell RW (2001) Effects of cidofovir on the pathogenesis of a lethal vaccinia virus respiratory infection in mice. *Antiviral Res* 52: 55–62

57 Bray M, Martinez M, Smee DF, Kefauver D, Thompson E, Huggins JW (2000) Cidofovir protects mice against lethal aerosol or intranasal cowpox virus challenge. *J Infect Dis* 181: 10–19
58 Smee DF, Bailey KW, Wong M, Sidwell RW (2000) Intranasal treatment of cowpox virus respiratory infections in mice with cidofovir. *Antiviral Res* 47: 171–177
59 Bray M, Martinez M, Kefauver D, West M, Roy C (2002) Treatment of aerosolized cowpox virus infection in mice with aerosolized cidofovir. *Antiviral Res* 54: 129–142
60 Robbins SJ, Jackson RJ, Fenner F, Beaton S, Medveczky J, Ramshaw IA, Ramsay AJ (2005) The efficacy of cidofovir treatment of mice infected with ectromelia (mousepox) virus encoding interleukin-4. *Antiviral Res* 66: 1–7
61 De Clercq E, Andrei G, Balzarini J, Leyssen P, Naesens L, Neyts J, Pannecouque C, Snoeck R, Ying C, Hocková D, Holý A (2005) Antiviral potential of a new generation of acyclic nucleoside phosphonates, the 6-[2-(phosphonomethoxy)alkoxy]-2,4-diaminopyrimidines. *Nucleosides Nucleotides Nucleic Acids* 24: 331–341
62 Smee DF, Wong M-H, Bailey KW, Beadle JR, Hostetler KY, Sidwell RW (2004) Effects of four antiviral substances on lethal vaccinia virus (IHD strain) respiratory infections in mice. *Int J Antimicrob Agents* 23: 430–437
63 Buller RM, Owens G, Schriewer J, Melman L, Beadle JR, Hostetler KY (2004) Efficacy of oral active ether lipid analogs of cidofovir in a lethal mousepox model. *Virology* 318: 474–481
64 Quenelle DC, Collins DJ, Wan WB, Beadle JR, Hostetler KY, Kern ER (2004) Oral treatment of cowpox and vaccinia virus infections in mice with ether lipid esters of cidofovir. *Antimicrob Agents Chemother* 48: 404–412
65 Lu S, Cheng L, Hostetler KY, Koh HJ, Beadle JR, Davidson MC, Freeman WR (2005) Intraocular properties of hexadecyloxypropyl-cyclic-cidofovir in Guinea pigs. J Ocul Pharmacol Ther 21: 205–209
66 Meadows KP, Tyring SK, Pavia AT, Rallis TM (1997) Resolution of recalcitrant molluscum contagiosum virus lesions in human immunodeficiency virus-infected patients treated with cidofovir. *Arch Dermatol* 133: 987–990
67 Ibarra V, Blanco JR, Oteo JA, Rosel L (2000) Efficacy of cidofovir in the treatment of recalcitrant molluscum contagiosum in an AIDS patient. *Acta Derm Venereol* 80: 315–316
68 Geerinck K, Lukito G, Snoeck R, De Vos R, De Clercq E, Vanrenterghem Y, Degreef H, Maes B (2001) A case of human orf in an immunocompromised patient treated successfully with cidofovir cream. *J Med Virol* 64: 543–549
69 Kile JC, Fleischauer AT, Beard B, Kuehnert MJ, Kanwal RS, Pontones P, Messersmith HJ, Teclaw R, Karem KL, Braden ZH, Damon I, Khan AS, Fisher M (2005) Transmission of monkeypox among persons exposed to infected prairie dogs in Indiana in 2003. *Arch Pediatr Adolesc Med* 159: 1022–1025
70 Anderson MG, Frenkel LD, Homann S, Guffey J (2003) A case of severe monkeypox virus disease in an American child: emerging infections and changing professional values. *Pediatr Infect Dis J* 22: 1093–1096
71 Abu-Daya A, Brown PM, Fox KR (1995) DNA sequence specificity of several AT-selective minor groove binding ligands. *Nucleic Acids Res* 23: 3385–3392

72 Broyles SS, Kremer M, Knutson BA (2004) Antiviral activity of distamycin A against vaccinia virus is the result of inhibition of postreplicative mRNA synthesis. *J Virol* 78: 2137–2141

73 Byrd CM, Bolken TC, Mjalli AM, Arimilli MN, Andrews RC, Rothlein R, Andrei T, Rao M, Owens KL, Hruby DE (2004) New class of orthopoxvirus antiviral drugs that block viral maturation. *J Virol* 78: 12147–12156

74 Byrd CM, Bolken T, Hruby DE (2002) The vaccinia virus I7L gene product is the core protein proteinase. *J Virol* 76: 8973–8976

75 Byrd CM, Bolken TC, Hruby DE (2003) Molecular dissection of the vaccinia virus I7L core protein proteinase. *J Virol* 77: 11279–11283

76 Yang G, Pevear DC, Davies MH, Collett MS, Bailey T, Rippen S, Barone L, Burns C, Rhodes G, Tohan S et al (2005) An orally bioavailable antipoxvirus compound (ST-246) inhibits extracellular virus formation and protects mice from lethal orthopoxvirus challenge. *J Virol* 79: 13139–13149

77 Husain M, Weisberg A, Moss B (2003) Topology of epitope-tagged F13L protein, a major membrane component of extracellular vaccinia virions. *Virology* 308: 233–242

78 Blasco R, Moss B (1991) Extracellular vaccinia virus formation and cell-to-cell virus transmission are prevented by deletion of the gene encoding the 37,000-dalton outer envelope protein. *J Virol* 65: 5910–5920

79 Seet BT, Johnston JB, Brunetti CR, Barrett JW, Everett H, Cameron C, Sypula J, Nazarian SH, Lucas A, McFadden G (2003) Poxviruses and immune evasion. *Annu Rev Immunol* 21: 377–423

80 van den Broek MF, Muller U, Huang S, Zinkernagel RM, Aguet M (1995) Immune defense in mice lacking type I and/or type II interferon receptors. *Immunol Rev* 148: 5–18

81 Huang S, Hendriks W, Althage A, Hemmi S, Bluethmann H, Kamijo R, Vilcek J, Zinkernagel RM, Aguet M (1993) Immune response in mice that lack the interferon-gamma receptor. *Science* 259: 1742–1745

82 Weimar W, Stitz I, Billiau A, Cantell K, Schellekens H (1980) Prevention of vaccinia lesions in Rhesus monkeys by human leucocyte and fibroblast interferon. *J Gen Virol* 48: 25–30

83 Liu G, Zhai Q, Schaffner DJ, Wu A, Yohannes A, Robinson TM, Maland M, Wells J, Voss TG, Bailey C, Alibek K (2004) Prevention of lethal respiratory vaccinia infections in mice with interferon-α and interferon-γ. *FEMS Immunol Med Microbiol* 40: 201–206

84 Moss B, Shisler JL (2001) Immunology 101 at poxvirus U: immune evasion genes. *Semin Immunol* 13: 59–66

85 Katze MG, He Y, Gale M Jr (2002) Viruses and interferon: a fight for supremacy. *Nat Rev Immunol* 2: 676–687

86 Symons JA, Tscharke DC, Price N, Smith GL (2002) A study of the vaccinia virus interferon gamma receptor and its contribution to virus virulence. *J Gen Virol* 83: 1953–1964

87 Ahmed CMI, Burkhart MA, Subramaniam PS, Mujtaba MG, Johnson HM (2005) Peptide mimetics of gamma interferon possess antiviral properties against vaccinia virus and other viruses in the presence of poxvirus B8R protein. *J Virol* 79: 5632–5639

Poxviruses
ed. by Andrew A. Mercer, Axel Schmidt and Olaf Weber

Environmental resistance, disinfection, and sterilization of poxviruses

Friedrich v. Rheinbaben[1], Jürgen Gebel[2], Martin Exner[2] and Axel Schmidt[1]

[1]Institute of Medical Microbiology and Virology, University Witten/Herdecke, Stockumer Str. 10, 58448 Witten, Germany; [2]Institute of Hygiene and Public Health, Rheinische-Friedrich-Wilhelms-Universität Bonn, Germany

Abstract

The virion of a poxvirus is an enveloped particle that differs significantly from other enveloped viruses. Apart from DNA, proteins and phospholipids, poxvirus virions also contain carbohydrates. They show a high environmental stability and remain contagious over a period of several months in an ambient environment. Poxviruses show an extraordinary high resistance to drying, which is further enhanced by materials in which they are released into the environment (e.g., dermal crusts, serum, blood residues and other excretions). Dried *Vaccinia virus* can be stored at 4°C over a period of more than 35 weeks without any loss of infectivity. Frozen in buffer at –20°C, a titer reduction of only 3 log-steps is observed within 15 years. In general, virus isolated from patients and/or environment is more resistant to environmental conditions than virus deriving from cell cultures. In addition, poxviruses show a high stability towards different pH values. Due to their low lipid content, they are less sensitive to organic solvents/disinfectants compared to other enveloped viruses. This is the reason for the considerably higher resistance of poxviruses to diethylether in comparison to other enveloped viruses. Despite all of these aspects, poxviruses are highly sensitive to all common approved disinfection regimens. Cell-bound poxvirus may show a higher stability than cell-free virus. This phenomenon is not observed if quaternary ammonium compounds are used. Due to the possible renewed importance of smallpox, e.g., in case of abuse in biological warfare, but also because of the impact of poxviruses in veterinary medicine, representatives of the poxvirus family have been chosen to test the efficacy of common disinfectants. The common sterilization procedures – thermal, chemical, an/or radiation – are usually effective against poxviruses.

Environmental resistance

Poxviruses (*Poxviridae*) are a very diversified family of viruses and still represent a potential danger to health, even for humans [1, 2]. They show a broad occurrence in nature and infect not only vertebrates down to fish, but also insects and even plants. The poxvirus virion is an enveloped particle that differs significantly from all other enveloped viruses. Poxviruses have only a comparably low content of lipids in their envelope, although there are considerable differences between the different subfamilies and genera of poxviruses. Avipoxviruses, for example, have a higher lipid content than that found in orthopoxviruses. Apart from DNA, proteins and phospholipids, poxviruses also contain small quantities of carbohydrates (about 3%) [3–5].

Poxviruses show an extraordinarily high resistance to drying [6–9]. This property is enhanced by the materials in which the virus is released into the environment, such as dermal crust, serum, blood and other excretions [10–12]. Already in the 18th century it was recognized that material from patients infected with smallpox stays contagious over a period of at least several months [13]. In particular, dust, blankets, bed linen and personal clothes remained contagious for several years [14] and as well as direct human-to-human transmission, transmission *via* personal belongings, clothes and even underwear was presumed to occur [14]. In the past, clothes and linen, especially, possessed a significantly higher commercial value than today. It was, therefore, common practice to pass them on to others even if they originated from severely ill or deceased persons.

A case reported from Galicia in 1912 provides evidence that the virus was, for example, transmitted *via* paper, specifically, by a letter. Its paper seemed to have been contaminated with *Variola virus* (VARV) and this was transported to Mühlacker in Baden (Germany), where an epidemic developed. From there it was reported to have spread to the cities of Pforzheim, Aue and Freiburg in Germany *via* person-to-person contact as well as *via* contaminated textiles [15].

Although the environmental resistance of poxviruses is high at ambient temperatures, it is even greater at lower temperatures. Dried *Vaccinia virus* (VACV) can be stored at 4°C over a period of more than 35 weeks without any decline of infectivity. Frozen in buffer at –20°C a titer reduction of only 3 log-steps was observed after 15 years. Virus isolated from patients and/or the environment is commonly more resistant than virus material derived from cell cultures. Cell-free or purified virus preparations isolated from supernatants of cell cultures are generally less resistant than the corresponding cell-bound virus [12].

Poxviruses show an increased temperature tolerance compared to most other enveloped viruses. A titer reduction of only 2 log-steps was observed for cell-bound virus on heating to 56°C for 15 min. Nevertheless, differences within the temperature stability for the subfamilies and genera seem to exist. For example, avipoxviruses have been reported to be inactivated by heating at 56°C for 60 min, whereas parapoxviruses need inactivation conditions of 2.5 h at 56°C or alternatively 1 h at 80°C. Therefore, a short exposure of even 90°C does not guarantee reliable inactivation of infectivity. Purified virus preparations are considerably easier to inactivate at 56°C for 15 min even in the presence of 2% fetal calf serum (FCS) with a titer reduction of 4 log-steps [16].

Disinfection

In addition to the high resistance to drying, poxviruses show a high stability across different pH values in the range between pH 4.5 and 10. Due to their low lipid content they are less sensitive to organic solvents compared to other enveloped virus families [17, 18]. This explains their considerably high diethylether resistance in contrast to their sensitivity to chloroform, phenol and ethanol, which has been described, for example, for the *Shope fibroma virus* [19]. Whereas 30–40% ethanol at 0°C for 1 h was sufficient to inactivate this virus, a concentration of 60–70% diethylether was necessary under the same experimental conditions [20].

Poxviruses are highly sensitive to commercial chemical disinfectants, as are all lipid-containing enveloped viruses, although cell-bound poxvirus can exhibit a remarkably high stability [21–23]. If 0.5% formaldehyde is used for a contact time of 5–15 min, a titer reduction of cell-free VACV of 3.5–4 log-steps can easily be achieved. In contrast, only a 1 log-step reduction could be obtained under the same conditions for cell-bound virus. If treated with sodium hydroxide, cell-free VACV can be inactivated in 15 min by a 0.1% solution (4 log-step reduction), whereas cell-bound virus titers could only be reduced by 1 log-step. Comparable results can be observed for peracetic acid: a working concentration of 0.1% (150 ppm active oxygen content) yields a reduction rate of 4–5 log-steps within a 30-min contact time for cell-free virus, but only a 1–2 log-steps of reduction could be obtained under the same conditions for cell-bound virus. If quaternary ammonium compounds (QAC) were used this significant difference was not observed: 0.2% *N*-cetylpiridinium chloride yielded a reduction factor of 4 log-steps for both cell-free and cell-bound virus with a contact time of 15 min (cell-bound virus: reduction factor 3.5–4.0; cell-free virus: 4.0) [24]. The efficacy of some further active ingredients for disinfection is presented in Table 1 [25].

Because of the importance of possible smallpox contamination [26], e.g., due to its exceptional epidemic impact and in terms of a potential abuse in case of biological warfare [27–29], as well as their impact in veterinary medicine, members of the poxvirus family have been chosen for efficacy testing of disinfectants. This has been laid down in several national and/or international guidelines [30–33]. The German Society of Veterinary Medicine (Deutsche Veterinärmedizinische Gesellschaft, DVG) uses samples of VACV both in a suspension for direct tests as well as on pieces of wood (poplar) to simulate carrier contamination [30]. In addition, the German National Health Authorities (Robert-Koch-Institute) together with the German Society for the Control of Virus Diseases (Deutsche Vereinigung zur Bekämpfung der Viruskrankheiten, DVV) employs VACV in their suspension test for the field of human medicine [31]. Orthopoxviruses are prescribed in the French AFNOR guidelines (Association Française de Normalisation) [33] for their suspension test for the human medical field [34]. Correspondingly, broad experiences of the efficacy of commercial chemical disinfectants are

Table 1. Efficacy of common active ingredients of disinfectants against poxviruses tested exemplarily against *Vaccinia virus* as a representative for most other poxviruses [38–49]

Substance	Concentration/contact time	Test conditions
Sodium hypochlorite	200 ppm/10 min	Suspension test WPL
H_2O_2	1%/5–10 min*	Suspension test WPL
$KMnO_4$	0.02%/5–10 min*	Suspension test WPL
Peracetic acid	0.1%/5–10 min*	Suspension test WPL
Formaldehyde	2%/5 min*	Suspension test WPL
Glutaraldehyde	0.02%/10 min**	Suspension test WPL
Phenol	2%/10 min**	Suspension test WPL
o-Phenylphenol	0.12%/10 min**	Suspension test WPL
Ethanol	40%/10 min**	Suspension test WPL
2-Propanol	30%/10 min**	Suspension test WPL
$HgCl_2$	0.02%/10 min**	Suspension test WPL
Formic acid	0.1%/30 min** 0.25%/15 min**	Suspension test WPL Suspension test with 0.2% BSA or 10% FCS
Propionic acid	1%/10 min** 1%/1 h**	Suspension test WPL Suspension test with 0.2% BSA or 10% FCS
Citric acid	1%/15 min** 1%/30 min**	Suspension test WPL Suspension test with 0.2% BSA or 10% FCS
Acetic acid	1%/30 min** 2%/15 min**	Suspension test with or WPL Suspension test with or WPL
Propionic acid Citric acid Acetic acid	0.5–2%/7.5–120 min**	Carrier test on wood and cotton (according to DVG)

BSA, bovine serum albumin; DVG, Deutsche Veterinärmedizinische Gesellschaft (German Society of Veterinary Medicine); FCS, fetal calf serum; WPL, without protein load.
* Reduction factor ≥ 5, ** reduction factor ≥ 4.

available [35], and the results show that poxviruses can be easily controlled by such commercial disinfectants. Table 2 summarizes the efficacy of some marketed disinfectant formulations. As smallpox was eradicated some while ago now, a large number of publications – also on the disinfection issue – derive from the time before the 1970s/1980s.

Sterilization

Every sterilization procedure used in the medical field is effective against viruses. Although poxviruses have a better tolerance against heat, they do

Table 2. Efficacy of some commercially available disinfectant formulations against pox viruses tested against *Vaccinia virus* according to the RKI (Robert Koch Institute) suspension test

Disinfectant formula (for 100 g concentrate)	Reduction Factor > 4 log-steps	
	Application concentration (%)	Contact time (min)
70 g 2-Propanol 0.05 g Chlorhexidine digluconate 0.45 g H_2O_2 (30%)	90	0.5
46 g Ethanol 27 g 2-Propanol 1 g Benzyl alcohol	90	1
10.4 g Ethanol 1.67 g H_2O_2 (30%) 1.5 g Chlorhexidine digluconate	90	1
38.4 g Ethanol 0.35 g Formaldehyde 0.066 g Glyoxal 0.018 g Glutaraldehyde	90	10
40 g Ethanol 10 g n-Propanol 0.018 g Glutaraldehyde 0.05 g Benzalconium chloride 0.01 g 5-Bromo-5-nitro (1,3)-dioxa-cyclohexane	90	5
11 g Formaldehyde 12 g Glyoxal 3.75 g Glutaraldehyde 2.7 g Benzalconium chloride 1 g Oligo-[di(iminoimidocarbonyl) imidohexamethylene]	0.5	5
15 g Benzalconium chloride 2 g Oligo-[di(iminoimidocarbonyl) iminohexamethylene] 2 g 2-Oxydiphenyl	0.8	5
4.5 g Glutaraldehyde 8.8 g Glyoxal	2	5
8 g Formaldehyde 8 g Glyoxal 4.5 g Glutaraldehyde	0.25	1
20 g Sodium perborate 15 g Tetraacetylethylene diamine (TAED)		
6 g Glutaraldehyde 5 g Quarternary ammonium compounds (QAV)	0.5	5
11.1 g Formaldehyde 12 g Glyoxal 3.75 g Glutaraldehyde 2.7 g Benzalconium chloride	1.5	5
25 g Glucoprotamine	1	< 5
4 g Peracetic acid 26 g H_2O_2 (30%)	3	2.5
35 g Sodium hypochloride	3	2.5
50 g Propylene glycol 5 g Potassium hydroxide	90	5
20 g o-Phenylphenol 10 g *p*-Chloro-*m*-cresol	2	5

not form an exception to this rule [36]. Dry heat and/or steam sterilization techniques are as effective as chemical sterilization procedures, such as exposure to formaldehyde or ethylene oxide, and radiation [37].

References

1 Steinborn A, Essbauer S, Marsch WC (2003) Human cowpox/catpox infection, a potentially unrecognized disease [Kuh-/Katzenpocken-Infektionen beim Menschen. Ein potenziell verkanntes Krankheitsbild]. *Dtsch Med Wochenschr* 128: 607–610

2 Committee on the Assessment of Future Needs for Variola Virus (1999) *Epidemiology: Assessment of Future Scientific Needs for Live Variola Virus.* Institute of Medicine, National Academic Press, Washington D.C., 33–35

3 Haas R, Vivell O (1965) *Human Viral and Rickettsial Infections [Virus- und Rickettsieninfektionen des Menschen].* JF Lehmanns, Munich, Germany

4 Tidona CA, Darai G (eds) (2001) *The Springer Index of Viruses.* Springer, Berlin, 863–921

5 Fenner F (1996) Poxviruses. In: BN Fields, DM Knipe, PM Howley, RM Chanock, P Monath, B Roizman, DE Griffin, RA Lamb, MA Martin, SE Straus (eds): *Fields Virology*, 3 edn. Lippincott/Raven, Philadelphia, 2673–2702

6 Mahnel H (1987) Experimental results on the stability of poxviruses under laboratory and environmental conditions [Experimentelle Ergebnisse über die Stabilität von Pockenviren unter Labor- und Umweltbedingungen]. *J Vet Med B* 34: 449–464

7 Downie AW, Meiklejohn M, St Vincent L, Rao AR, Sundara Babu BV, Kempe CH (1965) The recovery of smallpox virus from patients and their environment in a smallpox hospital. *Bull WHO* 33: 615–622

8 Sidwell RW, Dixon GJ, McNeil E (1966) Quantitative studies on fabrics as disseminators of viruses. I. Persistence of vaccinia virus on cotton and wool fabrics. *Appl Microbiol* 14: 55–59

9 Sidwell RW, Dixon GJ, McNeil E (1967) Quantitative studies on fabrics as disseminators of viruses. III. Persistence of vaccinia virus on fabrics impregnated with a virucidal agent. *Appl Microbiol* 15: 921–927

10 Noda M, Matsuda S, Kobayashi M (2000) Virucidal activity of disinfectants. Influence of the serum protein upon the virucidal activity of disinfectants. *Kasenshogaku Zasshi* 74: 664–669

11 Weber DJ, Barbee SL, Sobsey MD, Rutala WA (1999) The effect of blood on the antiviral activity of sodium hypochlorite, a phenolic, and a quaternary ammonium compound. *Control Hosp Epidemiol* 20: 821–827

12 Kraatz G (1984) *Comparative investigations on the infectious potential of free and cell-bound orthopoxviruses [Vergleichende Untersuchungen über die Tenazitaet freier und zellgebundener Orthopockenviren].* PhD Thesis, LMU Munich, Germany

13 Harper GJ (1961) Airborne micro-organisms: Survival tests with four viruses. *N Engl J Med* 339: 556–559

14 State Act (1850) *Report of a General Plan for the Promotion of Public and Personal Health.* State Archive of Massachusetts, Boston, 326–332
15 Greimer K (1922) *Handbook for Practicising Disinfectors [Handbuch des Praktischen Desinfektors]*, 2 edn. Steinkopff, Dresden/Leipzig, Germany
16 Rheinbaben F v, Wolff MH (2002) *Handbook of Antiviral Disinfectants [Handbuch der viruswirksamen Desinfektion].* Springer-Verlag, Berlin
17 Wallhäußer KH (1995) *Practice of Sterilization, Disinfection, Conservation [Praxis der Sterilisation, Desinfektion, Konservierung]*, 5 edn. Thieme, Stuttgart
18 Bellamy K (1995) A review of the test methods used to establish virucidal activity. *J Hosp Infect S* 30: 389–396
19 Rolle M, Mayr A (2002) *Medical Microbiology, Infectiology and Epidemiology of Infectious Diseases [Medizinische Mikrobiologie, Infektions- und Seuchenlehre]*, 7 edn. Enke, Stuttgart
20 Pontier G, Chaumont F (1954) Action of different antiseptics on Shope fibroma virus. *Ann Inst Past* 86: 532–534
21 Tanabe I, Hotta S (1976) Effect of disinfectants on variola virus in cell culture. *Appl Environ Microbiol* 32: 209–212
22 Joklik WK (1962) The purification of four strains of poxvirus. *Virology* 18: 9–12
23 Turner GS, Squires EJ, Murray HGS (1970) Inactivated smallpox vaccine. A comparison of inactivation methods. *J Hyg* 68: 197–202
24 Pöhn HP, Heicken K (1967) Evaluation of disinfectants on their virucidal properties against viruses of the pox-vaccinia-group [Prüfung von Desinfektionsmitteln auf Viruzidie gegenüber Virusarten der Pocken-Vaccine-Gruppe]. *Zentralbl Bakteriol I [Orig]* 202: 172–183
25 Ferier A, Garin D, Crane JM (2004) Rapid inactivation of vaccinia virus in suspension and died on surfaces. *J Hosp Infect* 57: 73–79
26 Baxby D (1988) Human poxvirus infection after the eradication of smallpox. *Epidemiol Infect* 100: 321–334
27 Henderson DS, Inglesby TV, Bartlett JG, Ascher MS, Eitzen E, Jahrling PB, Hauer J, Layton M, McDade J, Osterholm MT et al (1999) Smallpox as a biological weapon: Medical and public health management. Working Group on Civilian Biodefense. *JAMA* 281: 2127–2137
28 Cohen J (2001) Bioterrorism. Smallpox vaccinations: How much protection remains? *Science* 294: 985–987
29 Breman JG, Henderson DA (1998) Poxvirus dilemmas – monkeypox, smallpox, and biologic terrorism. *N Engl J Med* 339: 556–559
30 German Society of Veterinary Medicine (ed) (1984) *Guidelines for the Evaluation of Chemical Disinfectants [Richtlinien für die Prüfung chemischer Desinfektionsmittel].* Deutsche Veterinärmedizinische Gesellschaft, Gießen
31 German Federal Health Office (BGA) and German Society for the Control of Viral Diseases (DVV) (1990) Guidelines of German Federal Health Office and German Association for the Control of Virus Diseases for testing the effectiveness of chemical disinfectants against viruses. *Zentralbl Hyg Umweltmed* 189: 554–562
32 DVV, RKI (2005) Guideline of the German Society for the Control of Virus Diseases and the Robert-Koch-Institute on the evaluation of chemical dis-

infectants against viruses for purposes within human medicine, effective date: 15 June 2005 [Leitlinie der Deutschen Vereinigung zur Bekämpfung der Viruskrankheiten (DVV) e.V. und des Robert Koch-Instituts (RKI) zur Prüfung von chemischen Desinfektionsmitteln auf Wirksamkeit gegen Viren in der Humanmedizin, Fassung vom 15. Juni 2005]. *Hyg Med* 30: 460–467

33 Association Française de Normalisation, AFNOR (French Organization for Normation, AFNOR) (1986) *Liquid and Water-Soluble Antiseptics and Disinfectants. Determination of the Virucidal Activity within Vertebrates [Antiseptiques et désinfectants utilisé à l'état liquide, miscibles à l'eau. Détermination de l'activité virucide vis-à-vis des virus des vertébrés]*. T72-180, March 1986

34 Garrigue G (1984) *In vitro* virucidal activity of antiseptics and disinfectants. I. Draft of the AFNOR virucidal activity standard. *Pathol Biol Paris* 32: 640–642

35 Butcher W, Ulaeto D (2005) *Information to: Guide F: Environmental Control of Smallpox Virus/Smallpox Response Plan. March 20 2003*. Environmental Protection Agency, Washington D.C., 1–10

36 Kaplan C (1958) The heat inactivation of vaccinia virus. *J Gen Microbiol* 18: 58–61

37 Lea DE, Salman MH (1942) The inactivation of vaccinia virus by radiations. *Br J Exper Pathol* 23: 27–37

38 Dawson FW, Jenson RJ, Hoffman RK (1960) Virucidal activity of beta propiolactone vapor. II. Effect on etiological agent of smallpox, yellow fever, psittacosis and Q fever. *Appl Microbiol* 8: 39–41

39 Angeloff S, Panajotoff P, Manolova N, Nikoloff PN (1956) Efficacy of selected chemical substances against vaccinia virus and sheep-pox virus [Wirkung einiger chemischer Mittel auf das Vakzinevirus und auf das Virus der Schafpocken]. *Arch Exp Vet Med* 10: 365–369

40 Bingel KF, Hermann C (1966) Experimental disinfection against vaccinia virus as rationale for the clinical application in case of smallpox [Die experimentelle Desinfektion des Vakziniavirus als Grundlage für die klinische Pockendesinfektion]. *Med Welt* 17: 76–82

41 Großgebauer K (1967) Hand disinfection in case of hand-contamination with poxviruses [Zur Desinfektion der mit Pockenviren kontaminierten Hand]. *Gesundheitswes Desinfekt* 59: 1–4

42 Gildemeister E, Hailer E, Heuer G (1930) Efficacy of disinfectants against vaccinia virus [Das Verhalten des Vakzinevirus gegenüber keimtötenden Stoffen]. *Arch Hyg Bakteriol* 103: 132–135

43 Kewitsch A, Weuffen W (1970) Efficacy of chemical disinfectants against influenza-, vaccinia-, and poliomyelitis virus [Wirkung chemischer Desinfektionsmittel gegenüber Influenza-, Vakzinia und Poliomyelitisvirus]. *Z Ges Hyg* 16: 687–691

44 Schümann KO, Großgebauer G (1977) Evaluation of the efficacy of disinfectants against vaccinia virus in crusts deriving from rabbits and on the hand [Versuche zur Desinfektion von Vakziniavirus in Kaninchenborken bzw. an der Hand]. *Zentralbl Bakteriol Hyg I [Orig B]* 164: 45–63

45 Dunham WB, McNeal WJ (1943) Inactivation of vaccinia virus by mild antiseptics. *J Lab Clin Med* 28: 947–953

46 Kaplan C (1959) Inactivation of vaccinia virus by mercury. *Nature* 184: 1074–1078
47 Mahnel H, Herlyn, M (1976) Stability of Teschen-, HCC-, ND- and vaccinia-virus against 5 disinfectants [Stabilität von Teschen-, HCC-, ND- und Vacciniavirus gegenüber 5 Desinfektionswirkstoffen]. *Zbl Vet Med B* 23: 403–411
48 Micklem LR, Kaplan C (1958) The influence of thiomersolate on vaccinia virus. *Virology* 6: 775–777
49 Sidwell RW, Westbrook L, Dixon GJ, Happich WF (1970) Potentially infectious agents associated with shearling bedpads. I. Effect of laundering with detergent-disinfectant combinations on poliovirus and vaccinia viruses. *Appl Microbiol* 19: 53–59

Poxviruses
ed. by Andrew A. Mercer, Axel Schmidt and Olaf Weber

Early disease management strategies in case of a smallpox outbreak

Andrea Ammon[1], Julia Sasse[2] and Klaus Riedmann[2]

[1]*European Center for Disease Prevention and Control (ECDC), 17183 Stockholm, Sweden;*
[2]*Robert Koch-Institut, Seestrasse 10, 13353 Berlin, Germany*

Abstract

As a consequence of the threat of smallpox being potentially used as a means of bioterrorism, many countries have developed preparedness plans for smallpox in the past few years. This chapter summarizes some of the most important issues for the management of smallpox. Usually, the strategy for the management of clinical cases of poxviruses includes the early detection of cases, rapid laboratory diagnosis, an assessment of the risk of further spread and containment measures. For the early detection, different systems are being tested to identify suspected cases before a diagnosis is confirmed (e.g., syndromic surveillance). Also it is necessary to provide special training on the disease pattern, including differential diagnosis, to clinicians and practitioners. If a suspected case has been identified, rapid diagnostic tests are required. In addition to the national and international notifications based on given case definitions, certain measures are necessary to allow an initial risk assessment of the epidemic development. For a rapid risk assessment, the investigations should follow the algorithms of epidemiological outbreak investigation such as the tracing and identification of exposed contacts and the sources of infection. Further decisions have to be taken on the basis of a continuous risk assessment. Countermeasures can be divided into medical and non-medical ones. The choice of an adequate vaccination strategy as a medical countermeasure for the case of a re-emergence of smallpox very much depends on the epidemic scenario, and the general availability and quality of a vaccine. Logistic aspects of the vaccination strategies have to be considered in preparedness planning (e.g., resources necessary for the implementation of mass vaccinations), and also the prioritization of groups to be vaccinated. In addition non-medical measures to prevent the spread of infection, such as the isolation of cases and quarantining of exposed persons (e.g., contact persons of confirmed cases) have to be foreseen. The effectiveness of other measures like prohibition of mass gatherings or closure of institutions is often assessed in the light of historical events. However, they have to be considered within today's ethical and societal context, taking into account, in particular, the increased number of people who are immunocompromised. Since our knowledge of how the virus would behave today is limited to extrapolations from historical data and is therefore imperfect, these measures are still under discussion. All relevant groups should be involved in exercises to assure the effective operation of the plan mainly regarding communication and cooperation.

Introduction

After the eradication of smallpox, it was possible to cease the most successful strategy against smallpox, namely vaccination. Apart from rare events like the outbreaks of monkeypox in the Democratic Republic of Congo or in the USA [1, 2], there has been no need to think about the management of this disease anymore. However, the threat of smallpox being used as a means of bioterrorism has forced reconsideration of the need for smallpox vaccinations and other measures to manage potential cases or outbreaks of smallpox. In the past few years, many countries have developed preparedness plans for smallpox. In the following chapter we have tried to summarize some of the most important issues for the management of smallpox. A full description of all the necessary parts of the preparedness plans would go beyond the space available here.

Strategy

The strategy for the management of clinical cases of poxviruses (occurring sporadically or in outbreaks) usually includes the early detection of cases, rapid laboratory diagnosis, an assessment of the risk of further spread and containment measures.

Early detection

Early detection of a first smallpox case will be crucial for a successful management of any new outbreak. The earlier anti-epidemic countermeasures are initiated, the more likely the epidemic can be controlled or prevented in time and casualties can be limited.

Conventional surveillance systems like epidemiological surveillance of a well-defined set of clinically suspected diseases or laboratory confirmed agents are important to monitor and control the occurrence of infectious diseases. Yet, these systems usually detect outbreaks or unusual epidemic developments only with a certain time delay. Therefore, planning considerations include concepts that identify an attack as early as possible [3]. Among such systems are for example strategies to monitor the number of emergency department visits, over-the-counter medication sales or school absenteeism. Also, environmental monitoring systems like air samplers, which permanently test the air for threat agents to detect a biological agent before it causes symptoms, have been suggested. Since they only cover selected areas and have to be analyzed against a background noise, they do not necessarily guarantee a timely recognition of a biological threat [3]. After 11th September 2001, various models of syndromic surveillance have been established and tested in the United States for different syndromes (e.g., [4]), but they also still need to prove their value in detecting a bioterrorist attack in a timely manner. Most likely a deliberate release of smallpox would not be detected unless one or more human cases with clinical symptoms of the disease occurred.

The early clinical detection of a smallpox case requires familiarity with the disease pattern. The number of the actually practicing physicians who have clinical experience with smallpox patients is decreasing, and it is therefore necessary to provide special training on the disease pattern, including differential diagnosis to clinicians and practitioners.

The emergence of highly contagious diseases with high mortality and morbidity rates pose an immediate threat to public health and ask for a real time detection of the onset.

Laboratory diagnosis

As a separate chapter in this book describes poxvirus diagnostics, we will not go into specific diagnostic techniques. A very important issue is the necessity to confirm any suspicion of smallpox as fast as possible to avoid false alarms with far-reaching consequences. To ensure the safety of staff involved in taking samples and performing the diagnostics, good cooperation and agreed procedures between health authorities, clinicians and laboratory staff are required. Electron microscopy and nucleic acid detection are the fastest methods and can give results within 24 h. For culturing the virus, biosafety level 4 facilities are required.

Risk assessment

An initial suspected smallpox case triggers various notifications according to the requirements of national and international health legislation and regulations. Furthermore, if a deliberate release of the virus seems possible,[1] an actual threat to the affected state has to be presumed. In this case, disaster management and law enforcement agencies will assist the responsible health authorities to guarantee a comprehensive management in case of a confirmation and the likely spread of the disease. Epidemiological and criminal investigation should be coordinated.

In addition to the national and international notifications based on given case definitions, certain measures are necessary to allow an initial risk assessment of the epidemic development. These measures should follow the algorithms of epidemiological outbreak investigation, such as the tracing and identification of exposed contacts and the sources of infection. Further decisions have to be taken on the basis of a continuous risk assessment.

1 Something very likely in the case of an eradicated disease. The only alternative reason would be an accidental release of the agent.

Intervention

Immediate anti-epidemic measures are of considerable importance. A permanent monitoring of the epidemic is necessary to guarantee that the effectiveness of the measures taken can be accurately evaluated, which in turn can lead to new measures or to a modification of the actual strategy. The following target groups for intervention measures can be distinguished:

1. Measures concerning smallpox patients:
   Smallpox patients must be transferred immediately to a hospital with an isolation unit for further treatment. If no adequate infrastructure is available, isolation standards should be followed as well as possible (for requirements for isolation and isolation facilities see Tab. 1).
2. Measures concerning contacts of infected persons:
   Most important is the vaccination of the contact persons as soon as possible within the first 4 days after exposure and their isolation and observation either at home or in hospital. Contraindications, e.g., history of severe eczema or immunodeficiency have to be weighed against the risk of disease. The treatment of complications resulting from vaccination must be also taken into account.
3. Measures concerning the population:
   Even after a deliberate release, it is rather unlikely that a major epidemic or pandemic will occur if the appropriate countermeasures are taken in time. In the event of a smallpox outbreak the population can be protected by the prompt implementation of a vaccination campaign adapted to the epidemic realities. Due to the historical experience, a second eradication of the smallpox disease is possible on the basis of the known eradication measures. The bigger challenge will be the identification and elimination of the sources of the intentional release.

Further public measures

Furthermore, the spread of a smallpox epidemic can be counteracted by limiting access to public facilities and events and by restricting freedom of movement.

Risk communication

In addition, recommending appropriate protective measures and risk avoidance behavior to the population will be helpful. It is most important that all the measures taken are communicated to the public according to best practice of a consistent risk communication.

Table 1. Anti-epidemic measures

Measure	How	Who	Where
Segregation	Unspecified measure aiming at a locally and timely defined segregation of the target groups from each other and from susceptible and non-infected person	Persons who are ill, suspected of being ill, suspected of being infected	Usually in hospitals or specially equipped accommodations under permanent supervision
Segregation at home	Measure ordered by public health authorities, not to leave the home, home contacts are to be reduced to the absolute necessary level, or under protective precautions	Persons who are ill, suspected of being ill or being infected Suspected infection risk is low or the disease is not very dangerous	Home
Supervision	Regular presentation at the public health service or control by phone	Persons suspected of being ill or being infected without symptoms Suspected infection risk is low or the disease is not very dangerous	
Quarantine	Segregation	Persons suspected of being infected with a dangerous disease who need no treatment But: no ill persons or persons being suspected of being ill	At home with special obligations or in special quarantine facilities under permanent supervision
Isolation	In-patient treatment	Ill persons or persons suspected of being ill with highly contagious or very dangerous infection	Special isolation units

The general public has to be given consistent information adapted to target groups and the situation *via* the available media. Information of general relevance can be broadcast nationwide by television, for example, whereas information of regional or local relevance can be transmitted *via* other media (radio, local newspapers, cars with loudspeakers, leaflets, etc.). The information to be disseminated will include recommendations for protective measures as well as the announcement of restrictions on entry to events and facilities. The protection of the non-infected population will necessitate quarantine measures for suspect cases.

As viruses do not recognize national borders, international cooperation is also of decisive importance. This may include technical and personnel support as well as the exchange and coordination of information but also coordinated action.

International Health Regulations

In the revised International Health Regulations adopted by the World Health Assembly in 2005, smallpox is one of the four diseases (the other three are poliomyelitis due to wild-type poliovirus; human influenza caused by a new subtype; severe acute respiratory syndrome, SARS) for which just a single case case is considered unusual or unexpected with potentially serious public health impact, and thus must be notified (http://www.who.int/csr/ihr/WHA58_3-en.pdf, accessed 6th May 2006). WHO Member States have 5 years to implement the necessary systems for surveillance and response including national focal points, which have to be accessible at all times for communication with the WHO focal points.

Vaccination strategy

The choice of an adequate vaccination strategy for the case of a re-emergence of smallpox in a country very much depends on the epidemic scenario one has in mind and the general availability and quality of a vaccine. At the same time, logistic aspects of the vaccination strategies have to be considered in preparedness planning, i.e., the facility and personnel resources necessary for the implementation of mass vaccinations have to be determined and identified.

With the exception of the very unlikely situations of an accidental release or a natural re-emergence [caused, for example, by mutants of orthopoxviruses (camel- or monkeypox)], the only realistic scenario for a re-emergence of smallpox is a deliberate release of the agent, which does not necessarily have to follow historic patterns of epidemic spread. Simultaneous and multilocal outbreaks are possible and have to be included as possible scenarios for a comprehensive preparedness planning. Predictive modeling of the epidemic spread has to rely entirely on historic data and is of limited value.

The availability and quality of a vaccine has the most significant influence on the strategy, as there is no evidence of an effective therapy with antiviral drugs against a smallpox infection in humans. The chosen strategy will be determined by the particular epidemiological situation and consideration of the threat of further releases and the risk of secondary infections compared with the well-known adverse effects of the currently available vaccines. Unlike during a natural outbreak, the threat of additional intentional releases has to be considered for a vaccination policy.

Various models have been developed to assist in identifying the best use of the available vaccines (e.g., [5–8]), as well as other control measures like case isolation and contact tracing or combinations thereof [9, 10]. Since all these models have different assumptions for important parameters (like R_0), the conclusions also vary.

Following historical data from the last natural, in this case imported, smallpox cases in Europe in the decades before and during the eradication, the first step will be – after the immediate isolation measures have been initiated – the vaccination of contacts and simultaneous ring vaccinations.

There are efforts to predict the best anti-epidemic measures on the base of mathematic modeling [7, 9, 11–15]. Such models are fitted in such a way that they can reproduce historical outbreaks very well and try to predict the effects of different anti-epidemic measures on the basis of historical data. The quality and predictive value are limited and depend very much on the inclusion of a sufficient number of necessary and correct parameters. A slight change in a parameter can lead to exaggerated effects that do not follow the common sense experience. A lot of the decisive factors can only be roughly estimated, like transmission rate, population immunity or the effectiveness of a post-exposure vaccination.

Furthermore, as the re-emergence of smallpox is most likely to result from a deliberate release and multiple geographically unlinked outbreaks may be possible, this historically based vaccination strategy might seem idealistic. Public and political pressure and security considerations may quickly lead to the ultimate step, the mandatory vaccination of the entire population. Nevertheless, this should be done after a careful risk-benefit-calculation considering the serious adverse effects of the available vaccines.

Vaccination priorities: First responders, other priority groups

No matter which strategy is chosen the availability of vaccine is a key issue. Most industrialized countries have acquired a certain stockpile of first or second generation vaccine. The sizes of the stockpiles vary from country to country. Some countries have sufficient stockpiles to cover the whole population, some do not. Therefore, priority population groups have to be identified for vaccination – in accordance with epidemiological, political, ethical and societal necessities and based on a public consensus.

As long as there are no smallpox cases worldwide, obligatory prophylactic vaccinations especially of entire populations are not necessary. The re-emergence of smallpox has a limited likelihood, whereas the certainty of serious adverse effects due to vaccination is a proven fact. Nevertheless, it can be necessary if there is an increased likelihood of occupational exposure.[2] Prophylactic vaccination may seem useful for the staff of special isolation units, which are most likely to treat the first smallpox cases or of those laboratories designated for confirmatory diagnostics. In this phase also members of infectious disease task forces (interdisciplinary teams on any administrative level for the initial risk assessment and subsequent investigations) may be offered vaccination on a voluntary basis.

As soon as a first smallpox case is confirmed worldwide, and a real threat and exposure seem more likely, the offer of voluntary vaccination to all professional groups who are required to keep the necessary public services running during a smallpox epidemic has to be considered. These groups include mainly medical staff, fire brigades and disaster relief organizations, Red Cross etc., but also people working in critical infrastructures (power and water supply, public transportation and communication) or for public security and order or on the administration or political level, i.e. those population groups who are relevant for the maintenance of public life.

Once a smallpox case is confirmed, vaccination strategies should focus on the necessities of an anti-epidemic management. First of all the population being affected or at risk must be vaccinated. If the epidemic spread cannot be controlled, mandatory mass vaccinations will be necessary.

Isolation, quarantine

Smallpox can be spread by droplets and by direct or indirect contact with the pustules on the skin. This assumes that all primary contact persons of a confirmed smallpox case (see Tab. 2) may be infected and must be identified as soon as possible. The risk of infection for persons with an extended contact time or a close contact distance is much higher than for persons with a short contact time.

According to historical data, the highest risk of infection exists for household members or hospital contacts. The European outbreaks between 1950 and 1971 showed that 55% of the infected persons contracted smallpox at a hospital, 20% in the family, 14% at their working place or school and 3% of the infected persons were working in a laundry, while 8% were unidentified contacts. None of the 945 smallpox cases in Europe since the Second World War contracted it on an airplane, a train or a bus [16].

Yet, under special conditions, an airborne transmission may be possible. In a hospital in Meschede, Germany, patients and nurses from the two floors above the floor where a smallpox patient was treated were infected by air circulation [17, 18]. Based on publications on smallpox transmissions, Table 2 describes the risks of infection.

---

2 e.g. this may be the case for those who work in the field of vaccine development with infectious vaccinia virus or for veterinarians or keepers in zoos who have a higher risk of exposure to other poxviruses.

Table 2. Categories of the risk of being infected by a contact with a smallpox patient (National German smallpox plan, 2003, www.rki.de/Infektionskrankheiten A–Z, Pocken)

High risk
– Persons who are living in the same household with the patient and persons with a similar risk of infection (members of the family and household contacts, etc.) – Persons who have had „face-to-face-contact" with a sick person, which includes all persons, who have been so close to the patient that they could be infected by droplets, or who have touched the efflorescence of the skin [e.g., friends or neighbors who have taken care of the patient, physicians who have been consulted before the hospital, hospital staff (medical doctors, nurses, cleaning staff), persons in a public traffic system with direct contact, i.e., less than ca. 2 m to the infectious case of smallpox, etc.] – Persons who have been longer in the same (confined) room with a patient (e.g., work colleagues, transport staff of the ambulance, etc.) – Persons who have direct contact with the dead body of a smallpox patient (e.g., undertaker, pathologist, priest, etc.) – Persons who have worked with infectious samples of a smallpox patient without appropriate protection – Persons who have touched scabs of a smallpox patients without appropriate protection – Persons who have had direct, non-protected contact with the personal clothes, bed linen or other personal belongings, materials that a smallpox patient wore or used after the onset of fever
Medium risk
– Persons who are in the same building as a smallpox case, if this building has a ventilation system, air conditioning or comparable installation systems that circulate the air between different rooms in the building – Persons who have traveled in the same compartment of a public transportation system or airplane with a ventilation system, air conditioning or comparable installation systems to circulate the air
Low risk
– Persons with a short and/or not close contact to an infectious smallpox case (e.g., a short stay in the same room, or a longer stay in the same building without ventilation system, air conditioning or comparable installation systems to circulate the air; sharing the same public transportation system without ventilation system, air conditioning or comparable installation to circulate the air; distance to the index case >2 m) – Medical staff, if they have used appropriate personal protection equipment

It might be impossible to control an outbreak of smallpox using only vaccination, therefore isolation of cases and monitoring of the contacts may be necessary in addition [9, 19]. Quarantine in an isolation ward for all persons who were exposed seems to be the safest way, but it has some limitations, like the quantity of qualified isolation wards, the supply of the population with food, drinking water etc. and the cooperation of the population. Therefore, it will be helpful to adjust the anti-epidemic measures to the likelihood of developing the disease (Tab. 1) [20].

The isolation concept should be adapted to the epidemic situation, the requirements on effective isolation and the expected number of contact persons. The personnel in all hospitals/facilities must be vaccinated and trained, personal protective equipment (including gloves, masks, goggles, gowns) and means to follow the hygiene measures must be available. If primary contacts develop fever and other typical symptoms of smallpox, their transfer to a hospital with isolation ward is immediately necessary.

For contact persons with a low risk of infection and a timely, successful vaccination, segregation at home seems to be appropriate as long as they have not developed fever, all household contacts have been vaccinated and the local health authority has the capacity to observe them daily.

Nevertheless, it must be kept in mind that a vaccination, even when administered in time, does not yield 100% protection. According to historical data, the risk of infection for vaccinated household contacts of a smallpox patient in the past was 3.7% [21], in comparison to 65% of unvaccinated household contacts. These data did not give any information about when the contact persons had had their last vaccination.

Vaccination should also be offered to secondary contact persons. They must be registered because they will become primary contacts themselves if the originally primary contact develops the disease.

Other restrictions

Since transmission of smallpox is favored by close distance between persons, so-called "social distancing" measures are considered as further intervention measures to stop the spread. Whereas the isolation of cases or segregation of exposed persons (contacts) is not under debate, the effectiveness of other measures like prohibition of mass gatherings, closure of institutions or even curfews are often assessed in the light of historical events. However, they should be considered within today's ethical and societal context, taking into account differences in the society, in travel behavior, and the increased recognition of contraindications to vaccination [10]. Also, the number of people who are immunocompromised (due to HIV, chemotherapy, transplantations etc.) has increased [10]. These measures are still under discussion, since we have limited knowledge of how the virus would behave today.

Preparation of medical countermeasures

Vaccination

According to the vaccination strategy described above, the majority of vaccinations would be carried out in the case of the real event. Therefore, elaborate preparations have to be implemented in the pre-event phase. Smallpox vaccine and bifurcated needles have to be procured and stockpiled. Some governments have a national stockpile of smallpox vaccines, but not all of them have a stockpile covering the need of their entire population. Therefore, multi-lateral support in the case of an event has to be assured in time. Within the European Union, a Task Force on Bioterrorism was set up in May 2002 with the main objective of implementing the health security program [22]. The World Health Organization (WHO) has to convince some states to contribute to an international stockpile at WHO level.

For national stockpiles, the logistics for storage, transport and distribution have to be determined in advance as well. To allow immediate mass vaccinations, the required infrastructure, such as facilities or personnel, has to be identified and the latter informed and trained in time. The entire process should be tested and practiced in simulation exercises.

When choosing vaccination facilities important aspects have to be considered to enable the vaccination of a large number of people in a very short time, such as:

- Number and size of vaccination facilities according to population density
- Transport connections
- Easy access, also for handicapped people
- Water and energy supply
- Toilets
- Possibility of separate treatment of suspected cases
- Availability of rooms for personnel, first aid, treatment
- Phone
- Furniture

Material for documentation of the vaccinations and checking of contraindications (questionnaires, vaccination list/card) as well as information for the public has to be produced in advance and distributed to the authorities. They take care of the implementation of preparedness measures on the regional and local level. Other tasks have to be achieved or initiated in the pre-event phase as well: vaccination of the vaccinators, training of the necessary staff and provision of the material needed at the vaccination facilities.

Research on new vaccines

A survey of over 14 million vaccinations in the USA in 1968 showed that per million vaccinations there were 75 serious adverse effects, including 1 death [23]. Some of the known adverse effects that may arise from smallpox vaccination are post-vaccination encephalitis, progressive vaccinia, eczema vaccinatum or generalized vaccinia. Therefore, the production of modern and more compliant vaccines is under consideration.

A way to minimize the adverse events of smallpox vaccination might be the use of modified vaccinia virus Ankara (MVA), which was developed in the 1970s by more than 500 passages in chicken embryo fibroblasts [24]. However, smallpox had been eradicated before the efficiency of the protective effect of MVA could be tested. Experiments with animals indicate that there may be fewer complications after vaccination with MVA [25–27], and show also that MVA provokes a high antibody titer and a high concentration of IFN-γ-positive cells. Some data show that MVA-vaccinated animals are protected against smallpox infection [26, 28], but other results allow the interpretation that a MVA-vaccination alone can not guarantee a full protection against infection [25]. MVA might be a good candidate for a pre-immunization [25] or for persons with strong contraindications [26, 29]. Other replication-deficient VACV strains have also been developed for immunization [14, 30–32]. Some MVA strains currently under development require a higher virus titer as they do not replicate in the human body.

VACV strains have the potential to inducing post vaccination encephalitis. Derived from historical data with 1–2 cases per million, the vaccination of the entire population of a country like Germany would lead to 80–160 cases of severest adverse effects.

Finally, a lot of research is being performed to develop new vaccines. Experiments on a DNA basis are very promising, even if these vaccines do not fully protect from infection yet [33, 34]. All the vaccines under development are still in the pre-clinical state.

Vaccination: Legal issues

Usually, vaccination strategies are chosen on the basis of scientific evidence and national health legislation. For the special case of smallpox, the only vaccine which has proven its efficiency decades ago is known to produce serious side effects. Therefore, legal regulations for the financial compensation of vaccination damages have to be agreed upon and guaranteed before the implementation of vaccinations, no matter if they are being recommended for occupational safety reasons in the pre-event phase or as anti-epidemic measure in the case of an event.

Training, exercises

More than 20 years after the eradication of smallpox only very few health professionals have practical experience with the management of this disease. Therefore, all relevant professions involved in the management of a smallpox outbreak or epidemic have to be trained on the disease pattern and its specific consequences on their professional tasks.

Training must include the professional implementation of sampling techniques as well as safe transport, which have to be arranged in advance to avoid any unnecessary delay or hazard from improper handling or packaging. The laboratories selected for smallpox diagnostics have to guarantee that this can be done both rapidly and with assured quality. These laboratories have to immediately report a suspected or confirmed[3] laboratory diagnosis to the appropriate authorities.

Public health officers, clinicians and practitioners for example have to update their knowledge on the clinical picture to guarantee an early recognition of the disease and also get familiar with the treatment and therapy of smallpox cases. Laboratory personnel have to be trained in the diagnostics of smallpox on the basis of the Standard Operating Procedures. The validity of the diagnosis is improved by regular participation in a quality assurance system.

In general, if preparedness plans exist, they have to be evaluated among all the relevant groups by exercises to assure the effective operation of the plan mainly in the field of communication and cooperation. Public health services might test the implementation of mass vaccinations or the reporting systems for a smallpox alert; clinicians might check the clinics' preparedness plans for cases of highly contagious diseases, ambulance services might train for the transport of highly contagious patients and all together they might check the interaction between the relevant actors aiming at a harmonization of the preparedness planning.

References

1 Hutin YJF, Williams RJ, Malfait P, Pebody R, Loparev VN, Ropp SL, Rodriguez M, Knight JC, Tshioko FK, Khan AS et al (2001) Outbreak of human monkeypox, Democratic Republic of Congo, 1996–1997. *Emerg Infect Dis* 7: 434–438

2 CDC (2003) Update: Multistate outbreak of monkeypox – Illinois, Indiana, Kansas, Missouri, Ohio, and Wisconsin, 2003. *MMWR* 52: 561–564

3 Rotz LS, Hughes JM (2004) Advances in detecting and responding to threats from bioterrorism and emerging infectious diseases. *Nat Med* 10: S130–136

4 Heffernan R, Mostashari F, Das D, Karpati A, Kulldorff M, Weiss D (2004) Syndromic surveillance in public health practice, New York City. *Emerg Infect Dis* 10: 858–864

5 Kretzschmar M, van den Hof S, Wallinga J, van Wijngaarden J (2004) Ring vaccination and smallpox control. *Emerg Infect Dis* 10: 832–841

6 Legrand J, Viboud C, Boelle PY, Valleron AJ, Falhault A (2003) Modelling responses to a smallpox epidemic taking into account uncertainty. *Epidemiol Infect* 132: 19–25

7 Bozzette SA, Boer R, Bhatnagar V, Brower JL, Keeler EB, Morton SC, Stoto MA (2003) A model for a smallpox-vaccination policy. *N Engl J Med* 348: 416–425

8 Massoudi MS, Barker L, Schwartz B (2003) Effectiveness of a postexposure vaccination for the prevention of smallpox: results of a Delphi analysis. *J Infect Dis* 188: 973–976

3 A first smallpox case or first smallpox cases would need "official" confirmation in one of the two laboratories designated by WHO (CDC and VECTOR).

9 Eichner M (2003) Case isolation and contact tracing can prevent the spread of smallpox. *Am J Epidemiol* 158: 118–128
10 Kerrod E, Geddes AM, Regan M, Leach S (2005) Surveillance and control measures during smallpox outbreaks. *Emerg Infect Dis* 11: 291–297
11 Epstein JM, Cummings DAT, Chakravarty S, Singa RM, Burke DS (2005) Towards a containment strategy for smallpox bioterror: an individual-based computational approach. [cited 2005 Nov 21]; available from: URL: http://homepage.univie.ac.at/Franz.Vesely/ABC_Korneuburg/pdf/bio_terror_epstein.pdf
12 Halloran ME, Longini J, Nizam A, Yang Y (2002) Containing bioterrorist smallpox. *Science* 298: 1428–1431
13 Gani R, Leach S (2001) Transmission potential of smallpox in contemporary populations. *Nature* 414: 748–751
14 Edghill-Smith Y, Venzon D, Karpova T, McNally J, Nacsa J, Tsai WP, Tryniszewska E, Moniuszko M, Manischewitz J, King LR et al (2003) Modeling a safer smallpox vaccination regimen, for human immunodeficiency virus type 1-infected patients. In: Immunocompromised Macaques. *J Infect Dis* 188: 1181–1191
15 Meltzer M, I, Damon I, LeDuc JW, Millar D (2001) Modeling potential responses to smallpox as a bioterrorist weapon. *Emerg Infect Dis*7: 959–969
16 Mack TM (1972) Smallpox in Europe, 1950–1971. *J Infect Dis* 125: 161–169.
17 Mack T (2003) A different view of smallpox and vaccination. *N Engl J Med* 348: 460–463
18 Wehrle PF, Posch J, Richter KH, Henderson DA (1970) An airborne outbreak of smallpox in a German hospital and its significance with respect to other recent outbreaks in Europe. *Bull World Health Organ* 43: 669–679
19 Gelfand HM, Posch J (1971) The recent outbreak of smallpox in Meschede, West Germany. *Am J Epidemiol* 93: 234–237
20 Fock R, Finke EJ, Fleischer K, Gottschalk R, Graf P, Grünewald T, Koch U, Michels H, Peters M, Wirtz A et al (2005) Begriffsbestimmungen seuchenhygienisch relevanter Maßnahmen und Bezeichnungen. In: *Biologische Gefahren. Beiträge zum Bevölkerungsschutz*, 2nd edn. Bundesamt für Bevölkerungsschutz und Katastrophenhilfe, Bonn, 211–230
21 Fenner F, Henderson DA, Arita I, Jezek Z, Ladnyi ID (1988) *Smallpox and its eradication.* WHO, Geneva
22 Tegnell A, Bossi P, Baka A, van Loock F, Jendriks J, Wallyn S, Gouvras G (2003) The European Commission's Task Force on Bioterrorism. *Emerg Infect Dis* 10: 1330–1332
23 Lane JM, Ruben FL, Neff JM, Millar JD (1969) Complications of smallpox vaccination, 1968/National Surveillance in the United States. *N Engl J Med* 281: 1201–1208
24 Mayr A, Stickl H, Müller HK, Danner K, Singer H (1978) Der Pockenimpfstamm MVA: Marker, genetische Struktur, Erfahrungen mit der parenteralen Schutzimpfung und Verhalten im abwehrgeschwächten Organismus [The Smallpox Vaccinnation Strain MVA: Marker, Genetic Structure, Experience Gained with the Parenteral Vaccination and Effect in Immunocomprimised Organism]. *Zentralbl Bakteriol Hyg* 167: 375–390
25 Earl PL, Americo JL, Wyatt LS, Eller LA, Whitbeck JC, Cohen GH, Eisenberg

RJ, Hartmann CJ, Jackson DL, Kulesh DA et al (2004) Immunogenicity of a highly attenuated MVA smallpox vaccine and protection against monkeypox. *Nature* 428: 182–185

26 Wyatt LS, Earl PL, Eller LA, Moss B (2004) Highly attenuated smallpox vaccine protects mice with and without immune deficiencies against pathogenic vaccinia virus challenge. *Proc Natl Acad Sci USA* 101: 4590–4595

27 Stittelaar KJ, van Amerongen G, Kondova I, Kuiken T, van Lavieren RF, Pistoor FH, Niesters HG, van Doornum G, van der Zeijst BA, Mateo L et al (2005) Modified vaccinia virus Ankara protects macaques against respiratory challenge with monkeypox virus. *J Virol* 79: 7845–7851

28 Belyakov IM, Earl P, Dzutsev A, Kuznetsov VA, Lemon M, Wyatt LS, Snyder JT, Ahlers JD, Franchini G, Moss B, Berzofsky JA (2003) Shared modes of protection against poxvirus infection by attenuated and conventional smallpox vaccine viruses. *Proc Natl Acad Sci USA* 100: 9458–9463

29 McCurdy LH, Larkin BD, Martin JE, Graham BS (2004) Modified Vaccinia Ankara; potential as an alternative smallpox vaccine. *Clin Infect Dis* 38: 1749–1753

30 Ober BT, Bruhl P, Schmidt M, Wieser V, Gritschenberger W, Coulibaly S, Savidis-Dacho H, Gerencer M, Falkner FG (2002) Immunogenicity and safety of defective vaccinia virus lister: comparison with modified vaccinia virus Ankara. *J Virol* 76: 7713–7723

31 Legrand FA, Verardi PH, Jones LA, Chan KS, Peng Y, Yilma TD (2004) Induction of potent humoral and cell-mediated immune responses by attenuated vaccinia virus vectors with deleted serpin genes. *J Virol* 78: 2770–2779

32 Kidokoro M, Tashiro M, Shida H (2005) Genetically stable and fully effective smallpox vaccine strain constructed from highly attenuated vaccinia LC16m8. *Proc Natl Acad Sci USA* 102: 4152–4157

33 Enserink M (2004) Smallpox vaccines: looking beyond the next generation. *Science* 304: 809

34 Hooper JW, Thompson E, Wilhelmsen C, Zimmerman M, Ichou MA, Steffen SE, Schmaljohn CS, Schmaljohn AL, Jahrling PB (2004) Smallpox DNA vaccine protects nonhuman primates against lethal monkeypox. *J Virol* 78: 4433–4443

Poxviruses
ed. by Andrew A. Mercer, Axel Schmidt and Olaf Weber

Historic aspects and early smallpox management approaches in the New World

Axel Schmidt

Institute of Medical Microbiology and Virology, University Witten/Herdecke, Stockumer Str. 10, 58448 Witten, Germany

Abstract

Smallpox is an ancient burden of mankind. It was an established disease of the Old World brought into the New World in the post-Columbian era, although preventive efforts seem to have been made in non-European countries long before this time. After smallpox rapidly spread throughout the New World, outstanding achievements in early disease management were made there. During the Boston smallpox epidemic in 1721/1722, a clergyman, Cotton Mather, and a physician, Dr. Zabdiel Boylston, introduced immunization against smallpox into the New World against tremendous opposition. Boylston communicated his immunization experiences to the Royal College of Physicians and the Royal Society of London in 1726. The state of Massachusetts subsequently released a public health law, the "Act to Prevent the Spreading of Contagious Sickness". These important contributions to the control of smallpox are not sufficiently recognized. The work of these two "forgotten persons" in the history of smallpox was significant in its own right and it seems likely to have played an important part in the rapid acceptance of Jenner's vaccination approach to the control of smallpox initiated 70 years later in 1796.

"...for a man to infect a family in the morning with smallpox and to pray to God in the evening against the disease is blasphemy; that smallpox is 'a judgment of God on the sins of the people', and that 'to avert it is but to provoke him more'; that inoculation is 'an encroachment on the prerogatives of Jehova, whose right is to wound and smite'."

Press release, Boston, 1771 [1]

Smallpox in the New World

The quotation above exemplifies the deep impact of religion on medicine and sciences and in particular, on the history of smallpox in the New World. A disease engendering tremendous conflicts. How did everything start with this disease?

Smallpox seems to be a very "old" burden in the history of mankind. The first documented historical evidence of the prevalence of smallpox is based on the Egyptian king Ramesses V. He belonged to the 20th Dynasty

(1186–1070 B.C.); his regency is said to have lasted no more than 4 years, from 1147/1145 (?) to 1143/1142 (?) B.C. His mummy is kept in the Egyptian Museum in Cairo and shows lesions of smallpox. Thus, it is most probable that Ramesses V died of smallpox at an age of about 35 years. The 20th Dynasty was the end of kingdom in old Egypt, and there is much evidence that this change in the Egypt history is associated with severe outbreaks of smallpox within the Egyptian Royal Families [2–5].

Additionally, there is evidence that already around 1000 A.D. immunization against smallpox was carried out in China and India. Contagious material from dried crusts of smallpox lesions was, for example, inhaled or set into an artificially induced skin lesion [6]. Further, in ancient times, it appears that immunization against smallpox was more often performed for cosmetic purposes to preserve the beauty of the children, especially daughters, than for preserving lives [6].

Smallpox appears to be a characteristic disease of the Old World and was apparently first spread to the New World by the Spanish conquerors in the post-Columbian era; vice versa, syphilis is thought to have been brought back from the New World during this period. Thereafter, the smallpox expanded all over the American continent, also severely affecting millions of Indians. Most probably the last rulers of the Aztec and Inca Indians died of smallpox. Smallpox was also a significant scourge during the exploration of the northern parts of America and Canada [7] and caused huge numbers of deaths amongst the native population as well as the explorers, trappers and settlers. That fact is what makes directing this historical view towards this continent attractive, where smallpox is a rather recent disease. A very well-, probably the best, documented outbreak is the Boston smallpox epidemic of 1721/1722, which is therefore analyzed here more deeply.

In the early spring of 1721, a maritime fleet from Barbados arrived at Boston harbor, Massachusetts Bay Colony (New England). This fleet seems to have brought the smallpox that caused the Boston epidemic. By autumn 1721, the epidemic culminated and rapidly spread into the neighboring towns of Cambridge, Charleston and Roxbury [8]. Cotton Mather, an influential clergyman and politician, successfully approached Dr. Zabdiel Boylston, a physician, to "inoculate" the people of the city of Boston for disease prevention purposes. Herewith, the first prevention against this disease was introduced to the New World and finally gained public acceptance.

Cotton Mather

Cotton Mather (1663–1728) [9, 10] (Fig. 1) was an American Congregational Minister, author and a stringent supporter of the ruling clergy. He became one of the most celebrated persons of all New England Puritans. Three of the most eminent and influential Puritan clergymen in the Colonial

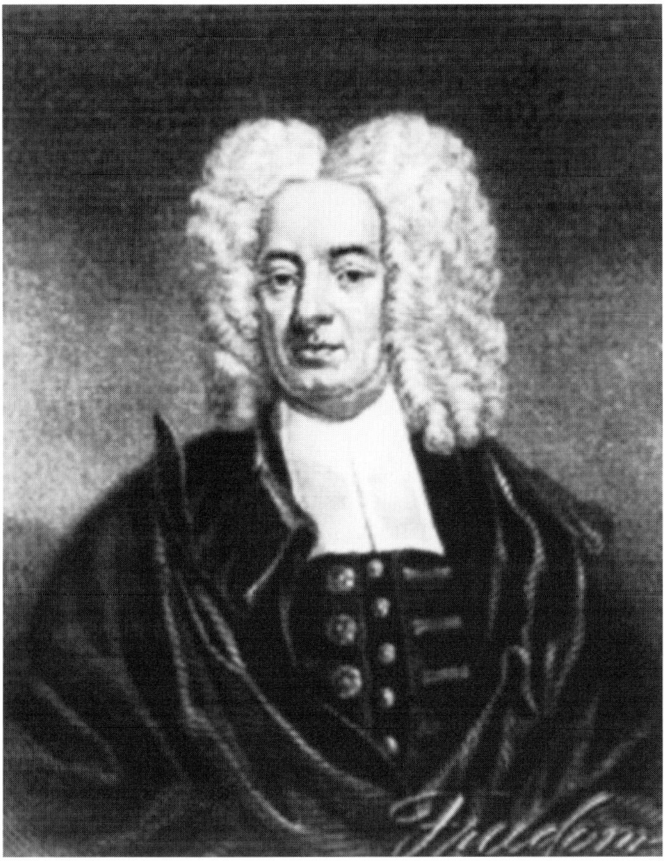

Figure 1. Cotton Mather (1663–1728).

Massachusetts were members of the Mather family, including his father. Mather spent his whole life within the city of Boston.

Mather received a college degree from Harvard and his interest in science prompted him also to become a physician. With his outstanding qualifications and reputation, he was the socially and politically influential Puritan Minister, prolific author, and pamphleteer of that time. After his post-graduate work, he joined his father as assistant Pastor, and it was not until his father's death that Mather assumed full responsibilities as Pastor.

Mather dominated the nation's moral tone, and also sounded the call for fundamental Puritanism in the New World [11, 12]. Despite acknowledging the importance of health and medicine, many religious fundamentalists were reluctant to accept medical help and followed the message: "*He hath torn, and he will heal us; he hath smitten, and he will bind us up*" (Hosea) [6].

Politically, after the fall of the English King James II, Mather was also amongst the most successful persons in the revolt against James' Governor, Sir Edmund Andros.

On the other hand Mather was very influential in early American science and apparently a person of inner contradictions. He combined the old mystical strain, e.g., believing in the existence of witchcraft, with modern scientific interests, e.g., in supporting the immunization against smallpox.

Mather had read of a technique employed in turkeys to prevent a kind of smallpox by transferring infectious material from an infected bird to a healthy bird to cause a mild form of this disease, and thereby preventing the healthy bird from subsequent severe disease. Further, he had a slave named Onesimus, who told him that he had been immunized against smallpox as a child in Africa and that immunization of man against smallpox with infectious material from man and animals such as cows was effective and commonly used in Africa to prevent a later, severe form of smallpox. Therefore, it is likely that immunization of man with infectious material, including material derived from animals, was already known at least in Africa and communicated to the New World, at the latest, by the early 1700s. Unfortunately, during these exploding epidemics of smallpox there was obviously no time to apply and/or optimize these techniques from the medical and ethical perspective.

Mather provided this information concerning immunization against smallpox to the Boston medical community in a pamphlet written by him, but there was absolutely no positive response and a huge amount of objection due to religious concerns [13].

Despite all resistance, Mather was extremely engaged in individually encouraging physicians in Boston to evaluate, optimize and apply immunization methods for prevention of smallpox in the very beginning of the Boston smallpox epidemic. The local physicians were generally not interested in this approach, and Mather's intentions and activities were even equated with murder by a lot of Boston's medical opinion leaders at this time. The only person Mather could interest in his idea was Dr. Zabdiel Boylston, a good friend of Mather's family and recognized physician and surgeon in Boston.

Dr. Zabdiel Boylston

Dr. Zabdiel Boylston (*1676/1679 (?), † 1766) [6, 8] was born in Brookline, Massachusetts Bay Colony (New England) and became a physician. Almost nothing is known about his career until the smallpox epidemic in Boston.

After many personal communications, Mather finally wrote an official letter to him on the immunization issue on June 24, 1721 [14], which may have prompted Boylston to immunize his 6-year-old son and two of his families of Afro-American servants/slaves 2 days after with material of human origin [15]. All developed mild cases of smallpox from which they completely recovered by early July 1721 and showed resistance to a "wild-type" smallpox infection. This was a real historic mark in American and medical history, introducing the practice of immunization against smallpox to the "New World" for the first time. Nevertheless, after his first "inoculation" against smallpox, the selectmen of Boston forbade him to repeat this "experiment". Boylston ignored this fact and, as a consequence, faced extreme public opposition [6].

Boylston was initially skeptical of Mather's suggestions, but he was rapidly convinced to think about Mather's proposal and to implement an immunization method. It is very likely that due to the urgency necessitated by the epidemic, contagious material of exclusively human origin was used for this purpose, as it was directly available and there was no time for the evaluation of any possible alternatives such as taking contagious material of non-human origin. By early 1722, Boylston had inoculated 247 persons, and two of his friends, who were also physicians (Dr. Emanuel Timonius and Jacobus Pylarinus) [16] had immunized an additional 39 persons. Of these 286 persons, 6 (2 %) died, which contrasts with the average mortality of 15–50% in case of the wild-type infection. Several of the inoculated individuals were said to or might already have been infected with smallpox prior to immunization [17]. As the Boston epidemic posed a severe threat to the population of this district, these contrasting mortality rates provided a significant justification of the Boylston/Mather strategy, despite the apparent ethical contrast with the religious belief of the "New England puritan attitude towards life" at this time.

Two years later, Boylston's success was finally recognized by the Puritans and to some extent also religiously and ethically tolerated. He was invited to London as the physician with the most extensive smallpox immunization experience in the world. As well as other honors from the Royal Family, he was accorded a lectureship at the Royal College of Physicians and elected to the Royal Society of London in 1726. There are also speculations that he was involved in attempts to inoculate members of the British Royal Family [17], which derive mostly from his economic wealth thereafter.

At the request of the Royal Society of London, Boylston recounted his clinical experiences with smallpox in a small treatise, published in London in 1726 [18]. This monograph was dedicated to her Royal Highness Caroline, the Princess of Wales, daughter of King George I, which may also be a hint to an immunization of the British Royal Family. Returning to Boston, Boylston prepared a second, corrected edition that was published in Boston in 1730 [19] (Fig. 2).

The controversy

There was a lot of opposition against the smallpox immunization approaches in "New England", and "The England Courant" published writers who opposed this method [6].

Outstanding in this issue is Dr. William Douglass' (better known under his nickname "Sawney") letter from 1722. Therefore, further details on this epidemic and prevention/immunization issues are given by quoting this letter, which is addressed to a physician, Dr. Cadwallader Colden of New York dated on May 1, 1722 [20, 21]. Douglass was a Scottish physician [22, 23] who wrote his dissertation about pros and especially cons of "inoculation" of smallpox [24] and at least initially was one of Boylston's foremost opponents.

"(...). Your reasons against inoculation of the smallpox are strong, and I return you thanks for the communication. Having the opportunity of my good friend Mr. Relf, I could not neglect writing, and your present entertainment shall be the general history of our smallpox in 1720 in Boston, and the inoculation thereof, without descending to particulars. I have by me some practical observations relating to the history and method of cure in this distemper, candidly communicate, providing you give a large allowance for the imperfections of a young practitioner. About eighty have died with purple spots and profuse hemorrhage, which cases I have particularly noted. The cases of the inoculated, as far as I have been able to learn and of which I am assured for fact, being either witness or from good information, shall also in due time communicate.

After nineteen years intermission we received, via Saltertudas from Barbados, the smallpox, middle of April 1721, and by the January following it was nearly over, having affected only Boston and two of three adjacent towns, which demonstrates that no condition of air, etc., can produce the smallpox without some real communication of infection from a smallpox illness. At first it makes but small progress, the month of May proving a cold, wet month and the infected houses being shut up and guards set over them. About the change of the moon, middle of June, it spread so much that the watches being of no use were removed; of this first parcel very few died. Beginning of July another and large parcel taken down whereof several die; thus in the beginning they were taken all in distinct parcels at about sixteen or eighteen days distance from seizure to seizure; but when the infection became universal this could not be so distinctly observed. Hence I made this remark, that the more decumbents, the infection was the more intense (abstracting from the influence of the weather and season, i.e., in October, though a fine autumn month, was the time of the greatest decumbiture and mortality) and more died than in proportion to the number of the sick. My second remark is, I have frequently observed all along our sick time that, if one of a family by some accidental infection was taken down, it proved generally sixteen to eighteen days there-

after before the rest of the family were ill (if the infection was received at home). I shall not pretend to account for this, only I observe first that about the eighth, ninth, or tenth day of decumbiture, the smallpox pustules begin to crack, run and smell, the infection then perspiring and making its way abroad; second, that the inoculated generally begin to sicken the seventh or eighth day from their inoculation; and of those who were taken ill of the smallpox at sea, having received the infection ashore, none, so far as I can learn, exceeded nine or ten days being from home.

Our smallpox burials were as follows: May, 1; June, 8; July, 20; August, 26; September, 101; October, 402; November, 249; December, 31; January, 6; in all 844 persons from Boston. Last February an exact scrutiny was made; it was found that Boston consisted of 10 565 souls, whereof 6000 have had the smallpox and of those 899 died; about 700 who never had it escaped and a few who remained in the country are free of it.

Having, something before the smallpox arrived, lent to a credulous vain preacher, Mather, Jr., the Philosophical Transactions, No. 339 and 337, which contain Timonius' and Pylermus' accounts of inoculation from the Levant, that he might have something to send home to the Royal Society, who had long neglected his communications as he complained, he sets inoculation to work in month of June. By 18th of November, 100 were inoculated, and by January, in all, some few more than 250 in town and country. Whereof some have been inoculated oftener than once before it took effect; with some it never wrought. They all complained much of head disorders, even with those who had but very few, and these imperfect, pustules; their incisions grew up in a few days, as in common superficial wounds of the skin. But about the seventh or eighth day generally they begin to complain (some few sooner or later), are feverish, their incisions inflame, open, and discharge profusely without a peculiar noisome fetor [stench], and continue running some weeks after their smallpox pimples are dried up; and they abroad about their affairs, infect wherever they go (this spreading the infection and consequently rendering it more intense is a great objection against inoculation practised at random in a place whose greatest part of people are liable to the distemper).

We all knew of nine or ten inoculation deaths, besides abortions that could not be concealed. We suspect more who died in the height of the smallpox, it being only known to their nearest relations whether they died of inoculation or in the natural way. Some had the confluent kind, many were very full of a distinct kind ; some had a large red burrow round every pustule, in some they appeared like red face pimples, but not of a determined round as in a natural distinct sort, some like the chicken pox, others so free and without pus that they can scarce be said to have had the smallpox. In some the running of their incision sores has been troublesome many months and endangered the loss of limbs; with some there still remains a crusty scab which falls and returns on the place of incision. Many have had a good genuine distinct kind.

What the consequences may be and if some of them may not be liable to the smallpox in the natural way, time only can determine. But to speak can-

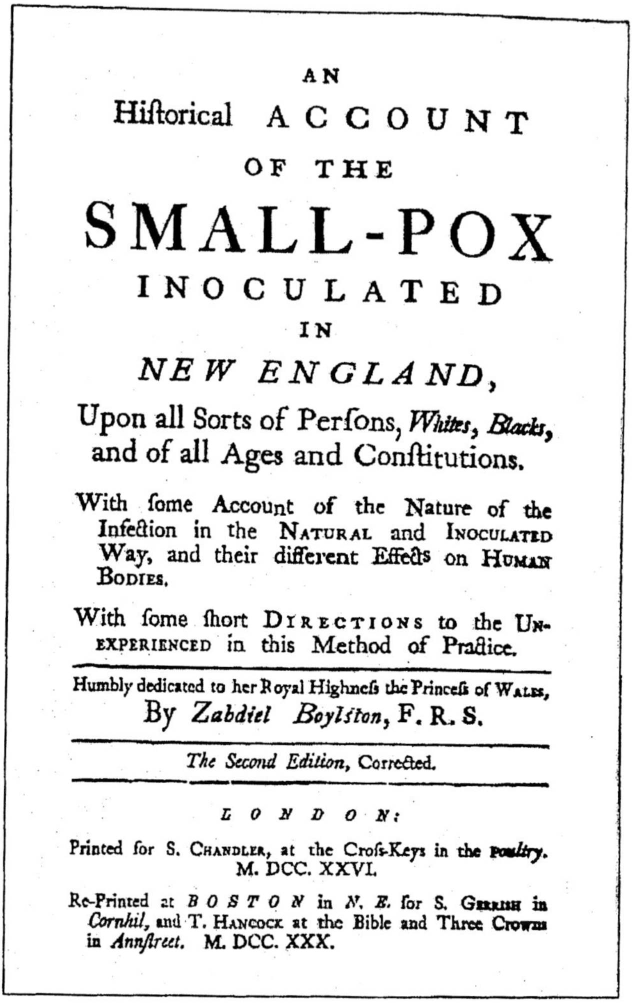

AN
Hiſtorical ACCOUNT
OF THE
SMALL-POX
INOCULATED
IN
NEW ENGLAND,
Upon all Sorts of Perſons, *Whites*, *Blacks*, and of all Ages and Conſtitutions.

With ſome Account of the Nature of the Infection in the NATURAL and INOCULATED Way, and their different Effects on HUMAN BODIES.

With ſome ſhort DIRECTIONS to the UN-EXPERIENCED in this Method of Practice.

Humbly dedicated to her Royal Highneſs the Princeſs of WALES,
By *Zabdiel Boylston*, F. R. S.

The Second Edition, Corrected.

LONDON:

Printed for S. CHANDLER, at the Croſs-Keys in the *Poultry*. M. DCC. XXVI.

Re-Printed at *BOSTON* in *N. E.* for S. GERRISH in *Cornhil*, and T. HANCOCK at the Bible and Three Crowns in *Annſtreet*. M. DCC. XXX.

Figure 2. Cover page of the treatise of Dr. Zabdiel Boylston [19] (MHSC-Collection Massachusetts Historical Society, Boston, USA).

didly for the present it seems to be somewhat more favourably received by inoculation than received by the natural way. I oppose this novel and dubious practice, not being sufficiently assured of its safety and consequences. In short, I reckon it a sin against society to propagate infection by this means and bring on my neighbor a distemper which might prove fatal and which perhaps he might escape (as many have done) in the ordinary way, and which he might certainly secure himself against by removal in this country, where it prevails seldom. However, many of our clergy had got into it and they scorn to retract; I had them to appease, which occasioned great heats (you may perhaps admire how they reconcile this with their doctrine of predestination). The enclosed pamphlets, which unwillingly I was obliged to publish, may inform you more at large of the controversy. They were calculated for New York, and I am afraid will scarce bear reading anywhere else. Our people at present are generally averse to it.

Favor me with the nature and cure of that distemper you call "pain in the side" in New York, as also of your dry bellyache."

This letter reflects (a) the Boston smallpox epidemic of 1721/1722, (b) the description of "inoculation" symptoms, and (c) the heavy concerns about this approach. Thirty years later also Douglass reversed his position and stated in 1751:

> *"The novel practice of procuring the smallpox by inoculation is a considerable and most beneficial improvement in that article of practice"* [21].

Reflection

After this experience of smallpox, the state of Massachusetts consecutively intensified state-wide health programs towards the end of the 18th century, and on June 22, 1797 the state legislature finally passed the comprehensive "Act to Prevent the Spreading of Contagious Sickness" [25, 26] as public health law (General Plan for the Promotion of Public and Personal Health). It has to be highlighted that the rationale for this law was mainly based on the smallpox experiences; a process of learning from history in a new country. This "State Act/Quarantine Act" consists of 13 sections and gives an excellent overview of an effective disease management program against the spread of infectious diseases at the end of the 18th century.

In conclusion, two almost "forgotten" persons, Cotton Mather and Dr. Zabdiel Boylston of Boston, deserve to be honored for introducing outstanding smallpox disease management and immunization strategies into Boston (Massachusetts Bay Colony), "The Colonies" and the New World in general in the face of tremendous opposition. Additionally, Boylston communicated these experiences to England, and thereby to the European continent, with presentations on the immunization issue to the Royal College of Physicians and the Royal Society of London. These contributions to smallpox management appear worthy of greater recognition than they have received. They were likely to have made a significant contribution to the rapid uptake of Sir Edward Jenner's (1749–1823) [5, 27, 28] vaccination approach to the control of smallpox initiated in 1796 [29, 30], some 70 years later.

Acknowledgement

I thank the staff of the State Archive of Massachusetts and the Massachusetts Historical Society for greatly supporting this study by giving access also to documents from the Massachusetts Historical Society Collection (MHSC). Further, I want to thank my brother, Dipl. theol. Holger H. Schmidt, for fruitful discussions on underlying religious and historical aspects of this issue and Dr. Beatrice Menz, Senior Editor BioSciences, Birkhäuser Publ. Ltd., for inspiring discussions on this topic.

References

1 White AD (1897) *A History of the Warfare of Science with Theology in Christendom*. Dover Publ, New York
2 Author unknown (2005) Links to the Pharaohs. http://users.skynet.be/egypt/images/kings.htm
3 Author unknown (2005) *Ramesses V*. http://touregypt.net/20dyn04.htm
4 Author unknown (2005) *Ramses V*. http://www.semataui.de/NR/20-04.htm
5 Kölbing HM (1992) Edward Jenner. In: P Wiench (ed): *Die großen Ärzte (Famous Physicians)*. Droemersche Verlagsanstalt Knaur Th Nachf, München, pp 216–229
6 Author unknown (2005) *Zabdiel Boylstone*. http://www.todayinsci.com/B/Boylston_Zabdiel/Boylston_Zabdiel.htm
7 Hackett P (2004) Averting disaster: The Hudsons's Bay Company and smallpox in western Canada during the late eighteenth and early nineteenth centuries. *Bull Hist Med* 78: 575–609
8 Author unknown (2005) *Biography of Zabdiel Boylston*. http://www.bookrags.com/biography/zabdiel-boylston/
9 Author unknown (2005) *Mather, Cotton*. http://www.britannica.com/eb/article?tocId=9051381
10 Author unknown (2005) *Cotton Mather*. <http://en.wikipedia.org/wiki/Cotton_Mather>
11 Author unknown (1976) Jeremiah Dummer: A defense of the New England Charters. In: Adler MJ, Doren C v, Ducas G, Moquin W, Stauffer T (eds): *The Annals of America, 1493–1754: Discovering a New World*, vol 1. Encyclopaedia Britannica, Chicago, 336–343
12 Author unknown (1976) John Winthrop: Life among the Puritans. In: MJ Adler, C v Doren, G Ducas, W Moquin, T Stauffer (eds): *The Annals of America, 1493–1754: Discovering a New World*, vol 1. Encyclopaedia Britannica, Chicago, 132–138
13 Barret JJ (1942) The inoculation controversy in puritan New England. *Bull Hist Med* 12: 169–190
14 Mather C (1721) *Letter of Cotton Mather Addressed to Zabdiel Boylston Dated on June 24 1721*. MHSC – Collection Massachusetts Historical Society, Boston
15 Schuster N (1965) Edward Jenner: The history of a medical myth. Comments on PE Razzell's paper. *Med Hist* 9:381–383

16 Boylston Z (1721) *Some Account of What is Said of Inoculating or Transplanting the Small Pox, by the Learned Dr. Emanuel Timonius, and Jacobus Pylarinus; With Some Remarks Thereon: To Which Are Added, a Few Quaeries in Answer to the Scruples of Many About the Lawfulness of This Method.* Gerrish S, Boston. MHSC – Collection Massachusetts Historical Society, Boston
17 Rutkow IM (2001) Zabdiel Boylston and smallpox inoculation. *Arch Surg* 136: 1213
18 Boylston Z (1726) *An Historical Account of the Small-Pox Inoculated in New England, Upon All Sorts of Persons, Whites, Blacks, and of All Ages and Constitutions; With Some Accounts of The Nature of the Infection in the Natural and Inoculated Way, and Their Different Effects on Human Bodies. With Some Short Directions to the Unexperienced in This Method of Practice, Humbly Dedicated to Her Royal Highness the Princess of Wales by Zabdiel Boylston, F.R.S.* Chandler S, London. MHSC – Collection Massachusetts Historical Society, Boston
19 Boylston Z (1730) *An Historical Account of the Small-Pox Inoculated in New England, Upon All Sorts of Persons, Whites, Blacks, and of All Ages and Constitutions; With Some Accounts of the Nature of The Infection in the Natural and Inoculated Way, and Their Different Effects on Human Bodies. With Some Short Directions to the Unexperienced in This Method of Practice, Humbly Dedicated to Her Royal Highness the Princess of Wales by Zabdiel Boylston, F.R.S.* Gerrish S & Hancock T, Boston. MHSC – Collection Massachusetts Historical Society, Boston
20 Douglass W (1795) *Original Letter From May 1 1722.* MHSC – Collection Massachusetts Historical Society, Boston
21 Author unknown (1976) William Douglass: Against Inoculation for Smallpox. In: MJ Adler, C v Doren, G Ducas, W Moquin, T Stauffer (eds): *The Annals of America, 1493–1754: Discovering a New World*, vol 1. Encyclopaedia Britannica, Chicago, 348–350
22 Author unknown (1976) William Douglass: The New England Confederation. In: MJ Adler, C v Doren, G Ducas, W Moquin, T Stauffer (eds): *The Annals of America, 1493–1754: Discovering a New World*, vol 1. Encyclopaedia Britannica, Chicago, 172–175
23 Walter T (1722) *A Friendly Debate; or, a Dialogue, Between Academicus; and Sawney & Mundungus, Two Eminent Physicians, About Some of Their Late Performances.* Green B, Boston. MHSC – Collection Massachusetts Historical Society, Boston
24 Mather S (1730) *A Letter to Doctor Zabdiel Boylston; Occasion'd by a Late Dissertation Concerning Inoculation.* Henchman D and Hancock T, Boston. MHSC – Collection Massachusetts Historical Society, Boston
25 State Act (1850) *Report of a General Plan for the Promotion of Public and Personal Health.* State Archive of Massachusetts, Boston, 326–332
26 Author unknown (1976) William Douglass: Against Inoculation for Smallpox. In: MJ Adler, C v Doren, G Ducas, W Moquin, T Stauffer (eds): *The Annals of America, 1797–1820: Domestic Expansion and Foreign Entanglements*, vol 4. Encyclopaedia Britannica, Chicago, 13–18
27 Lücke MH (1991) Edward Jenner. In: D v Engelhardt, F Hartmann (eds):

Klassiker der Medizin: Von Hippokrates bis Christoph Wilhelm Hufeland (Famous Physicians: From Hippokrates to Christoph Wilhelm Hufeland), vol 1. CH Beck, München, pp 309–327

28 Mellanby E (1949) Jenner and his impact on medical science. *BMJ* 1: 921–926

29 Jenner E (1798) *An Inquiry into the Causes and Effects of the Variolae Vaccinae, a Disease Discovered in Some of the Western Counties of England, Particularly Gloucestershire, and Known by the Name of the Cow Pox*. Low S, London

30 Jenner E (1978) *An Inquiry into the Causes and Effects of the Variolae Vaccinae, a Disease Discovered in Some of the Western Counties of England, Particularly Gloucestershire, and Known by the Name of the Cow Pox*. Low S, London. Reprint: The Classics of Medicine Library, Gryphon, Birmingham, AL

Index

The BAID-Series

Birkhäuser Advances in Infectious Diseases

Infectious diseases remain a substantial drain on human well-being and economies despite the availability of modern drugs. New pathogens emerge and known pathogens change their geographical distribution and their susceptibility to the available drugs. An understanding of the structure and function of infectious disease pathogens is a major scientific challenge with important potential applications.

This new cross-disciplinary monograph series will provide up-to-date information on the latest developments in infectious disease research. The multi-authored volumes will cover basic biology and biochemistry of pathogens as well as applied medical aspects and implications for public health and policy.

The contributions are written by leading infectious disease researchers and pharmaceutical scientists with a wide range of expertise.

The envisaged readership includes academic and industrial researchers in medicine and infectious diseases as well as clinicians and others involved in diagnostics and drug development.

Forthcoming volumes:

Pediatric Infectious Diseases Revisited, H. Schroten, S. Wirth (Editors), 2007

Available volumes:

Coronaviruses with Special Emphasis on First Insights Concerning SARS, A. Schmidt, M.H. Wolff, O. Weber (Editors), 2005

The Grand Challenge for the Future. Vaccines for Poverty-Related Diseases from Bench to Field, S.H.E. Kaufmann and P.-H. Lambert (Editors), 2005

Community-Acquired Pneumonia, N. Suttorp, T. Welte, R. Marre (Editors), 2007